Dedication

We dedicate this book to our husbands and children who have supported us throughout this endeavor. We always have and always will cherish the love you have shown us.

Kate A. Barba
Terry Mahan Buttaro

Nursing Care of the Hospitalized Older Patient

Edited by

Terry Mahan Buttaro
and Kate A. Barba

W WILEY-BLACKWELL

A John Wiley & Sons, Inc., Publication

Editorial Offices
2121 State Avenue, Ames, Iowa 50014-8300, USA
The Atrium, Southern Gate, Chichester, West Sussex, PO19 8SQ, UK
9600 Garsington Road, Oxford, OX4 2DQ, UK

For details of our global editorial offices, for customer services and for information about how to apply for permission to reuse the copyright material in this book please see our website at www.wiley.com/wiley-blackwell.

Library of Congress Cataloging-in-Publication Data

Nursing care of the hospitalized older patient / edited by Terry Mahan Buttaro and Kate A. Barba.
    p. ; cm.
  Includes bibliographical references and index.
  ISBN 978-0-8138-1046-1 (pbk. : alk. paper)
  I. Buttaro, Terry Mahan.   II. Barba, Kate A.
  [DNLM: 1. Geriatric Nursing-methods.   2. Aged.   3. Hospitalization.
WY 152]
  618.970231-dc23

                                          2012004865

A catalogue record for this book is available from the British Library.

Cover design by Buffy Clatt

Set in 9/12.5pt Interstate by SPi Publisher Services, Pondicherry, India
Printed and bound in Singapore by Markono Print Media Pte Ltd

1   2013

Contents

Contributors

Editors

Terry Mahan Buttaro, PhD, ANP-BC, GNP-BC, FAANP, DPNAP
Assistant Clinical Professor
Simmons College
Boston, Massachusetts

Lecturer
University of Massachusetts Boston
Boston, Massachusetts

Nurse Practitioner
Coastal Medical Associates
Salisbury, Massachusetts

Kate A. Barba, RN, MS, GNP-BC
Clinical Nurse Specialist
Massachusetts General Hospital
Boston, Massachusetts

Contributors

Susan Bardzik, RN-BC, MSN
Massachusetts General Hospital
Boston, Massachusetts

Eva Beliveau, RN, MSN
Associate Professor
Department of Nursing
Northern Essex Community College
Lawrence, Massachusetts

Margaretta Byrne, MPH, MS, FNP-BC
Master's in Nursing Student
Simmons College
Boston, Massachusetts

Lesley Caracci, RN, MSN, ACNS-BC
Massachusetts General Hospital
Boston, Massachusetts

Chelby Cierpial, RN, MSN, ACNS, BC
Clinical Nurse Specialist/Ellison 11
Cardiac Interventional Unit
Massachusetts General Hospital
Boston, Massachusetts

Anita M. Coppola-Ash, RN, BSN, MSN, ANP-BC, LCSW, MSW
Anna Jacques Hospital
Newburyport, Massachusetts

Constance Cruz, RN, MSN, PMHCNS
Psychiatric Clinical Nurse Specialist
Inpatient Psychiatric Unit
Massachusetts General Hospital
Boston, Massachusetts

Deborah A. D'Avolio PhD, BC-ACNP, ANP
Associate Professor
School of Nursing
Northeastern University
Boston, Massachusetts

Melissa Donovan, MSN, RN
Massachusetts General Hospital
Boston, Massachusetts

Theresa E. Evans, MS, ANP-BC
Clinical Nurse Specialist
Massachusetts General Hospital
Boston, Massachusetts

Jean B. Fahey, MSN, RN, ACNS-BC, CCRN, CNRN, CWS
Neuroscience Clinical Nurse Specialist
Massachusetts General Hospital
Boston, Massachusetts

Sara A. Fisher, MSN, RN, PMHCNS-BC
Psychiatric Clinical Nurse Specialist
Massachusetts General Hospital
Boston, Massachusetts

Patricia Fitzgerald, RN, MSN, ACNS, BC
Clinical Nurse Specialist
Massachusetts General Hospital
Boston, Massachusetts

Susan R. Gavaghan, ACNS-BC
Clinical Nurse Specialist
Massachusetts General Hospital
Boston, Massachusetts

Ashley Moore Gibbs, RN, MSN, ANP/GNP-BC, CHFN
Faculty, School of Nursing
University of Southern Maine
Portland, Maine

Donna M. Glynn, PhD, RN, ANP-BC
Assistant Clinical Professor
Simmons College
School of Nursing and Health Sciences
Boston, Massachusetts

Grace A. Good, APRN, BC
Acute Care Nurse Practitioner
Massachusetts General Hospital
Boston, Massachusetts

Hallie S. Greenberg, MS-PREP, BSN, BC
Adjunct Faculty,
Simmons College
Nurse Educator
Brigham and Women's Hospital
Boston, MA

Jennifer R. Howard, MSN, APRN, BC
Clinical Instructor
Simmons College
Boston, Massachusetts

Marian Jeffries, MSN, ACNS, BC, FNP-C
Clinical Nurse Specialist, Thoracic and Laryngeal Surgery
Massachusetts General Hospital
Boston, Massachusetts

Nancy A. Kelly, GNP-BC, DNP
Patient Care Services
Massachusetts General Hospital
Boston, Massachusetts

Arlene J. Lowenstein PhD, RN
Professor and Director
Health Professions Education Doctoral Program
School of Nursing and Health Sciences
Simmons College
Boston, Massachusetts

Mary Lussier-Cushing, MS, RN/PC, PMHCNS
Psychiatric Clinical Nurse Specialist
Psychiatric Nursing Consultation Service
Massachusetts General Hospital
Boston, Massachusetts

Rosemarie Marks, RN, MSN
Clinical Nurse Educator
Signature Healthcare
Brockton, Massachusetts

Mary L. McDonough, RN, MSN
Clinical Practice Manager
Department of Urology
Massachusetts General Hospital
Boston, Massachusetts

Deanne C. Munroe, JD, MSN, APRN-BC
Risk Management Coordinator
The Queen's Medical Center
Honolulu, Hawaii

Linda Olson, RN, BSN, CWON
Wound, Ostomy Nurse
UMass Memorial Medical Center
Worcester, Massachusetts

Marion Phipps, RN, MS, CRRN, FAAN
Clinical Nurse Specialist, Neuroscience
Massachusetts General Hospital
Boston, Massachusetts

Jennifer Repper-DeLisi, RN, MSN, PMHCNS-BC
Clinical Nurse Specialist
Psychiatric Nursing Consultation Service
Massachusetts General Hospital
Boston, Massachusetts

Kate Roche, MS, RN, ANP-BC
Clinical Nurse Specialist
Massachusetts General Hospital
Boston, Massachusetts

Sharon R. Smart, MS, APRN, FNP
Vital Care Services
New England Community Medical Services
Methuen, MA

Nichole Spencer, MSN, ARNP-C
Assistant Professor
Department of Nursing
William Jewell College
Liberty, Missouri
Adult Nurse Practitioner
Shawnee Mission Internal Medicine
Overland Park, Kansas

Monica G. Staples, RN-BC, MSN
Clinical Nurse Specialist
General Medicine
Massachusetts General Hospital
Boston, Massachusetts

Susan Stengrevics, MSN, RN, ACNS, BC, CCRN
Clinical Nurse Specialist/Ellison 10
Cardiac Arrhythmia Stepdown Unit
Massachusetts General Hospital
Boston, Massachusetts

Caroline Sturm-Reganato, RN, BSN, ACRN
AIDS Clinical Trial Unit
New York School of Medicine
New York, New York

Carol A. Tyksienski, RN, DNP, APRN, BC
Clinical Nurse Specialist
Nurse Practitioner
Hemodialysis Unit
Massachusetts General Hospital
Boston, Massachusetts

Vince M. Vacca, Jr., RN, MSN, CCRN
Clinical Nurse Educator
Neuroscience Intensive Care Unit
Brigham & Women's Hospital
Boston, Massachusetts

Kristina N. Wickman, MSN, RN
Adjunct Faculty
Simmons College
Boston, Massachusetts

Susan L. Wood, RN, MSN, ANP, BC
Clinical Nurse Specialist, Adult Medicine
Massachusetts General Hospital
Boston, Massachusetts

Sharon Zisk, MSN, RN, ACNS-BC
Clinical Nurse Specialist
Cardiac Surgery and Interventional Cardiology
Beth Israel Deaconess Medical Center
Boston, Massachusetts

Preface

Worldwide, older adults constitute the fastest growing demographic cohort and comprise a large percentage of all hospitalized patients. Compared to younger patients, older adult patients have higher acuity, use more healthcare resources, experience more complications, and have longer length of stay when hospitalized. Older patients are also at higher risk for experiencing an iatrogenic event such as an adverse reaction to medication, falls, functional decline, delirium, malnutrition, dehydration, pressure ulcers, urinary incontinence, constipation and depression.

The complexity of caring for older adults, especially in the hospital setting, cannot be understated. In addition to their presenting acute process, many elders have multiple comorbid illnesses and are confronted with aging changes that include visual and hearing impediments as well as cognitive, functional, and health literacy challenges. At the same time, there are ongoing societal and medical care changes. Today, children can live far away from their older parents. Hospital care is often provided by hospitalists rather than the patient's primary care provider. In addition, patients are often quickly discharged from the acute care setting to home or to rehabilitation, sub-acute care or long-term care facilities.

The changes in health care delivery also present challenges for health care providers and particularly so for nurses caring for older adults. Despite the growing emphasis on geriatric care, many healthcare providers are not attuned to the atypical presentation of illness in elders, nor are all providers skilled in assessing the impact of illness on function and well-being in elders. Illness presentations in this cohort can be subtle and precipitate a cascade of events that result in temporary or permanent functional and cognitive changes. Elders have complex needs and the nursing care of older adults is highly specialized. The care of the hospitalized older adult requires not only focus and attentiveness, but also a working knowledge of the common geriatric syndromes and illnesses affecting older adults.

This book was primarily designed for nurses caring for older patients in hospitals and acute care settings, but it is a valuable reference for nurses caring for older patients across varied health care environments. The organized format provides easy access to the common disorders encountered when caring for ill elders and provides nurses with specific information related to geriatric care. The text is organized into four sections. The first section describes normal aging changes and the impact of illness and hospitalization on older adults. The second section is concerned with health assessment in the geriatric patient. Guidance on obtaining an accurate patient history and a review of laboratory values are discussed in this chapter. The third and major section of the book provides an overview of the commonly encountered health issues that can affect the older patient during a hospitalization. These health issues are organized by systems and the format of these chapters is consistent. The sections are often bulleted affording the reader quick and easy access to pertinent information. Each chapter gives a brief description of the illness or disorder. Risk factors, clinical presentation, physical examination, common diagnostics, differential diagnosis and physician consultation are discussed to aid the nurse in the collaborative care of each patient. In addition, the common treatment modalities and patient/family education concerns for patients will these illnesses or disorders are described, though we realize that organizations may have specific guidelines for the management of some disorders and that research and evidence are continually evolving affecting patient care management.

The final section of this book is concerned with those considerations that commonly concern nurses caring for older patients. These include palliative care, pain management, safety issues, and discharge planning.

Acknowledgments

Each patient teaches us more about the best way to care for ourselves and our patients. Through them, we become better clinicians. Our colleagues generously contributed their time, experience and wisdom in writing chapters. In addition, many other clinicians collaborated with us on this text. Their knowledge and experience are evident and we appreciate their expertise and guidance. Without them, this book would not be complete.

Nursing Care of the Hospitalized Older Patient

Chapter 1

Introduction

Terry Mahan Buttaro

Demographics

There are currently 39.6 million Americans older than age 65; most are women (Administration on Aging [AOA], 2010). In another 20 years it is expected that about one fifth of all Americans (72.1 million) will be older than age 65 and by 2050, the number of elders living in this country will likely double (AOA, 2009; Vincent & Velkoff, 2010). This seemingly sudden onset of older citizens is related to the aging of the "baby boomers". The "boomers" were born between 1946 and 1964 and are a racially and ethnically diverse population that includes healthy elders, as well as elders with a variety of co-morbidities and disabilities. Many are foreign born; some are Vietnam War veterans. Many are still working (AOA, 2011).

Older adults are the fastest growing cohort in the US and though these elders often describe themselves as being in good health, they frequently have many co-morbid disorders, such as hypertension, arthritis, or hyperlipidemia. Almost one-third (30%) live alone (AOA, 2011). Some are dependent on Social Security for income, but some have private or government pensions or carefully saved for their retirement (AOA, 2011).

The average income for older females was $15,282 in 2009; for men $25,877 that same year (AOA, 2011).

Other countries are experiencing a similar change in aging demographics. In some of these countries, the life expectancy, especially of women, is longer than in the US (Federal Interagency Forum on Age-Related Statistics, 2010). It has been known for some time that women lived longer than men worldwide, but this, too, is changing as life expectancy for men is projected to improve in the future (Vincent & Velkoff, 2010).

Persons between age 55 and 75 are thought of as "young old" while those over age 75 are considered "old old". Some elders are referred to as "frail elders". Frail elders are more dependent, because they are less able to care for themselves and perform their own activities of daily living (ADLs). Frail elders are often older than 75 years of age, though illness and comorbidity can cause frailty in any age cohort.

Nursing Care of the Hospitalized Older Patient, First Edition. Edited by
Terry Mahan Buttaro and Kate A. Barba.
© 2013 John Wiley & Sons, Inc. Published 2013 by John Wiley & Sons, Inc.

Patients over age 65 represent more than one third of all hospital admissions and more than half of all hospital days (CDC, 2007). Men and women in the US have similar health care disorders, though the percentages for each disorder are quite different.

Heart disease, malignancy, and cerebrovascular disease are the top three causes of death for all elders (Xu *et al.*, 2009).

Theories of aging

There are numerous theories about aging. Some are biologic or programmed theories that address physiological changes that occur over time (Jin, 2010). Biologic theories suggest that aging is programmed in some way. It could be built in senescence or a gradual decrease in gene or immunologic function (Jin, 2010). Wear and tear theory is an example of damage theory, another biologic theory of aging. In wear and tear theory, it is proposed that over time, cells fatigue and eventually cannot function appropriately. This theory can explain some aging changes (e.g., degenerative bone disorders) and is another example that considers aging a preprogrammed rather than random process.

Other common theories associated with aging include psychological and sociological theories. Psychosocial theories are primarily concerned with explaining human personality and behavior. Erikson, a developmental theorist, described human stages of development that ranged from infancy to old age. In Erikson's theory, at each stage of development there are specific tasks that individuals must master. Infants learn to trust themselves and others, while at the opposite end of the life spectrum, elders prepare for the end of life by reviewing one's life – the achievements and disappointments. This theory is commonly considered when planning end of life care, but a different theory (Activity Theory) encourages active, healthy engaged elders (Roy & Russell, 2005). There are many other psychosociological theories of aging. Some theorize that our personalities really do not change as we age (i.e., the Continuity theory) while other theorists describe how roles and activities change as we age (i.e., Disengagement theory) (Roy & Russell, 2005).

No one theory addresses the complexity of aging, as growing older involves physiologic changes as well as personality and attitude changes. For nurses, understanding the interplay of these theories is very important because it helps understand the many changes that occur with aging.

Healthy aging

Healthy aging is dependent on many factors. Genetics and lifestyle play a significant role, but people who had fewer acute and chronic illnesses over their lifetime may also be healthier as they age. Other factors that contribute to healthy aging include:

- Ideal weight for height
- Normal blood pressure, blood sugar, and cholesterol
- Daily exercise
  - 10,000 steps per day *or* 30 minutes a day
  - Weight training twice weekly to strengthen abdomen, back, chest, arms, shoulders, hip and leg muscles
- Balance training each day
- Low fat, low cholesterol, low calorie diet, that includes:
  - lean meats
  - fruits, fiber, and vegetables
  - adequate calcium and vitamin D
  - 1 glass red wine per day
- Fewer medications
- Smoking cessation
- Stress reduction
  - Breathing exercises
  - Meditation
  - Yoga
- Socialization

Many of the elements associated with healthy aging are appropriate for elderly patients. Adults older than age 65 still need exercise, but the physician always needs to determine if an older patient is healthy enough for exercise. In general, if a person over age 65 is healthy and has no limiting health disorders, physical exercise guidelines continue to recommend 150 minutes of moderate intensity exercise (e.g., brisk walking) each week and exercise that strengthens muscles twice weekly (CDC, 2011). Even for frail elders exercise can be beneficial. Researchers learned that exercise in these patients improves well being, sleep, decreases pain, increases mobility and helps prevent falls (Heath & Stuart, 2002).

It is also never too late for people to learn about healthier foods, and it is never too late to begin an exercise regimen. The Nurses' Health Study and other research studies provided evidence that proper diet and exercise at any age are beneficial, maintaining telomere length on chromosomes and increasing cellular lifespan as well as decreasing the risk of physical or cognitive problems (Baer *et al.*, 2011; Hu *et al.*, 2003).

In addition to the healthy behaviors described above, there are other components of healthy or successful aging. Socialization or engagement in life and a positive outlook on life impact quality of life and possibly cognition. Elders themselves describe the importance of being adaptable to aging changes and losses as they grow older.

Normal aging changes

Numerous issues affect aging and not all are physiologic. Financial concerns, family stressors, and the loss of family and friends are important considerations that impact all of us. Some physiologic changes do occur over time despite proper diet and exercise, in most, if not all, body systems. These changes are linear, occurring over time and starting around age 45. In addition, co-morbid disorders and illness can impact aging significantly in some people. Though not all changes affect all elders, common changes associated with normal aging include:

- Decreased body water
- Increased body weight
- Homeostasis easily affected by illness
- Temperature regulation impacted over time
- Gait changes especially after age 80 may be multifactorial
  - Increased double stance time; decreased gait speed
- Cellular changes
  - Diminished cell mediated immunity
  - Decreased number of receptors and diminished receptor sensitivity impact medication pharmacodynamics
- Skin: initial aging changes are seen in skin changes
  - Epidermis thins, becomes dryer and less elastic
  - Decreased subcutaneous fat
  - Sweat glands, blood vessels, melanocytes, and nerve cells decrease in number
  - Absorption of topical medications is more rapid
- Head, ears, eyes, nose, throat (HEENT)
  - Visual and hearing changes
  - Decreased thirst
  - Diminished sense of smell and taste
- Cardiac
  - Cardiac and arterial muscle stiffening results in some cardiac enlargement, hypertension
  - Decreased baroreceptor sensitivity
  - Decreased cardiac output affects blood flow to all organs and can affect medication absorption, distribution, first pass effect, biotransformation, and elimination
- Respiratory
  - Possible increase in AP chest diameter
  - Decreased bronchiolar smooth muscle
  - Vital capacity decreases, residual volume increases
  - Increased risk aspiration
- Gastrointestinal
  - Atrophic gastritis
  - Decreased absorption medication/nutrients is possible.
  - Diminished esophageal motility
  - Functional changes in swallowing (usually related to medications or neurological disorder)
  - Decreased hepatic blood flow
- Genitourinary
  - Decreased blood flow can cause decreased glomerular filtration and tubular secretion; diminished creatinine clearance.

- Decreased number of nephrons
- Diminished bladder capacity
- Prostate enlargement
- Incontinence
- Musculoskeletal
  - Decreased muscle mass and strength
  - Increased bone loss
- Neurological
  - Brain atrophy
  - Increased fragility of blood vessels
  - Neurodegenerative changes include decreased nerve impulse conduction
  - Decreased cerebral blood flow
  - Decreased proprioception (spacial awareness).

Impact of hospitalization on older adults

Older adults are at increased risk for injury when hospitalized for any reason. Some risks are related to aging changes (e.g., organ changes that increase the risk for pharmacodynamic or pharmacokinetic drug interactions). Other risks are related to the hospital environment and/or social isolation. For nurses, a primary goal for this population is patient safety. Particular concerns for elders include:

- Adverse drug reactions
- Alteration in mobility
- Alteration in skin integrity (i.e., pressure ulcers)
- Anxiety
- Cognitive changes: delirium, unmasking of dementia
- Constipation
- Deconditioning
- Depression
- Falls
- Fluid and electrolytes disorders (e.g., dehydration, fluid overload)
- Functional changes
- Iatrogenic injury
- Incontinence
- Malnutrition
- Nosocomial infections

Ageism

Ageism or age discrimination is rampant in the United States. In a culture that worships youth and beauty, older adults are often portrayed as helpless or demented, a characterization that is far from the truth. Many older adults continue to be successful, contributing members of society. They range from grandparents caring for their grandchildren to successful businessmen and women. Although in many societies elders were valued for their prestige and wisdom, ageism has likely always existed in one form or another. Like other types of discrimination, there are different facets to ageism. Age discrimination can be witnessed in many forms: abuse, neglect, prejudice and injustice in the workplace and, unfortunately in healthcare. Healthcare providers may not realize that they are discriminating against elders, but decreased healthcare screenings and preventative care are common examples of elderly discrimination.

Health literacy

Many patients do not understand health information. For some patients, health literacy is compromised because of language or poor reading or writing skills. However, even well-educated people may not understand the language that we as healthcare providers speak. If we think about the language that doctors and nurses use everyday (e.g., NPO, PICC line, angiocath, etc.) it is no wonder our patients do not understand us. For patients over age 60 and for other vulnerable populations, health literacy is an acute problem. According to The National Patient Safety Foundation:

- Health literacy skill affects health status more than age, income, ethnicity, or race.
- 20% of Americans read at the 5th grade level.
- Most health care education information is written at the 10th grade level.
- 66% of patients over age 60 have negligible literacy skills.
- 50% of patients take medications incorrectly because of medical misunderstanding.
- Low health literacy increases hospitalizations by 50%.
- For patients with low health literacy, healthcare costs are four times higher than for patients with high health literacy.

Health literacy in US elders is less than in any other age group in this country. It takes older patients longer to understand health care information and their understanding decreases with age (Federal Interagency Forum on Age-Related Statistics, 2010). Additionally, older adults may have cognitive deficits and functional changes that prevent them from navigating the health care system successfully Yet, older patients usually have more health problems, see more doctors, and take more medications. For elders whose primary language is not English, the concern about their health literacy is increased. Unfortunately, it is sometimes difficult to determine health literacy. Patients may feel uncomfortable asking providers for more information about their instructions and healthcare providers may be embarrassed to ask questions that help assess health literacy.

Nurses are the primary caregivers in hospitals and other health care facilities. Nurses also teach patients about illness and health, thus have an opportunity to assess patient literacy and work with other health care providers to create patient education tools and improve patient understanding of their health. In addition, patients often feel more comfortable with nurses and rely on nurses to interpret physician information.

To effectively educate patients, nurses need to determine each patient's health literacy as part of the nursing assessment. Older patients may not be able to assess their literacy accurately and asking patients their highest level of education may not be helpful because of the cognitive changes that occur with aging (Safeer & Keenan, 2005).

Varied assessment tools are available, but the *Rapid Estimate of Adult Literacy in Medicine* (http://www.ahrq.gov/populations/sahlsatool.htm) is effective and simple to use, plus quick and easy to use (Safeer & Keenan, 2005). Other suggestions to improve patient understanding include:

- Take time to establish a relationship with the patient (and/or family):
  - Be respectful and attentive.
  - Do not allow prejudice to interfere with the nurse-patient relationship.
- Sit opposite the patient and make eye contact.
- Begin the encounter by explaining what you are about to do.
- Limit distractions and focus on the patient.
- Assess patient health literacy skills.
- Use simple language and pictures.
- Provide small amounts of information at a time.
- Encourage patient to ask questions and participate.
- Have the patient "Teach back" to evaluate understanding.
- Provide written information at 3rd grade level and include pictures:
  - Microsoft Word Auto-Summarize and Readability will simplify language (Pugliese & Janowski, 2009).
- For patients who speak a language other than English, written instructions (with pictures) should be provided in the patient's primary language.

References

Administration on Aging (2009) Profile of Older Americans. Online. Available from http://www.aoa.gov/AoARoot/Aging_Statistics/Profile/2009/4.aspx (accessed 8 March 2012).

Administration on Aging (2010) Profile of Older Americans. Online. Available from http://www.aoa.gov/aoaroot/aging_statistics/Profile/2010/docs/2010profile.pdf (accessed 20 June 2011).

Administration on Aging (2011). A Profile of Older Americans. Available from http://www.aoa.gov/aoaroot/aging_statistics/Profile/2011/docs/2011profile.pdf (accessed 22 May 2012).

Baer, H.J., Glynn, R.J., Hu, F.B. *et al.* (2011) Risk factors for mortality in the nurses' health study: a competing risks analysis. *American Journal of Epidemiology* **173**(3), 319–329.

Centers for Disease Control and Prevention and The Merck Company Foundation (CDC). (2007) The State of Aging and Health in America 2007. Online. Available from http://www.cdc.gov/aging/pdf/saha_2007.pdf (accessed 8 March 2012).

Centers for Disease Control and Prevention (2011) How much physical activity do older adults need? Online. Available from http://www.cdc.gov/physicalactivity/everyone/guidelines/olderadults.html (accessed 8 March 2012).

Federal Interagency Forum on Aging-Related Statistics (2010) Older Americans 2010: Key Indicators of Well-Being. US Government Printing Office, Washington, DC. Online. Available from http://www.agingstats.gov/agingstatsdotnet/Main_Site/Data/2010_Documents/Docs/OA_2010.pdf (accessed 23 April 2012).

Heath, J.M. & Stuart, M.R. (2002) Prescribing exercise for frail elders. *Journal of the American Board of Family Practice* **15**, 218–228.

Hu, F.B., Li, T.Y., Colditz, G.A., Willett, W.C. & Manson, J.E. (2003) Television watching and other sedentary behaviors in relation to risk of obesity and Type 2 diabetes mellitus in women. *JAMA* **289**(14), 1785–1791.

Jin, K. (2010). Modern biological theories of aging. *Aging and Disease* **1**(2), 72–74.

Pugliese, M. & Janowski, K. (2009) Supporting patient literacy using technology. In *Teaching Strategies for Health Education and Health Promotion: Working with Patients, Families, and Communities* (Lowenstein, A., Foord-May, L., & Romano, J., eds). Jones & Bartlett, Boston, MA.

Roy, H. & Russell, C. (2005). The Encyclopedia of Aging. Available from http://www.medrounds.org/encyclopedia-of-aging/2005/12/activity-theory.html

Safeer, R.S. & Keenan, J. (2005) Health literacy: The gap between physicians and patients. *American Family Physician* **72**(3), 463–468.

Vincent, G.K. Velkoff, V.A. (2010) The Next Four Decades. The Older Population in the United States: 2010–2050. Online. Available from http://www.aoa.gov/AoARoot/Aging_Statistics/future_growth/DOCS/p25-1138.pdf (accessed 8 March 2012).

Xu, J., Kochanek, K.D. & Tejada-Vera, B. (2009) National Vital Statistics: Deaths, Preliminary Data 2009. *National Vital Statistics* **58**(1). Online. Available from http://www.cdc.gov/nchs/data/nvsr/nvsr59/nvsr59_04.pdf (accessed 8 March 2012).

Further reading

Institute of Medicine (2004) Health literacy: A prescription to end confusion. Online. Available from http://www.nap.edu/openbook.php?record_id=10883&page=302#p2000a60a9970302001 (accessed 8 March 2012).

Kleinpell, R., Fletcher, K. & Jennings, B.M. (2008) Reducing functional decline in hospitalized elderly. In *Patient Safety and Quality: An Evidence-Based Handbook for Nurses* (Hughes, R.G., ed.). Agency for Healthcare Research and Quality (US). Online. Available from http://www.ahrq.gov/qual/nurseshdbk/docs/KleinpellR_RFDHE.pdf (accessed 23 April 2012).

Chapter 2
Health Assessment

Kate A. Barba

Introduction

Adults age 65 and older comprise approximately 38% of all hospitalized patients (DeFrances et al., 2008). This percentage will continue to increase as the population ages. Compared to younger patients, older adult patients have higher acuity, use more healthcare resources, experience more complications, and have longer length of stay (Russo & Elixhauser, 2003). Older adults are also at higher risk for experiencing an iatrogenic event such as an adverse reaction to medication, falls, functional decline, delirium, malnutrition, dehydration, pressure ulcers, urinary incontinence, constipation and depression (Francis, 2005).

The health assessment of older adults is a process of collecting and analyzing data. Nurses perform health assessments on older adults when they are first admitted to the hospital and as needed during each nursing shift. The data obtained from the health assessment will guide the nurse in developing a patient plan of care. It is important that the nurse establish an older adult's baseline early on in the admission so that acute changes can be identified either during the initial health assessment or when changes occur during hospitalization.

The health assessment of an older adult focuses on the health history, physiological findings, psychological data, functional abilities and cognitive function of the older adult. Special focus should be placed on the most prevalent problems experienced by hospitalized older adults. These include sleep disorders, eating difficulties, incontinence, confusion, falls and skin breakdown (Fulmer, 1991; Wallace & Fulmer, 2007). Early recognition, prevention and treatment of these problems can decrease complications and plan for the continuation of care either at home or in a rehabilitation facility. Standardized assessment tools can help the nurse to identify these disorders.

When assessing an older adult, it is important that the nurse to be able to distinguish between normal changes of aging and illness. For example, a change in mental status may mistakenly be contributed to old age when in fact it could be a sign of an underlying health issue. In addition, in older adult

Nursing Care of the Hospitalized Older Patient, First Edition. Edited by Terry Mahan Buttaro and Kate A. Barba.
© 2013 John Wiley & Sons, Inc. Published 2013 by John Wiley & Sons, Inc.

patients, clinical features of a disorder may present differently than those in a younger patient. For example, not all older adults will have a high fever with an infection. Other symptoms of infection may include falls, incontinence, or confusion (Amella, 2004). Many disorders in older adults present solely as a functional decline.

Ideally, all hospitalized older adults would be assessed by a geriatric interdisciplinary team (GIT). This team usually consists of a physician, nurse, pharmacist, nutritionist, physical therapist, occupational therapist, and social worker. Each GIT member would be assigned a component of the assessment based upon their area of expertise. After all components of the assessment are complete, the team would meet to analyze assessment results and to develop a single patient plan of care. Treatment plans developed by a GIT have been shown to be more comprehensive and effective in managing the complex care of older adults (Fulmer *et al*., 2005). Alternatively, if no GIT is available, after completing the health assessment the nurse should include in the patient's plan of care appropriate consults to other healthcare providers. For example, the older adult with a poor appetite and weight loss should be referred to the registered dietician.

The goals of the health assessment include:

- Establish a patient's baseline physical, mental, functional, nutritional and social support system.
- Distinguish between normal changes of aging and illness.
- Determine an older adult's specific symptoms of an illness.
- Identify older adults at risk for an iatrogenic event. Determine the older adult's specific risk factors.
- Develop an individualized patient plan of care that includes strategies to eliminate or diminish the risk of experiencing an iatrogenic event.
- Early identification and treatment of common syndromes that are more prevalent in the older adult.
- Early consultation with other healthcare providers.

Geriatric assessment

Nurses may need to spend more time performing a health assessment on older adult patients than on younger patients. Sensory deficits, cognitive impairments and functional limitations can prolong the assessment process. For example, an older adult with right-sided weakness will require additional time and assistance to turn in bed for a skin assessment. In addition, many older adults may not have the stamina to complete the assessment all at once. It is important that that the older adult does not feel rushed. If needed, the nurse should perform the assessment in increments.

When meeting the older adult patient, the nurse should clearly state their name and role and the purpose of the health assessment. Out of respect, the older adult should be addressed by their last name and title. First names or nicknames may be used upon the patient's request. If the patient is a poor historian or lacks the strength to answer questions, the nurse may need to engage the older adult's family or significant other in completing the assessment. Although family members may assist in answering questions, the focus of the assessment should remain on the patient. The older adult's per-mission should be asked before questions are directed to others in the room. Other healthcare providers (e.g., primary care providers, visiting nurse, or nursing home staff) should also be contacted if accurate information is unable to be obtained from the older adult patient or family. In addition, the nurse should always make sure she has some time alone with the older adult patient so that any concerns can be discussed in privacy. The patient must be alone when questions of safety (i.e., "do you ever feel unsafe at home") are asked.

The health assessment should be performed in a room with a climate comfortable to the patient. The room should be free from distraction and background noise. TVs and radios should be turned off and the door to the room closed to diminish outside sounds. Clutter in the room should be removed to diminish diversions and to allow space for any adaptive devices used by the older adult. Doors and curtains should be closed to allow for privacy. Lightening should be adequately bright but indirect to compensate for decreased visual acuity and accommodation. Fluorescent lightening and window glare should be avoided. If the nurse does not speak the older adult's primary language, a medical interpreter should be utilized. Family members should not be used as the primary interpreter since medical information may be incorrectly interpreted by untrained translators. The nurse should be sensitive to cultural differences.

Many older adults have a vision or hearing impairment, which can affect their ability to communicate clearly and participate in the health assessment. Therefore, the nurse should not begin the health assessment until any sensory deficits in the older adult are addressed. The older adult with a vision deficit should be asked if glasses are usually worn and if so for what activities. If needed, glasses should be placed on the patient before the assessment begins. The older adult with a hearing deficit should be asked if hearing aids are used. If yes, the nurse should assure that the hearing aids are on and working properly. Also, determine if the older adult can read lips and what ear has the best hearing. If available, assistive devices, such as a lighted magnifying glass or listening device (e.g., PocketTalker) may be used. If the older adult wears dentures, they should be worn to help facilitate clearer pronunciation. Aphasic patients may be able to communicate with a pen and paper.

Health assessment techniques may need to be adapted to better accommo-date the older adult with a sensory deficit. Some techniques include (Wallhagen *et al.*, 2006a, b):

● Get the older person's attention and face them before speaking to assist the individual with lip reading. This is a common compensatory mechanism for older adults.
● Do not shout at people with hearing impairments.

- Speak using the lower tones of your voice. Many older adults have difficulty hearing high pitched sounds.
- Avoid your face from being backlit.
- Talk slowly and clearly.
- State when the subject is changing.
- Allow adequate time for the patient to answer questions.
- Utilize visual cues, body language and gestures.
- Provide written instructions if needed. Use a large black marker on white paper if a person is visually impaired. At least 24 point print should be used.

Health history

A thorough health history, including the reason for hospitalization, past medical and surgical history, immunizations, allergies, cultural background, spirituality, advance directive preferences, pain, social and financial support, occupation, education, learning needs, bowel and urinary patterns, skin issues, sleep patterns, and sexuality should be obtained.

Medication review

The nurse should complete a comprehensive review of all prescribed and over the counter medications the older adult is taking. If possible, medication containers or a current list of medications should be provided by the patient or family. Once the review is complete, all medications should be returned to the family to take home or securely locked-up until discharge.

The focus of the medication review should be on reconciliating home medications with hospital medication orders. Any medication that was recently started should be carefully noted and ruled out as causing the symptoms that brought the older adult to the hospital. Also, the nurse should identify any potential polypharmacy, drug interactions, inappropriate medications, and needed therapeutic medication levels. A pharmacist should be consulted if necessary.

History of substance abuse

When taking a substance abuse history, the nurse must be sure to use a nonjudgmental and straightforward approach. Unfortunately, substance abuse is often missed in the older adult because healthcare providers may not expect the older adult to abuse, may not ask the older adult about abuse, or symptoms of abuse may be misinterpreted as being normal changes of aging.

Older adults should be asked about prior or current tobacco use. If the patient stopped smoking, learning when the patient stopped smoking as well as the number of years the patient smoked and the number of packs per day, is important to assess pack year history. Older adults who currently smoke should be counseled to quit and nicotine replacement therapy offered throughout the hospitalization.

Older adults should also be asked about their alcohol consumption. Even small amounts of alcohol consumption in older adults can contribute to liver disease, cognitive impairment, falls, dizziness, insomnia, depression, anxiety, poorly controlled diabetes, and exacerbation of heart disease (Lewis, 2008; Awan, 2010). The older adult's frequency of alcohol use, quantity and last drink should be assessed. You can screen an older adult using the CAGE questionnaire:

- Have you every felt that you should Cut down on your drinking?
- Have people ever Annoyed you by criticizing your drinking?
- Have you ever felt Guilty about your drinking?
- Have you every had a drink (Eye opener) first thing in the morning to steady your nerves or get rid of a hangover?
- Scoring: A score of one or more positive answers indicates a possible alcohol use disorder.

Questions about use of other recreational drugs or other substances of abuse, including prescription medications, should also be asked. The nurse should consider potential or actual alcohol or other substance withdrawal if the history of substance abuse is positive.

Nutrition history

The older adult should be asked about the number and type of meals they consume, appetite, diet restrictions, meal preparation, eating disorders, and swallowing, chewing or choking difficulties. Also, oral health (i.e., cavities, gum disease, and missing teeth) and xerostomia, or dry mouth, should be addressed. Xerostomia impairs an older adult's ability to lubricate, masticate, and swallow food. These conditions may lead to unintentional weight loss. Any older adult with an unintentional weight loss greater than 4.5 kg (10 pounds) or equal to 10% of body weight or decreased food intake should be referred to the registered dietician. Decreased appetite in an older adult may indicate that other problems are developing.

Skin assessment

The older adult should be asked if they have any skin problems including rashes, pressure ulcers, wounds, edema or itchiness. Pressure ulcers are a particularly serious concern for hospitalized older adults and thus pressure ulcer prevention should begin immediately on admission. The Braden scale for predicting pressure score risk (Bergstrom et al., 1987) (Table 2.1) was developed to help nurses determine a patient's risk of developing a pressure ulcer. This scale evaluates a patient's sensory perception, moisture, activity, mobility, nutrition, and friction/shear risks. The nurse uses the results of the Braden Scale to develop interventions to minimize an older adult's specific risk factors.

Table 2.1 Braden Scale for assessing pressure sore risk.

Patient's Name	Evaluator's Name			Date of Assessment			
SENSORY PERCEPTION ability to respond meaningfully to pressure-related discomfort	**1. Completely Limited** Unresponsive (does not moan, flinch, or grasp) to painful stimuli, due to diminished level of consciousness or sedation. OR limited ability to feel pain over most of body	**2. Very Limited** Responds only to painful stimuli. Cannot communicate discomfort except by moaning or restlessness OR has a sensory impairment which limits the ability to feel pain or discomfort over ½ of body.	**3. Slightly Limited** Responds to verbal commands, but cannot always communicate discomfort or the need to be turned. OR has some sensory impairment which limits ability to feel pain or discomfort in 1 or 2 extremities.	**4. No Impairment** Responds to verbal commands. Has no sensory deficit which would limit ability to feel or voice pain or discomfort.			
MOISTURE degree to which skin is exposed to moisture	**1. Constantly Moist** Skin is kept moist almost constantly by perspiration, urine, etc. Dampness is detected every time patient is moved or turned.	**2. Very Moist** Skin is often, but not always moist. Linen must be changed at least once a shift.	**3. Occasionally Moist** Skin is occasionally moist, requiring an extra linen change approximately once a day.	**4. Rarely Moist** Skin is usually dry, linen only requires changing at routine intervals.			
ACTIVITY degree of physical activity	**1. Bedfast** Confined to bed.	**2. Chairfast** Ability to walk severely limited or non-existent. Cannot bear own weight and/or must be assisted into chair or wheelchair.	**3. Walks Occasionally** Walks occasionally during day, but for very short distances, with or without assistance. Spends majority of each shift in bed or chair.	**4. Walks Frequently** Walks outside room at least twice a day and inside room at least once every two hours during waking hours.			
MOBILITY ability to change and control body position	**1. Completely Immobile** Does not make even slight changes in body or extremity position without assistance.	**2. Very Limited** Makes occasional slight changes in body or extremity position but unable to make frequent or significant changes independently.	**3. Slightly Limited** Makes frequent though slight changes in body or extremity position independently.	**4. No Limitation** Makes major and frequent changes in position without assistance.			

	1. Very Poor	2. Probably Inadequate	3. Adequate	4. Excellent	
NUTRITION usual food intake pattern	Never eats a complete meal. Rarely eats more than ⅓ of any food offered. Eats 2 servings or less of protein (meat or dairy products) per day. Takes fluids poorly. Does not take a liquid dietary supplement OR is NPO and/or maintained on clear liquids or IV's for more than 5 days.	Rarely eats a complete meal and generally eats only about ½ of any food offered. Protein intake includes only 3 servings of meat or dairy products per day. Occasionally will take a dietary supplement. OR receives less than optimum amount of liquid diet or tube feeding.	Eats over half of most meals. Eats a total of 4 servings of protein (meat, dairy products per day. Occasionally will refuse a meal, but will usually take a supplement when offered). OR is on a tube feeding or TPN regimen which probably meets most of nutritional needs.	**4. Excellent** Eats most of every meal. Never refuses a meal. Usually eats a total of 4 or more servings of meat and dairy products. Occasionally eats between meals. Does not require supplementation.	
	1. Problem	**2. Potential Problem**	**3. No Apparent Problem**		
FRICTION & SHEAR	Requires moderate to maximum assistance in moving. Complete lifting without sliding against sheets is impossible. Frequently slides down in bed or chair, requiring frequent repositioning with maximum assistance. Spasticity, contractures or agitation leads to almost constant friction.	Moves feebly or requires minimum assistance. During a move skin probably slides to some extent against sheets, chair, restraints or other devices. Maintains relatively good position in chair or bed most of the time but occasionally slides down.	Moves in bed and in chair independently and has sufficient muscle strength to lift up completely during move. Maintains good position in bed or chair.		
					Total Score

Functional

When an older adult experiences the onset of disease, function and cognitive changes are often the first symptoms experienced. Therefore, a geriatric health history must always include function and cognitive assessments.

Functional assessment is a systemic evaluation of an older adult's ability to perform activities of daily living (ADLs) and instrumental activities of daily living (IADLs). ADLs are the basic activities of daily living and include bathing, dressing, toileting, continence, mobility, grooming and feeding. IADLs are the more complex skills older adults need to live independently. IADLs include shopping, cooking, telephone use, laundry, housekeeping and managing medications, finances, and transportation. The Katz Index of Independence in Activities of Daily Living (Katz ADL) is a reliable and commonly used tool to assess older adults' ability to perform ADLs independently (Wallace & Shelkey, 2007). The Lawton Instrumental Activities of Daily Living (Lawton IADL) measures the amount of help needed to perform IADLs and is often used in rehabilitation settings and for the assessment of patients to be discharged home.

All older adults should be assessed for a history of falls and other fall risk factors on admission to the hospital, daily, and in any change in condition. Interventions based on specific fall risks should be initiated on admission to the hospital.

Cognition and health literacy assessment

The goals of a cognitive assessment are to determine an older adult's cognitive abilities, to recognize early the presence of impairment in cognitive functioning, and to monitor an older adult's cognitive response to various treatments (Braes et al., 2009). The routine assessment of cognitive function is the foundation for early detection and prompt treatment of a change in cognition. Undetected impairment in cognition is associated with greater morbidity and mortality (Inouye et al., 2001).

The Mini-Mental State Examination (MMSE) (Folstein et al., 1975) is one tool that is commonly used to screen for or monitor cognitive changes symptomatic of dementia. However, performance on the MMSE is adversely influenced by education, age, language, and verbal ability. The MMSE also is criticized for taking too long to administer and score. The Mini-Cog (Borson et al., 2000) also can be used to screen and monitor cognitive function. This tool is not adversely influenced by age, language, or education and it takes about half as much time to administer and score as the MMSE. The Mini-Cog consists of a three-item recall with a clock drawing test (CDT). To administer:

- Tell the patient that you will say three words.
- Ask the patient to remember the three given words.
- Tell the patient to listen carefully.
- Say the three words and ask the patient to repeat after you.
- Instruct the patient to put numbers on a sheet with the clock circle already drawn.

- Ask the patient to draw the hands of the clock to read 11:10 or 8:20. Allow three minutes to complete the task.
- After 3 minutes, ask the patient to recall the three previously presented words.
- Score: Score 0–3 for recall (1 point for each word recalled after CDT distractor). Give 2 points for normal CDT and 0 points for abnormal CDT. A score of 0–2 out of 5 means a positive screen for dementia.

Other screening tools, such as the Confusion Assessment Method (CAM) assess for the symptoms of delirium.

Limited health literacy is associated with a decreased ability to manage medications appropriately resulting in increased adverse events, hospitalizations, and mortality (Agency for Healthcare Research and Quality, 2011). Determining health literacy is particularly important for vulnerable elders, as researchers previously estimated that a majority of older adults have limited health literacy skills (National Network Libraries of Medicine, 2010; Singleton & Krause, 2009). The Rapid Estimate of Health Literacy in Medicine Tool Short-Form (REALM-ST) and the Newest Vital Sign are validated tools that are quick and easy screening instruments that can provide nurses with more information to tailor patient teaching to patient understanding (Weiss *et al.*, 2005; ahrq.gov/populations/sahlsatool.htm).

Physical assessment

A complete physical examination should follow the health history and a review of symptoms. Emphasis should be placed on distinguishing common age-related changes from symptoms of an illness.

The physical assessment of the older adult begins by observing how they present to the hospital. Are they having difficulty breathing or in pain? Are they well groomed or appear disheveled? Are they able to independently ambulate to the bed or do they need assistance? Tremors, skin pallor, total body edema, gait instability, agitation and sensory loses can also be detected through observation.

Vital signs should be checked including respiratory rate, heart rate, blood pressure, temperature, oxygen saturation, weight and height. All older adults admitted to the hospital should be checked for orthostatic hypotension upon admission and daily during the hospital stay. It is estimated that one-third of adults older than 65 have orthostatic changes in blood pressure that can result in falls and morbidity (Awan, 2010). Blood pressure should be checked lying, sitting, and standing with 3 to 5 minute intervals between positions. A 20-mmHg drop in systolic blood pressure is positive for orthostatic hypotension. A normal temperature or a low-grade fever in an older adult may actually indicate a temperature increase since older adults tend to have lower core body temperatures at baseline. A baseline weight and height will help determine malnutrition and also provide a reference point for an older adult's fluid balance.

The skin should be assessed for any lesions, pressure ulcers, rashes, tissue ischemia, and signs of trauma or physical abuse. Since many older adults present to the hospital with dehydration, a dry mouth or lips and poor skin turgor should be noted. The chest should be assessed for kyphosis and tenderness. All lobes of the lungs should be percussed and ascultated. Atelectasis may produce bibasilar crackles but often these will disappear once the older adult takes a few deep breaths. Other adventitious sounds should be noted. The heart rate, rhythm, and the presence of S3, S4 or murmurs should be determined during the cardiac exam. A S3 may indicate congested heart failure while a S4 is not necessarily an abnormal finding in older adults (Awan, 2010).

During the abdominal exam note if the abdomen is soft, firm, or distended. Determine if bowel sounds are present in all four quadrants. Note the quality of bowel sounds (tinkling or diminished). Note any tympany or dullness with percussion. Determine if there is abdominal tenderness and its location. Rebound tenderness or guarding are ominous signs and should be reported to the physician upon discovery. The suprapubic area is assessed for tenderness and evidence of urinary retention. Discomfort with percussion in the costovertebral angles should be assessed for kidney tenderness.

Lower extremities should be assessed for edema, heel erythema or bogginess, wounds, and poor perfusion. Pedal pulses should be palpated and signs of peripheral and sensorimotor neuropathy determined. In older adults with arterial disease and/or edema it may be necessary to assess pulses using a Doppler. Patients with foot problems (i.e., overgrown toenails) should be referred to a podiatrist. Mobility and gait can be assessed by the Timed "Get up-and Go" Test (Podsiadlo & Richardson, 1991). It measures, in seconds, the time it takes to rise from a standard chair, walk 3 m (10 feet), turn, walk back to the chair, and sit down. A normal time is less than 20 seconds. If an older adult takes longer than 20 seconds, a physical therapy consult should be considered.

Clinical presentation

Older adults may not present with the classic symptoms of an illness. Often, non-specific symptoms such as confusion, self-neglect, falls, incontinence, apathy, anorexia, dyspnea, and fatigue may be the only indicator of the onset of an acute illness (Flaherty, 2005). It is important that the nurse be aware of the different clinical presentations that older adults may have so that early diagnosis and treatment can occur (Table 2.2).

Laboratory interpretation

The high prevalence of disease in those 65 and older combined with age-related physiologic changes, alterations in nutrition and fluid intake, and medication regimens can make the interpretation of laboratory values in older

Table 2.2 Atypical presentation of illness in older adults.

Illness	Atypical presentation
Infection	• Absence of fever • Sepsis without leukocytosis and fever • Confusion • Decrease in food and fluid intake • Decreased functional ability • Falls
Pneumonia	• Increased respiratory rate with decreased appetite and functioning
Urinary tract infections	• May not have urinary burning • Incontinence • Confusion • Falls
Skin infections	• May be missed in older adults with less ability to undress or move. • Early signs may be missed in people with chronic edema.
Myocardial infarction	• May not have the classic crushing chest pain. • Often presents with a sudden onset of dyspnea which may be accompanied by anxiety and confusion. • Vague symptoms of fatigue, nausea and a decrease in functional ability. • Decreased urine output due to decreased renal perfusion.
Heart failure	• May not experience classic symptoms such as paroxysmal nocturnal dyspnea or coughing • Decreased appetite. • Weight gain of 2–3 pounds. • Complaints of poor sleep.
Type 2 diabetes	• Hyperglycemia: May not experience polyuria, polydipsia, and polyphagia. May present with dehydration, confusion, and incontinence due to glycosuria, and weight loss. • Hypoglycemia: Confusion is an early symptom.
Thyroid disease	• Fatigue and tremor (two common symptoms of thyroid problems) may be absent or missed. • Hyperthyroidism may present with new onset atrial fibrillation, weight loss, proximal muscle weakness, and confusion. • Hyperthyroidism may present as "apathetic thyrotoxicosis" i.e. fatigue and slowing down • Hypothyroidism may have no symptoms or present with confusion and agitation. • Both hypothyroidism and hyperthyroidism may be mis-diagnosed as depression.
Gastrointestinal bleed	• May present with signs of dehydration and crampy abdominal pain that is difficult to localize.

(Continued)

Table 2.2 (*Continued*)

Illness	Atypical presentation
Gastrointestinal obstruction	• May be absence of usual board-like abdomen. • May present with cramps, dehydration, stringy stool or diarrhea, and vague complaints of feeling unwell.
Diverticulosis	• Diffuse abdominal pain and a low-grade fever
Depression	• Lack of sadness • Somatic complaints • Hyperactivity • Assumed as a normal part of aging

Sources: Amella, E. (2004) Presentation of illness in older adults. *American Journal of Nursing* **104**, 40-52. Flaherty, E. (2005). Atypical presentation. Online. Available from http://consultgerirn.org/topics/atypical_presentation/want_to_know_more (accessed 9 March 2012).

adults complicated. Normal laboratory ranges are often based on samples taken from healthy individuals age 20 to 40 and are not always pertinent to patients that are older. When interpreting laboratory values in older adults a geriatric reference range should be used. Nurses must recognize that there is no singular trend for changes in laboratory values in older adults: Some values increase, some decrease, and others remain unchanged with aging. Laboratory values should be interpreted with the full assessment of an older adult in mind. (Edwards & Baird, 2005). Routine assessment of the older patient's renal status (i.e. glomerular filtration rate) is essential since many medications require renal dosing.

References

Agency for Healthcare Research and Quality (2011) Health literacy measurement tools. Online. Available from http://www.ahrq.gov/populations/sahlsatool.htm (accessed 24 April 2012).

Amella, E. (2004) Presentation of illness in older adults: If you think you know what you are looking for, think again. *American Journal of Nursing* **104**, 40-52.

Awan, K. (2010) Caring for the geriatric patient: The initial visit. *The Clinical Advisor* **13**(1), 29-34.

Bergstrom, N., Braden, B., Laguzza, A. & Holman, A. (1987) The Braden Scale for predicting pressure sore risk. *Nursing Research* **36**(4), 205-210.

Borson, S., Scanlan, J.M., Brush, M., Vitaliano, P. & Dokmak, A. (2000) The Mini Cog: A cognitive 'vital signs' measure for dementia screening in multi-lingual elderly. *International Journal of Geriatric Psychiatry* **15**, 1021-1027.

Braes, T., Milisen, K. & Foreman, M.D. (2009) Assessing cognitive function. Online. Available from http://consultgerirn.org/topics/assessing_cognitive_function/want_to_know_more (accessed 9 March 2012).

DeFrances, C.J., Lucas, C.A., Buie, V.C. & Golosinskly, A. (2008) 2006 National hospital discharge survey. *National Health Statistic Reports* **5**, 1-20.

Edwards, N. & Baird, C. (2005) Interpreting laboratory values in older adults. *MEDSURG Nursing* **14**(4), 220-229.

Flaherty, E. (2005) Atypical presentation. Online. Available from http://consultgerirn.org/topics/atypical_presentation/want_to_know_more (accessed 9 March 2012).

Folstein, M.F., Folstein, S.E. & McHugh, P.R. (1975) "Mini-MentalState": A practical method for grading the cognitive state of patients for the clinician. *Journal of Psychiatric Research* **12**, 189-198.

Francis, D.C. (2005) Iatrogenesis. Online. Available from http://consultgerirn.org/topics/iatrogenesis/want_to_know_more (accessed 9 March 2012).

Fulmer, T.T. (1991) The geriatric nurse specialist role: A new model. *Nursing Management* **22**(3), 91-3.

Fulmer, T., Hyer, K., Flaherty, E., *et al.* (2005) Geriatric interdisciplinary team training program: Evaluation results. *Journal of Aging and Health* **17**(4), 443-470.

Inouye, S.K., Foreman, M.D., Mion, L C., Katz, K.H. & Cooney, L.M., Jr. (2001) Nurses' recognition of delirium and its symptoms: Comparison of nurse and researcher ratings. *Archives of Internal Medicine* **161**, 2467-2473.

Lewis, T.P. (2008) Assessing an older adult for alcohol use disorders. *Nursing2008* **38**(6), 60-61.

National Network Libraries of Medicine (2010) Health literacy. Online. Available from http://nnlm.gov/outreach/consumer/hlthlit.html (accessed 24 April 2012).

Podsiadlo, D. & Richardson, S. (1991) The timed "Up and Go": A test of basic functional mobility for frail elderly persons. *Journal of the American Geriatrics Society* **39**(2), 142-148.

Russo, C.A. & Elixhauser, A. (2003) Hospitalization in the elderly population.

Singleton, K. & Krause, E. (2009) Understanding cultural and linguistic barriers to health literacy. *The Online Journal of Issues in Nursing* **14**(3). Online. Available from http://www.nursingworld.org/MainMenuCategories/ANAMarketplace/ANAPeriodicals/OJIN/TableofContents/Vol142009/No3Sept09/Cultural-and-Linguistic-Barriers-.aspx (accessed 24 April 2012).

Wallace, M. & Fulmer, T. (2007) Fulmer SPICES: An overall assessment tool for older adults. Try This Assessment Series: The Hartford Institute for Geriatric Nursing. Online. Available from http://consultgerirn.org/uploads/File/trythis/try_this_1.pdf (accessed 9 March 2012).

Wallace, M. & Shelkey, M. (2007) Try this. Katz Index of Independence in activities of daily living (ADL). Online. Available from http://consultgerirn.org/uploads/File/trythis/try_this_2.pdf (accessed 9 March 2012).

Wallhagen, M.I., Pettengill, E. & Whiteside, M. (2006a) Sensory impairment in older adults: Part 1: Hearing loss. *American Journal of Nursing* **106**(10), 40-47.

Wallhagen, M.I., Pettengill, E. & Whiteside, M. (2006b) Sensory impairment in older adults: Part 2: Vision loss. *American Journal of Nursing* **106**(11), 52-61.

Weiss, B.D., Mays, M.Z., Martz, W. *et al.* (2005) Quick assessment of literacy in primary care: The newest vital sign. *Annals of Family Medicine* **3**(6), 514-522.

Chapter 3
Clinical Issues

Unit 1: Skin Disorders

Terry Mahan Buttaro

Skin disorders in elders occur for varied reasons. Skin cellular regeneration decreases, subcutaneous tissue is lost and the skin becomes dry and less elastic (causing wrinkling). Skin and blood vessels also thin with aging and become more fragile. As a result, elders bruise easily, and purpura and skin tears occur with minimal trauma.

■ Risk factors
- Medications
- Multiple co-morbidities
- Decreased immune system
- Decreased vision and other sensory changes
- Diminished reaction time
- Decreased mobility
- Cognition changes
- Increased risk for falls

■ Clinical presentation
Skin disorders can have an acute (e.g., skin tear) or more gradual onset (e.g., a fungal infection). Learning the onset, progression, associated symptoms, and recent exposures to medications, soaps, or other potential irritants is important (see Table 3.1.1.1). If an injury caused the skin problem then it is essential to know the mechanism or injury cause. For example, a skin tear that occurs

Nursing Care of the Hospitalized Older Patient, First Edition. Edited by
Terry Mahan Buttaro and Kate A. Barba.
© 2013 John Wiley & Sons, Inc. Published 2013 by John Wiley & Sons, Inc.

Table 3.1.1.1 Morphology of skin lesions.

> Macule: flat lesion, less than 10 mm, with change in skin color (e.g., a freckle, port wine stain, or drug reaction)
> Papule: a palpable, raised lesion less than 10 mm (e.g., wart)
> Plaque: palpable lesion greater than 10 mm (e.g., psoriasis)
> Nodule: firm lesion extends into dermis (e.g., cyst, lipoma)
> Vesicle: small blister less than 10 mm filled with clear fluid (e.g., herpes zoster)
> Bullae: large blister greater than 10 mm filled with clear fluid (e.g., bullous pemphigoid)
> Pustule: a vesicular lesion containing pus (folliculitis)
> Cyst: defined, soft, palpable lesion
> Urticaria: a raised localized lesion with defined borders (hives)
> Scales: dead cells that are dry, flaking (seborrheic dermatitis, psoriasis)
> Crusts/eschars: dried blood, serum or purulent material often found in wound bed or with infectious processes (e.g., impetigo)
> Fissures: cracks/crevices found in athlete's foot or xerosis

Created from information found in The Merck Manuals Online Medical Library (http://www.merckmanuals.com/professional/index.html).

because the patient fainted is often more serious (because the fainting suggests a serious underlying problem) that a skin tear caused by a bump into a counter. Other important information includes:

- Allergies
  - A sulfa allergy prohibits the use of silver sulfadiazine cream for burns.
- Current medications including creams, herbal ointments, and over the counter medications
- Review of symptoms
  - Did the patient have a recent illness?
  - Are there associated symptoms?
- Past medical history
  - Has the patient had this skin problem in the past?
  - What treatments were used and successful?
- Family history
  - Do other family members have a similar skin problem?

Physical examination

A head to toe skin exam is thorough and provides information about the skin problem as well as other important physical findings. Examine the scalp hair, mouth, torso, extremities (including the plantar surfaces of the feet), skin folds, and nails. Skin findings should be documented noting the location, size (in millimeters or centimeters), and characteristics (e.g., morphology of skin lesions, erythema, scaling, exudate, tenderness) (see http://www.merck.com/mmpe/sec10/ch109/ch109b.html).

Reference

The Merck Manuals On Line Medical Library. Description of Skin Lesions. Available from http://www.merck.com/mmpe/sec10/ch109/ch109b.html (accessed 12 March 2012).

PART 2: BURNS

Terry Mahan Buttaro

Burn injuries in elders occur for a variety of reasons: trauma, scald/flame injuries, and occasionally chemical injuries (Gomez *et al.*, 2008). Women incur more burns than men and most burns occur in the home in the kitchen or bath (Gomez *et al.*, 2008). Unfortunately, co-morbidities and aging changes complicate wound healing and patient recovery.

■ Risk factors

- Cognitive dysfunction
- Decreased reaction time in older adults
- Disability
- Immobility

■ Clinical presentation

Most burns that occur in older adults are related to trauma or an accident in the home. Often these are related to a flame or scalding injury, though electrical injuries or chemical burns are also common causes of burns in all age groups. Scald burns can also occur in hospitals or nursing facilities. These burns are usually from hot liquid spills, hot bath or shower water, and hot or cold packs. However, acquired burns can be related to chemotherapeutics, surgical procedures (e.g., cauterization), defibrillation, radiation, or medical equipment (e.g., a nitroglycerin patch left on a patient in an MRI machine). Determining the cause of the burn is important in guiding treatment as electrical burns may cause significant internal injuries rather than visible skin injury.

■ Nursing assessment

Burn assessment is based on the classification (Table 3.1.2.1) of the burn as well as the amount of body surface affected (Table 3.1.2.2). Body surface is assessed by the "rule of nines", but it is essential also to assure that the patient's airway has not been affected by fire and smoke inhalation (Table 3.1.2.2). Important considerations include:

- Vital signs
- Airway assessment:
  - Is there cyanosis?

Table 3.1.2.1   Burn classification.

First degree burns: Superficial injury, painful, erythematous, without skin loss

Second degree: Partial thickness skin loss, erythematous areas with vesicles, painful

Third degree: Painless full thickness skin loss with possible tissue destruction into subcutaneous tissue and/or muscle

Table 3.1.2.2   Burn percentage body surface estimate for adults.

● Head	● 9%
● Arm	● 9% each arm
● Anterior torso	● 18%
● Posterior torso	● 18%
● Leg	● 9% each leg
● Genitals	● 1%

  ○ Is the patient coughing?
  ○ Is there sooty appearing sputum?
● Respiratory:
  ○ Are lung sounds clear or wheezing?
● Cardiac:
  ○ Are peripheral pulses symmetrical in all extremities?
● Skin:
  ○ Head to toe assessment of body surfaces including scalp, eyelashes, palms, soles or feet.

■ Diagnostics

For minor burns, diagnostic testing may not be necessary. For major burns, arterial blood gases, CBC/differential, serum electrolytes, (blood urea nitrogen) and creatinine.

■ Differential diagnosis

● Chemical burn
● Contact burn
● Electrical burn
● Flame burn
● Scald burn
● Scalded skin syndrome
● Toxic epidermal necrolysis

■ Treatment

- Individualized for each patient
- Tetanus update if indicated
- Pain management
- Keep patient adequately hydrated, monitor intake/output.
- Some burns can be left uncovered, others will require dressing with non-adherent dressing, then DSD.
- Avoid using tape on elderly skin. Wrap wounds with Kerlix to prevent further skin damage.
- General burn care
  - Clean with normal saline or mild soap and water.
  - Keep wound beds clean.
  - Discuss with physician accumulation of debris or eschars in wound.
  - Superficial burn treatment
    - Discuss with physician:
      - Thin film silver sulfadiazine (Silvadene) cream in non-sulfa allergic patients
        - Thin film mupirocin (Bactroban) cream or Aquaphor dressing in sulfa allergic patients.
  - Cover with Telfa or other non-adherent dressing, then a DSD.

■ Collaborative consultation

Burn care requires continual assessment and evaluation of treatment and pain management. Daily consultation with the physician is necessary. Additionally, any deleterious change in the patient's condition should be immediately discussed with the physician.

■ Complications

- Cellulitis
- Fluid and electrolyte abnormalities
- Infection
- Scarring
- Sepsis

■ Prevention

- Education is paramount in preventing burns. Unfortunately, patient teaching on burn prevention does not often occur until after the injury. Since older patients are at risk for scald injuries, reminding patients to decrease the water temperature may be helpful. Other reminders include:
  - Avoid flame burns by not using candles, not wearing loose clothing while cooking.
  - Avoid contact burns with hot water bottles, heating pads, and ice packs by reminding patients to wrap these devices in a towel and using only for 15 minutes, then waiting 15 minutes before applying the device again. Patients should be reminded not to take heating pads, hot water bottles or ice packs to bed.

- Turn off electrical current before making repairs.
- Remind patients to "stop, drop, and roll" if clothes begin to burn.
- Avoid the use of microwaves to warm soaks as uneven distribution of heat can occur.

■ Patient/family education

- Burn care and potential complications and sequelae should be carefully explained to the patient and family.
- Fire Prevention for Older Adults (http://www.usfa.dhs.gov/downloads/pdf/publications/fa-221.pdf)
  - Family members should be encouraged to do a safety check of electrical equipment (including smoke alarms) and water temperature for older patients unable to do this themselves. A home safety evaluation by the local Visiting Nurses Association is another consideration.
  - If the older adult smokes or lives in a home with a smoker, education needs to include how to dispose of smoking materials appropriately, importance of not smoking in bed or while sleepy. If oxygen is in the home, no one in the home should smoke.
  - While cooking, use pot holders, turn pot handles in toward the back of the stove , and do not wear loose clothes.
  - Have heating equipment inspected yearly.

References

Gomez, M., Cartotto, R. & Fish, J. (2008) Survival following burn injury among 12,434 older adults: a ten-year analysis of the National Burn Repository of the American Burn Association. *Journal of Burn Care & Research* **29**(1), 130–137.
US Fire Administration (2010) Fire Safety Checklist for Older Adults. Online. Available from http://www.usfa.dhs.gov/downloads/pdf/publications/fa-221.pdf (accessed 12 March 2012).

Further reading

Deignan, E.M. & Carrougher, G. (2008) Burns (minor). In Buttaro, T.M., Trybulski, J., Bailey, P.P. & Sandberg-Cook, J. (eds). *Primary Care: A Collaborative Practice*, 3rd edition. Mosby, St. Louis.
Hettiaratchy, S. & Dziewulski, P. (2004) ABC of burns. *British Medical Journal*, **328**(7452), 1366–1368.

PART 3: CELLULITIS

Terry Mahan Buttaro

Commonly caused by staphylococci or group A beta-hemolytic streptococci, cellulitis is a skin infection that affects the deep dermis and subcutaneous tissue as well as the epidermis. Skin infections both in hospitals and in the community are increasing , often caused by methicillin resistant staphylococcus aureau (MRSA) (Hersh *et al.*, 2008). There is often no specific point of entry identified, but older adults are particularly vulnerable because of associated comorbid disorders and dry skin.

Periorbital cellulitis occurs around the eyes or in the lacrimal system (tear ducts). These infections can be related to insect bites also, or from conjunctivitis, blepharitis, inflammation of lacrimal sac, impetigo, sinusitis, or other facial infections.

■ Risk factors

- Any alteration in skin integrity: falls, fracture, trauma
- Chronic skin irritation
- Edema
- Fungal skin infection
- Heart failure
- History of falls, fractures
- Hyperglycemia
- Immunocompromised
- Intravenous lines, medications
- Lymphedema
- Obesity
- Poor hygiene
- Venectomy
- Venous stasis

■ Clinical presentation

Onset is often acute. Patients may be asymptomatic or complain of a recent rash, insect bite, injury, infection, or joint stiffness. Associated symptoms can include change in mental status, fever, chills, edema, fatigue, nausea, vomiting, malaise, and/or myalgias. History should also include patient allergies, current medications, associated symptoms, time of onset, and past medical history.

■ Nursing assessment

Common clinical signs of cellulitis include:

- Erythema with well-defined borders
- Edema (may have stretched shiny appearance to skin)
- Warmth
- Tenderness
- Lymphadenitis (red streaking) (possible finding)
- Vesicular lesions (possible finding).

Findings associated with periorbital cellulitis include erythema, edema, and tenderness of eyelids or areas around the eye. Possible vesicular eruption around eye can suggest herpes zoster infection.

Other signs important to determine include:

- Vital signs:
  - Fever
  - Tachypnea
  - Tachycardia
  - Hypotension
- Cardiovascular evaluation
- Lymph glands: Check for lymphadenopathy near area of infection
- Skin assessment for bites, burns, lacerations, decubiti, fungal infections (tinea, intertrigo), rashes, recent surgical procedures, ulcerations
  - Check between fingers/toes for fissures, cracks.

■ Diagnostics

Often, cellulitis is a clinical diagnosis and diagnostic testing is not indicated. For patients with a high fever, systemic symptoms (anorexia, nausea, vomiting), or concerns about osteomyelitis or dehydration related to the infection, the following diagnostics tests might be indicated:

- Complete blood count/differential
- Serum electrolytes
- Blood urea nitrogen (BUN), creatinine
- Uric acid (if gout is considered in the differential diagnosis)
- Blood cultures, if sepsis is suspected
- X-rays if hand, foot, or joint involvement is suspected
- Wound cultures (not often indicated)
- Sedimentation rate (ESR) if suspected osteomyelitis
- Non-cardiac C-reactive protein (CRP) if suspected osteomyelitis
- Bone biopsy (for suspected osteomyelitis)

■ Differential diagnosis

- Deep vein thrombophlebitis
- Erysipelas (rapidly spreading bacterial infection with lymphadenitis [red streaking])
- Folliculitis
- Gout
- Localized reaction to insect bite
- Necrotizing fasciitis
- Ruptured Baker's cyst
- Vasculitis
- Venous stasis dermatitis

■ Treatment

- Antibiotic therapy is usually indicated and will depend on patient presentation and comorbidities, recent antibiotic therapy, allergies, and current medications.

- Good daily hygiene
- Dressing care if indicated (for weeping, exudates)
- Tetanus prophylaxis if indicated

■ Collaborative consultation

- Consult with physician for all suspected skin or bone infections. Some patients can be treated with oral antibiotics, but many require hospitalization for intravenous therapy.
- When discussing potential antibiotic treatment with the physician or other health care provider, be certain to review patient allergies, antibiotic therapy within the past 3 to 6 months, concurrent medications (especially warfarin), and comorbidities.

■ Complications

- Brain abscess
- Joint infections
- Infective endocarditis
- Meningitis
- Osteomyelitis
- Sepsis
- Tissue necrosis

■ Prevention

- Arm and leg protectors for patients in wheelchairs
- Clear areas around bed, bathroom and halls to prevent injuries
- Falls prevention
- Foot care with proper fitting slippers/shoes
- Good nutrition
- Hydration
- Hygiene (especially foot, nail, and skin care)
- Hyperglycemic control
- Monitor and care for intravenous sites
- Nail care (nails cut regularly)
- Skin care with daily lotion application to prevent skin cracking

■ Patient/family education

- Explain cause and treatment of infection as well as potential side effects of antibiotic therapy.
- Discuss the importance of taking medications as prescribed to prevent complications.
- Discuss preventive care to avoid falls, trauma, and subsequent infection.
- Explain how to contact physician after discharge for medication side effects or increase in fever, pain, or other concerning symptoms.

Reference

Hersh, A.L., Chambers, H.F., Maselli, J.H. & Gonzales, R. (2008) National trends in ambulatory visits and antibiotic prescribing for skin and soft-tissue infections. *Archives of Internal Medicine* **168**(16), 1585-1591.

Further reading

Chung-Hsin, Y., Wen-Chao, C., Lin, M., Hwa, Tzu, H., Shih Chun, C. & Yi-Chen, L. (2010) Intracranial brain abscess preceded by orbital cellulitis and sinusitis. *Journal of Craniofacial Surgery* **21**(3), 934-936.

PART 4: CONTACT DERMATITIS

Terry Mahan Buttaro

A skin reaction caused by a substance that causes a rash and pruritus, allergic contact dermatitis is associated with poison ivy or poison oak, but some jewelry, perfumes, soaps, cleansing agents, creams, topical medications, latex, or other allergens can also cause this irritating skin disorder. Allergic contact dermatitis is a Type IV (delayed) hypersensitivity reaction (Pichler, 2003).

Irritant contact dermatitis affects patients with a history of chronic exposure to irritants that can include friction, soap and water or harsh irritants such as chemicals that cause erythema, edema, and burns (Habif *et al.*, 2006).

■ Risk factors

- Allergen exposure
  - Metals, gloves, skin products, neomycin or other topical medications, tape
  - Poison ivy, oak, or sumac
- Irritant exposure
  - Airborne irritants (chemicals, resins, solvents, sawdust)
  - Chronic friction
  - Chronic hand washing or continued exposure to moisture (e.g., childcare, food service or healthcare workers)
  - Airborne irritants (chemicals, resins, solvents, sawdust)
  - Soaps, detergents
- Personal or family history of eczema

■ Clinical presentation

Patients will complain of a recent or chronic, pruritic rash after exposure to allergen. The history is important to determine the allergen as well as previous personal history.

■ Nursing assessment

A careful and thorough skin exam is necessary to determine and document the appearance as well as locations and extent of the lesions.

- Allergic contact dermatitis:
  - Poison ivy, oak and sumac: pruritic, vesicular lesions on erythematous base at site(s) of point of contact. Lesions often have a linear appearance.
- Irritant contact dermatitis:
  - Burning, cracking, fissuring, scaling, erythema and tenderness acutely. After time, chronic skin changes occur, causing hyperkeratosis.
  - Irritant diaper dermatitis.

■ Diagnostics

Contact dermatitis is usually based on patient history and physical exam findings. Skin (patch) testing is considered for patients with continued episodes of pruritus and skin irritation despite therapy. Other tests include:

- RAST testing
- Skin scraping if scabies is a consideration
- Culture if tinea is suspected
- Scratch test

■ Differential diagnosis

- Allergic contact dermatitis
- Atopic dermatitis
- Dyshidrotic eczema
- Impetigo
- Irritant contact dermatitis
- Psoriasis
- Scabies
- Tinea

■ Treatment

- Allergic contact dermatitis:
  - Identifying offending allergens is helpful to prevent future reactions.
  - Wearing gloves, cleanse skin with tepid water, mild soap, rinse, pat dry, and apply topical corticosteroid as prescribed. Do not use other skin products while using topical corticosteroids unless prescribed by the doctor.
  - Systemic corticosteroids may be necessary for facial and/or hand involvement and in severe cases. Oral steroids are best taken in the morning with food.
  - Hydroxyzine may be indicated for severe pruritus, but use carefully in elders.
  - Monitor for signs of infection, improvement.

- Irritant contact dermatitis:
  - Friction or other physical irritant (e.g., constant moisture) should be avoided.

■ Collaborative consultation

Discuss with physician: patient history and nursing assessment for treatment recommendations.

■ Complications

- Secondary infection
- Lichenification (dry, thickened skin)

■ Prevention

- Avoiding substances that cause the reaction is crucial. If contact is unavoidable wearing gloves can be helpful though for some chemical products specific glove and protective clothing is often indicated.
- For moisture associated irritant contact dermatitis, it is important to keep moisture contact with the skin to a minimum. Vaseline or other protective skin cream can also be helpful.

■ Patient/family education

Patients and families need to understand the cause of the reaction and how best to prevent reoccurrence. It is also useful for patients and families to know when and how to contact the healthcare provider when dermatitis occurs.

Reference

Pichler, W.J. (2003) Delayed drug hypersensitivity reactions. *Annals of Internal Medicine* **139**(8), 683-693.

Further reading

Habif, T.P., Campbell, J.L., Chapman, M.S., Dinulos, J.G.H. & Zug, K.A. (2006) *Dermatology*. Mosby, St. Louis.

PART 5: HERPES ZOSTER

Terry Mahan Buttaro

More than a million people are afflicted with herpes zoster each year (Weaver, 2007; CDC, 2010). This skin disorder occurs rather acutely and is caused by a reactivation of the varicella (chicken pox) virus which remains dormant in ganglion after chicken pox infection. Commonly known as shingles, herpes zoster is associated with a unilateral painful rash that can occur in any body dermatome. The rash and pain does resolve, but many patients develop postherpetic neuralgia, which can be disabling and surprisingly may not be diagnosed (Dworkin *et al.*, 2007). Elders seem to be at risk for shingles, though people in any age group can be affected.

Herpes zoster ophthalmicus is a herpetic infection involving the ophthalmic nerve, the first division of cranial nerve 5 (the trigeminal nerve) (Liesegang, 2008). Symptoms of herpes zoster ophthalmicus are similar to herpes zoster. Some patients do not develop the rash. Often the only sign is a vesicular lesion near the tip of the nose, but a typical herpes zoster ophthalmicus rash would extend from the forehead to the eye to the nose.

■ Risk factors

- Increased age
- Immunosuppression from disease or medications
- Previous history chickenpox
- Radiation
- Stress
- Trauma

■ Clinical presentation

Up to 3 days prior to the rash eruption, patients may note a prodrome: discomfort, pruritus, a burning sensation and/or fever, generalized malaise or headache. When the rash occurs it is unilateral involving one or two dermatomes.

■ Nursing assessment

Some patients will not have an obvious skin eruption, but will have pain or discomfort along a dermatome.

Rash characteristics include:

- Pruritic, painful macular-papular eruption on erythematous base becomes vesicular:
  - Vesicles occur in clusters and can be varied in size.
  - Initially vesicles contain clear fluid, but fluid appears purulent in a few days.
  - Vesicles rupture and crust.
- Unilateral on one-two dermatomes
- Vesicles on the forehead, nose, or near the eye suggest ophthalmic herpes

■ Diagnostics

Herpes zoster is a clinical diagnosis, so diagnostics are not usually necessary. Diagnostics that might aid in determining if rash is herpes zoster include:

- Varicella-zoster virus (VSV) culture from vesicular lesion fluid
- VSV serology

- Direct fluorescent antibody staining
- VZV polymerase chain reaction

■ Differential diagnosis

- Shingles pain usually precedes the rash, so that the pain caused by herpes zoster can be mistaken for angina, appendicitis, ulcer, colic or other disorder.
- Contact dermatitis
- Drug allergy
- Eczema herpeticum
- Folliculitis
- Impetigo
- Herpes simplex
- Coxsackie virus infection

■ Treatment

- Lesions should be kept clean, dry, and covered (CDC, 2008).
- Antiviral treatment is most beneficial if started within 48 hours (Habif, Zug et al., 2006):
  - Acyclovir (Zovirax), valacyclovir (Valtrex), or famciclovir (Famvir) can be used to treat shingles. Dosing depends on the patient's renal status as patients with renal insufficiency will need lower dosing (CDC, 2008).
- Pain medication:
  - Oxycodone may be more helpful than gabapentin in the acute phase (Dworkin et al., 2009), though some elders will become confused on opioids.
  - For post herpetic pain:
    - Lidocaine 5% patches 1-3 applied once daily
    - Acetaminophen
    - Opiates
    - NSAIDs (cautiously because of GI bleeding risks and fluid retention concerns)
    - Gabapentin (Neurontin)
- Appropriate infection control precautions should be initiated:
  - A person who has never had chickenpox can get chickenpox from a patient who has shingles (herpes zoster) through direct contact with drainage from the lesions or by contact with items that have been contaminated by drainage from the lesions.
  - An immunocompromised patient who has disseminated herpes zoster can transmit chickenpox by the airborne route as well as by contact.
  - Patients suspected of having disseminated herpes zoster or localized zoster in an immunocompromised patient should be placed in a private room with negative air pressure on Airborne Precautions and Contact Precautions.

■ Collaborative consultation

- It is important to notify the physician whenever herpes zoster is suspected. The sooner shingles is treated the less likely the patient will develop postherpetic neuralgia.
- Immediate consultation with the physician is necessary for suspected ophthalmic involvement (if the patient has vesicles on the forehead, nose, or close to the eye).

■ Complications

- Aseptic meningitis
- Chronic encephalitis
- Contralateral hemiparesis
- Encephalomyelitis
- Infection
- Guillain-Barré syndrome
- Hearing problems
- Myelitis
- Necrosis
- Ocular complications with ophthalmic zoster
  - Blindness
- Peripheral nerve palsies
- Pneumonia
- Postherpetic neuralgia
- Ramsay Hunt syndrome
  - Vesicles/pain in external auditory canal
  - Facial palsy (ipsilateral)
  - Diminished taste sensation anterior aspect tongue (ipsilateral)
- Direct contact with the rash can result in transmission to others who never had chickenpox or varicella vaccine.
- Scarring

■ Prevention

Varicella virus vaccine (Varivax)

■ Patient/family education

All older patients should be educated about shingles and shingles prevention. Patient education should include the following:

- Cause of shingles and progression to postherpetic neuralgia
- Risk factors
- Symptoms and need to call doctor as soon as possible after symptom onset
- Preventing shingles transmission
- Vaccine prevention

References

Centers for Disease Control and Prevention (2010) Shingles disease-questions and answers. Online. Available from http://www.cdc.gov/shingles/about/index.html (accessed 12 March 2012).

Centers for Disease Control and Prevention (2008) Prevention of herpes zoster: recommendations of the Advisory Committee on Immunization Practices. *MMWR* **57**(5), 1-20.

Dworkin, R.H., Barbano, R.L., Tyring, S.K., *et al.* (2009) A randomized, placebo controlled trial of oxycodone and gabapentin for acute pain in herpes zoster. *Pain* **142**, 209-217.

Dworkin, R.H., White, R., O'Connor, A.B., Baser, O. & Hawkins, K. (2007) Healthcare costs of acute and chronic pain associated with a diagnosis of herpes zoster. *Journal of the American Geriatrics Society* **55**(8), 1168-1175.

Habif, T.P., Campbell, J.L., Chapman, M.S., Dinulos, J.G.H. & Zug, K.A. (2006) *Dermatology*. Mosby, St. Louis.

Liesegang, T.J. (2008) Herpes zoster opthalmicus natural history, risk factors, clinical presentation and morbidity. *Opthalmology* **115**(2 Suppl), S3-S12.

Weaver, B.A. (2007) The burden of herpes zoster and postherpetic neuralgia in the United States. *Journal of the American Osteopath Association* **107**(3 Suppl 1), S2-S7.

PART 6: PURPURA

Terry Mahan Buttaro

Purpura is an area of hemorrhage in the skin or mucous membranes. Initially the lesions, which can be flat or palpable, are a slightly erythematous color, but as the lesions resolve they turn brownish (Sandberg-Cook, 2008). Purpura are approximately 3mm to 1cm in size (Sandberg-Cook, 2008). Petechiae look similar to purpura but are smaller, less than 3mm (Sandberg-Cook, 2008). Ecchymoses are larger lesions (>1cm) (Sandberg-Cook, 2008). Purpura and ecchymoses occur frequently in older adults. Ecchymoses are usually related to trauma and purpura can be caused by trauma also. Older adults are particularly susceptible because the dermis of their skin is thinner, they have less subcutaneous tissue, and their blood vessels are thinner. Purpura are often benign (e.g., senile purpura), but purpura are associated with more serious conditions also: tickborne diseases, medications, autoimmune disorders, leukemia, lymphoma, and vasculitis (Sandberg-Cook, 2008; Warkentin, 2007).

There are two distinct types of purpura:

- Inflammatory (palpable) purpura (Sandberg-Cook, 2008)
  - A vascular response causes blood vessel wall inflammation (vasculitis) and hemorrhage resulting in a raised, palpable lesion
    - Henoch–Schönlein purpura
    - Schamberg purpura
- Noninflammatory purpura (Molise *et al.*, 2007; Sandberg-Cook, 2008)

○ Categorized by the hemostatic defect as nonpalpable purpura or vascular purpura
- ○ Allergic
  - ■ Drug induced vasculitis
- ○ Coagulation or platelet abnormality
- ○ Embolic
  - ■ Atheroembolic
- ○ Impaired blood vessel integrity
  - ■ Senile purpura
  - ■ Steroid therapy
  - ■ Vitamin C deficiency
- ○ Infection
  - ■ Meningococcemia
  - ■ Tick borne (Lyme disease, Rocky Mountain spotted fever), Viral
- ○ Neoplastic
  - ■ Leukemia
  - ■ Lymphoma
- ○ Thrombotic
  - ■ Antiphospholipid syndrome
  - ■ Disseminated intravascular coagulation
  - ■ Idiopathic thrombocytopenic purpura
  - ■ Purpura fulminans
- ○ Trauma

■ Risk factors

Risk factors may differ depending on the underlying etiology of the purpura. Potential risk factors can include the following:

- Age
- Antiphospholipid antibody syndrome or other coagulation disorder
- Autoimmune disorder
- Cardiopulmonary bypass surgery
- Infectious process
- HIV infection
- Malignancy
- Medications
- Splenomegaly
- Trauma
- Vitamin C deficiency

■ Clinical presentation

The onset of purpura can be sudden and noticed by the patient or caregiver. Senile purpura, isolated lesions seen on an elder's hands/upper extremities, are benign and can occur after minor trauma. Other causes of purpura can be quite serious and related to a medication, illness, or a clotting or platelet disorder. A careful history should include:

- Current medications
- Past medical history plus history of recent infection, tick bite, travel, trauma
- A thorough review of any associated patient symptoms (i.e., headache; bleeding; easy bruising; menometrorrhagia; fever; chills; arthralgias; abdominal, joint, scrotal, or lesion pain) helps differentiate the type of purpura.

■ Nursing assessment

A careful skin exam plus evaluation of the mucous membranes may reveal multiple purpura. The lesions may be pinpoint or larger. They may be isolated and discrete or begin to coalesce. Depending on the type of purpura, the lesions may or may not be palpable, pruritic, symmetric, and located on buccal mucosa, hands, upper or lower extremities, buttocks, or back (Habif *et al.*, 2006). Lesion color ranges from a bright erythema in new lesions to a brownish tone in older lesions. The lesions can be scale-like in appearance. Further assessment is necessary to determine lymphadenopathy, hepatomegaly, splenomegaly, Lower extremity edema is possible in some types of purpura (Habif *et al.*, 2006).

■ Diagnostics

- CBC/differential
- Platelets
- PT/PTT/INR
- Bleeding time
- BUN, creatinine
- LFTs
- ESR
- Rheumatoid factor, if indicated
- Antinuclear antibodies, if indicated
- Antineutrophil cytoplasmic antibody, if indicated
- Serum protein electrophoresis, if indicated
- Immunoglobulin levels, if indicated
- Bone marrow aspiration, if indicated
- Biopsy, if indicated
- Dermoscopy

■ Differential diagnosis

The differential diagnosis is extensive. Purpura can be benign, related to a number of medications, subacute endocarditis, sepsis or other infection, transfusions, lymphoproliferative disorders, HIV, DIC, embolization, vitamin C deficiency, and varied other disorders.

Medications associated with purpura include:

- Allopurinol
- Antibiotics

- Aspirin
- Cimetidine
- Cytotoxic agents
- Estrogen
- Ethanol
- Gold
- Heparin
- Hydralazine
- Ketoconazole
- NSAIDs
- Phenytoin
- Propylthiouracil
- Quinidine
- Quinine
- Steroids
- Thiazides
- Vancomycin
- Warfarin

■ Treatment

Treatment depends on the cause of the purpura. If a medication is the cause, stopping the medication, if possible, will be helpful. Consultation with a hematologist or other specialist may be necessary for new onset platelet disorders. NSAIDs are helpful for managing the pain associated with Henoch-Schönlein purpura. Steroids and/or possibly immunosuppressive medications are usually used for the treatment of idiopathic thrombocytopenia and some other purpuras.

■ Collaborative consultation

The doctor should be consulted for any new rash or oral lesions particularly if the patient has a fever. Obtaining the patient history, reviewing recent and current medications, and doing a thorough physical exam will help determine the cause of the purpura so treatment can be initiated.

■ Complications

Complications differ depending on the etiology of the purpura. Bleeding is associated with idiopathic thrombocytopenic purpura. Kidney damage is possible with Henoch-Schönlein purpura (Habif *et al.*, 2006).

■ Prevention

It is not possible to know which patients will develop petechiae or purpura from medications, but being alert and performing a daily skin check is helpful in identifying untoward drug reactions and preventing more serious complications. For patients with senile purpura, avoiding injury is paramount. Keeping the patient's arms and legs covered is helpful. It is also important to try to keep the area in the patient's room and hallways as clear as possible.

■ Patient/family education

Explaining the cause of the purpura and treatment helps allay patient and family anxiety. If a medication is found to be the cause of the purpura avoidance of that medication and others in that category may be necessary. However, in some instances (e.g., for patients taking anticoagulants or antiplatelet medications) it may not be possible to stop the medication.

References

Habif, T.R., Campbell, J.L. Jr., Chapman M.S., Dinulos, J.G.H. & Zug, K.A. (2006) *Dermatology DDx Deck*. Mosby, St. Louis.

Molise, T.A., Tunick, P.A. & Kronzon, I. (2007) Complications of aortic stenosis: atheroemboli and thromboemboli. *Current Treatment Options in Cardiovascular Medicine* **9**, 137-147.

Sandberg-Cook, J. (2008) Purpura. In: Buttaro, T.M., Trybulski, J., Bailey, P.P. & Sandberg-Cook, J. (eds) *Primary Care: A Collaborative Practice*. St. Louis, Mosby.

Warkentin, T.E. (2007) Drug induced immune mediated thrombocytopenia: from purpura to thrombosis. *New England Journal of Medicine* **356**, 891-893.

PART 7: PRURITUS

Terry Mahan Buttaro

Older patients seem to develop pruritus or itching easily. Often the need to scratch is related to xerosis (dry skin), but soaps, medications, systemic illnesses, insect bites, or malignancy are also common causes of pruritus.

■ Risk factors

- Age
- Air conditioning
- Environmental allergens

■ Clinical presentation

The history is very important in determining the cause. Often an acute onset is associated with a new medication, exposure to soaps or fragrances, or a pathological cause. A complete review of medications, allergies, and possible exposures (e.g., pets, heat, humidity, skin care products) is necessary. Learning the patient's family history and past medical history (alcohol use, comorbid illnesses, previous episodes of pruritus) is also helpful.

■ Nursing assessment

A thorough skin examination includes the scalp, finger and toe web spaces as well evaluating the torso and extremities for dry skin, cracking and/or scaling as well as jaundice, insects, rashes, and scratch marks (Norman, 2008). Additional physical assessment should focus on the presence of lymphadenopathy, organomegaly, and cognitive changes (Buttaro *et al.*, 2006).

■ Diagnostics

Diagnostics are not always indicated. If the pruritus is related to an obvious cause (e.g., fungal infection, xerosis) treatment is usually administered without diagnostic testing. If, however, the patient does not respond to initial treatment or the etiology is unclear, then diagnostics may be necessary but are based on each patient's history and clinical presentation. Possible diagnostics can include:

- Blood urea nitrogen/creatinine: evaluate renal function
- Complete blood count/differential to determine if allergies, anemia, or polycythemia is potential cause
- Chemistry panel: evaluate serum glucose and electrolytes
- Erythrocyte sedimentation rate (ESR): measures inflammatory response
- Iron studies
- Liver function tests
- Skin biopsy
- Stool for occult blood
- Stool for ova and parasites
- Thyroid stimulating hormone (TSH)
- If malignancy is suspected:
  - Chest X-ray
  - Serum protein electrophoresis
  - 24 hour urine for 5-Hydroxy indoleacetic acid (5HIAA)

■ Differential diagnosis

There are many causes of pruritus. Some causes will seem obvious if the patient has a skin rash, but often an elder will complain of pruritus and there is no obvious skin disorder. Potential causes include:

- Bullous pemphigoid
- Contact dermatitis
- Drug reaction
- Endocrine disorder: diabetes, hypothyroid
- Folliculitis
- Fungal infection
- Hematologic disorder: iron deficiency anemia, polycythemia vera
- HIV infection

- Infestation (lice, scabies)
- Insect bite
- Lichen simplex dermatitis
- Liver disease
- Malignancy
- Medications
- Neurologic disorders (affecting sweating)
- Nutritional deficiencies
- Parasitic infection
- Psoriasis
- Psychogenic
- Renal disease
- Seborrheic dermatitis
- Systemic illness
- Urticaria
- Xerosis

■ Treatment

Patient comfort is paramount, though treatment is aimed at the cause of the patient's pruritus. If a rash is not present, the approach includes:

- Eliminate environmental allergens
- Adequate hydration and humidification
- Cool environment
- Decrease number of baths
- Tepid water
- Mild soaps (e.g., Cetaphil, Dove unscented)and/or oatmeal baths
- Emollient creams (Lac-hydrin, Eucerin) applied to damp skin
- Unbleached linen
- Cotton clothing
- Topical steroids
- Medication to control itching

■ Collaborative consultation

Patients with pruritus associated with a rash require evaluation by the physician. For patients who do not have a rash associated with pruritus, tepid water baths with a mild soap and an emollient cream to the affected areas may resolve the itching. However, if the pruritus does not resolve within 2 weeks, physician evaluation is necessary (Norman, 2005).

■ Complications

- Scratches
- Infection

■ Prevention

Pruritus associated with dry skin can usually be prevented or at least controlled with adequate hydration, humidification, mild soaps, tepid water, and emollient creams. Prevent scratches and possible infection by keeping nails well trimmed.

■ Patient/family education

All older patients need to understand the importance of adequate hydration, environmental control of heat and humidification, and skin care with mild soaps and emollient creams. Further patient teaching is related to the underlying cause of the pruritus.

References

Buttaro, T.M., Aznavorian, S., & Dick, K. (2006) Clinical Management of Patients in SubAcute and Long-Term Care Settings. Mosby, St. Louis.

Norman, R.A. (2005) Xerosis and pruritus in elderly patients. Part 1. Ostomy Wound Management. Online. Available from http://www.o-wm.com/article/5240 (accessed 12 March 2012).

Norman, R.A. (2008) Xerosis and pruritus in the elderly: Recognition and management. In: Norman, R.A. (ed.) Diagnosis of Aging Skin Diseases. Springer-Verlag, London, pp. 151-160.

PART 8: ACNE ROSACEA

Terry Mahan Buttaro

Rosacea or adult acne starts when people are in their mid 20s or 30s, but then persists throughout adulthood affecting both men and women. The exact etiology of rosacea is unknown, though potential causes include genetics, inflammation, and varied microorganisms (Buechner, 2005). The result is a symmetric erythematous, papular- pustular facial rash with telangiectasia (Buechner, 2005). Warm weather, stress, spicy foods, alcohol, and warm beverages cause vasodilation exacerbating the rash.

■ Risk factors

- Celtic heritage

■ Clinical presentation

Older patients will likely have a past medical history of facial flushing or rosacea, but currently may not be receiving treatment. Alcohol, emotions, sunlight, environmental factors (i.e., heat, humidity), medications, cosmetics/

creams, and foods (e.g., spicy or hot foods) can trigger eruptions, but patients usually have consistent facial erythema (National Rosacea Society, 2010). Some patients will complain of a burning sensation in affected areas, eye discomfort, or a "gritty" sensation in their eyes.

■ Nursing assessment

Facial areas (i.e., forehead, cheeks, and nose) are erythematous with scattered clusters of papular-pustular eruptions. Occasionally the ears, neck, scalp and upper torso will have similar areas of erythema and lesions. Some patients will have telangiectasias (small, visible dilated blood vessels) or rhinophyma (ruddy colored bulbous appearance to nose). Patients with ocular involvement may have conjunctival telangiectasia, lacrimation and/or conjunctivitis (Habif *et al.*, 2006).

■ Diagnostics

Not usually indicated as diagnosis of rosacea is based on clinical presentation and physical exam findings.

■ Differential diagnosis

- Acne
- Perioral dermatitis
- Seborrheic dermatitis
- Carcinoid syndrome – facial flushing without papular/pustular lesions
- Lupus erythematosus – facial flushing without papular/pustular lesions

■ Treatment

- Trigger avoidance
- Sunscreen when outside
- Topical medications
  - Metronidazole 0.75% cream or lotion *or*
  - Sodium sulfacetamide 10% (contraindicated if sulfa allergy)
- Oral antibiotics for severe rosacea
  - Tetracycline 250 milligrams PO twice a day *or*
  - Doxycycline 20-100 milligrams PO daily to twice a day *or*
  - Erythromycin 500 milligrams PO twice a day
- Surgery or laser treatment may be necessary for severe cases

■ Collaborative consultation

- Older patients who complain of new onset facial flushing without lesion eruptions should be evaluated by the physician for possible lupus or carcinoid syndrome.

- For patients with a history of rosacea, physician consultation is indicated if trigger avoidance does not control symptoms.

■ Complications

- Ocular complications are the most serious, but the facial disfigurement can cause patients to feel self-conscious.

■ Prevention

- Trigger prevention is key to controlling flushing and lesion eruption
- Avoid harsh skin products (e.g., soaps, cleansers, cosmetics)
- Avoid skin products with fragrances, alcohol
- Sun protection
  - Hats to shield face from sun
  - Sunscreen

■ Patient/family education

Understanding how trigger prevention can control symptoms is helpful.

References

Buechner, S.A. (2005) Rosacea: an update. *Dermatology* **210**(12), 100-108.
Habif, T.P., Campbell, J.L., Chapman, M.S., Dinulos, J.G.H. & Zug, K.A. (2006) *Dermatology*. Mosby, St. Louis.
National Rosacea Society (2010) Information for patients. Online. Available from http://www.rosacea.org/patients/materials/triggersindex.php (accessed 12 March 2012).

PART 9: SEBORRHEIC DERMATITIS

Terry Mahan Buttaro

Seborrheic dermatitis affects varied age groups, but older patients may be more at risk because of changes in immune function. It is a fairly common condition that may be related to a yeast infection (Habif *et al.*, 2006). *Malassezia* spp., a commonly found yeast, may play a role in this disorder, but the pathology is unclear and the organism is not a direct cause of the inflammation in seborrheic dermatitis (Zisova, 2009). Associated with Parkinson's disease as well as with other neurological disorders and some medications, seborrheic dermatitis can be worse in colder climates and some patients, there may be a familial predisposition (Berk & Scheinfeld, 2010). Several areas can be affected, but when the scalp is affected this disorder is more commonly known as dandruff.

■ Risk factors

- Immune dysfunction (e.g., age, cancer, diabetes mellitus, human immuno-deficiency virus/acquired immune deficiency syndrome)
- Familial amyloidosis
- Medications
  - Buspirone (Buspar)
  - Chlorpromazine
  - Haloperidol (Haldol)
  - Lithium
- Trisomy 21

■ Clinical presentation

Although the rash can be pruritic, some patients themselves may not complain of the rash or scaling associated with seborrheic dermatitis. Family members may comment on it or when caring for the patient, you may notice erythematous patches and scaling on the scalp, forehead, eyebrows, eyelids, and beard area (Naldi & Rebora, 2009). The chest and back area can also be affected. With eyelid involvement (blepharitis) the patient may complain of crusting and eye irritation especially in early morning. Tearing, pruritus, and decreased or blurry vision are other possible complaints.

■ Nursing assessment

The patient's skin may be oily with erythematous scaly patches especially notable on the scalp and forehead. Other potentially affected areas include the auricular area, eyebrows, eyelids, nasal bridge, lacrimal folds, sternal area and upper back (Buttaro et al., 2006; Habif et al., 2006).

If the eyelids are involved, they may be edematous and irritated with a crusting on the lids and lashes.

■ Diagnostics

- Diagnostics are usually not necessary. A skin scraping with potassium hydroxide or biopsy may be indicated for patients who do not respond to usual therapies.
- In eyelid involvement, a culture may be necessary if there is no response to treatment.

■ Differential diagnosis

- Acne rosacea
- Atopic dermatitis
- Contact dermatitis
- Dermatomyositis

- Erythrasma
- Impetigo
- Langerhans cell histiocytosis
- Pityriasis versicolor
- Psoriasis
- Rosacea
- Scabies
- Tinea capitis
- Vitamin B deficiency
- Wiskott-Aldrich cutaneous lupus
- Zinc deficiency

Physician consultation

- If no response to vigilant skin care and over-the counter shampoos
- If increased symptoms/severity with treatment
- For pruritus, consult the physician for prescription for hydrocortisone cream 1%, *thin* film applied twice daily to affected scalp and facial lesions for 2 weeks.

■ Treatment

Treatment begins initially with over-the counter agents and a daily hygiene regimen.

- Scalp: shampoo daily with Head & Shoulders™ shampoo or selenium sulfide (Selsun™) shampoo
  - For dense plaque-like areas on scalp, mineral oil rubbed into scalp, covered with shower cap will help loosen scale before shampooing.
  - For pruritus, discuss with physician: hydrocortisone cream 1%, *thin* film applied twice daily to affected scalp and facial lesions for 2 weeks.
  - In severe cases, consultation with a dermatologist may be necessary for treatment with tar based shampoo.
- Facial and skin plaques: zinc pyrithione (ZnP soap) or Head & Shoulders™ shampoo
- Blepharitis (inflammation of eyelids)
  - Warm packs to the crusted areas will loosen crusts.
  - Wash eyes daily with ½ strength baby shampoo.
  - Blephamide ophthalmic ointment or eye drops (contraindicated if sulfa allergy or suspected herpetic infection)

For patients who do not respond to the above therapies, antifungal agents or antibiotics may be considered.

- Antifungal medications (e.g., ketoconazole, terbinafine, ciclopirox, butenafine) are available in varied formulations (i.e., foams, creams, gels and oral agents). Topical agents can be used in older adults, but oral agents are rarely used as they are metabolized through the P450 system increasing the risk of serious drug-drug interactions.

- Antibiotics (e.g., metronidazole gel)

■ Complications

- Vision can be affected if eyes are affected.
- Pruritus and scratching can result in superimposed infection.
- Liberally applied hydrocortisone cream for long periods of time can cause skin atrophy and systemic absorption.
- Severe pruritus can cause difficulty sleeping.

■ Prevention

Seborrheic dermatitis and blepharitis cannot be prevented but can be controlled with daily treatments.

■ Patient/family education

- Once seborrheic dermatitis or blepharitis improves, patients/families frequently discontinue treatment and the disorder returns. Explaining the importance of regular skin and eye care to control the disorder is essential.
- Patients and families also need to know that liberal application of topical corticosteroids can be harmful.

References

Berk, T. & Scheinfeld, N. (2010) Seborrheic dermatitis. *Pharmacy & Therapeutics* **35**(6), 348-352.

Buttaro, T.M., Aznavorian, S., & Dick, K. (2006). *Clinical Management of Patients in SubAcute and Long-Term Care Settings*. Mosby, St. Louis.

Habif, T.P., Campbell, J.L., Chapman, M.S., Dinulos, J.G.H. & Zug, K.A. (2006) *Dermatology*. Mosby, St. Louis.

Naldi, L. & Rebora, A. (2009). Seborrheic dermatitis. *New England Journal of Medicine* **360**, 387-396.

Zisova, L.G. (2009) *Malassezia* species and seborrheic dermatitis. *Folia Med (Plovdiv)* **51**(1), 23-33.

Further reading

Deignan, E.M. (2008) Fungal infections (superficial). In: Buttaro, T.M., Trybulski, J., Bailey, P.P., & Sandberg-Cook, J. (eds) *Primary Care: A Collaborative Practice*. Mosby, St. Louis.

PART 10: THRUSH

Terry Mahan Buttaro

Thrush, a mucous membrane infection caused by yeast (*Candida albicans*), occurs in people of all ages. Antibiotic therapy sometimes causes thrush, but it is also associated with inhaled steroid therapy. Thrush can also be a sign of immunosuppression. Babies can have thrush because their immune system has not fully developed, but in elders thrush may be a sign of diminishing immunity, diabetes, cancer, or even an human immunodeficiency virus infection. Although commonly seen in the mouth, thrush can affect the esophagus and lower gastrointestinal system also.

■ Risk factors

- Advanced age
- Antibiotic therapy
- Cancer
- Chemotherapy
- Dentures
- Diabetes
- Iron deficiency anemia
- Nutritional deficiency
- Poor oral hygiene
- Radiation therapy
- Steroid therapy
  - Inhaled, oral, or intravenous steroids

■ Clinical presentation

Patients may complain of white patches in their mouth, pain or burning on the tongue, difficulty swallowing (especially with esophageal candida) or taste changes. Some patients may not complain of any discomfort, but simply stop eating.

■ Nursing assessment

For all hospitalized patients it is important to check the mouth daily. Good oral hygiene is essential to help prevent aspiration pneumonia and to promote good nutrition. The presence of white patchy exudates on the tongue, upper palate, or buccal mucosa suggests a *Candida* infection. In some cases, the tongue and posterior pharynx are erythematous and this requires evaluation by the physician.

■ Diagnostics

Usually thrush is a clinical diagnosis based on the patient's history and the physical exam. Microscopic evaluation of the lesion scraping may reveal pseudohyphae, indicating a yeast infection. Lesion cultures can also be obtained if the diagnosis is uncertain (Munsell, 2008). Patients with esophageal candidiasis may require endoscopy.

■ Differential diagnosis

Most often the white exudates on the mucous membranes of the mouth indicate thrush. Other oral infections include:

- Aphthous ulcers
- Condyloma lata
- Gluten sensitivity
- Leukoplakia
- Lichen planus
- Secondary syphilis (mucous membrane lesions)
- Stomatitis
- Trauma
- Vitamin B12 of folate deficiency

■ Treatment

Treatment includes good oral hygiene, denture care, and anti-fungal therapy. Patient dentures should be removed prior to using clotrimazole troche or nystatin suspension.

- Oral candidiasis
    - Clotrimazole troche, 10 milligrams, 5 times a day for 7-14 days (Pappas *et al.*, 2009)
    - Nystatin suspension, 400,000-600,000 units swish and swallow four times a day 7-14 days (Pappas *et al.*, 2009)
    - Fluconazole 100-200 milligrams PO daily 7-14 days (Pappas *et al.*, 2009)
        - Fluconazole may substantially increase PT/INR and bleeding risk if patient is on warfarin (Coumadin).
        - Fluconazole may increase risk of rhabdomyolysis for patients taking HMG-CoA reductase inhibitors or red rice yeast.
- Esophageal candidiasis
    - Fluconazole 200-400 milligrams PO daily for 14-21 days or fluconazole 6 milligrams/kilogram IV daily (Pappas *et al.*, 2009)
- Prophylaxis
    - For neutropenic patients receiving chemotherapy, fluconazole 400 milligrams PO daily may be considered (Pappas *et al.*, 2009).

■ Collaborative consultation

- Discuss any oral lesions or patient pain with the physician.
- Consult dietician if PO intake is limited by swallowing difficulties.

■ Complications

- Candidemia and other invasive fungal infections (e.g., endocarditis, septic arthritis, etc.)
- Dehydration
- Esophageal candidiasis
- Malnutrition

■ Prevention

- For cancer patients being treated with radiation or chemotherapy, prophylaxis may help prevent oral candidiasis.
- Instruct patients to rinse their mouth after the use of a steroid inhaler.

■ Patient/family education

- Explain the possible causes of the oral or esophageal candida.
- Explain and demonstrate good oral and denture care.
- Discuss how to use troches and swish and swallow medications appropriately.

References

Munsell, D.S. (2008) Oral Infections. In: Buttaro, T.M., Trybulski, J., Bailey, P.P. & Sandberg-Cook, J. (eds) *Primary Care: A Collaborative Practice*. Mosby, St. Louis.

Pappas, P.G., Kauffman, C.A, Andes, D., *et al.* (2009) Clinical Guidelines for the Management of Candidiasis: 2009 Update by the Infectious Diseases Society of America. *Clinical Infectious Diseases* **48**, 503–535. Online. Available from http://www.guideline.gov/content.aspx?id=14174 (accessed 15 March 2012).

PART 11: TINEA

Terry Mahan Buttaro

Tinea is a fungal infection caused by a variety of dermatophytes that include *Epidermophyton*, *Microsporum* and *Trichophyton* and affect the skin and/or nails (Weinstein & Berman, 2002). Other fungal organisms and/or yeast are also implicated. Most of these infections are spread either by contact with an infected person or animal or by touching infected clothing, towels, or bedding (Deignan, 2008). The organism that causes Tinea versicolor is commonly found on human skin. However, heat, humidity, and patient resistance are factors implicated in activation of organism and subsequent infection. The varied superficial fungal infections include:

- Tinea capitis: scalp
- Tinea barbae: beard
- Tinea versicolor: affects the torso, neck, and arms usually in warm weather. Patients with fair complexions may not notice the lesions in winter (Habif *et al.*, 2006).
- Tinea curis, a fungal infection of the groin
- Tinea manuum: the hands
- Tinea pedis: the feet
- Tinea unguium (onychomycosis): a fungal infection of the nails, most frequently affects the toenails but fingernails are also affected.

■ Risk factors

- Tinea capitis
  - Age: more common in children
  - History of diabetes or immunologic disorder
  - Poor hygiene
  - Sharing combs or brushes with someone with this tinea infection
  - Touching with a pet with this tinea infection
- Tinea barbae
  - Immunologic disorder
  - Poor hygiene or sanitation
  - Warm, moist environment
- Tinea versicolor:
  - Age: more common in adolescents and young adults
  - May be more common in people with oily skin
  - Warm, moist environment
- Tinea curis
  - Contamination from other areas of the body that are infected with tinea organisms
  - Sharing towels contaminated with fungus
  - Wearing tight clothing that promotes a warm, humid environment
- Tinea manuum:
  - Hand infection usually results from contact with an infected area of the body, or an infected pet or individual
- Tinea pedis
  - Age : more common in children
  - Contamination from another area of the body
  - Diabetes
  - Easily spread in communal showers/locker rooms
  - Immunologic disorder
  - Warm, damp environments (including damp shoes, sneakers, boots)

- Tinea unguium (onychomycosis)
  - Age: more common in older adults
  - Contamination
  - Diabetes
  - Immunologic disorder
  - Peripheral vascular disease
  - Warm, humid environment (e.g., sneakers, shoes, boots)

■ Clinical presentation

Tinea and other superficial fungal infections are fairly prevalent in all populations, but for patients with preexisting co-morbidities or immunosuppression, there is increased risk. Patients may complain of pruritus or a rash or the infection may be noted by the nurse or nursing assistant while providing patient care.

■ Nursing assessment

Patients require an admission assessment and daily skin assessment by nurses throughout their hospitalization or admission to other nursing care facility. Important clues to the dermatophyte infections are as following:

- Tinea capitis: scaling, patchy areas on the scalp. Some lesions may appear erythematous and pustular (Deignan, 2008). Areas of hair loss may be present.
- Tinea barbae: ring like lesions beneath the beard or mustache area. Occasionally there are papular/pustular lesions that can appear infected.
- Tinea corporis: also known as ringworm, tinea corporis presents as plaque like, circular lesions that occur most anywhere on the body, but often on the more exposed areas. The outer aspect of the lesion is erythematous and ring like in appearance, while the center area is lighter in color.
- Tinea cruris: erythematous patches in the groin area and gluteal folds. The borders are raised and scaling may be present (Deignan, 2008).
- Tinea pedis: also known as athlete's foot, this tinea infection primarily affects the web spaces between the toes, but it can spread to other areas of the foot. The areas affected are usually macerated and scaly. Erythema and fissuring also are possible (Deignan, 2008).
- Tinea manuum can also affect the feet (Deignan, 2008). The lesions are plaque-like, dry and scaly.
- Tinea unguium (onychomycosis): yellowed or discolored nails. Nails often are often quite thick.

■ Diagnostics

Diagnosis of a fungal infection is offer based on the clinical presentation. Skin scrapings can be obtained and examined microscopically with a KOH preparation (Deignan, 2008). Cultures or biopsy may be helpful in some situations.

■ Differential diagnosis

- Bacterial pyodermas
- Dermatitis
- Psoriasis
- Secondary syphilis
- Skin cancer
- Urticaria

■ Treatment

- Tinea versicolor will usually respond to a 2 week application of selenium sulfide lotion 2.5% or a selenium shampoo (e.g., Selsun™ Blue or Pert® Plus) to neck, torso, and extremities, then washed off 10 minutes (Deignan, 2008; Habif *et al.*, 2006). Zinc pyrithione soap applied in a similar fashion, allowed to dry 5 minutes, and then rinsed off is another treatment (Habif *et al.*, 2006). Other treatments include antifungal creams applied topically at bedtime for 2 to 4 weeks or in some cases oral antifungal medications such as fluconazole (Diflucan) or griseofulvin (Habif *et al.*, 2006).
- Onychomycosis is often not treated because the medications can affect the liver and/or kidneys. However, sometimes ciclopirox (Penlac), solution can be applied to the nails and surrounding skin once a day, but must be removed weekly with alcohol (LexiComp., 2010).
- Other fungal infections: Treatment is based on lesion appearance, but the goal is to remove the causative dermatophyte or yeast. Drying agents (e.g., Domeboro's solution) are used for wet lesions, while scales must be removed with a peeling agent (Deignan, 2008). Topical antifungals (e.g., clotrimazole or nystatin) are then used twice a day. The recommendation is to continue the topical antifungal until the lesions are gone for at least one week (Deignan, 2008).

■ Collaborative consultation

Discuss any skin eruption with the physician describing the appearance and location of the lesions. Further consultation may be necessary if the lesions are not resolving or if there is a change suggesting a superimposed infection.

■ Complications

- Medication side effects or adverse effects
- Reoccurrence is common even with appropriate treatment.
- Superimposed bacterial infection

■ Prevention

There are varied dermatophyte infections, but generalized recommendations for prevention include:

- Keep body folds, areas between toes, and other moisture prone body areas clean and dry.
- Wear cotton or other absorbent clothing. Change socks or clothing if sweaty.
- Wear sandals or flip-flops in community bathing areas.
- Do not share towels, clothing, combs, brushes and other grooming products.
- Use antifungal powders on feet daily.
- Discuss with patient the importance of not scratching infected areas to prevent superinfection or infection spread.

■ Patient/family education

Patients need to understand the common triggers associated with superficial fungal infections so that environmental factors (e.g., heat, humidity) that contribute to these infections can be controlled.

References

Deignan, E.M. (2008) Fungal infections (superficial). In: Buttaro, T.M., Trybulski, J., Bailey, P.P., & Sandberg-Cook, J. (eds) *Primary Care: A Collaborative Practice*. Mosby, St. Louis.

Habif, T.P., Campbell, J.L., Chapman, M.S., Dinulos, J.G.H. & Zug, K.A. (2006) *Dermatology*. Mosby, St. Louis.

Penlac (2010) Lexi-Comp. http://www.lexi.com/institutions/products/online/ (accessed 27 August 2010).

Weinstein, A. & Berman, B. (2002) Topical treatment of common superficial tinea infections. *American Family Physician* **65**(10), 2095–2103.

PART 12: PRESSURE ULCERS

Linda Olson

Pressure ulcers have been a concern for the health care industry since October of 2008. At that time the Centers for Medicare and Medicaid services took steps to make hospitals more accountable for the care they give by not reimbursing for stage 3 or 4 pressure ulcers that were acquired during the hospital stay. The cost to treat one full-thickness pressure ulcer can be over $70,000 with an estimated annual cost in the United States to be as high as $11 billion (Cunningham, 2009). It is also estimated that 60,000 patients die each year from complications related to pressure ulcers (Ratliff & Tomaselli, 2010).

This is causing health care organizations to take a more conscientious approach to skincare in order to prevent pressure ulcers from developing.

Pressure ulcers are a particular problem for the older adult population. It is noted that 15% of older patients develop pressure ulcers within the first week of hospitalization and over half of the patients noted to have pressure ulcers are 65 years of age or older (Ratliff & Tomaselli, 2010). Age-related changes that occur in other body systems make the skin more vulnerable to breakdown, delayed healing, and potential complications.

According to the National Pressure Ulcer Advisory Panel a pressure ulcer is defined as localized injury to the skin and/or underlying tissue usually over a bony prominence, as a result of pressure, or pressure in combination with shear (Ratliff & Tomaselli, 2010). Decubiti, decubitus ulcers, or bed sores are other names associated with pressure ulcers, however, since the underlying cause is pressure, the term pressure ulcer best describes the cause of skin breakdown and has become the more preferred term (Bryant & Nix, 2007).

The primary cause of a pressure ulcer is pressure from an external source. Though pressure ulcers commonly occur over a bony prominence, they can develop anywhere on the body. The intensity of the pressure can cause tissue injury if the force is applied at a high intensity for a short period of time or a low intensity for a long period of time (Morison, 2001). The force of pressure disrupts blood flow to the tissues by occluding the capillaries resulting in oxygen and nutrient deprivation as well as metabolic waste accumulation in the tissue. The resulting damage to the capillaries causes increased permeability and leakage into the interstitial space, causing localized tissue edema, decreased perfusion, inflammation, increased hypoxia and eventually cell death (Hess, 2005). Contrary to what one would expect, pressure ulcers develop from the inside out. The tissues closest to the bone are usually damaged first. Conversely, the first notable sign of a pressure ulcer may be nonblancheable erythema which indicates a lack of blood flow to the area and probable tissue ischemia (Revis & Caffee, 2006).

■ Risk factors

- Acute illness/critical care patients
- Advanced age
- Chronically ill patients
- Comorbid conditions
- Decreased or impaired consciousness
- Decreased mobility or immobility
- Dehydration
- Incontinence/moisture
- Malnutrition
- Presence of vascular disease
- Previous history of a pressure ulcer
- Previous history radiation to area
- Sensory impairment

■ Clinical presentation

The most widely used classification system for pressure ulcers comes from the National Pressure Ulcer Advisory Panel (NPUAP) (Hess, 2005). The stages are defined by level of tissue injury and can only be accurately staged after necrotic tissue has been removed to allow visualization of the wound bed (see Figure 3.1.12.1). Once a pressure ulcer has been staged it cannot be downgraded in stage (reversed staging) because the original tissue has been destroyed and will be replaced by

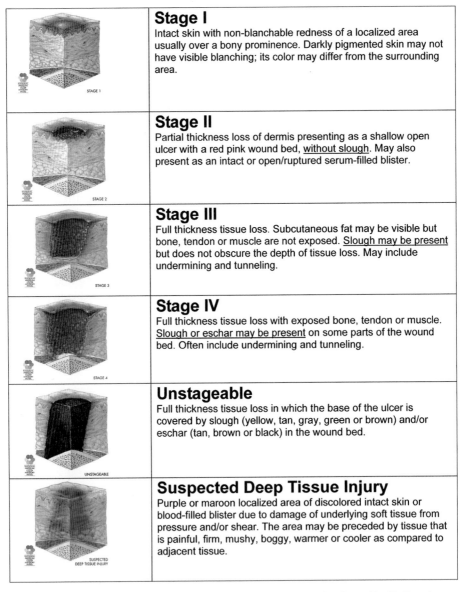

Stage I
Intact skin with non-blanchable redness of a localized area usually over a bony prominence. Darkly pigmented skin may not have visible blanching; its color may differ from the surrounding area.

Stage II
Partial thickness loss of dermis presenting as a shallow open ulcer with a red pink wound bed, <u>without slough</u>. May also present as an intact or open/ruptured serum-filled blister.

Stage III
Full thickness tissue loss. Subcutaneous fat may be visible but bone, tendon or muscle are not exposed. <u>Slough may be present</u> but does not obscure the depth of tissue loss. May include undermining and tunneling.

Stage IV
Full thickness tissue loss with exposed bone, tendon or muscle. <u>Slough or eschar may be present</u> on some parts of the wound bed. Often include undermining and tunneling.

Unstageable
Full thickness tissue loss in which the base of the ulcer is covered by slough (yellow, tan, gray, green or brown) and/or eschar (tan, brown or black) in the wound bed.

Suspected Deep Tissue Injury
Purple or maroon localized area of discolored intact skin or blood-filled blister due to damage of underlying soft tissue from pressure and/or shear. The area may be preceded by tissue that is painful, firm, mushy, boggy, warmer or cooler as compared to adjacent tissue.

Figure 3.1.12.1 Pressure ulcer stages. Reprinted with permission from the National Pressure Ulcer Advisory Panel (NPUAP).

granulation tissue and new epithelium. This new tissue has a tensile strength that is 15-20% less than the normal tissue. It is not the same and thus cannot be classified as if the damage had never occurred. A stage 3 pressure ulcer cannot become a stage 2. It would be classified as a "healing stage 3".

Nursing assessment

- Head to toe skin assessment to determine risk of pressure ulcer development as well as presence of pressure ulcers
- If pressure ulcer present note:
  - Location
  - Stage
  - Size (length × width × depth)
  - Tissue type
  - Wound bed and periwound skin appearance
  - Presence of undermining/tunneling or sinus tract
  - Exudate (amount and type)
  - Odor
  - Pain
  - Signs or symptoms of infection (erythema, warmth, tenderness)
  - Dressing type
- Nutritional status

Diagnostics

- Albumin
- Prealbumin
- Complete blood count/differential
- C-reactive protein, if osteomyelitis is suspected
- Erythrocyte sedimentation rate (ESR), if osteomyelitis is suspected
- Wound culture
- X-ray or MRI, if indicated
- Bone biopsy, if indicated

Differential diagnosis

- Diabetic/neuropathic ulcers
- Moisture-associated skin damage/incontinence-associated dermatitis
- Skin tears
- Vascular ulcers

Treatment

Treatments should be focused on maintaining the goals of the patient to optimize healing or provide comfort.

- Pressure relief is essential.
- Provide appropriate support surface.
- Optimize nutrition.
- Choose wound dressings which promote a moist wound environment and manage exudate.
- Debride and/or irrigate wound as needed.
- Treat infections.
- Manage incontinence, keeping wound and other skin areas clean and dry.
- Manage pain.
- Surgery as needed
- Consider negative pressure wound therapy, if indicated.
- Hyperbaric oxygen, if indicated
- Ultrasonography
- Electrical stimulation, if indicated

■ Collaborative consultation

- Primary care physician
- Certified Wound Care Nurse
- Surgery if surgical debridement needed
- Dietician for recommendations on nutritional supplements and/or vitamins
- Physical therapy for positioning recommendations
- Occupational therapy

■ Complications

- Pain
- Infection
- Osteomyelitis
- Death

■ Prevention

The Institute for Healthcare Improvement recommends six components to prevent hospital-acquired pressure in their 5 Million Lives campaign on ulcers.

(1) Assess patient risk:
   a. There are several risk assessment scales (Norton, Braden, Gosnell & Waterlow). Each scale has categories with numbers assigned that describe parameters of risk that have been associated with pressure ulcer development. The numbers are tallied and a risk level is identified. A plan of care should be put in place based on the level of risk. If the tool is used correctly, the patients will have individualized treatment plans. For example: the Braden Scale (see Table 2.1) identifies 5 subgroups to be evaluated with defined parameters. A number is assigned to each subgroup parameter. The nurse chooses the number that best describes the patient. The subgroups are added together to determine the overall risk associated

with that patient. Proper interventions can then be implemented based on the total risk score. Specific interventions should then be put in place based on the individual subcategory results. For example, if a patient scores low for the subgroup mobility, measures should be established that concentrate on overcoming (or decreasing) that area of risk. Refer to Table 3.1.12.1 for interventions based on the specific risk subgroup.

(2) Reassess patient risk daily-patient's condition can change quickly and interventions should be adjusted accordingly.

(3) Inspect skin daily- patient's skin can deteriorate in a matter of hours.

(4) Manage moisture:
  a. Underpads to wick away moisture
  b. Barrier creams
  c. Toileting program
  d. Containment devices:
    i. Fecal incontinent collectors
    ii. Urinary or condom catheters
    iii. Rectal pouches

(5) Optimize nutrition and hydration:
  a. Consult dietician.
  b. Offer supplements and vitamins.
  c. Monitor intake and output

(6) Minimize pressure:
  a. Appropriate support surface
  b. Reposition at least every 2 hours.
  c. Float heels off pillows.
  d. Protect bony prominences/pressure points.
  e. Assistive devices

■ Patient/family education

- Explain potential causes and risk factors for pressure ulcer development.
- Discuss interventions to decrease risk factors.
  - Regular toileting
  - Assist with repositioning.
  - Prompt cleansing.
- Importance of regular skin inspections
  - Look for signs of pressure.
  - Look for change in tissue temperature.
- Skin care
  - Lubricating/hydrating with skin creams
  - Mild soap and warm water-avoid hot water
  - Moisture barrier creams for incontinent patients
- Measures to reduce friction and shear
  - Lifting instead of dragging
  - Use of a lift sheet
  - Use of a trapeze

Table 3.1.12.1 Pressure ulcer prevention interventions by the Braden Subgroup.

Sensory-perception	Activity/mobility	Moisture	Nutrition	Friction & shear
• Reposition q2hrs in bed & q1 hr in chair • 30 degree lateral rotations • Monitor mental status/ check LOC • Consider pressure redistribution surface • Protect bony prominences from each other with pillows or wedges • Medicate for pain as needed • Elevate heels with pillows under calves lengthwise or specialty boots • Avoid wrinkled sheets • Avoid lying on tubes or equipment • Avoid lying on pressure ulcer • Protect contractures • Remove and check restraints • Remove devices (stockings, SCDs) Q shift for skin inspection	• OT/PT eval • Encourage OOB • Reposition q2hrs in bed & q1 hr in chair • 30 degree lateral rotations • Keep HOB <30 degrees • Use lift device • Medicate for pain as needed • Use chair cushion when OOB • Perform ROM • Avoid restraints • Do not use sheep skins or donuts • Obtain a trapeze for the bed	• Protect potential incontinent patients with barrier creams • Use containment devices: foley, FMS, rectal pouch, condom catheter • Cleanse after each episode of incontinence • Avoid diapers • Offer toileting q2hrs • Use absorbent pads • Pouch leaking drain site, tubes or wounds	• Encourage well balanced diet • Offer supplements • Dietary consult • Offer sips of water or other fluids with repositioning • Ensure proper hydration • Assist with meals • Monitor NPO status • Monitor I & Os • Speech and swallow eval	• Do not rub bony prominences • Use Allkare Barrier wipes on elbows and heels • Use protective lotion after bathing • Use elbow pads • Prevent slumping in a chair • Keep HOB <30 degrees • Obtain a trapeze for the bed • Use draw sheets • Bowel/bladder program

* Assess all patients for appropriate Pressure Redistribution Surface.

- Dressing care
- When to notify physician/signs and symptoms of infection
- Importance of routine turning and repositioning
- Use of pressure redistribution surfaces
- Avoid donut cushions.
- Importance of adequate nutrition and hydration
  - Provide fluids on a regular basis.
  - Provide eating assistance.
  - Provide frequent small well balanced meals and snacks.
- Monitor weight loss, appetite and gastrointestinal changes.

References

Bryant, R. & Nix, D. (2007) *Acute & Chronic Wounds Current Management Concepts*. Mosby Elsevier, St. Louis.

Cunningham, B. (2009) Pressure ulcers are preventable: Medicare and Medicaid agree. Online. Available from www.injuryboard.com/printfriendly.aspx?id=255006 (accessed 12 March 2012).

Hess, C.T. (2005) *Wound Care*. Lippincott Williams & Wilkins, Philadelphia.

Morison, M. (2001). The Prevention and Treatment of Pressure Ulcers. Mosby, Edinburgh..

Ratliff, C. & Tomaselli, N. (2010) *Guideline for Prevention and Management of Pressure Ulcers*. WOCN, Mount Laurel.

Revis, D. & Caffee, H. (2006) *Pressure Ulcers, Nonsurgical Treatment and Principles*. Online. Available from http://www.emedicine.com/plastic/topic424.htm (accessed 12 March 2012).

Further reading

Catania, K., Huang, C., James, P., Madison, M., Moran, M. & Ohr, M. (2007) PUPPI: The pressure ulcer prevention protocol interventions. *American Journal of Nursing* **107**(4), 44-52.

European Pressure Ulcer Advisory Panel and National Pressure Ulcer Advisory Panel (2009) *Pressure Ulcer Prevention and Treatment of: Quick Reference Guide*. National Pressure Ulcer Advisory Panel, Washington, DC.

Gray, M., Bohacek, L. & Zdanuk, J. (2007) Moisture vs pressure. *Journal of Wound Ostomy and Continence Nursing* **34**(2), 134-142.

Krasner, D. & Kane, D. (1997) *Chronic Wound Care: A Clinical Source Book for Healthcare Professionals*. Heath Management Publications, Inc., Wayne.

Milne, C., Corbett, L. & Dubuc, D. (2003) *Wound, Ostomy, and Continence Nursing Secrets*. Hanley & Belfus, Inc., Philadelphia.

National Pressure Ulcer Advisory Panel (2009) *Treatment of Pressure Ulcers: Quick Reference Guide*. National Pressure Ulcer Advisory Panel, Washington, DC.

National Pressure Ulcer Advisory Panel and European Pressure Ulcer Advisory Panel. (2009) *Pressure Ulcer Prevention and Treatment: Clinical Practice Guideline*. National Pressure Ulcer Advisory Panel, Washington, DC.

Institute for Healthcare Improvement (2007) *Relieve the Pressure and Reduce Harm*. Online. Available from http://www.ihi.org/knowledge/Pages/ImprovementStories/RelievethePressureandReduceHarm.aspx (accessed 4 May 2012).

Stoelting, J., McKenna, L., Taggart, E., Mottar, R., Jeffers, B.R., & Wendler, M.C. (2007) Prevention of nosocomial pressure ulcers: A process improvement project. *Journal of Wound Ostomy Continence Nursing* **34**(4), 382-388.

Stolowski, L. (Feb 5) *In this Corner: The Unavoidable Pressure Ulcer*. Online. Available from www.medscape.com/viewarticle/715969.

PART 13: LOWER EXTREMITY ULCERS

Linda Olson

There are 2.5 million people affected by lower extremity ulcers in the United States (Bryant & Nix, 2007) with 600,000 new cases diagnosed each year (Khachemoune & Kauffman, 2002). Lower extremity ulcers are classified by location, appearance, and etiology and generally fall into three categories: venous, arterial, and neuropathic. Patients may exhibit symptoms of a single etiology or have mixed disease in which they exhibit symptoms of two different types of ulcers. This can be challenging for the clinician since proper identification of the type of ulcer is imperative for effective treatment. Patient education in all aspects of care is an important component for ensuring patient compliance and treatment success.

Venous ulcers are typically related to abnormalities of the veins, valves and the calf muscle. There are two main mechanisms that impact the development of venous ulcers: (1) the calf muscle that pumps the blood toward the heart and (2) valves that maintain a one-way flow of blood by preventing backflow. Improper functioning of the valves in the veins and ineffective calf pumping leads to reflux and venous pooling (*Leg Ulcers*, 2010). The high venous pressure caused by this results in fibrin deposits and leakage of fluid into the extracellular space causing local edema and inflammation (Bryant & Nix, 2007). This edema and inflammation inhibits the delivery of oxygen and nutrients necessary for tissue function and ultimately causes cellular death and ulceration.

Arterial ulcers result from poor blood circulation to the lower extremities. This is often caused by atherosclerosis, in which deposits of cholesterol, lipids and calcium are deposited in the arteriolar wall causing the vessels to narrow and lose elasticity (Hess, 2005). This narrowed blood vessel impedes the delivery of oxygen and nutrients to the tissue and can lead to tissue ischemia and cell death (*Leg Ulcers*, 2010). For patients with the slightest arterial compromise even minimal trauma can result in a chronic nonhealing ulcer due to the body's inability to meet the demands necessary for tissue healing (Bryant & Nix, 2007).

Neuropathic ulcers are most commonly associated with the diabetic patient, although neuropathy can occur in other disease processes (e.g., spina bifida, Hansen's disease, systemic lupus erythematosus, human immunodeficiency virus/acquired immune deficiency syndrome, cancer, vitamin B deficiency, multiple sclerosis, uremia and vascular disease). The neuropathic process is poorly understood and there are different theories regarding its etiology. Many believe that neuropathy is caused by hyperglycemia which is why tight glucose control is important in diabetics to reduce the severity of neuropathy. The trineuropathy (sensory, autonomic, and motor) that occurs in a neuropathic foot contributes to the development of neuropathic ulcers (Elftman & Conlan, 2007).

■ Risk factors

Although many of the risk factors for the development of venous, arterial or neuropathic lower extremity ulcers overlap, there are specific risk factors associated with each type of ulcer (see Table 3.1.13.1).

■ Clinical presentation

Venous ulcers

Venous ulcers typically occur in the gaiter area, from the lower calf to the ankle. They are generally shallow, irregularly shaped wounds that are clean or have a fibrinous base. Unless there is mixed disease (venous and arterial) the patient will have a normal ankle/brachial index and a normal pedal pulse. The patient's legs will typically have edema which causes moderate to heavy wound drainage. Patients usually feel more comfortable with their legs elevated. The patient may have skin discoloration of the gaiter area or hemosiderin staining caused by the leaking of the blood into the surrounding tissue. There may be dry flaking skin surrounding the wounds or there may be signs and symptoms of cellulitis.

Arterial ulcers

Arterial ulcers occur on the feet, heels, on the tips of toes or on the malleolus. They are typically round, deep punched out wounds with well-defined wound margins. The wound beds are dry and pale or necrotic with minimal to no exudate. Pedal pulses are usually diminished or absent and the Ankle/Brachial index is abnormal. The legs may appear shiny and without hair. Patients may feel more comfortable when their legs are dangled. There may also be redness in the foot and leg when the leg is dangled which is known as dependent rubor. The patient may also complain of leg discomfort when walking that is relieved with rest. Known as intermittent claudication this disorder is caused by a decrease in oxygenation to the leg. Because blood flow is so impaired in arterial vascular disease, signs or symptoms of infection may be undetectable.

Neuropathic/diabetic ulcers

Diabetic ulcers are found on the pressure points of the foot, typically the plantar surface of the metatarsal head or toes. Also called neuropathic ulcers, these wounds characteristically present as round, deep punched out ulcers with well-defined wound margins. They have a red or necrotic wound bed with

Table 3.1.13.1 Lower extremity ulcer comparison chart.

	Venous	Arterial	Neuropathic
Risk factors	Thrombosis Postphlebitic syndrome Incompetent valves Congestive heart failure Obesity Pregnancy Muscle weakness d/t paralysis/arthritis Varicose veins Malnutrition Trauma Advanced age	Smoking Diabetes Hyperlipidemia Hypertension Cardiovascular disease Peripheral vascular disease Advanced age Intermittent claudication: esp. after exertion and leg elevation	Diabetic pt with peripheral neuropathy Long term poorly controlled diabetes h/o numbness, paresthesias Spinal cord injury Advanced age Obesity
Location	Gaiter area-between malleolus and lower calf Usually medial malleolus over distal bony prominences	Feet Between or on tips of toes Malleolus	Plantar aspect of foot Pressure areas on toes and metatarsal heads Plantar heel
Clinical presentation	Normal pulse Dull ache pain with dependency- relieved with leg elevation Generalized edema	Weak or absent pulse Pain at night with elevation Localized edema	Diminished or absent pulse- not reliable indicator No pain d/t neuropathy Localized edema
Wound characteristics	Moist wound bed Ruddy appearance-or may be covered with a thin yellow fibrin tissue Superficial/shallow wounds Irregular wound margins Moderate to heavy exudate	Dry wound bed Pale or necrotic wound bed Deep punched out-Round, well defined wound margins Minimal exudate	Dry or necrotic wound bed Red/pink or necrotic wound bed Deep, calloused Well defined wound margins Low to moderate exudate

Nursing assessment	Hemosiderin– staining caused by leakage of blood into tissues Ankle flare-edema Venous dermatitis may be present Normal ABIs	Hair loss of lower limb Thickened toenails Cyanosis Elevational pallor Dependent rubor Coolness of lower limb Delayed capillary refill Abnormal ABIs	Dry cracked foot Insensate Foot deformities: claw toes, Charcot's ABIs unreliable d/t possible noncompressible vessels
Treatment	Eliminate edema Moist wound healing Control underlying medical issues: CHF, HTN, edema, nutrition Treat infection Protect from trauma Elevation Hydrate skin 4 layer compression bandages UNNA boot Flexible nonelastic wrap Extremity pumps Manage dermatitis-steroid creams Ligation & stripping of superficial veins Diuretics to remove excess fluid Pharmacologic agents-pentoxifylline Pt education and support	Moist wound healing for moist wounds Keep dry stable eschar intact Revascularization-bypass grafting Angioplasty, stents Amputation Protect wound-only debride with infection Do not compress No elevation Reduce caffeine(constrictor) Treat infection Hyperbaric oxygen Bio-engineered skin equivalents Pharmacologic agents-ASA, vasodilators, antiplatelets, hemorheologics, antilipids Pt education and support	Tight glucose control Offloading-may need custom fitted boot Orthotics Treat infection Moist wound healing Total contact casting Debridement of necrotic tissue Inspection Bioengineered skin equivalents Electrical stimulation Surgery Amputation Osteotomy Tendon release Pt education and support

low to moderate drainage. The wounds generally have surrounding callus. The ankle/brachial index and the pedal pulse are unreliable possibly because of incompressible vessels. The patient may present with a dry, cracked insensate foot that has structural deformities. Any new areas of pain, erythema, or swelling on the foot or toenail are frequently early signs of infection and should be addressed promptly to prevent complications such as amputation.

Patients with diabetes also commonly have some level of sensory, motor and/or autonomic neuropathy, though the patient may be asymptomatic (Baranoski & Ayello, 2004). Sensory nerve damage causes a decrease in sensation to pain, pressure, heat or injury (*Leg Ulcers*, 2010). There can be partial or total numbness in which the patient is unaware of the damage to the tissue thus potentially leading to ulceration (Hess, 2005). This is generally referred to as the loss of protective sensation (Baranoski & Ayello, 2004). With autonomic neuropathy there is a decrease in the function of the sweat and oil glands causing cracks and fissures in the skin which increase the risk of wounds and infection (*Lower Extremity Ulcers*, n.d.). There is also muscle wasting in motor neuropathy which can cause balance deformities that change the weight bearing surfaces and predispose the patient to ulceration (Hess, 2005). Patients typically present with varying degrees and combinations of the above neuropathies increasing their susceptibility for ulcer development.

■ Nursing assessment

- Head to toe skin assessment
- Palpation of bilateral pulses: Femoral, popliteal, dorsalis pedis, and posterior tibial artery pulses. A consistent system should be used to grade pulses (see Table 3.1.13.2).
- Presence of ulcers
- If ulcer present note:
  - Location
  - Stage
  - Size (length × width × depth)
  - Tissue type
  - Wound bed appearance
  - Periwound skin
  - Presence of undermining/tunneling or sinus tract

Table 3.1.13.2 Grading pulses.

4+	Bounding
3+	Normal pulse
2+	Diminished
1+	Barely felt
0	No pulse

- Exudate (amount and type)
- Odor
- Pain
- Signs or symptoms of infection
- Dressing type
- Nutritional status
  - Albumin
  - Prealbumin
  - Intake and output

■ Diagnostics

Diagnostic testing depends on the type of ulcer and if there is suspected infection or other complications. Possible diagnostics include the following:

- Albumin or prealbumin
- Complete blood count with differential
- HgBA1c
- Ankle/brachial index (see Box 3.1.13.1)
- Tourniquet tests
- Plethysmography
- Duplex imaging
- Doppler waveforms
- Segmental pressure measurement
- Magnetic resonance angiography
- Venography
- Arteriography
- Angiography
- Pulse volume recordings
- Transcutaneous oxygen pressure measurement
- X-ray and/or magnetic resonance imaging to rule out osteomyelitis

■ Differential diagnosis

Less common but other causes of lower extremity ulcers include:

- Calciphylaxis
- Cryoglobulinemia
- Drug reaction
- Hypercoagulable states
- Kaposi's sarcoma
- Microemboli
- Pressure ulcers
- Raynaud's phenomenon

Box 3.1.13.1 Ankle brachial index (ABI)

The ABI is an noninvasive test used to identify large vessel peripheral artery disease in lower extremities by comparing the ankle systolic pressure to the highest arm systolic pressure.

Procedure:
(1) Take brachial pressures bilaterally using a Doppler.
   - Record the highest arm pressure.
(2) Take the ankle pressures bilaterally with a Doppler:
   - Place cuff around ankle 2.5 cm above the malleolus.
   - Measure both the dorsalis pedis and posterior tibial pressures in both legs.

Formula:
Calculate the ABI for each lower extremity by dividing the higher of the dorsalis pedis or the posterior tibial systolic pressures for each ankle by the higher of the 2 upper extremity brachial systolic pressure.

$$ABI = \frac{\text{highest ankle pressure}}{\text{highest brachial arm pressure}}$$

ABI values:

ABI	Diagnosis	Compression
<0.5	Arterial insufficiency Severe ischemia	No compression
0.5–0.8	Mixed etiology Borderline	Low compression
0.8–1	Venous disease	Compression
1–1.2	Normal	None or maintenance compression
1.3 or higher	Abnormal Calcification	Further testing needed

Adapted from Fleck, C.A. (2007).

Special Considerations:
In diabetic patients, the ABI can be falsely elevated. This is due to noncompressible vessels secondary to calcification of the inner layer of the artery.

- Sickle cell disease
- Skin cancer
- Traumatic skin injury
- Vasculitis

■ Treatment

Treatment of lower extremity ulcers is based on the type of ulcer, appearance of ulcer, amount of exudate and goal of care (see Table 3.1.13.1). Treatment of lower extremity ulcers should include thorough daily (and prn) cleaning of the ulcer, protection of surrounding skin from maceration, and weekly measurements of the ulcer to assess progression. Overall, accurate diagnosis and correction of underlying conditions are critical to the lifelong management of the lower extremity ulcer.

Venous ulcers

Treatment for the venous ulcer focuses on the control of the causative under-lying disease process, elimination of edema, moist wound healing and the management of exudate. Compression therapy is an important part of managing venous ulcers and the chronic swelling. This can be accomplished through the use of elastic graduated compression hosiery, UNNA boots or lay-ered compression bandage systems that are applied from the toes to just below the knee. The frequency of the dressing/stocking changes may depend on the condition of the wound and/or the amount of exudate. The type of dressing will be determined by the appearance of the wound bed and the amount of exudate.

Arterial ulcers

Patients should consult with a vascular surgeon to help determine the severity of the disease as diminished circulation impacts perfusion and treatment (Lower Extremity Ulcers, n.d.) The key focus of arterial wound treatment is to protect dry, stable eschar, provide moist wound healing to moist wounds, and prevent infection. Reperfusion can be accomplished through surgery, pharma-cologic agents, lifestyle changes and adjunctive therapies.

Neuropathic/diabetic ulcers

Treatment of the diabetic ulcer focuses on maximizing wound healing through a moist wound environment, debriding necrotic tissue, eliminating pressure, improving muscle strength and preventing infection. The patient should be seen regularly by the treating physician to ensure appropriate treatment. The type of dressing will be determined by the appearance of the wound bed and the amount of exudate. Offloading the wound is essential to the success of wound healing. There are many modalities to facilitate this depending on the location of the wound and the resources available to the patient and facility. Some examples are custom fitted boots, diabetic shoes or total contact casting, as well as, the use of a wheel chair or crutches (Baranoski & Ayello,

2004). Patients may need to follow up with a Physical Therapist to assist with overcoming gait changes that predispose patients to the development of an ulcer (Hess, 2005). Treating an infection is essential for the preservation of the foot and to prevent amputations.

■ Collaborative consultation

- Certified wound nurse
- Dietician to assess nutritional status and make recommendations for nutritional and vitamin supplements.
- Endocrinologist for diabetic patients
- Physical therapist
- Plastic surgeon
- Podiatrist
- Primary care physician
- Vascular surgeon if arterial disease is suspected

■ Complications

- Amputation
- Chronic leg ulcers
- Death
- Infection
- Osteomyelitis

■ Prevention

(See Table 3.1.13.3)

General prevention for lower extremity ulcers

- Control contributing factors (congestive heart failure, diabetes, hypercholesterolemia, hypertension, renal failure).
- Avoid trauma/injury.
- Avoid prolonged sitting or standing.
- Exercise regularly.

Table 3.1.13.3 Specific prevention strategies for lower extremity ulcers.

Venous	Arterial	Neuropathic
Use compression stockings	Remove irritant	Adequate glycemic control
Elevate feet	Control cholesterol and triglycerides	Appropriate footwear selection
Limit salt intake	Keep warm	Check for signs or symptoms of infection
Exercise calf muscles	Prevent hypothermia	Regular podiatry visits

- Maintain a healthy weight.
- Avoid extreme temperatures.
- Check feet regularly for blisters, cracks, sores or changes in color – use a mirror if necessary.
- Avoid sitting cross-legged.
- Avoid restrictive clothing.
- Avoid heating pads.
- Avoid cream between toes.
- Appropriate foot care
  - Wash feet daily.
  - Do not soak feet.
  - Moisturize daily.
  - Trim nails straight across.
  - Do not go barefoot.
- Seek treatment for corns and calluses.
- Avoid smoking.
- Inspect shoes before putting them on.
- Wear comfortable well fitting shoes and socks.

■ Patient/family education

- Importance of adequate glycemic control
- Implication of losing protective sensation
- Risk factors for development of lower extremity ulcers
- Measures to reduce/control risk factors
- How to make appropriate footwear selections
- Correlation between dependency and edema
- Importance of daily foot inspection
- Self assessment skills
- Dressing care
- When to notify physician/signs and symptoms of infection
- Importance of proper fitting shoes:
  - No thongs
  - No shoes made from non-breathable material
  - Adjustable shoes

References

Baranoski, S. & Ayello, E. (2004) *Wound Care Essentials – Practice Principles*. Lippincott Williams & Wilkins, Springhouse.

Bryant, R. & Nix, D. (2007) *Acute & Chronic Wounds Current Management Concepts*. Mosby Elsevier, St. Louis.

Elftman, N. & Conlan, J.E. (2007) Management of the neuropathic foot. In: C. Sussman & B. Bates-Jensen (eds) *Wound Care: A Collaborative Practice Manual for Health Professionals*, 3rd edn. Lippincott Williams & Wilkins, Baltimore, MD.

Fleck, C.A. (2007) Measuring ankle brachial pressure index. *Advances in Skin & Wound Care* **20**(12), 645–649.

Hess, C.T. (2005) *Wound Care*. Lippincott Williams & Wilkins, Philadelphia.

Khachemoune, A. & Kauffman, C.L. (2002) *Diagnosis of Leg Ulcers*. The Internet Journal of Dermatology ISSN. 1531-3018 Vol 1. Number 2. Available from http://www.ispub.com/ostia/index.php?xmlFilePath=journals/ijd/vol1n2/ulcer1.xml (accessed 12 March 2012).

Leg Ulcers (Feb 27, 2010) Online. Available from http://dermnetnz.org/site-age-specific/leg-ulcers.html (accessed 12 March 2012).

Lower Extremity Ulcers (n.d.) Online. Available from http://my.clevelandclinic.org/disorders/Pressure_Ulcers/hic_Lower_Extremity_Ulcers.aspx (accessed 5 May 2012).

Milne, C., Corbett, L. & Dubuc, D. (2003). *Wound, Ostomy, and Continence Nursing Secrets*. Hanley & Belfus, Inc., Philadelphia.

PART 14: SKIN TEARS

Linda Olson

It is because skin tears are often considered accidents that their prevalence and significance is overlooked. In fact, each year 1.5 million skin tears occur in institutionalized adult patients (LeBlanc & Baranowski, 2009) with 80% occurring in the upper extremities (Baranoski, 2003). A skin tear is defined as a traumatic wound that occurs as a result of friction and/or shear which separates the epidermis from the dermis or separates both the epidermis and the dermis from underlying structures (Roberts, 2007). Sometimes the cause of the skin tear is undeterminable, however, most result from routine care activities or trauma.

Skin tears occur more frequently in the older adult due to skin changes that happen over time increasing their risk of tears or blisters. As we age, the skin's ability to stretch diminishes due to a decrease in elastin fibers. There is also a decrease in sweat and oil glands which can cause dry skin and lead to scratching and trauma (*Aging Changes in Skin*, n.d.). A 20% decrease in dermal thickness and a thinning of the subcutaneous layer may result in less cushioning, and may limit the body's ability to protect from trauma. These changes, among others, contribute to the increased susceptibility of the older adult to skin tears.

■ Risk factors

There are many risk factors that make a patient susceptible to skin tears.

- Age (advanced or very young)
- Co-morbidities: diabetes, liver failure, kidney failure, cardiac disease
- Dependency with care
- Edema /third spacing
- Impaired mobility

- Impaired nutrition
- Medication: steroids, anticoagulants, diuretics, sedatives, analgesics
- Previous history of a skin tear
- Sensory and cognitive deficits

■ Clinical presentation

Skin tears present as irregularly shaped, partial or full thickness wounds that are in the form of a laceration or skin flap with the separation of the epidermis and/or dermis. They typically occur on an extremity with or without ecchymosis (Morey, 2007; Bryant & Nix, 2007).

■ Nursing assessment

- Head to toe skin assessment
  - Presence of ecchymosis
  - Presence of skin tears
- Assess for risk of skin tears (previously noted)
- If skin tear present note:
  - Location
  - Size (length × width × depth)
  - Drainage
  - Wound bed appearance
  - Presence of skin flap
  - Odor
  - Periwound skin
  - Signs or symptoms of infection
  - Type of dressing/treatment

■ Diagnostics

Payne and Martin (1993) established a classification system for skin tears. Although generally accepted, the Payne-Martin classification system is not widely incorporated into practice. The system identifies three main categories with subcategories that are based on wound characteristics and volume of tissue loss (see Table 3.1.14.1).

■ Differential diagnosis

- Pressure ulcer
- Venous stasis ulcer

■ Treatment

- Physician consultation might be indicated for extensive skin tears.
- Tetanus immunization should be updated if indicated.

Table 3.1.14.1 Payne and Martin classification system for skin tears.

Category 1
A: Linear type, skin tear without tissue loss; the epidermis and dermis are separated as if an incision has been made.
B: Flap type, epidermal flap completely covers the dermis to within 1mm of the wound margin.

Category 2
A: Skin tears with partial tissue loss, scant tissue loss, 25% of the epidermal flap is lost.
B: Skin tears with partial tissue loss, moderate to large tissue loss, >25% of the epidermal flap is lost.

Category 3
Skin tear with complete tissue loss, epidermal flap is absent.

Adapted from Leblanc, K. & Baranoski, S. (2009).

- Treatment should focus on local wound care that promotes moist wound healing, manages exudate and prevents new skin tears from occurring. Dressings should be held in place with flexible netting, gauze rolls or other wraps. Tape should usually be avoided, but if tape is necessary a skin sealant or barrier wafer should be used to avoid skin stripping with their removal. For skin tears that are open and draining, consider covering them with a primary dressing that will allow drainage into an absorbent pad. Other treatment suggestions depend on the appearance of the wound and are noted below.
- Approximation of the skin flap. Wound closure strips or topical liquid films can be used when appropriate.
- 3M™ Tegaderm™ absorbent clear acrylic dressing
- Petroleum-based gauze
- Hydrofiber/calcium alginate
- Foam dressing
- Petroleum-based protective ointment
- Hydrogel
- Non-adherent dressing
- Avoid:
  - Tapes or adherent dressings
  - Hydrocolloids
  - Plain transparent film

■ Collaborative consultation

- Primary care physician
- Certified Wound Care Nurse
- Collaborate with dietician for the initiation of more aggressive nutritional therapy such as the addition of protein, calories, and fluid if a skin tear shows only limited improvement after 7-14 days (Posthauer, 2007).

■ Complications

- Chronic wound
- Infection
- Pain

■ Prevention

- Identify patients at risk.
- Ensure adequate nutrition and hydration by assisting with meals as necessary and offering fluids between meals if medically appropriate.
- Utilize proper patient handling:
  - Use open handed movements, do not grab the patients.
  - Use a pull/draw sheet or lift device to prevent shear and friction.
  - Pat dry the skin and avoid scrubbing.
  - Minimize force and friction with cleansing.
- Ensure proper removal of tape and adhesive dressings – remove by pushing down on the skin while pulling up on the tape or for some adhesive dressings the manufacturer may recommend pulling at an angle to break the adhesive seal of the dressing.
- Use petroleum-based creams to hydrate skin.
- Consider skin sealants under adhesive dressings or tapes.
- Consider skin barrier wafers for tape anchoring.
- Pad bedrails to protect from potential trauma.
- Avoid the use of hot water which can dehydrate the skin.
- Use flexible netting, gauze rolls other wraps to hold dressings in place.
- Avoid the use of tapes and adhesive dressings-if tape must be used, protect the skin with skin prep prior to using tape.
- Consider using full length arm or leg protective sleeves such as Geri sleeves or NONSLEEVES, to protect patient's arms and legs.
- Have the patient wear long sleeves and pants for extra protection.
- Control the environment-lighting, rugs, and location of furniture, wheelchairs to prevent falls which can result in a skin tear.

■ Patient/family education

Education for patients and families should focus on the preventatives measures listed above that reduce the risk of getting a skin tear. There should be a focus on techniques that prevent pulling and friction through the use of proper patient handling techniques. The education should also include measures to help treat and heal the wounds, signs and symptoms of infection and when to notify their physician.

References

Aging Changes in Skin (n.d.) Online. Available from http://www.umm.edu/ency/article/004014.htm (accessed 12 March 2012).

Bryant, R. & Nix, D. (2007) *Acute & Chronic Wounds Current Management Concepts*. Mosby Elsevier, St. Louis.

Baranoski, S. (2003) How to prevent and manage skin tears. *Advances in Skin & Wound Care* **16**(5), 268–270.

Leblanc, K. & Baranoski, S. (2009) Prevention and management of skin tears. *Advances in Skin & Wound Care: The Journal for Prevention and Healing* **22**, 325–332.

Morey, P. (2007) Skin tears: A literature review. *Primary Intention* **15**(3), 122–129.

Payne R.L. & Martin M.L. (1993) Defining and classifying skin tears: need for a common language. *Ostomy Wound Management* **39**(5), 16–20, 22–24, 26.

Posthauer, M.E. (2007) Nutrition al assessment and treatment. In: Sussman, C. & Bates-Jensen, B. (eds). *Wound care: A Collaborative Practice Manual for Health Professionals*, 3rd edn. Lippincott Williams & Wilkins, Baltimore, MD.

Roberts, M. (2007) Preventing and managing skin tears. *Journal of Wound Ostomy Continence Nursing* **34**(3), 256–259.

Further reading

Baranoski, S. & Ayello, E. (2004) *Wound Care Essentials – Practice Principles*. Lippincott Williams & Wilkins, Springhouse.

Ratliff, C. & Fletcher, K. (2007) Skin Tears: a review of the evidence to support prevent and treatment. *Ostomy Wound Management* **53**(3), 32–34, 36, 38–40.

Unit 2: Cardiovascular Disorders

PART 1: ACUTE CORONARY SYNDROME

Sharon Zisk

Acute coronary syndrome (ACS) is an "umbrella term" that encompasses any condition characterized by signs and symptoms of sudden myocardial ischemia (Overbaugh, 2009). ACS includes the following conditions: unstable angina, non-ST elevation myocardial infarction (MI) (NSTEMI) and ST elevation MI (STEMI). ACS is directly related to coronary artery disease (CAD), a disease in which atherosclerotic plaques build up inside the coronary arteries and restrict blood flow to the heart. Unstable angina and NSTEMI normally result from a partially or intermittently occluded coronary artery; whereas STEMIs typically result from a fully occluded coronary artery (Overbaugh, 2009).

Up to 7 million patients present to emergency departments every year complaining of chest pain (Agostini-Miranda & Crown, 2009; Kelly, 2007). There are many causes of chest discomfort, and in order to decrease morbidity and mortality, it is imperative that patients be diagnosed accurately and quickly. Life-threatening causes (identified below) must first be excluded. In older adults, an atypical presentation can make acute coronary syndrome more difficult to identify.

Although chest pain is a common complaint, elders (Kelly, 2007) often present with non-specific symptoms and physical findings. This increases the risk of misdiagnosis making an accurate patient history and detailed physical assessment essential for accurate diagnosis of the patient's chest discomfort.

ACS is the end result of CAD progression. The precipitating cause of ACS is usually the rupture of an atherosclerotic plaque causing first, formation of a thrombus, and then partial or complete occlusion of the involved coronary artery (DeVon & Ryan, 2005). The thrombus is what is responsible for preventing myocardial perfusion, not the plaque itself. Angina is described as the pain or discomfort the patient experiences when atherosclerosis causes narrowing of an artery. A myocardial infarction occurs when there is a plaque rupture and a thrombus develops, thus blocking the artery.

■ Risk factors

For ACS

Non-modifiable:

- Increased age
  (1) Men older than 45
  (2) Women older than 55

- Family history of premature CAD especially:
  - (1) A first degree male who developed CAD before 55
  - (2) A first degree female who developed CAD before 65
- Ethnicity/race: African Americans have a higher risk of hypertension
- Premature menopause
- Women with diabetes

Modifiable:

- Elevated serum cholesterol
- Elevated low-density lipoprotein cholesterol (LDL)
- Elevated triglycerides
- Type II diabetes
- Cigarette smoking
- Obesity
- Sedentary lifestyle
- Hypertension
- Stress

For atherosclerosis
- High cholesterol
- Diabetes mellitus
- Arterial hypertension
- Cigarette smoking
- Systemic inflammatory disease
- Chronic infections

■ Clinical presentation

Chest pain is the classic symptom of ACS, in which the quality of the discomfort may be described as a heaviness, aching, crushing, burning, or squeezing. The pain may radiate to the jaw, neck, arms, or back. In unstable angina, chest pain normally occurs at rest or with exertion and results in limited activity. Chest pain associated with NSTEMI is usually longer in duration and more severe than chest pain associated with unstable angina (Overbaugh, 2009). Older patients are more likely to describe their pain as an ache, pressure, discomfort, or heaviness, and will often report the pain originating from other areas of the body, such as the neck, shoulders, back, and arms (Kelly, 2007).

Unfortunately, many patients having an acute cardiac event are asymptomatic and elders do not seek always medical care when symptoms occur (ACC/AHA, 2011). Symptoms of myocardial infarction include (ACC/AHA, 2011):

- Chest discomfort that can feel like pressure, squeezing, fullness, or pain
- Discomfort in the jaw, arms, back, neck, or stomach

Associated symptoms:

- Shortness of breath
- Dyspnea
- Cold sweat
- Nausea
- Lightheadedness
- Extreme fatigue

For any patient with chest pain, a detailed history (if patient is hemodynamically stable and not in acute distress) is necessary. The history should include specific risk factors for ACS, pulmonary emboli (PE), and aortic dissection. Determining the following will assist in proper diagnosis and treatment.

- *Onset of the chest pain*: important in interpreting cardiac biomarkers
- *Location of chest pain*: may distinguish between other potential diagnosis, such as a PE or aortic dissection
- *Duration of the chest pain*: important in differentiating unstable angina from acute myocardial infarction
- *Aggravating factors*: What makes the pain worse? Pain worsened by activity, stress, or exposure to cold suggests myocardial ischemia. Pain worsened by deep breathing or change in position may be more indicative of a pneumothorax or pericarditis. Musculoskeletal pain tends to be reliably and exactly reproducible.
- *Alleviating factors*: Does anything improve the pain? Antacids and sublingual nitroglycerine may improve the pain of a patient with ACS, so it is important to not exclude these patients based on relief from these medications.
- *Associated symptoms*: Does the patient have any other symptoms? Nausea, vomiting, diaphoresis may be present. Older patients often report belching, indigestion, or generalized fatigue when suffering from an acute MI. The most common presenting symptom of angina in a patient >85 years old is dyspnea (Kelly, 2007).
- *Radiation*: Pain associated with an acute MI may radiate to the neck, shoulder, arm or jaw. If the pain radiates widely, as to both arms, suspicion of acute MI increases.
- *Severity*: Pain associated with myocardial ischemia generally comes on gradually, with intensity increasing over a 5-10 minute period.

■ Nursing assessment

Vital sign changes usually are associated with a cardiac event. These changes may include tachypnea, hypertension/hypotension, decreased oxygen saturation and cardiac rhythm abnormalities.

Hypotension, tachycardia, impaired cognition, cool, clammy, and pale color are signs of systemic hypoperfusion, and cardiogenic shock must be considered.

In addition to changes in vital signs, there are other key components in the assessment of a patient having chest pain. These include (adapted from Kelly, 2007):

- *General appearance*: Is the patient pale, clammy, anxious, or diaphoretic? These patients need immediate attention.
- Rapid survey of airway, breathing, circulation

■ Diagnostics

Clinical assessment, laboratory tests, electrocardiogram findings, combined with patient history are essential in diagnosing ACS.

ECG findings

- Unstable angina: ST depression may not be present in affected leads.
- NSTEMI: there is typically ST depression, T wave inversion, or nonspecific ST changes.
- STEMI: there is ST elevation in affected leads (note: ECG is a poor predictor of MI in patients with a left bundle branch block).

Electrocardiograms identify up to 65% of all myocardial infarctions, but may be of little value in diagnosing unstable angina or NSTEMIs.

Laboratory tests

The following laboratory tests are necessary in all patients experiencing signs and symptoms of ACS:

- Complete blood count/differential
- Serum glucose, electrolytes, blood urea nitrogen, creatinine
- Liver function tests
- Thyroid function
- Total cholesterol

Lab tests specific to MI (cardiac markers):

- Troponins
- Creatine kinase (CK-MB)
- Myoglobin
- Lactate dehydrogenase

The most frequently used cardiac markers are CK-MB and troponins. The value of the troponin and CK-MB will vary depending on the assay used (see Table 3.2.1.1). An elevation in the concentration of these two markers is required for the diagnosis of an acute MI. If a troponin value is normal, while the CK-MB

Table 3.2.1.1 Cardiac markers.

	Creatine-kinase-total and MB	Troponins	Myoglobin	Lactate dehydrogenase
Onset	3–12 hours	3–12 hours	1–4 hours	6–12 hours
Peak	18–24 hours	18–24 hours	6–7 hours	24 hours
Duration	36–48 hours	Up to 10 days	24 hours	6–8 days

Adapted from Reeder & Kennedy, 2011.

is elevated, MB is likely due to release from non-cardiac tissue (Reeder & Kennedy, 2011).

■ Differential diagnosis

There are many causes of chest pain so the following differential diagnoses need to be considered.

- Anxiety
- Costochondritis
- Esophageal rupture
- Gallstones
- Gastroesophageal reflux (GERD)
- Pancreatitis
- Pericarditis
- Pleurisy
- Pneumonia
- Ulcers

Life-threatening causes of chest pain:

- Dissecting aortic aneurysm
- Pulmonary embolism
- Pneumothorax
- Trauma

■ Treatment

- Oxygen: supplemental oxygen should be given to patients with oxygen saturation <90 %, respiratory distress, or hypoxia.
- Aspirin: most patients experiencing acute coronary syndrome are given a 325 milligram aspirin to chew. Discuss with physician.
- Morphine is given (SQ or IV) for relief of chest pain and/or anxiety.
- Beta blockers: universal treatment for all patients with acute STEMI. Some contraindications include heart failure, low cardiac output, high risk

for cardiogenic shock, bradycardia, heart block, or reactive airway disease (Reeder *et al.*, 2011).
- Nitrates dilate coronary arteries, cause systemic vasodilation and are helpful in alleviating persistent chest pain. However, nitrates must be used cautiously (if at all) in patients with hypotension and are contraindicated in patients with critical aortic stenosis.
- Calcium channel blockers: a second medication used in management of angina, also causes vasodilation.
- Anticoagulant therapy: many agents are available for anticoagulation. Selected agent is dependent upon overall treatment strategy.
- Fibrinolytic therapy: may be considered for a patient who presents with a STEMI within 12 hours of onset of symptoms and has no contraindications for fibrinolysis. Percutaneous coronary intervention (PCI); may be considered for a patient presenting with an acute STEMI who can undergo the procedure within 90 minutes of first medical contact by people skilled in the procedure (ACC/AHA 2008).
- Coronary artery bypass surgery: may be indicated in urgent cases if fibrinolysis or PCI fails, or in patients with cardiogenic shock, or life threatening arrhythmia associated with left main or three-vessel disease (Reeder *et al.*, 2011).
- Antiplatelet therapy: prevents the formation of a thrombus.
- Lipid-lowering medications (statins)
- Cardiac rehabilitation

■ Collaborative consultation

The American College of Cardiology/American Heart Association recommended that all hospitals establish multidisciplinary teams to develop guideline-based protocols, specific to the institution, that will result in effectively triaging and managing patients who present with symptoms of myocardial ischemia (Reeder *et al.*, 2011). There are an increasing number of institutions that use structured algorithms, checklists, or pathways to screen patients with suspected ACS.

■ Complications

- Patients >75 years old have a higher in hospital mortality, often due to electrical and mechanical complications (Reeder *et al.*, 2011).
- Older patients are more likely to have severe bleeding secondary to fibrinolytic therapy, thus increasing their risk for hemorrhagic stroke.
- Due to the sometimes atypical presentation of older patients with acute coronary syndrome, there is often a delay in diagnosis and treatment.
- Development of heart failure post MI
- Stroke/transient ischemic attack
- Angina
- Adverse drug interactions, in older adults: ADRs are frequently related to metabolic changes and decreased drug clearance associated with aging, as well as the risk of interactions due to polypharmacy.

■ Prevention
- Medications to lower cholesterol
- Improved glucose control for diabetic patients
- Smoking cessation
- Weight reduction if obese
- Exercise
- Medications to control hypertension
- Stress management

■ Patient/family education
- Discuss with patient and family the importance of proper medication management and instruct them to call their health care provider with any questions.
- Explain each medication and ensure the patient and family understand the rationale for each drug, dosing, and side effects.
- Explain to the patient and family the reason for admission to the hospital, what it means for their health, and when to call the doctor after discharge.
- Encourage the patient to modify their lifestyle if necessary utilizing the modifiable risk factors.

References

Agostini-Miranda, A.A. & Crown, L.A. (2009) An approach to the initial care of patients with chest pain in an emergency department located in a non-cardiac center. *American Journal of Clinical Medicine* **6**(1), 24–29.

ACC/AHA (2008) 2007 Focused Update of the ACC/AHA 2004 Guidelines STEMI FOCUSED UPDATE or the Management of Patients With ST-Elevation Myocardial Infarction. *Circulation* **2**(117), 296–329.

ACC/AHA (2011). ACC/AHA Practice Guideline 2011. ACCF/AHA Focused Update Incorporated Into the ACC/AHA 2007 Guidelines for the Management of Patients With Unstable Angina/Non-ST-Elevation Myocardial Infarction. A Report of the American College of Cardiology Foundation/American Heart Association Task Force on Practice Guidelines.

DeVon, H. & Ryan, C. (2005) Chest pain and associated acute coronary syndromes. *Journal of Cardiovascular Nursing* **20**, 232–238.

Kelly, B. (2007) Evaluation of the elderly patient with acute chest pain. *Clinics in Geriatric Medicine* **23**, 327–349.

Overbaugh, K. (2009) Acute coronary syndrome. *American Journal of Nursing* **109**(5), 42–52.

Reeder, G. & Kennedy, H. (2011) Criteria for the diagnosis of acute myocardial infarction. Online. Available from http://www.uptodate.com/contents/criteria-for-the-diagnosis-of-acute-myocardial-infarction (accessed 13 March 2012).

Reeder, G., Kennedy, H. & Rosenson, R. (2011) Overview of the acute management of acute ST elevation myocardial infarction. Online. Available from http://www.upto-date.com/contents/overview-of-the-acute-management-of-acute-st-elevation-myocardial-infarction (accessed 13 March 2012).

Further reading

ACCF/AHA (2011) Focused Update Incorporated Into the ACC/AHA 2007. *Circulation* **123**, e426-e579.

Conway, B. & Fuat, A. (2007) Recent advances in angina management: implications for nurses. *Nursing Standard* **21**, 38, 49-56.

Tough, J. (2004) Assessment and treatment of chest pain. *Nursing Standard* **18**, 45-53.

Zitkus, B. (2010) Take chest pain to heart. *The Nurse Practitioner* **September**, 41-47.

PART 2: ATRIAL FIBRILLATION

Theresa E. Evans

Atrial fibrillation (AF) is the most common type of arrhythmia affecting an estimated 2.66 million people in 2010 and as many as 12 million by the year 2050 (American Heart Association, 2012). With each passing decade the prevalence doubles and by 80 years of age, AF affects approximately 10% of people age 80 and older (Kannel & Benjamin, 2009). According to Kannel and Benjamin (2009) by 2050 those 80 years and older will constitute half of the AF cases.

Fibrillation is defined as the rapid, irregular and unsynchronized contracting of heart muscle fibers. In AF, electrical impulses no longer originate in the sinus node (pacemaker of the heart) but are initiated from other parts of the atria. These impulses do not travel through the normal pathway and can spread through the atria in a rapid and chaotic manner, causing the upper heart chambers to fibrillate. The atrioventricular (AV) node, or "gatekeeper" is subsequently flooded with impulses. Although the AV node does not allow all impulses to be conducted through to the ventricles (lower heart chambers), the ventricles do begin to beat faster in an attempt to meet the demand of the atria, with rates of 100-200 beats per minute. Because atrial squeeze is compromised, blood begins to pool in the atrial chambers and is not pumped into the ventricles, causing inconsistencies in amounts of blood pumped to the body with each beat. In addition to varying cardiac output, this pooling may lead to clot formation in the atria. The rapid ventricular response is often the ultimate cause of symptoms, although many people are asymptomatic, at least initially.

A recurrent AF episode that begins and terminates independent of external intervention is called paroxysmal AF. These episodes may produce mild to severe symptoms, if at all, and last minutes, hours, or days. If the arrhythmia requires termination with medicine or cardioversion, it is categorized as persistent atrial fibrillation. Ultimately both paroxysmal and persistent AF may lead to permanent AF in which the usual treatments do not restore normal rhythm.

■ Risk factors

- Advanced age
- Alcohol excess or withdrawal
- Chronic obstructive pulmonary disease
- Diabetes
- Heart disease (coronary artery disease, heart failure, valvular disease)
- Hyperlipidemia
- Hypertension
- Hyperthyroidism
- Hypoxia
- Infection especially when associated with fever
- Obesity
- Pericarditis
- Sleep apnea
- Steroid use, chronic high dose

■ Clinical presentation

AF, especially in elders, can cause only mild symptoms and as a result often goes undetected. Often, it is found during a physical examination or a workup for other disease processes (e.g., stroke). Symptoms associated with AF include:

- Angina (particularly in patients with underlying coronary disease)
- Anxiety
- Chest pain
- Dizziness or fainting
- Dyspnea
- Fatigue
- Palpitations
- Shortness of breath or dyspnea (congestion related)
- Syncope
- Weakness
- Angina (particularly with underlying coronary disease)

■ Nursing assessment

A thorough medical history, review of systems and family history are essential, especially given the subtle nature of symptoms. Determining if the AF are new in onset or chronic is also important.

Physical exam findings may include the following:

- Vital signs:
  - Determine presence of fever
  - Heart rate: irregularly irregular rhythm with auscultation, often tachycardic with ventricular rates of 100-200

- Blood pressure: elevated heart rates often lead to vasodilation of systemic vessels to meet oxygen needs, thus decreasing blood pressure.
- Respiratory rate: rapid breathing to meet oxygen demands; seen most with pulmonary congestion associated with heart failure.
- Oxygen saturation levels: patients with heart failure/pulmonary congestion often have decreased oxygen saturation levels.
- Assess for recent unintentional weight gain.
- Neurologic:
  - Changes in mental status related to hypoxia are common, but in older patients with dementia or delirium, cognitive changes may be difficult to assess.
  - Complete neurologic exam to exclude possibility of stroke:
    - It is important to be aware of a history of previous stroke and residual effects.
- Cardiac:
  - Auscultation of heart sounds is imperative to assessment.
    - Findings may include irregular rhythm and rapid heart rates.
    - Assess for murmurs that may be related to underlying valvular disease.
- Respiratory:
  - Adventitious lung sounds (i.e., rales or cardiogenic wheezes) may indicate heart failure.
- Peripheral vascular:
  - Lower extremity edema, cyanosis, or clubbing may indicate heart failure.
  - Absence of peripheral pulses may indicate peripheral vascular compromise.

■ Diagnostics

- Electrocardiogram (ECG): simple and accurate test for determining arrhythmia if patient is experiencing signs or symptoms at the time of exam.
  - Portable ECG can record rhythm for extended time and most helpful if paroxysmal AF is suspected
    - Events monitor: set to record changes in rhythm.
    - Holter monitor: set to continuously record for particular timeframe.
- Echocardiogram (ECHO):
  - Transthoracic: non-invasive, provides images of size, shape of heart and how the heart valves and chambers are working.
  - Transesophageal: invasive (through esophagus): visualizes atria better and may also detect clots.
- Chest X-ray: assists to determine lung involvement with heart failure.
- Laboratory:
  - Complete blood count/differential
  - Serum electrolytes, blood urea nitrogen, creatinine
  - Thyroid panel
  - Cardiac enzymes (especially if suspected acute coronary event)
  - Brain natriuretic peptide (BNP) (if heart failure is suspected)
  - Arterial blood gases if indicated
  - Ethanol level if indicated

■ Differential diagnosis

Narrow QRS tachycardia including:

- Atrial flutter
- Atrioventricular nodal reentry tachycardia
- Multifocal atrial tachycardia
- Paroxysmal tachycardia
- Premature atrial contractions
- Premature junctional contractions
- Sinus tachycardia

■ Treatment

- Careful consideration should be taken by the healthcare provider when determining treatment goals of rate versus rhythm focus. All factors including risks and benefits must be included when deciding treatment course and will vary with each patient. The initial goal of treatment is to determine if the patient is hemodynamically stable or unstable (i.e., chest pain, hypotensive, acute pulmonary congestion, change in mental status). Patients who are unstable require emergency treatment such as synchronized cardioversion (120-200 J). For patients who are stable, treatment goals are to control the rate and, if possible restore normal sinus rhythm.
- Rate control: goal is to slow heart rate and decrease patient symptoms. Rate control does not convert arrhythmia to normal sinus rhythm, but attempts to moderate rate. It is important to assess vital signs prior to and after medication administration to titrate medications accurately to meet the needs of each individual. Commonly used medications include:
  - Beta-blockers (e.g., metoprolol)
  - Calcium channel blockers (e.g., diltiazem)
  - Digitalis: imperative to monitor patients for anorexia, nausea, vomiting or other symptoms associated with digoxin toxicity as well as monitor therapeutic level with blood tests.
- Rhythm control: goal is to regain normal sinus rhythm; most often attempted and successful with new onset AF. May be used if traditional rate control methods have not improved function.
  - Electrical cardioversion: usually performed using conscious sedation and essential to monitor patient comfort. It is important to rule out clots prior to performing.
  - Anti-arrhythmic drugs (e.g., Amiodarone, calcium channel blocker [i.e., diltiazem or verapamil] or a beta blocker). These medications must be monitored and titrated closely.
- Catheter ablation: destroys electrical connections that are disrupting normal flow of signals.
- MAZE procedure: blocks spread of disruptive impulses.
- Pacemaker placement

- Stroke prevention: decreasing chances of forming blood clots is imperative to stroke prevention with patient affected with AF.
  - Administering anticoagulant therapy is a vital intervention but these medications must be monitored closely and risk/benefit ratio assessed especially in older adults.
    - Heparin: traditional short-term bridge to long-term regime. Administered IV with close monitoring of partial thromboplastin time (PTT) levels to maintain therapeutic range.
    - Low-molecular weight heparins (e.g., Lovenox): newer short-term treatment options ideal for outpatient settings and administered subcutaneously.
    - Warfarin (Coumadin): long-term treatment of AF that must be monitored and titrated closely using international normalized ratio (INR) goals.
    - Dabigatran Etexilate (Pradaxa), an oral anticoagulant, 75 to 150 milligrams PO twice a day depending on renal function, was approved by the FDA in nonvalvular AF to prevent emboli (Nagarakanti *et al.*, 2011; LexiComp, 2012).
    - Rivaroxaban (Xarelto), a Factor Xa inhibitor, 15 to 20 milligrams by mouth once a day depending on renal function (Patel *et al.*, 2011; LexiComp, 2012).
  - Safety evaluation and assessment of risk of falls is essential in elders and must be factored into treatment goals. According to a study done by Poli *et al.* (2009) even in older adults, rates of bleeding complications can be kept low as long as careful anticoagulation management was maintained.
  - Left atrial appendage exclusion: prevents blood clots by sealing off the left atrial appendage.

■ Collaborative consultation

- Consider consultation with the cardiologist and/or electrophysiologist.
- Dietician consultation if dietary restrictions are imposed due to anticoagulation therapy with warfarin.

■ Complications

The greatest complication of atrial fibrillation is a thromboembolism. Because the atria are not efficiently pumping blood into the ventricles, the blood pools in the atria increasing the chances of clot formation. When a clot travels out of the atria it is called an embolus. These clots can travel to various parts of the body including the brain, lungs, and kidneys resulting in:

- Stroke
- Pulmonary embolus
- Renal embolus

The American Heart Association's most recent data suggests that someone suffers a stroke in the United States every 40 seconds (AHA, 2011). Atrial fibrillation is considered a strong, independent risk factor for thrombolitic event, increasing the risk of stroke about five-fold. With advancing age the percent of atrial fibrillation attributed strokes increases markedly (AHA, 2012).

According to Hardin and Steele (2008) the average rate of ischemic stroke among older adults with atrial fibrillation is 5% per year and further note that in women in particular, atrial fibrillation is the primary cause of debilitating strokes.

Acute rapid atrial fibrillation can be complicated by decreased cardiac output, hypotension and acute heart failure.

■ Prevention

- Healthy diet
  - Low sodium (especially in hypertension)
  - Decreased caffeine intake
- Smoking cessation
- Treatment of underlying causes (thyroid or sleep apnea).
- Stress reduction
- Weight maintenance
- Alcohol reduction
- Tight blood glucose control (especially in diabetes).
- Medication adherence for patients with underlying heart disease or hypertension.
- Regular physical exams and follow up.

■ Patient/family education

- Educating patients and families on ways to maintain healthy lifestyle including diet
- Educating patients and families on prevention of disease
- Educating and continued monitoring of medications
  - When to call their health care provider
  - How to monitor vital signs and what they mean
  - Identify signs of stroke.
  - Identify signs of heart failure.
- Anticoagulation therapy
  - How to manage medications (Warfarin)
    - Educate about diet, specifically vitamin K intake and maintenance.
    - Educate about the numerous drug interactions (e.g. antibiotics).
    - Educate on importance with compliance with meds and introduce calendar to assist with complicated regimes.
  - Highlight importance of good follow up and compliance with INR checks.

References

American Heart Association (2011) Facts. A Serious and Worsening Problem: Stroke in the US. Online. Available from http://www.heart.org/idc/groups/heart-public/@wcm/@adv/documents/downloadable/ucm_305054.pdf (accessed 6 May 2012).

American Heart Association (2012 updates) Heart disease and stroke statistics. Online. Available from http://circ.ahajournals.org/content/125/1/e2.full#sec-1 (accessed 7 May 2010).

Hardin, S.R. & Steele, J.R. (2008) Atrial fibrillation among older adults. *Journal of Gerontological Nursing* **34**(7), 26–33.

Kannel, W.B. & Benjamin, E.J. (2009) Current perceptions of the epidemiology of atrial fibrillation. *Cardiology Clinics* **27**, 13–24.

Nagarakanti, R., Ezekowitz, M.D., Oldgren, J. *et al.* (2011) Dabigatran versus warfarin in patients with atrial fibrillation undergoing cardioversion: An analysis of patients undergoing cardioversion. *Circulation* **123**, 131–136.

Patel, M.R., Mahaffey, K.W., Garg, J. *et al.*; and the ROCKET AF Steering Committee, for the ROCKET AF Investigators (2011) Rivaroxaban versus warfarin in nonvalvular atrial fibrillation. *New England Journal of Medicine* **385**(10), 883–891.

Poli, D., Antonucci, E., Grifoni, E., Abbate, R., Gensini, G.F. & Prisco, D. (2009) Bleeding risk during oral anticoagulation in atrial fibrillation patients older than 80 years. *Journal of the American College of Cardiology* **54**(11), 999–1002.

PART 3: VENOUS THROMBOEMBOLISM

Eva Beliveau

Venous thromboembolism (VTE) is the presence of a blood clot (thrombus) in the venous circulation. The thrombus can remain stagnant as a deep vein thrombosis (DVT) causing minor or no symptoms at all, or it can travel to the lung to form a pulmonary embolism (PE), leading to major illness and/or death. Although a thrombus can occur in any large vein, they occur most commonly in the proximal or distal leg veins. The elderly population, due to their decreased activity level and affinity for coagulation abnormalities, are particularly vulnerable.

The United States Department of Health and Human Services estimates 350,000 to 600,000 Americans suffer from VTE annually, which directly or indirectly result in 100,000 deaths (US Department of Health and Human Services, 2008). Because VTE can be difficult to diagnose, it is conceivable that the morbidity and mortality may actually be much higher. Other cohort studies have concluded that approximately 30% of those who have a DVT in a given year will experience a recurrence within 10 years, as well a marked increase occurrence of VTE with age and in males. And, of particular mention, a large study also found that the diagnosis of PE in nursing home residents was missed up to 70% of the time and confirmed only on autopsy (US Department of Heath and Human Services, 2008). Further DVT morbidity includes chronic venous insufficiency, encompassing chronic venous hypertension causing leg pain, edema, hyperpigmentation, venous ulcers and lipodermatosclerosis (scarring of the skin and fat). These DVT manifestations can be difficult to differentiate from other disorders such as cellulitis, lymphedema, torn calf muscles, lower leg fracture and hematoma (Tovi & Wyatt, 2003).

In 2006, these alarming statistics and diagnostic challenges associated with VTE's led to a Surgeon General Workshop designated specifically for VTE prevention and treatment. The outcome was the commitment to develop a consistent plan to better recognize and treat VTE in order to reduce the morbidity and mortality. The National Heart, Lung, and Blood institute (NHLBI) under the umbrella of the National Institute of Health (NIH) has been given generous funding to conduct research to develop consistent evidence-base practice guidelines in the treatment of VTE, and provide education to both heath care providers and the general public. More specific guidelines to assess and treat VTE are now present at most heath care facilities. And, the Joint Commission, the agency that certifies healthcare facilities for safety standards, is now looking at the methods acute care hospitals use to screen and implement VTE prophylaxis when validating certification (Joint Commission Annual Conference, 2009).

Pathophysiology

In order to understand the consequences and sequelae of presentation of a VTE, it is necessary to understand how the thrombus develops. Normally, the venous circulation is slow, especially in the deep veins of the lower extremities. Together the valves in the veins and contractions of the calf and thigh muscles promote the upward flow of the venous blood back to the heart. In addition, in the body's effort to maintain free flow, the blood vessel walls secrete a number of substances that prevent the adherence of platelets and/or activation of the clotting cascade. These regulatory mechanisms, along with the body's blood clotting factors, continuously maintain a balance between hemorrhage and clotting (Fitzpatrick & Wood, 2010). Any disruption in these complex physiological functions can lead to venous stasis and potential thrombus formation. If the thrombus dislodges and travels, it can travel to the lungs and cause a PE. Identifying risk factors and proving good prophylactic treatment can prevent VTEs from developing.

■ Risk factors

- Past history of VTE
- Trauma patients
- Advanced age
- Pregnancy (PE is the most common cause of maternal death.)
- Cancer (pancreatic has the highest incidence.)
- Cigarette smoking
- Medications
    - Estrogen-based contraceptives (especially the transdermal route)
    - Hormone replacement medication
- Family history of VTE
- Inherited blood clotting disorders (protein C, protein S, and antithrombin deficiencies)
- Nursing home residency

The risk of developing a VTE is cumulative and increases in magnitude with the number of contributing risk factors. Many VTE events can be correlated to specific triggering events which include:

- Hospitalization
- Major surgery
- Trauma
- Prolonged periods of immobility such as during illness and long airplane travel

◼ Clinical presentation

VTEs can manifest as either a DVT, PE, or both, and symptoms may be subtle or absent. Recognizing presenting symptoms therefore, is particularly challenging for heath care providers. Patients with a DVT may present with the following in the affected extremity:

- Edema
- Warmth to touch
- Pain
- Lipodermatosclerosis (brownish discoloration and taut shiny skin)
- Erythema

A patient with a PE may present with some or all of the following:

- Chest pain
- Tachypnea
- Tachycardia
- Cough (with or without hemoptysis)

The onset of symptoms, if present, can occur quickly or gradually and as previously stated, can often be difficult to differentiate from other disorders such as:

- Cellulitis
- Orthopedic injuries
- Exacerbation of chronic obstructive pulmonary disease (COPD)
- Acute coronary artery disease (CAD)

Identifying those patients at risk for VTE is of paramount importance in recognizing and preventing VTE. This is especially true in older adults since they commonly have co-morbid illnesses that can present with VTE symptomatology. Since prophylactic treatment is initiated in patients at risk for VTE, accurate patient history, including family history, past medical and surgical history, and history of present illness together must be considered.

■ Nursing assessment

Along with patient history, the physical exam is extremely important both to identify patients who have or are at risk of developing VTE. Specific assessment considerations include:

- **Neurological**
  - Mental status changes; confusion and or dementia can impede both subjective and objective data collection.
  - Sudden increased restlessness or loss of consciousness could indicate a PE.
- **Vital signs**
  - Temperature may be elevated.
  - Blood pressure: increased or decreased blood pressure can be occur when PE partially or completely occludes the pulmonary artery.
  - Respirations: tachypnea (very rapid respiratory rate) is the most frequent sign of a PE. This along with other signs of respiratory distress such as cough with or without hemoptysis strongly indicate the presence of a PE.
  - Heart rate: tachycardia is one of the first signs of a PE.
  - Pulse oximetry: decreased O_2 saturation.
- **Respiratory**
  - Increased rate and depth of respirations
  - Productive cough with blood-tinged or frothy sputum
  - Chest pain with inspiration may occur with a PE.
- **Cardiac**
  - Substernal chest pain is often present with a PE.
  - Shock: If the outflow tract of the pulmonary artery is heavily or completely occluded, signs of shock will be present including increased heart rate, decreased blood pressure and multi system organ failure.
- **Skin**
  - Erythema or discoloration of the extremity
  - Edema of the effected extremity may be increased distal to the occlusion.
  - Ulceration of the skin distal to the occlusion.
  - Lipodermatosclerosis: brownish discoloration and smoothness above the ankles

■ Diagnostics

Diagnosing a VTE is challenging and complex. Prevention, with early prophylactic treatment, is now the primary goal. The standard practice is to separate the diagnostic methods into three categories: prophylaxis, DVT, and PE.

Prophylaxis

Use screening tools to identify patients at risk for VTE on all acute and chronic patient admissions. Wells Criteria is now commonly used by practitioners (http://mdcalc.com/wells-criteria-for-dvt).

DVT
- Contrast venography (involves injection of a dye) to identify size and location.
- Ultrasonography (three types) to identify size and location:
  (1) Compression ultrasound
  (2) Duplex ultrasound
  (3) Colour flow duplex imaging.
- Computerized tomography (CT) scan or magnetic resonance imaging (studies show results to have low reliability)
- D-dimer blood test, if positive suggests presence of blood clot.
- Clotting blood studies (prothrombin time (PT), partial thromboplastin time (PTT), fibrinogen, etc.) to identify clotting deficiencies
- Anticoagulation profile: (protein S, protein C, lupus anticoagulant, Antithrombin III, Factor V Leiden)-all preferably drawn before anticoagulation is started, to identify hereditary deficiencies.

PE
- Lung scan to locate the thrombus and determine size and potential effects.
- Ventilation-perfusion scan differentiate the diagnosis from other pulmonary events.
- Chest CT scan to locate the thrombus and determine size and potential effects.
- Arterial blood gases (ABG) to assess potential respiratory failure.

■ Differential diagnosis
- DVT
  - Cellulitis
  - Edema: dependent or related to fluid overload
  - Lymphedema or lymphangitis
  - Musculoskeletal injury
  - Popliteal cyst (Baker's cyst)
  - Superficial thrombophlebitis
  - Venous insufficiency
- PE
  - Anxiety
  - Aortic aneurysm
  - Asthma or COPD
  - Chest pain: costochondritis or chest trauma
  - Gastroesophageal reflux disease
  - Heart failure
  - Lung cancer
  - Myocardial infarction
  - Pericarditis
  - Pleural effusion

- Pneumonia
- Pneumothorax

■ Treatment

- Anticoagulation drug therapy, unless contraindicated, is initiated as soon as possible. The type and dosage are dependent on if the treatment is prophylactic, for an acute or suspected DVT or an acute or suspected PE. Coagulation blood studies are carefully monitored and doses are adapted as needed according to patient response. Newer therapies are being used for some patients (e.g., dabigatran), but the most common anticoagulants are:
  - Subcutaneous low molecular weight heparin
  - Intravenous unfractionated heparin
  - Subcutaneous unfractionated heparin
  - Oral vitamin K antagonist (i.e., Warfarin)
- Vena cava filters are not routinely used but are often considered with patients who cannot receive anticoagulation therapy.
- Mechanical compression is often used to prevent venous pooling and promote venous return. They can be divided into three types:
  - Graduating compression stockings
  - Intermittent pneumonic compression device
  - Venous foot pump
- Early ambulation if tolerated
- Leg exercises while in bed
- Oxygen therapy (for patients with PE) according to ABG

Nursing care

- Carefully monitor lab values:
  - (PT/International Normalized Ratio (INR)) if the patient is on warfarin:
    - Establish desired INR goals for each patient:
      - INR goal for DVT is commonly 2.0–3.0 with 2.5 the ideal.
      - For recurrent DVT/PE the goal INR may be as high as 3.5.
  - PT/ PTT for patients on intravenous unfractionated heparin and fibrinogen levels
- Assess patient response to medication and oxygen therapy as indicated.
- Carefully apply the mechanical compression device utilized.
- Encourage leg exercises and ambulation.
- Assess for signs and symptoms associated with the DVT and or PE.
- Monitor for signs of heparin-induced thrombocytopenia:
  - Decreased platelet count
  - Increased bruising (ecchymosis and hematoma)
  - Oozing from puncture sites
- Monitor for signs of bleeding:
  - Decreased hematocrit and hemoglobin levels
  - Hypotension
  - Tachycardia

■ Collaborative consultation

- It is important for the nurse to work collaboratively with the physician to monitor the patient's coagulation studies and be prepared to adapt therapy as needed.
- If the patient is on an oral vitamin K antagonist (i.e., warfarin) a nutritionist should be consulted to review with the patient dietary restrictions.

■ Complications

- Bleeding from over anticoagulation
- Chronic venous insufficiency from prolonged DVT
- Heparin induced thrombocytopenia
- Venous stasis ulcers
- Death from PE

■ Prevention

- Screen all acute and chronic hospitalized patients for VTE and VTE risk.
- Encourage physical activity.
- Prevent sitting for long periods.
- Encourage and administer prophylactic treatment.
- Public education about VTE prevention

■ Patient/family education

- Avoid sitting for long periods and the importance of leg exercises if unavoidable (i.e., on long flights).
- Review symptoms that should be reported right away such as: leg pain, swelling and warmth or pulmonary changes.
- Discuss the importance of taking anticoagulation therapy as ordered.
- Explain specific medications ordered including potential side effects, dietary restriction and follow up monitoring.

References

Fitzpatrick, L. & Wood, B. (2010) A review of prevention and treatment of venous thromboembolism. Online. Available from http://formularyjournal.modernmedicine.com/formulary/Feature+Articles/A-review-of-the-prevention-and-treatment-of-venous/ArticleStandard/Article/detail/662029 (accessed 7 May 2012).

Joint Commission Annual Conference on Quality and Safety Papers Titles and Abstracts: Screening and Implementation of a DVT Prophylaxis Program for Medical/Surgical Populations in Acute Care Settings. (2009) Online. Available from www.jcrinc.com/Thehttp://jrcrine.com (accessed 7 May 2012).

Tovi, C. & Wyatt, S. (2003) Diagnosis, investigation, and management of deep vein thrombosis. Online. Available from http://www.bmj.com/content/326/7400/1180 (accessed 7 May 2012).

US Department of Health and Human Services (2008) Surgeon General's Call to Action to Prevent Deep Vein Thrombosis and Pulmonary Embolism. Online. Available from www.surgeongeneral.gov/topics/deepvein (accessed 13 March 2012).

PART 4: HEART FAILURE

Theresa E. Evans

Heart failure occurs when the heart is no longer able to pump enough blood to meet the needs of the body. It is a chronic, progressive disease with no known cure. Heart failure can be caused by numerous cardiac conditions (e.g., myocardial infarction and hypertension) that damage or overwork the heart. With treatment of underlying conditions and symptom management people are now living longer, more active lives with the diagnosis of heart failure.

Heart failure is thought to affect over 5 million Americans resulting in over 1,000,000 hospitalizations and 300,000 deaths each year (Riegel *et al.*, 2009). It was estimated that the cost of direct and indirect care for heart failure patients in the US in 2010 was close to 40 billion dollars (Lloyd-Jones *et al.*, 2010).

The left ventricle of the heart pumps oxygenated blood to the entire body. In left-sided failure the left ventricle either loses it ability to contract and becomes too weak to pump blood to the body (systolic dysfunction) or becomes too stiff and cannot relax properly to fill with adequate blood (diastolic dysfunction). In systolic heart failure the ejection fraction (EF) is decreased while in diastolic heart failure there may be a normal ejection fraction. Left-sided failure is tied closely with pulmonary backup or congestion. Right-sided heart failure is commonly a result of left-sided failure. Over time the increased demand and pressure on the pulmonary system exerts additional demand on the right heart, leaving these muscles weakened and unable to pump blood to the lungs to be oxygenated. The blood may build up in the peripheral circulatory system causing lower extremity edema and venous distention. Chronic heart failure is often a combination of both left and right-sided failure.

■ Risk factors

- Age
- Arrhythmia (e.g., atrial fibrillation)
- Chemotherapeutics
- Coronary artery disease
- Diabetes
- Heart valve disease
- Hypertension
- Medications (history of ephedra)

- Myocardial infarction
- Race
- Radiation
- Thyroid disease

■ Clinical presentation

Heart failure symptoms may be subtle in the initial stage of the disease and worsen as the disease progresses. According to the ACC/AHA, Stage A and B candidates may not have active symptoms but meet criteria and be at high risk for developing symptoms as they progress to Stages C and D. The most common symptoms often result from the volume overload associated with failure. Symptoms of heart failure include:

- Anorexia
- Anxiety
- Change in mental status
- Chest pain
- Cough
- Depression
- Difficulty sleeping
- Dizziness or syncope
- Fatigue
- Lower extremity swelling
- Orthopnea
- Paroxysmal nocturnal dyspnea
- Shortness of breath or dyspnea on exertion
- Weight gain
- Wheezing

Older adults may delay seeking treatment for the early signs of heart failure because they relate the symptoms to normal aging. It is also possible that decreased functional ability in elders may limit their capacity to detect changes in breathlessness, dyspnea or fatigue. The chronic symptoms may become a part of normal life and not be detected as increasing in severity (Jurgens *et al.*, 2010).

■ Nursing assessment

A thorough medical history, review of systems and family history is essential, especially given the subtle nature of symptoms early in the disease. The history must include alcohol and drug use, lifestyle behaviors (e.g., nutrition, smoking) as well as alternative therapies and any history of chemotherapeutic treatments. A thorough assessment of the patient's functional ability with activities of daily living is imperative to determine baseline activity levels.

- Physical exam
  - Assess height, weight and body mass index (BMI):
    - Determine if recent unintentional weight gain which can indicate volume overload.
    - If patient was previously taking diuretics determine goal "dry weight".
  - Vital signs:
    - Blood pressure: may be elevated as part of patient's history.
      - Orthostatic blood pressure is also important to determine volume status.
    - Pulse: assess rate and regularity of rhythm.
    - Respiratory rate: rapid breathing may be present to meet oxygen demands.
    - Oxygen saturation levels
  - Neurologic:
    - Change in mental status in elder may represent hypoxia.
    - Patient may seem anxious or depressed.
  - Cardiac:
    - Auscultation of heart sounds. Assess for heart rate and rhythm as well S3, an early sign of heart failure and murmurs that may be related to underlying valvular disease.
    - Determine presence of jugular vein distention or hepatic jugular reflex.
  - Respiratory:
    - Adventitious lung sounds may include rales and wheezes indicating possible heart failure.
      - Assess for rhonchi which suggest pneumonia, a possible precipitant or consequence of heart failure.
  - Abdomen: Assess for ascites
  - Peripheral vascular:
    - Lower extremity edema, cyanosis, clubbing

■ Diagnostics

- Electrocardiogram (ECG):
  - Simple and non-invasive test assists to determine rate and rhythm.
  - Assesses for wall thickening and previous myocardial event.
- Imaging:
  - Echocardiogram (ECHO):
    - Transthoracic: non-invasive:
      - Provides images of size and shape of heart, wall thickness and how the valves and chambers are working (i.e., left ventricular ejection fraction).
    - Transesophageal: invasive (through esophagus):
      - May also detect clots.
  - Chest X-ray: may detect heart chamber enlargement and assists to determine lung involvement with heart failure.

- Cardiac magnetic resonance imaging: provides more detailed and accurate information and may be helpful in finding early signs of heart failure, prior to symptoms appearing.
- Stress test: may help determine ischemia.
- Cardiac catheterization/angiography: possibly indicated if patient has angina or when results of previous testing suggest ischemia.
  - Laboratory
    - B-type natriuretic peptide (BNP) levels help determine if a patient has heart failure or pulmonary disease. BNP levels are elevated in patients with heart failure, though the BNP may be higher in patients with reduced EF than in patients with preserved left ventricle function
    - Complete blood count/differential
    - Electrolytes including calcium and magnesium
    - Renal and hepatic function tests
    - Lipid panel
    - Cardiac enzymes (especially if suspected cardiac event)
    - Thyroid function tests

■ Differential diagnosis

The differential diagnosis is concerned with determining the cause of the heart failure (i.e., anemia, infection, infarction, ischemia, thyroid abnormality). Other causes of patient symptoms that are considered in the differential diagnosis include:

- Acute respiratory distress syndrome
- Asthma
- Cardiogenic shock
- Chronic obstructive pulmonary disease
- Myocardial infarction
- Pneumonia
- Pulmonary embolism
- Pulmonary fibrosis

■ Treatment

The goals of treatment should be to treat the underlying precipitant of the patient's heart failure, reduce symptoms and progression of failure, and ultimately improve quality of life. The plan of care will depend on the stage and severity of failure, but treatment of comorbid disorders (e.g., coronary artery disease, hypertension and diabetes) is also necessary.

Lifestyle modification to enhance healthy heart living is an important part of managing heart failure. Smoking cessation, weight loss when indicated, and avoidance of alcohol or illegal drugs will benefit all patients (Jessup et al., 2009). Maintaining proper fluid and sodium intake and eating a balanced diet are also helpful.

Pharmacologic therapy
- Stage A (at risk for heart failure):
  - Treat hypertension:
    - Angiotensin converting enzyme inhibitors (ACEI): indicated for patients who have history of vascular disease, diabetes or hypertension
    - Angiotensin II receptor blockers (ARB): Indicated for patients who cannot take ACEI and/or patients with a history of vascular disease, diabetes or hypertension
  - Treat hyperlipidemia.
  - Control associated endocrine/metabolic disorders (e.g., diabetes, thyroid).
- Stage B (cardiac structural abnormalities or remodeling without failure symptoms):
  - Treatment goals are the same as Stage A, but consider addition of one of the following beta blockers (i.e., bisoprolol, carvedilol, or sustained release metoprolol succinate) particularly in patients with a history of MI or those with reduced EF (Jessup *et al.*, 2009).
  - Digitalis is usually not indicated for patients with a low EF, normal sinus rhythm and no symptoms of heart failure.
- Stage C (patients with current or prior symptoms):
  - Treatment goals include Stage A and B goals.
  - Diuretics: with evidence of fluid retention
  - Aldosterone antagonist may be considered in select patients with moderate to severe symptoms of failure and reduced EF. Frequent and careful monitoring of renal function and electrolyte levels is imperative.
  - Digitalis may be used for symptomatic patients with decreased EF.
  - Hydralazine and nitrate may be used if patient does not tolerate ACEI or ARB or has persistent symptoms even with these therapies.
- Stage D (end-stage heart failure):
  - Intravenous inotropic agents delivered continuously may be considered if awaiting transplant or palliation with goal for patient to die comfortably at home.

■ Treatments
- Revascularization may be considered for patients with underlying heart disease, but without heart failure symptoms.
- Valve repair or replacement may be considered in asymptomatic patients who have underlying valve disease.
- Cardiac resynchronization alone or in combination with defibrillator may be considered in right bundle branch block, atrial fibrillation or other conduction issues.
- Placement of implantable cardioverter-defibrillator may reduce incidence of sudden death but could exacerbate failure symptoms and therefore the decision to implant device must be made with the individual patient in mind.

- Left ventricular assist device may be a bridge to transplant or as a "destination therapy" for end-stage heart failure patients.
- Cardiac transplantation.

■ Collaborative consultation

- Consider consultation of Cardiologist and Heart Failure Specialist/Team.
- Nutritionist
- Physical therapy
- Smoking cessation counselor
- Consider introducing palliative care in early stages of disease.

■ Complications

- Cardiac arrhythmias
- Pulmonary congestion
- Stroke
- Heart attack
- Valvular disease
- Kidney/liver failure
- Death

■ Prevention

All patients need reminders about a heart healthy lifestyle. Important considerations when discussing prevention of coronary artery disease and associated cardiac illnesses include:

- Patient and family awareness of cardiac risk factors, including family history.
- The importance of adhering to recommended treatment and medication regimes.
- Healthy heart living:
  - Diet: fluid intake and sodium restriction
    - Alcohol in moderation
    - Avoidance of street drugs
    - Control of hypertension, hyperlipidemia and hyperglycemia
  - Daily exercise: ideally 30 minutes a day or more
- Smoking cessation
- Immunizations

■ Patient/family education

- Discuss with patient/family the importance of a healthy diet and exercise.
- Encourage patients to take blood pressure and lipid-lowering agents as prescribed.
  - Patients should understand uses and side effects of medications.

- Encourage patient to follow closely with health care providers and be aware of when to call provider if symptoms occur or worsen. Keep all appointments.
- Discuss with patient the importance of smoking cessation and additional lifestyle modifications to enhance healthy heart living.
- Provide long-term emotional support and discuss feelings of fear, anxiety and depression.
- Introduce palliative care in early stages of illness and encourage conversation about advanced care planning.

References

Jessup, M., Abraham, W.T., Casey, D.E., *et al.* (2009) Focused Update: ACCF/AHA Guidelines for the Diagnosis and Management of Heart Failure in Adults. A Report of the American College of Cardiology Foundation/American Heart Association Task Force on Practice Guidelines. *Circulation* **119**, 1977-2016.

Jurgens, C.Y., Shurpin, K.M. & Gumersell, K.A. (2010) Challenges and strategies for heart failure symptom management in older adults. *Journal of Gerontological Nursing* **36**(11), 24-33.

Lloyd-Jones, D., Adams, R.J., Brown, T.M., *et al.* (2010) Heart disease and stroke statistics 2010 Update: Report from the AHA. *Circulation* **121**, e46-e215.

Rich, M. (2006). Heart failure in older adults. *The Medical Clinic of North America* **90**, 863-885.

Riegel, B., Moser, D.K., Anker, A.D., *et al.* (2009). State of the science: promoting self-care in persons with heart failure: a scientific statement from the AHA. *Circulation* **120**, 1141-1163.

PART 5: HYPERTENSION

Chelby Cierpial and Susan Stengrevics

Hypertension or high blood pressure is defined as two or more consecutive office readings of 140/90 (JNC-7). Hypertension has been shown to increase with age and its prevalence in individuals age 65 and over is 67% (NCHS Data Brief, Ostchega, *et al.*, 2008). There is a lifetime risk of more than 90% of developing hypertension in people aged 55-60 who do not have hypertension. Patients with hypertensive disease may have combined systolic and diastolic hypertension or isolated systolic hypertension. Isolated systolic hypertension occurs most commonly in elders and is characterized by a systolic blood pressure (SBP) above 160 mmHg and diastolic blood pressure (DBP) below 90 mmHg . These rising systolic and pulse pressures may be predictors of outcome in this age group.

It is estimated that more than 1 billion individuals worldwide are hypertensive. More than 7 million deaths per year are attributed to hypertension related cerebrovascular disease and ischemic heart disease (WHO, 2002). The Systolic Hypertension in the Elderly Program (SHEP) and other trials showed there are benefits in treating hypertension in elders even beyond age 80 (SHEP, 1991).

The risk of cardiovascular (CV) disease events is directly related to blood pressure. The higher the BP, the greater the risk of end organ damage (kidneys, heart, brain blood vessels) and/or of an event (e.g., myocardial infarction, heart failure, renal disease or stroke). When other risk factors such as elevated cholesterol level, low high density lipoproteins, smoking, diabetes and left ventricular hypertrophy are added, the CV risks become greater still.

■ Risk factors

Primary, essential or idiopathic hypertension may have no known specific cause but in fact affects most individuals with hypertension (90–95%). Genetic and environmental causes are thought to be responsible for the development of hypertension. Factors associated with the development of hypertension include:

- Excess body weight
- Excess dietary sodium intake
- Excess alcohol intake
- Inadequate intake of fruits, vegetables, and potassium
- Reduced physical activity

Secondary hypertension is due to altered hemodynamics related to a primary disorder. These predisposing problems may include:

- Acute stress
- Drugs and other substances
- Endocrine disorders
- Neurologic disorders
- Renal disorders
- Vascular disorders

■ Clinical presentation

- Often there is an absence of symptoms and hypertension goes undiagnosed until the patient presents for evaluation of another problem.
- Symptoms may not present until after years of living with hypertension.
- Most common symptom: waking with a headache (with severe hypertension).
- Other symptoms depend on target organ damage:
  - Ophthalmologic: blurred vision
  - Central nervous system: dizziness, memory loss, unsteady gait, fatigue, slow tremors,
  - CV: chest pain, signs of heart failure (dyspnea, peripheral edema), impotence, nosebleeds
  - Gastrointestinal: nausea, vomiting
  - Genitourinary: nocturia, hematuria

Table 3.2.5.1 Taking an accurate blood pressure measurement.

Do	How?	Why?
Choose appropriate cuff size:	Length of the bladder encircles 80% of the patients upper arm	**False high:** Cuff is too small/ large/loose
	Width covers 33–50% of the upper arm	Patient was physically active, had taken caffeine or is emotionally upset just prior to BP
Ensure appropriate timing of BP	The patient has been at rest for at least five minutes prior to the BP	Cuff deflation is too slow
Place patient in correct position	Have the patient sit supine with both feet on the floor and back and arm supported	**False low:** Inappropriate position of patient
	Extend arm so it is at the level of the heart	
	Use bare arm or a loosely rolled sleeve without constriction	

Don't use an arm: on the same side as a mastectomy or with an AV fistula for hemodialysis

- Orthostatic hypotension: a decrease in standing SBP ≥20 mmHg or DBP ≥10 mmHg within 3 minutes of standing, when associated with dizziness or fainting

■ Nursing assessment

- Obtain a detailed history of symptoms.
- Record all current and prior antihypertensive medications, as well as other prescribed and over-the-counter medications. Document allergies.
- Assess adherence, tolerance and any allergic reactions.
- Accurate blood pressure measurement is essential to ensure appropriate treatment (see Table 3.2.5.1).
- Blood pressure should be measured in both arms and the one with the higher reading should be used thereafter.
- In older adults, blood pressure should be taken both standing and sitting.
- Accurate BPs are more difficult in older adults due to more blood pressure variability, vasculature structural changes leading to noncompressibility of the brachial artery (false high), higher prevalence of "white coat" phenomenon, exaggerated BP response to environmental factors (activity, caffeine, tobacco, stress).
- Older patients are at an increased risk for the adverse effects of antihypertensives, especially orthostatic hypotension. They may need lower doses. Avoid volume depletion and rapid dose titration.

Table 3.2.5.2 Changes in blood pressure classification.

JNC-6 Category	SBP/DBP	JNC-7 Category
Optimal	<120/80	Normal
Normal	120–129/80–84	Prehypertensive
Borderline	130–139/85–89	
Hypertension	>140/90	Hypertensive
Stage 1	140–159/90-99	Stage 1
Stage 2	>160/100	Stage 2
Stage 3	>180/110	

Source: Chobanian *et al.*, 2003.

■ Diagnostics

- Complete history and physical exam
- Calculation of body mass index (BMI)
- Auscultated BP
- Exam of optic fundi
- Palpation of the thyroid
- Exam of heart and lungs including 12 lead ECG
- Exam of the abdomen for enlarged kidneys, masses, distended urinary bladder, abdominal aortic pulsation, bruits
- Auscultation for carotid, abdominal and femoral bruits
- Lower extremity assessment for edema and pulses
- Neurological exam
- Laboratory and other diagnostic procedures including: urinalysis, blood glucose, hematocrit, serum potassium, creatinine, glomerular filtration rate, calcium, lipid profile
- More extensive testing for identifiable causes if BP control is not achieved or if clinical or laboratory testing indicates a secondary cause:
  - White coat effect
  - Secondary causes: chronic kidney disease, coarctation of the aorta, Cushing's syndrome and other glucocorticoid excess states including chronic steroid use, drugs related effects, obstructive uropathy, pheochromocytoma, primary aldosteronism, renovascular hypertension, sleep apnea, thyroid or parathyroid disease

■ Differential diagnosis

The Seventh Report of the Joint National Committee on Prevention, Detection, Evaluation, and Treatment of High Blood Pressure (Chobanian *et al.*, 2003) includes the following blood pressure chart (see Table 3.2.5.2).

■ Treatment

- There is no cure for essential hypertension but it can be controlled with by pharmacologic and non-pharmacologic interventions.

Table 3.2.5.3 Life style changes.

Modification	Recommendation
Weight reduction	Maintain normal body weight (BMI 18.5–24.9)
Adopt DASH eating plan	Consume a diet rich in fruits, vegetables and low fat dairy products with a reduced content of saturated and total fat.
Dietary sodium reduction	Reduce dietary sodium intake to no more than 100 mmol per day (2.4 g sodium or 6 g sodium chloride).
Physical activity	Engage in regular aerobic physical activity such as brisk walking (at least 30 min per day, most days of the week).
Moderate consumption of alcohol	Limit consumption to no more than consumption 2 drinks (1 oz or 30 ml ethanol; e.g., 24 oz beer, 10 oz wine, or 3 oz 80-proof whiskey) per day in most men and to no more than 1 drink per day in women and lighter weight persons.

Adapted from Chobanian *et al.*, 2003.

- Treatment of secondary hypertension includes correcting the underlying cause and controlling hypertensive effects.
- Choice of initiation and progression of treatment depends on hypertension severity.
- Lifestyle change (exercise, weight reduction, limit sodium, stress reduction, quitting smoking) is one of the first interventions.
- Initial drug therapy should be thiazide-type diuretics followed by combination therapy with the addition of another drug class: angiotensin converting enzyme inhibitors (ACE inhibitors), angiotensin II receptor blockers (ARB), beta blockers, calcium channel blockers. Therapy is individualized and depending on patient co-morbidities may be different.

▪ Collaborative consultation

- Nutritionist to support adoption of dietary changes
- Nurse case manager or social worker to assist with obtaining medication
- Physicians to simplify med regimen to promote adherence

▪ Complications

- Hypertensive emergency and urgency (see Table 3.2.5.3)
- Target organ damage:
  - Eyes
    - Retinopathy
  - Heart
    - Left ventricular hypertrophy
    - Angina/myocardial infarction
    - Heart failure

- Brain
  - Stroke or transient ischemic attack
- Chronic kidney disease
- Peripheral artery disease

Hypertensive emergency and hypertensive urgency

(The following situations affect about 1% of hypertensive patients.)

- *Hypertensive emergency*. Severe hypertension (SBP ≥180 mmHg and/or DBP ≥120 mmHg) that can lead to acute, life-threatening complications such as encephalopathy, retinal hemorrhages, papilledema and acute renal failure.
- *Hypertensive urgency*. Equivalent degree of hypertension as in an emergency but patients are relatively asymptomatic (other than possible headache) and also are without end organ damage.

■ Treatment

Hypertensive emergency

BP reduction with vasodilators (e.g., sodium nitroprusside, nitroglycerine, hydralazine hydrochloride, fenoldopam mesylate, nicardipine hydrochloride, or enalaprilat).

Goal initially is to reduce mean arterial BP by 25% (within 1 hour) and to 160/100-110 within the next 2-6 hours. If well tolerated, further gradual reduction toward normal can occur within the next 24-48 hours (Chobanian *et al.*, 2003).

Hypertensive urgency

BP reduction using oral, short-acting medications (e.g., captopril, labetalol or clonidine). It is recommended that medication administration be followed by several hours of observation.

A follow-up visit within several days of discharge from the ER is *essential*.

Aggressive use of intravenous agents or oral agents is not recommended to rapidly lower severe uncomplicated hypertension.

■ Prevention

- Lifestyle changes (see Table 3.2.5.3)

■ Patient/family education

- Hypertension:
  - Describe the effects of uncontrolled hypertension.
  - Explain that treatment is lifelong.
  - Teach how to self monitor BP and importance of follow up.
- Medications:
  - Support establishment of a medication plan to support adherence.
  - Discuss importance of not stopping medications abruptly.
  - Teach patients and families about each of their medications, what they are for, how they work and potential side effects.
  - Explain the importance of continuing medication despite the absence of symptoms.
- List specific symptoms patients should report to their provider:
  - Side effects of medications
  - Signs and symptoms of stroke or heart attack
  - Signs and symptoms of orthostatic hypotension
- To prevent accidents such as falls, warn the patient not to sit up or get out of bed too rapidly. Instruct the patient to call for assistance in walking if they feel dizzy or faint.

References

Chobanian AV, Bakris GL, Black HR, *et al*. (2003) The Seventh Report of the Joint National Committee on Prevention, Detection, Evaluation, and Treatment of High Blood Pressure. The JNC-7 Report. *JAMA* **289**, 2560-2572.

National Center for Health Statistics (NCHS) Data Brief, Ostchega *et al*., (2008) Hypertension Awareness, Treatment, and Control—Continued Disparities in Adults: United States, 2005-2006. Online. Available from http://www.cdc.gov/nchs/data/databriefs/db03.pdf (accessed 9 May 2012).

SHEP Cooperative Research Group (1991) Prevention of stroke by antihypertensive drug treatment in older persons with isolated systolic hypertension. Final results of the Systolic Hypertension in the Elderly Program (SHEP). *JAMA* **265**(24), 3255-3264.

Wold Health Organization (2002) World Health Report 2002: Reducing risks, promoting healthy life. WHO, Geneva. Online Available from http://www.who.int/whr/2002/ (accessed 13 March 2012).

Further reading

Aronow, W.S. (2008) Treatment of hypertension in older adults. *Geriatrics and Aging* **11**(8), 457-463.

Hajjar, I. (2007) Hypertension. In: Duthie, E.H. Jr., Katz, P.R. & Malone, M. (eds) *Practice of Geriatrics*, 4th edition. WB Saunders, Philadelphia, pp. 429-436.

Hajjar, I. & Kotchen, T.A. (2003) Trends in prevalence, awareness, treatment, and control of hypertension in the United States, 1998–2000. *JAMA* **290**, 199–206.

Marik, P.E. & Varon, J. (2007) Hypertensive crises, challenges and management. *Chest* **131**, 1949–1962.

Smith-Temple, J. & Johnson, J. (eds) (2006) Nurses' Guide to Clinical Procedures. Lippincott, Williams & Wilkins, Philadelphia.

Stockslager, J.L. & Shaeffer, L. (eds) (2003) Hypertension. In: *Handbook of Geriatric Nursing Care*, 2nd edition. Lippincott, Williams & Wilkins, Philadelphia, pp. 334–337.

Tomlinson, B.U. (2010) Accurately measuring blood pressure: factors that contribute to false measurement. *MEDSURG Nursing* **19**(2), 90–94.

PART 6: PERIPHERAL VASCULAR DISEASE

Ashley Moore Gibbs

Peripheral vascular disease (PVD) refers to the gradual narrowing and occlusive process within the vascular system that results from progressive atherosclerosis. Nine to 12 million Americans have a diagnosis of PVD; 19% are 70 years or older (Almahameed, 2006). As populations around the world continue to age, the prevalence of this disease will increase significantly, though in the US the prevalence of PVD among ethnic groups is varied. Non-Hispanic blacks are disproportionately affected with a two- to three-fold increase in risk compared with Caucasians. Conversely, Hispanics and Asians have a similar or slightly lower risk than Caucasians (Aslam *et al.*, 2009).

Although PVD is common, it is often underdiagnosed and undertreated as only 25% of diagnosed patients are receiving treatment (Aslam *et al.*, 2009). The disease often goes undiagnosed in older adults as many experience no leg pain (Almahameed, 2006). Others do not report symptoms because they attribute the need to slow or decrease their activity with advancing age.

Prevalence of PVD increases twofold per decade of life. Both diabetes and smoking each independently increase the risk by three to fourfold. All patients with PVD should be treated with the same secondary prevention goals as those with coronary artery disease. Risk factor modification is essential in this patient population, with the two most important interventions being smoking cessation and a walking program (Gornik & Creager, 2006).

PVD is a major cause of lifestyle limitations, disability, and loss of work and income. Mortality rates are almost three times higher than in those with no vascular disease. While many patients are concerned with the possibility of a limb-related event, the greatest threat to the health of patients with PVD is myocardial infarction or stroke. The risk of a major cardiovascular event is increased in patients with PVD regardless if they experience symptoms and is highest among those with severe disease (Gornik & Creager, 2006).

■ Risk factors

- Advanced age*
- Cigarette smoking*
- Chronic kidney disease
- Diabetes mellitus*
- Dyslipidemia
- Family history of coronary artery disease*
- Hypertension*
- Inflammatory marker elevation (C-reactive protein, fibrinogen, leukocytes)

*Risk factors similar to those for coronary artery and cerebrovascular disease

■ Clinical presentation

Many patients have few or no symptoms and do not seek medical attention until the disease is advanced. Intermittent claudication (IC) is the most common symptom of PVD. It is defined as exercise-induced lower extremity pain caused by ischemia that is relieved with rest. Approximately 10% of patients report a classic pattern of IC while 50% will describe a variety of other leg complaints such as fatigue, numbness, tightness, or heaviness.

IC typically occurs distal to an arterial obstruction. The typical site of obstruction varies with age. In those over 40 years, 65% of obstructions are within the femoral or popliteal arteries (Mukherjee & Yadav, 2001). This typically causes symptoms in the distal thigh and/or lower leg. The pain often occurs at night when the legs are elevated in bed and improves by dangling the affected leg over the bed. This maneuver will occasionally cause edema and rubor of the dependent extremity.

With disease progression, obstructions worsen and critical limb ischemia may occur. Acute limb ischemia includes some or all of the following clinical features:

- Pain at rest
- Pallor
- Paresthesia
- Paralysis
- Pulselessness
- Poikilothermia (inability to regulate temperature)
- Ischemic ulcers
- Gangrene

Paresthesias and paralysis generally indicate irreversible ischemic injury (Almahameed, 2006). IC should be distinguished from pseudoclaudication which is caused by stenosis in the lumbar spinal canal and differs from IC in its onset, character, and relief of pain.

■ Nursing assessment

The physical examination findings may be as subtle as the clinical history. Assessment considerations include:

- Vital signs:
  - Blood pressure: check in upper extremities bilaterally.
  - Pulses: check for quality (diminished or absent). Auscultate for bruits (carotid, abdominal, renal, and femoral). An abnormal femoral pulse has a high specificity and positive predictive value, but low sensitivity for large vessel disease.
- Skin: assess for unilateral cool extremity, prolonged venous filling time, skin atrophy, or shiny color of skin. Assess for hair loss and thickened and brittle toenails.
- Capillary refill (prolonged in significant vascular disease)
- Neurologic exam: evaluate visual disturbance, speech disturbance, dizziness, syncope, ataxia, numbness or paralysis indicating possible occlusion of a carotid artery.
- Cardiovascular:
  - Check carotid upstroke comparing the pulse timing with the cardiac point of maximum impulse.
- Abdomen: auscultate for an abdominal bruit. Check for renal bruits in older patients with history of hypertension.
- Genitals: assess for discomfort, pain or impotence.
- Musculoskeletal: skeletal muscle groups may show atrophy in patients with chronic PVD.

■ Diagnostics

- Ankle-brachial index (ABI):
  - Simple, noninvasive test having 95% sensitivity and 99% specificity for detecting PVD.
  - ABI readings are obtained by dividing the systolic BP from the brachial artery into either the posterior tibial or dorsalis pedis arteries.
  - Normal ABI is >0.90–1.30; <0.90 indicates disease. Lower readings indicate severe disease. Readings >1.30 are not reliable and usually indicate noncompressible vessels due to diabetes, advanced age, and/or chronic renal insufficiency.
- Duplex ultrasonography
- Exercise treadmill testing
- Computed tomographic scan
- Computed tomographic angiography

- Magnetic resonance angiography (MRA)
- Contrast angiography

■ Differential diagnosis

- Chronic venous insufficiency
- Degenerative disk disease
- Diabetic neuropathy
- Osteoarthritis
- Spinal stenosis
- Venous thrombosis

■ Treatment

- Goals of treatment:
  - Reduce/eliminate ischemic symptoms.
  - Prevent progression of disease.
  - Prevent cardiovascular complications.
- Monitor VS and pulses regularly.
- Monitor for bleeding if patient receiving anticoagulation therapy.
- Pain management.
- Notify physician if patient develops acute limb pain or pulselessness in the involved limb.

■ Collaborative consultation

- When treating a patient with known atherosclerosis (symptomatic and asymptomatic) discuss the need for receiving antiplatelet therapy if none are prescribed.
- Screen patients at high-risk for PVD including those with known atherosclerotic disease, diabetes mellitus, age >70, and age >50 with one or more cardiovascular risk factors.

■ Complications

- Thrombosis
- Embolism
- Ulcers
- Gangrene
- Amputation

■ Prevention

- Dietary strategies (low fat, low cholesterol diet)
- Smoking cessation

- Antiplatelet therapy: all patients with evidence of atherosclerosis (symptomatic and asymptomatic) in any circulatory beds should be prescribed antiplatelet therapy:
  - Aspirin is the antiplatelet therapy of choice, but clopidogrel may be used if aspirin is not tolerated.
- Lipid control (diet, exercise, and medications as needed)
- Blood glucose control (diet, exercise, and medications as needed)
- Blood pressure control (diet, exercise, and medications as needed)
- Weight reduction (diet and exercise)
- Increase activity and engage in supervised walking program.
- Screen high-risk patients including those with known atherosclerotic disease, diabetes mellitus, patients age >70, and age >50 with one or more cardiovascular risk factors.

■ Patient/family education

- Smoking cessation: Smoking is the most important modifiable risk factor:
  - Smoking cessation reduces the severity of limb symptoms and the progression of disease and increase the survival rate.
- Exercise program:
  - Patients should walk at least three to five times a week for 30 to 45 minutes.
  - Instruct them to walk until the pain begins, rest, and then keep walking.
- Monitor blood pressure.
- Weight loss
- Take medications as prescribed:
  - Instruct patient to contact their healthcare provider if unable to tolerate prescribed medications prior to discontinuing:
    - Antiplatelet therapy is recommended for all patients (symptomatic and asymptomatic) with PVD and reduces the risk of limb loss and the need for surgical revascularization in patients with intermittent claudication.
    - Antiplatelet therapy reduces the risk of myocardial infarction, stroke, or death.

References

Almaameed, A. (2006) Peripheral arterial disease: Recognition and medical management. *Cleveland Clinic Journal of Medicine* **73**(7), 621-638.

Aslam, F., Haque, A., Foody, J. & Lee, L.V. (2009) Peripheral arterial disease: current perspectives and new trends in management. *Southern Medical Journal* **102** (11), 1141-1149.

Gornik, H.L. & Creager, M.A. (2006) Contemporary management of peripheral arterial disease: I. Cardiovascular risk-factor modification. *Cleveland Clinic Journal of Medicine* **73**(4), S30-S36.

Mukherjee, D. & Yadav, J.A. (2001) Update on peripheral vascular diseases: From smoking cessation to stenting. *Cleveland Clinic Journal of Medicine* **68**(8), 723-733.

PART 7: HEART VALVE DISEASE

Theresa E. Evans

With the aging population it has been speculated that the United States will continue to see an increasing number of cases of heart valve disease. Historically, congenital anomalies or rheumatic fever were considered the primary causes but advancing age coupled with longer life expectancy is now increasing the number of patients with valvular heart disease. In a study published in *The Lancet* in 2006, researchers from the Mayo Clinic found that the prevalence increased with age, from 0.7% in 18-44-year-olds to 13.3% in the 75 years and older group. The researchers went on to find a disparity between the prevalence of such diseases in the population and the percentage of people diagnosed with valvular heart diseases in the community, citing undiagnosed valve diseases. It was also noted that women were less likely than men to be diagnosed with this disorder (Nkomo *et al.*, 2006).

Each chamber of the heart is separated by one of the four heart valves. The *aortic valve* is located between the left ventricle and the aorta and the *pulmonary valve* is located between the right ventricle and pulmonary artery. The *triscupid valve* separates the right atria from the right ventricle while the *mitral valve* does the same on the left side of the heart.

As the atria begin to fill, the pressure forces the tricuspid and mitral valves open, allowing blood to flow down into the ventricles. Once complete the valves close, inhibiting backflow into the atria. The ventricles contract forcing open the pulmonary and aortic valves to allow forward blood flow out of the heart. Valvular heart disease is a disease in which one or more of the heart valves do not work correctly.

The backward flow of blood, termed regurgitation, occurs when the valve does not close tightly. A prolapsed valve is often the likely reason for regurgitation, particularly with the mitral valve. This means that the valve flaps "flop" or "bulge" backwards (NHLBI, 2011). Aortic regurgitation can also occur where blood backflows into the left ventricle. It can be either a chronic condition, with minimal symptoms, or acute, which requires immediate attention (Otto & Bonow, 2008).

Valves may become thick and stiffen, especially with advancing age. Called stenosis, the thickening causes narrowing of valve passage and complicates the valves' ability to open completely, impeding blood flow. Stenosis can affect any valve but most often affects the aortic valve (NHLBI, 2011).

Congenital valve disease occurs as the fetal heart is developing. Valve anomalies may result from any number of genetic or chromosomal disorders or occur without a known cause. Two common congenital abnormalities include a bicuspid aortic valve, which affects about 2% of population and pulmonary valve stenosis, with symptoms ranging from mild to severe (NHLBI, 2011).

In older adults, the most common valvular disorders are aortic stenosis and mitral regurgitation (Kupper & Mitchell, 2011). The causes are varied, but cardiovascular disease is the primary reason.

Table 3.2.7.1 Heart murmurs.

	Location	Radiation	Intensity	Pitch	Quality
Midstystolic murmurs					
Pulmonic stenosis	2nd and 3rd left intercostal space (ICS)	Left shoulder and neck if loud	Soft to loud; if loud may have thrill	Medium	Frequently harsh
Aortic stenosis	Right 2nd ICS	Neck and left sternal border; can extend to apex.	Soft to loud with thrill	Medium; may be higher at apex	Often harsh; may be more musical at apex.
Pansystolic murmurs					
Mitral regurgitation	Apex	Left axilla; sometimes to the left sternal border	Soft to loud; if loud may have apical thrill	Medium to high	Blowing
Tricuspid regurgitation	Lower left sternal border	Right of sternum, xiphoid area, left midclavicular line but not into axilla	Variable	Medium	Blowing
Diastolic murmurs					
Aortic regurgitation	2nd to 4th left ICS	If loud, to apex or right sternal border	Grade 1 to 3	High (use diaphragm of stethoscope)	Blowing; may sound like breath sounds.
Mitral stenosis	Usually limited to apex.	Little or none	Grade 1 to 4	Low (use bell of stethoscope)	

Created from information in Mehta, M. (2003). Cardiac assessment: A sensory experience. *Nursing Made Incredibly Easy* **1**(1), 6–9.

■ Risk factors

- Acquired immune deficiency syndromes (e.g., rheumatoid arthritis, systemic lupus erythematosus)
- Age
- Congenital abnormalities
- Coronary artery disease
- Diabetes
- Heart failure
- Hyperlipidemia
- Hypertension
- Infections: rubella, group A beta hemolytic streptococci, syphilis
- Infective endocarditis
- Marfan's syndrome
- Medications (e.g., fenfluramine and phentermine, cabergoline, pergolide, thalidomide, lithium, phenytoin (Dilantin))
- Myocardial infarction
- Obesity
- Radiation therapy
- Rheumatic fever (streptococcal infection)
- Smoking

■ Clinical presentation

Valvular disease is often asymptomatic and may only be appreciated on physical exam when ascultating for a murmur, an unusual heart sound. Not all heart murmurs indicate valvular disease so further evaluation is warranted prior to diagnosing a valve disease (see Table 3.2.7.1). Often valve disease worsens over time, with the clinical presentation changing as the patient ages. These symptoms most commonly relate to heart failure and include:

- Angina/chest pain
- Dizziness or syncope
- Fatigue
- Jugular vein distention
- Lower extremity swelling
- Palpitations
- Shortness of breath or dyspnea on exertion

■ Nursing assessment

A thorough medical history, review of systems and family history are essential, especially given the subtle nature of symptoms (ACC/AHA, 2006).

- Physical exam
- Vital signs:
  - Assess for recent unintentional weight gain: can indicate volume overload with failure.

- Blood pressure: may be elevated as part of patient's history
- Respiratory rate: rapid breathing to meet oxygen demands; seen most often with underlying congestion due to heart failure
- Oxygen saturation levels: when coupled with heart failure/pulmonary congestion, decreased oxygen saturation levels are common.
- Cardiac:
  - Auscultation of heart sounds is imperative to assessment.
    - Assess for murmurs that may be related to underlying valve disease.
  - Murmur description includes:
    - *Timing*
      - Systolic (between S1 and S2)
      - Diastolic (between S2 and S3)
    - *Location*
      - Where murmur is loudest
        - Aortic area, 2nd right intercostal space
        - Pulmonic area, 2nd left intercostal space
        - Erb's point, 3rd left intercostal space
        - Tricuspid area, 4th left intercostal space
        - Mitral area, 5th left intercostal space
    - *Radiation*
      - Transmission to surrounding areas from area of maximum intensity
    - *Quality*
      - Musical
      - Blowing
      - Harsh
      - Rumbling
    - *Pitch*
      - High
      - Medium
      - Low
    - *Shape* (described by intensity over time)
      - Crescendo - murmur grows louder
      - Decrescendo - murmur grows softer
      - Crescendo-decrescendo - murmur rises in intensity then falls
      - Plateau - murmur has same intensity throughout
    - *Loudness* (intensity of murmur)
      - Grade 1 - barely audible
      - Grade 2 - clearly audible but faint
      - Grade 3 - moderately loud; easy to hear
      - Grade 4 - loud with a palpable thrill
      - Grade 5 - very loud; heard with one side of stethoscope lifted off chest wall
      - Grade 6 - can be heard with entire stethoscope lifted off chest wall; loudest murmur
- Respiratory:
  - Adventitious lung sounds may indicate subsequent heart failure (rales).

- Peripheral vascular:
  - Lower extremity edema, cyanosis, clubbing may indicate failure.
  - Assess for jugular vein distention.

■ Diagnostics

- Electrocardiogram: assess for arrhythmias, ischemia, ventricular hypertrophy.
- Echocardiogram (ECHO):
  - Transthoracic: noninvasive:
    - provides images of size, shape of heart
    - shows how the valves and chambers are working
  - Transesophageal: invasive (through esophagus):
    - visualizes heart valves better
    - may also detect clots
- Chest X-ray: may detect heart chamber enlargement, which valve is diseased and assists to determine lung involvement with heart failure.
- Cardiac MRI: provides more detailed and accurate information.
- Stress test: may help determine likelihood of symptoms when heart is working.
- Cardiac catheterization: may be used especially when results of previous testing are inconsistent and/or related to other heart disease.
- Laboratory:
  - Baseline complete blood count/differential, serum electrolytes, blood urea nitrogen, and creatinine are usually obtained
  - Cardiac enzymes (especially if suspected event)
  - Brain natriuretic peptide (BNP) (if heart failure is suspected)
  - Blood cultures, if concern for active endocarditis (ACC/AHA, 2008)

■ Differential diagnosis

Other heart disease processes that manifest as heart failure should be considered. These include but are not limited to cardiac arrhythmias, coronary artery disease, and myocardial infarction.

A preliminary diagnosis of a specific heart valve disorder may be identified through the presence and description of a murmur (see Table 3.7.2.1).

■ Treatment

Lifestyle modification to enhance healthy heart living is ultimate goal of preventing complications of heart valve disease. At present, medication management focuses on treatment of concurrent heart disease with antihypertensives and lipid lowering agents. Diuretics are used when heart failure symptoms increase.

Surgical repair or replacement using both synthetic and biological valves may be necessary when symptoms become severe and/or are life-threatening.

- Heart valve repair:
  - Lowers risk of infective endocarditis
  - Ideally preserves function of cardiac muscle
  - Commonly done on mitral valve but less frequently done on aortic or pulmonary valves
- Valvuloplasty:
  - May be used with stenosed valves
  - May relieve symptoms for period of time
  - Used often with mitral stenosis
  - Often used on infants and children whose defect is congenital
- Heart valve replacement:
  - Mechanical valves often placed in younger population as these devices do not require replacement:
    - Require lifelong anticoagulation
    - Higher risk of infective endocarditis
  - Biological valves (human, pig or cow) may need to be replaced at 10-15 years:
    - Do not require immunotherapy or lifelong anticoagulation
  - New techniques are being explored but little research remains available. One such technique is the Ross operation:
    - During the Ross operation a diseased aortic valve is replaced with the patient's native pulmonary valve while a homograft valve replaces the pulmonary valve.
      - Much more complex and greater risk of complications
      - Validity continues to be debated.
      - May be most useful in children

■ Collaborative consultation

Consultation with cardiologist and cardiac surgeon is usually indicated.

■ Complications

- Heart failure
- Cardiac arrhythmias
- Stroke
- Blood clots
- Sudden cardiac arrest
- Endocarditis

■ Prevention

- See your doctor if you develop fever, sore throat and/or are exposed to streptococcal infection.
- Complete all courses of antibiotics for known infections.

- Healthy heart living:
  - Diet
  - Exercise
  - Cholesterol control
  - Blood pressure control
- Maintain good dental hygiene.
- Smoking cessation

■ Patient/family education

- Discuss with patient/family the importance of a healthy diet and exercise.
- Encourage patients to take blood pressure, lipid-lowering agents, and when necessary, anticoagulants as prescribed.
- Encourage patient to follow closely with health care providers.
- Discuss with patient the importance of smoking cessation and additional lifestyle modifications to enhance healthy heart living.

References

ACC/AHA (2006) Guidelines for the Management of Patients With Valvular Heart Disease. A Report of the American College of Cardiology/American Heart Association Task Force on Practice Guidelines (Writing Committee to Revise the 1998 Guidelines for the Management of Patients With Valvular Heart Disease). *Circulation* **114**, e84-e231. Online. Available from http://circ.ahajournals.org/content/114/5/e84.full.pdf+html (accessed 13 March 2012).

ACC/AHA (2008) Guideline Update on Valvular Heart Disease: Focused Update on Infective Endocarditis. A Report of the American College of Cardiology/American Heart Association Task Force on Practice Guidelines. *Journal of the American College of Cardiology* **52**, 676-678. Online. Available from http://content.online-jacc.org/cgi/content/full/j.jacc.2008.05.008 (accessed 13 March 2012).

Kupper, N. & Mitchell, D.F. (2011) Inflammatory and structural heart disorders. In: Lewis, S.L., Dirksen, S.R., Heitkemper, M.M., Bucher, L. & Camera, I.M. (eds) Medical Surgical Nursing: Assessment and Management of Clinical Problems 8th edition. Mosby, St. Louis.

Mehta, M. (2003) Cardiac assessment: A sensory experience. *Nursing Made Incredibly Easy* **1**(1), 6-9.

National Institute of Health: National Heart, Lung and Blood Institute Fact Sheet: revised October 2009b. Online. Available from www.nhlbi.nih.gov (accessed 13 March 2012).

Nkomo VT, Gardin JM, Skelton TN, *et al.* (2006) Burden of valvular heart diseases: a population-based study. *Lancet* **368**, 1005-1011.

Otto, C.M. & Bonow, R.O. (2008) Aortic regurgitation section of valvular heart disease. In: Libby, P. *et al.* (eds) *Braunwald's Heart Disease: A Textbook of Cardiovascular Medicine*, 8th edition, Saunders Elsevier, Philadelphia, pp. 1635-1646.

Unit 3: Respiratory Disorders

PART 1: ASTHMA

Marian Jeffries and Rosemarie Marks

Asthma is a chronic, intermittent, obstructive airway disorder that is characterized by airway inflammation and hyper-responsiveness. Individuals tend to have brief attacks followed by periods between episodes when they are symptom free. Interestingly, it has been shown that even symptom-free asthmatic individuals still have some degree of increased airway inflammation present (McCance & Huether, 2006; Huether & McCance, 2008). Unlike chronic obstructive pulmonary disease (COPD), asthma is considered to be a reversible airway disorder even though there are some asthmatic individuals who will have permanent structural changes with loss of lung function that cannot be reversed (National Asthma Education and Prevention Program, 2007). In 2008, it was estimated that 23.3 million Americans currently have asthma. Of these, 12.7 million Americans (4.1 million children under 18) had an asthma attack (CDC, 2008). It is one of the most common chronic diseases of childhood and there is considerable evidence that exposure to high levels of certain allergens during childhood increases the risk. In adults, episodes are more often triggered by inhalation of irritants and upper respiratory viral infections (Sommers *et al.*, 2007). Asthma attacks can present either acutely or slowly over several hours or days. Most acute events are triggered by allergen or irritant exposure, exercise, or stress. Slow onset episodes tend to follow an upper respiratory infection. Viral respiratory infections are a major precipitant for asthma exacerbations and may even contribute to the development of asthma (National Asthma Education and Prevention Program, 2007). Persons with asthma are at a high risk for influenza-related complications, such as pneumonia. The CDC advises that children and adults with asthma receive annual influenza vaccination (http://www.cdc.gov/asthma/healthcare.html). Adults over age 50 with any chronic lung disease should also receive pneumococcal immunization unless there is a compelling contraindication (CDC, 2012).

Airway hyper-responsiveness is the major feature of asthma (Huether & McCance, 2008). Exposure to allergens results in a cascade of inflammatory events beginning with the contraction and spasm of smooth muscle in the airway lumen. This decreases the airway lumen size leading to airflow obstruction. The body will produce antibodies such as immunoglobulin E (IgE). The next time that the allergen is encountered, the body will respond by releasing these IgE antibodies. These antibodies bind to tissue mast cells, lymphocytes and basophils in the airway mucosa. These cells will degranulate and release inflammatory mediators such as histamine, prostaglandins, and leukotrienes. Irritants will also stimulate mast cell degranulation. This inflammatory process results in swelling (edema) of the airway mucosa caused by increased capillary permeability and also stimulates the mucous glands to multiply, hypertrophy, and secrete thick mucus. Neutrophils and eosinophils will also respond and infiltrate the airways adding to the inflammatory response and airway obstruction.

Airway obstruction will cause a reduction of the forced expiratory volume in 1 second (FEV1) as well as a reduction in the FEV1 to FVC (forced vital capacity) ratio. This impaired exhalation will cause hyperinflation in the distal airways as measured by an increase in residual volume (RV) and functional residual capacity (FRC). The patient will have increased work of breathing and a sensation of breathlessness. Often the patient will assume a position of comfort that allows for maximum air flow.

Asthma is classified into four categories based on clinical severity: mild intermittent; mild persistent; moderate persistent; and severe persistent (Sommers *et al.*, 2007). Individuals who desire to learn more about asthma are encouraged to read the Expert Panel Report 3: *Guidelines for the diagnosis and management of asthma* that was published in 2007 by the US Department of Health and Human Services and the National Heart, Lung, and Blood Institute (National Asthma Education and Prevention Program, 2007, http://www.nhlbi.nih.gov/guidelines/asthma/asthgdln.htm).

■ Risk factors

- Allergen exposure-especially animal fur, dust mites, cockroaches, pollen, and mold
- Aspirin or sulfite allergy
- Cold weather
- Exercise
- Exposure to cigarette smoke
- Family history
- Inhalation of irritants such as air pollution and smoke from wood burning
- Personal history of other allergic reactions such as atopic dermatitis and eczema
- Respiratory infections – especially viral
- Urban dwelling/exposure to air pollution and cockroaches

■ Clinical presentation

- Anxiety
- Breathlessness
- Chest tightness
- Cough
- Decreased breath sounds
- Dyspnea
- Hypercapnia in severe asthma attacks – signaling impending respiratory failure
- Hypoxemia and cyanosis

- Increased respiratory effort with use of accessory muscles for breathing
- Wheezing – inspiratory and/or expiratory

■ Nursing assessment

- Obtain a detailed history, including prior allergic reactions and family history.
  - Assess recent exposure to allergens.
  - Assess recent history of respiratory infections – especially viral.
- Vital signs:
  - Determine presence of fever and/or tachycardia.
  - Respiratory inspection, palpation, percussion, and auscultation:
    - ○ Inspection for increased respiratory rate and work of breathing.
    - ○ Palpation may reveal fremitus.
    - ○ Percussion may reveal hyper-resonance.
    - ○ Auscultate for decreased breath sounds and inspiratory and expiratory wheezing.
  - Pulse oximetry at rest and with exertion.
- Obtain peak flow measurements – look for decreased FEV1.

■ Diagnostics

- Physical assessment with thorough history of potential exposures
- Oxygen saturation
- Chest X-ray, if indicated
- Arterial blood gases (if O_2 saturation <90%), if indicated
- Serum IgE
- Pulmonary function tests including peak expiratory flow measurement. Peak flow measurements can be used to guide and evaluate patient response to treatment.

■ Differential diagnosis

- Congestive heart failure
- Cough secondary to drugs – especially angiotensin-converting enzyme (ACE) inhibitors
- Exacerbation of chronic obstructive pulmonary disease (COPD)
- Mechanical obstruction of the airway (tumor, foreign objects)
- Pulmonary embolism
- Upper respiratory infection
- Vocal cord dysfunction

■ Treatment

- *Goals of management of asthma include*:
  - Assess and monitor episodic incidence.
  - Provide pulmonary hygiene measures.

- ⊙ Educate patient and family:
  - ○ Monitor daily peak flow assessments.
  - ○ Manage daily care and exacerbations.
  - ○ Reduce risk factors and improve health.
  - ○ Prevent respiratory infections.
- Supplemental oxygen as indicated.
- Rhinitis/sinusitis treatment with antihistamine, if indicated
- Inhaled bronchodilators - metered dose inhaler (MDI) or nebulizers:
  - ⊙ Short-acting beta$_2$-adrenergic agonists, such as albuterol
  - ⊙ Long acting beta-agonists, if indicated
- Inhaled anticholinergics-MDI or nebulizer:
  - ⊙ Ipratropium bromide
- Inhaled and/or systemic corticosteroids
- Leukotriene antagonists
  - ⊙ Mast cell stabilizers (cromolyn sodium and nedocromil)
- Methylxanthines:
  - ⊙ Theophylline: intravenous or oral
- Immunomodulators:
  - ⊙ Monoclonal antibody: omalizumab (anti-IgE)
- Allergy avoidance
- Immunotherapy
- Patient education
- Annual vaccination for influenza

■ Collaborative consultation

- Pulmonologist
- Respiratory therapist
- Case management

■ Complications

- Respiratory failure requiring ventilation (noninvasive positive pressure ventilation or invasive ventilation with intubation)
- Pulmonary fibrosis

■ Prevention

- Education/avoidance of allergens and environmental irritants
- Moderation of physical activity that provokes attacks
- Prophylactic use of bronchodilator MDI before physical activities that provoke attacks

■ Patient/family education

- Teach patient and family how to monitor and manage symptoms and avoid triggers.

- Medication teaching and evaluation of patient ability to use MDI, dry powder inhaler or nebulizer therapy appropriately.
- Teach patient to use spacer if needed.
- Daily peak flow monitoring with specific indications to notify primary care provider.
- Use of home nebulizer equipment as needed.
- Teach the patient to use the bronchodilator MDI before using the steroid inhaler.
- Teach patient to rinse the mouth and spit out after using the steroid inhaler to avoid thrush infection.
- Teach patient and family to identify and eliminate environmental allergens.
- Teach patient and family when to seek emergency care.

References

Centers for Disease Control and Prevention: National Center for Health Statistics (2008) National Health Interview Survey Raw Data. Analysis by the American Lung Association Research and Program Services Division using SPSS and SUDAAN software. Online. Available from http://www.cdc.gov/asthma/health-care.html (accessed 13 March 2012).

Centers for Disease Control and Prevention (2012) Recommended Adult Immunization Schedule – US 2012. *Morbidity and Mortality Weekly*. Online Available from http://www.cdc.gov/mmwr/preview/mmwrhtml/mm6104a9.htm (accessed 14 May 2012).

Huether, S. & McCance, K. (2008) *Understanding Pathophysiology*, 4th edition. Elsevier Mosby, St. Louis, MO.

McCance, K. & Huether, S. (2006) *Pathophysiology: The Biologic Basis for Disease in Adults and Children*, 5th edition. Elsevier Mosby, St. Louis, MO.

National Asthma Education and Prevention Program (2007) *Expert Panel Report 3: Guidelines for the Diagnosis and Management of Asthma*. US Department of Health and Human Services & National Heart, Lung, and Blood Institute (NHLBI). Online. Available from http://www.nhlbi.nih.gov/guidelines/asthma/asthgdln.pdf (accessed 13 March 2012).

Sommers, M., Johnson, S., & Beery, T. (2007) Diseases and Disorders, 3rd edition. FA Davis Company, Philadelphia.

PART 2: CHRONIC OBSTRUCTIVE PULMONARY DISEASE (COPD)

Marian Jeffries and Rosemarie Marks

Chronic obstructive pulmonary disease (COPD) is the fourth leading cause of death (Gold Report, 2011) and the 12th leading cause of disability in the United States (Smeltzer *et al.*, 2008). COPD is characterized by chronic airflow limitation, mucus hypersecretion, and air trapping due to pathological changes in the airways and/or lung parenchyma. The three primary symptoms of COPD are chronic cough, sputum production, and shortness of breath on exertion

(Smeltzer *et al.*, 2008). COPD is usually progressive, especially when left unchecked, and is associated with an abnormal inflammatory response throughout the airways, parenchyma, and pulmonary vasculature (Smeltzer *et al.*, 2008). The two most common forms of COPD are chronic bronchitis and emphysema. Most individuals with COPD will have some degree of both chronic bronchitis and emphysema present. Eliminating or reducing risk factors can help attenuate the signs and symptoms of COPD however, once COPD is present, it cannot be fully reversed (ATS, 2004).

With chronic bronchitis the symptoms of the inflamed bronchi and bronchioles predominate. The lining of the airways thickens. There is scarring and narrowing of the airway lumens. The bronchioles are chronically inflamed and thick mucus is produced, which can result in mucus plugging of the airways. The impaired ciliary function also compromises clearing the mucus from the airway and the patient becomes chronically susceptible to pulmonary infection (Huether & McCance, 2008). Chronic bronchitis is defined as the presence of a cough with sputum production for at least 3 months in each of 2 consecutive years.

With emphysema, the inflammatory process has caused destruction of the lung parenchyma. There is marked, permanent enlargement and destruction of the alveolar sacs with loss of lung elasticity and air trapping that leads to further enlargement of the remaining alveoli. The expiratory phase of the respiratory cycle is increased. There is reduced gas exchange due to the reduced number of air sacs. With advanced emphysema there will be marked hypoxia and hypercapnia present.

People with COPD usually start to become symptomatic in middle age and signs and symptoms usually progress and worsen with aging. Normal lung function changes that occur with aging will accentuate and accelerate this progression of illness. These normal changes include loss of elastic recoil, stiffening of the chest wall, weakening of the respiratory muscles, decreased vital capacity, increased residual volume and decreased forced expiratory volume in one second (FEV1) (McCance & Huether, 2006).

COPD can be classified in four stages based on the results of pulmonary function testing (spirometry) to measure airflow limitation: stage I mild, stage II moderate, stage III severe, and stage IV very severe (Gold Report, 2011). Spirometry is considered to be the best test to measure airflow limitation for diagnosing and assessing the severity of COPD. Individuals will often not seek medical care until they are in stage II or greater COPD.

■ Risk factors

- Tobacco smoking is the number one risk factor for COPD.
- Inherited deficiency of the enzyme α1-antitrypsin (primary emphysema)
- Environmental:
  - Exposure to secondhand cigarette smoke
  - Exposure to occupational dusts and chemicals
  - Indoor pollution especially in developing countries that use wood burning for heating and cooking

◼ Clinical presentation

- "Barrel chest" due to chronic hyperinflation
- Chest tightness
- Chronic cough with mucus production
- Chronic fatigue
- Exercise intolerance
- Frequent respiratory infections
- Shortness of breath (dyspnea) that worsens with exertion
- Shortness of breath (dyspnea) that worsens with exertion
- There is often concurrent a Anorexia and weight loss
- Wheezing

◼ Nursing assessment

- A thorough patient and family history is necessary.
  - Smoking: pack/year history; filtered or unfiltered cigarettes?
    - Still smoking?
  - Cough: if present ask about duration and mucus production.
    - Volume of mucus production
  - Assess pattern of dyspnea
    - Is there dyspnea at rest? With exertion?
    - Can the person climb one flight of stairs? Two or more?
    - Nocturnal? How many pillows needed to sleep?
    - Snoring at night? Wheezing? History of obstructive sleep apnea? CPAP or oxygen needs at home
  - Appetite concerns, anorexia
    - Has patient lost weight?
- Vital signs with special attention to the respiratory pattern:
  - Heart rate: tachycardia?
  - Respiratory rate, rhythm, and increased expiratory time
  - Pulse oximetry at rest and with ambulation
    - Since the presence and degree of hypercapnia and hypoxia are different in each patient, it is important that the nurse be aware of the oxygen saturation goals for each individual with COPD. As the degree of hypercapnia increases, the patient with COPD may require a level of hypoxia in order to maintain a respiratory drive. These patients would thus have a lower oxygen saturation goal than other patients.
  - Assess for signs of cyanosis and clubbing of the fingers.
- *Inspect, palpate, percuss and auscultate.*
  - Inspect chest for anteroposterior (AP) diameter. With aging there is a normal increase in this AP diameter that becomes more pronounced in the presence of COPD. This condition is referred to as a barrel chest.
  - On percussion there may be hyper-resonance.
  - There may be decreased breath sounds, wheezing and crackles present.
  - Peripheral edema and neck vein distention – signs of right-sided heart failure secondary to pulmonary hypertension (cor pulmonale).

- Note if there is anxiety (dyspnea), restlessness (hypoxia), or somnolence (hypercapnia) present. Anxiety may also be secondary to medication therapy (steroids and beta$_2$ adrenergic medications).
- Assess for depression. Depression may be present due to the degree of invalidism that the individual is experiencing.
  - Note the presence of pursed-lip breathing during expiration.
  - Observe for use of accessory muscles of respiration.
- DiagnosticsPulse oximetry (baseline at rest and with activity)
- EKG
- Pulmonary function testing – FEV1/FVC ratio (spirometry with bronchodilators)
- Sputum cultures and Gram stain
- Chest X-ray, if indicated.
- Arterial blood gases, if indicated

■ Differential diagnosis

- Acute coronary syndrome
- Asthma
- Bronchiectasis
- Congestive heart failure
- Interstitial lung disease
- Pneumonia
- Pneumovax
- Pulmonary embolus
- Tuberculosis

■ Treatment

- Goals of management of COPD include:
  - Assess and monitor disease progression.
  - Reduce risk factors.
  - Manage stable COPD symptoms.
  - Improve exercise tolerance.
  - Improve overall health status.
  - Prevent respiratory infections.
- Manage exacerbation episodes. Remove occupational or environmental air pollution/exposure.
- Vaccination: influenza and pneumococcal (PPV-23) vaccines as per CDC recommendations.
- Smoking cessation therapy:
  - Counseling: individual and/or group
  - Pharmacotherapy
    - Nicotine replacement
    - Bupropion SR
    - Nortriptyline
    - Varenicline (Chantix)

- Medications:
  - Bronchodilators (nebulized or per metered dose inhaler)
    - Beta$_2$ adrenergic agents
    - Anticholinergic agents
      - Ipratropium bromide MDI or nebulized or tiotropium inhalation
  - Inhaled corticosteroids
  - Systemic corticosteroids
  - Methylxanthines:
    - Aminophylline
    - Theophylline
  - Antibiotics if infection is present
  - Phosphodiesterase E4 (PDE4) inhibitors in severe disease:
    - Roflumilast (Daliresp)
- Hydration to assist in liquefying secretions
- Humidification to assist in liquefying secretions
- Oxygen therapy- usually low flow to treat hypoxia without worsening the hypercapnia:
  - Nasal cannula to allow for hydration and intake
- Noninvasive positive pressure ventilation (NPPV):
  - CPAP - Continuous positive airway pressure
  - BiPAP - Bi-level positive airway pressure: usually reserved for acute exacerbations in hospital environment

Pulmonary rehabilitation
Selected individuals may benefit from lung reductive surgery or lung transplantation.

■ Collaborative consultation
- Pulmonologist
  - Pulmonary function testing
- Pulmonary rehabilitation program. These programs are multidisciplinary. Program goals include symptom management, improved quality of life, and increased physical, mental, and emotional well-being.
- Respiratory therapy:
  - Bronchodilator therapy, education r/t oxygen therapy, pulmonary hygiene techniques and appliances, purse-lip breathing techniques.

Nutritionist to assess the caloric needs of the patient with anorexia, weight loss, or diminished capacity to eat due to shortness of breath and fatigue.

■ Complications
- Chronic respiratory infections including pneumonia
- Respiratory failure characterized by hypoxia and carbon dioxide retention
- Pulmonary hypertension (cor pulmonale)
- Pneumothorax

■ Prevention

- Encourage people not to smoke.
- Discuss the benefit of smoking cessation with patients currently smoking.
- Environmental controls over air pollution

■ Patient/family education

- Adequate rest and rest periods (HOB elevation and body positioning for maximum chest expansion at rest)
- Avoid crowds and individuals with respiratory infections.
- Coughing and deep breathing exercises; pursed lip breathing exercises
  - Use of flutter valve for coughing.
- Dietary teaching to include adequate protein intake and hydration
- Exercise training in moderation and with pulmonary rehabilitation support
- Flu vaccinations for family members
- Lifestyle teaching to accommodate the need for moderating activities along with the inclusion of rest periods to conserve the patient's energy
- Medication teaching including the proper use of inhalers and nebulizers
- Oxygen therapy: delivery devices. Home compressor vs. tank for mobilization outside
- Safety teaching: related to oxygen in the home and delivery to patient
- Smoking cessation for *all* members of household

References

American Thoracic Society (2004) Standards for the diagnosis and management of patients with COPD. Online. Available from http://www.thoracic.org/clinical/copd-guidelines/resources/copddoc.pdf (accessed 14 March 2012).

Global Initiative for Chronic Obstructive Lung Disease (GOLD) (2011) *Global strategy for the diagnosis, management, and prevention of chronic obstructive pulmonary disease*. Bethseda, MD, World Health Organization (WHO) & National Heart, Lung and Blood Institute (NHLBI). Online. Available from http://www.goldcopd.org (accessed 14 March 2012).

Huether, S. & McCance, K. (2008) *Understanding Pathophysiology*, 4th edition. Elsevier Mosby, St. Louis, MO.

McCance, K. & Huether, S. (2006) *Pathophysiology: The Biologic Basis for Disease in Adults and Children*, 5th edition. Elsevier Mosby, St. Louis, MO.

Smeltzer, S., Bare, B., Hinkle, J., & Cheever, K. (2008) *Brunner & Suddarth's Textbook of Medical Surgical Nursing*, 11th edition. Lippincott Williams & Wilkins, Philadelphia.

Web links to guidelines to diagnosing and managing COPD

All websites correct as of March 2012.

Several professional organizations have compiled guidelines, which are useful for medical professionals in diagnosing and managing COPD. Guidelines from the

American Thoracic Society (ATS), European Respiratory Society (ERS), Global Initiative for Chronic Obstructive lung Disease (GOLD), and American College of Physicians (ACP) are included below for your use. (Please note that by clicking on the below links, you will be directed to an offsite website.)

ACP Guidelines www.acponline.org/clinical_information/guidelines/guidelines
ATS Guidelines www.thoracic.org/clinical/copd-guidelines/resources/copddoc.pdf
ERS Guidelines http://dev.ersnet.org/275-guidelines.htm
GOLD Guidelines http://www.goldcopd.org

PART 3: INFLUENZA

Marian Jeffries and Rosemarie Marks

Influenza (the flu) is a contagious respiratory infection that is viral in origin and spreads rapidly through populations causing mild to severe symptoms of discomfort and in some cases death. Epidemics and pandemics can result in great loss of life. In the United States, it is estimated that approximately 200,000 individuals are hospitalized with flu complications annually. An average of 23,600 patients die each year from complications related to influenza (Sommers *et al.*, 2007) and 90% of these flu-related deaths and more than half of flu-related hospitalizations occur in people aged 65 and older (www.flu.gov/individualfamily/seniors/index.html).

In the US influenza is more common in the colder months from fall (October) to early spring, but it occurs worldwide in a seasonal pattern. Symptoms usually develop within 24 to 96 hours after contact with the virus in susceptible individuals. In most cases influenza is a self-limiting disease that can last from 2 to 7 days.

Influenza is believed to spread primarily by droplets that are formed when an infected individual coughs, sneezes, or speaks. Nearby individuals then inhale these droplets. It is also possible for an individual to touch a contaminated surface and then transfer the virus to his mouth or nose through touch (Seasonal Influenza, 2010). An infected individual can infect anyone within a 2 m (6-foot) radius.

The incidence of flu is highest in school age children. Infants and young children, the elderly, infirmed individuals, and women in the third trimester of pregnancy have the highest risk for developing complications secondary to influenza.

Three types of myxovirus influenzae (influenzavirus A, B, and C) are responsible for the strains that cause the flu. Influenza viruses can infect birds and mammals. Infection with a specific strain confers immunity only to that strain which is why it is important for susceptible individuals to receive an annual flu vaccine. Each year a new vaccine is developed based on the virus strains that are anticipated to be prevalent for the upcoming season. All individuals over the age of 65 and those with chronic illnesses should be strongly encouraged to get an annual influenza vaccination (unless the individual has an egg allergy).

■ Risk factors

- Exposure to person with active influenza
- Exposure to school school-age children
- Failing to receive the influenza vaccination
- Having a chronic illness such as asthma, chronic obstructive pulmonary disease (COPD), congestive heart failure (CHF), cancer, sickle cell anemia, etc.
- Healthcare providers
- Immunocompromised state (human immunodeficiency virus (HIV) infection, diabetes, chemotherapy, etc.)
- Very young or elderly (over age 65)

■ Clinical presentation

- Body aches
- Chills
- Cough
- Fatigue
- Fever (not always)
- Headache
- Rhinitis
- Sore throat
- Vomiting and diarrhea, especially in children

■ Nursing assessment

- Assess patient for recent contact with an infected person.
- Ask about yearly influenza immunization.
- Obtain vital signs, temperature, heart rate, respiratory rate, blood pressure and baseline pulse oximetry.
- Auscultate breath sounds noting any adventitious crackles, rales, wheezes.
- Institute droplet precautions.

■ Diagnostics

- Diagnosis is usually made based on clinical presentation and physical assessment. Nasal or throat swab for rapid flu testing. Can have false negative results with this testing so if patient has signs and symptoms that are highly suggestive of influenza he/she should be presumed to have it despite having a negative rapid flu test.
- Chest X-ray, if indicated

■ Differential diagnosis

- A common cold or upper respiratory infection vs. different microorganism
- Bronchitis

- COPD exacerbation
- HIV disease
- Legionnaires disease
- Pneumonia
- Viral infection

■ Treatment

- Antiviral medications may be prescribed. They are most effective when given at the time of exposure or at the first sign of infection. The two most common antivirals used during the 2009-2010 influenza season were oseltamivir (Tamiflu®) and zanamivir (Relenza®).
- Treatment is supportive and includes rest, hydration, and temperature regulation.
- Antibiotics may be given if a secondary bacterial infection is suspected.
- Place patient on droplet precautions (1m, 3ft clearance).
- Limit visitors and encourage handwashing and face masks.

■ Collaborative consultation

- Infection control specialist
- Respiratory therapy if underlying pulmonary issues escalate
- Complications-Dehydration
- Ear infections
- Exacerbation of asthma and COPD
- Myositis
- Pneumonia from secondary infections (Huether & McCance, 2008)
- Reye's syndrome
- Sinus infections

■ Prevention

- Avoid the spread of healthcare-associated infections: use personal protective equipment, signage, hand hygiene and droplet precautions in health care settings.
- The single best preventative measure is receiving an annual influenza vaccination. In 2010 the CDC's Advisory Committee on Immunization Practices (ACIP) voted for universal flu vaccination of every person in the United States. Any individual residing in the United States who is willing to receive the influenza vaccination and does not have a contraindication should receive it.
- CDC recommends that everyone 6 months of age and older should be vaccinated.

■ Patient/family education

- Educate the patient and family on the importance of yearly flu vaccination.
- Discuss infection control measures to prevent the spread of illness within the family and community.
  - Avoiding large crowds during peak incidences especially in enclosed spaces
  - Wash your hands often with soap and water.
  - Disposal of contaminated materials and disinfection of high touch areas
  - Sneeze into the bend of your arm or a tissue, not into your hands.
  - If you're sick, stay home except to get medical care.
  - Take antiviral drugs only if prescribed.

Some people should NOT be vaccinated. They include:

- People who have a severe allergy to chicken eggs.
- People who have had a prior severe reaction to an influenza vaccination.
- People with a history of developing Guillain–Barré syndrome (GBS) within 6 weeks of getting an influenza vaccine.
- Children younger than 6 months of age (influenza vaccine is not approved for use in this age group).
- People who are febrile or with severe illness should consider waiting to get vaccinated until their symptoms abate.
- Influenza vaccine is available in varied forms. Adults over age 49 should have flu injection, an inactivated form of the influenza virus strains. There is also a nasal spray which is a live attenuated vaccine, indicated only for children age 5 and older and non-pregnant adults up to age 49.

References

Flu.gov. Online. Available from http://www.flu.gov/ (accessed 14 March 2012).

Huether, S., & McCance, K. (2008) *Understanding Pathophysiology*. 4th edition. Elsevier Mosby, St. Louis, MO.

Seasonal Influenza. Online. Avaialble from Centers for Disease Control and Prevention (CDC): http://www.cdc.gov/flu/ (accessed 14 March 2012).

Sommers, M., Johnson, S., & Beery, T. (2007) *Diseases and Disorders*, 3rd edition. F.A. Davis Company, Philadelphia.

Web links for further information

All websites correct as of March 2012.

US Government

www.pandemicflu.gov

Nongovernmental organizations

Association of State and Territorial Health Officials (ASTHO) www.astho.org
Infectious Disease Society of America www.idsociety.org
National Foundation for Infectious Diseases www.nfid.org
Institute of Medicine (IOM) www.iom.edu
World Health Organization (WHO) www.who.org

Influenza background information

CDC. Presents information on the symptoms, treatment, and complications of the disease, prevention and control, the types of influenza viruses, questions and answers on symptoms, vaccination and myths. www.cdc.gov/flu

National Vaccine Program Office. Presents a historical overview of pandemics that occurred throughout the past century (Spanish Flu, Asian Flu, Hong Kong Flu), and three influenza scares (Swine Flu, Russian Flu, and Avian Flu). http://www.flu.gov/pandemic/about/index.html

World Health Organization. Defines an influenza pandemic, explains how a new influenza virus can cause a pandemic, presents the consequences of an influenza pandemic, explains the global surveillance systems, and provides links to other pandemic plans from other nations. http://www.who.int/topics/influenza/en/

PART 4: PNEUMONIA

Marian Jeffries and Rosemarie Marks

Pneumonia is an infection in the lower respiratory tract involving the lung parenchyma. Pneumonia may be caused by bacteria, viruses, fungi, protozoa, or parasites. As organisms multiply in the lung tissue the inflammatory response is provoked, which causes increased capillary permeability. This increased permeability causes fluid and blood cells to escape from the capillaries and fill the alveoli. White blood cells phagocytose organisms adding cellular debris to the alveolar secretions. Fluid filled alveoli cannot exchange oxygen and carbon dioxide so venous blood passing by these alveoli returns to the left atrium unoxygenated. This inflammatory process leads to stiffening of the lung tissue with a decrease in lung compliance, which causes an increase in the work of breathing.

An infectious agent can enter the lungs through either inhalation of microorganisms that were released from a nearby, infected individual who coughed or sneezed; aspiration of oropharyngeal secretions that contain the organism (this is the most common route, especially in the elderly); or via the bloodstream from bacteremia. Usually pneumonia is confined to one or two lobes and it is called lobular pneumonia. When pneumonia affects an entire lung it is termed lobar pneumonia.

Pneumonia is the sixth leading cause of death in the United States (McCance & Huether, 2006). Older adults have the highest incidence and mortality rate for pneumonia (Rhew, 2000). Aging affects the mechanical aspects of ventilation by decreasing chest wall compliance and elastic recoil of the lungs. Changes in these properties reduce ventilatory reserve (Huether & McCance, 2008). The natural physiological changes in the elderly along with comorbid conditions of disease make the advanced aged patient highly susceptible to respiratory compromise. For these reasons, it is imperative that the elderly client receives the pneumococcal and influenza vaccines per the recommendations of the Centers for Disease Control (CDC, 2008).

Pneumonia is classified as either community-acquired pneumonia (CAP) or nosocomial or hospital-acquired pneumonia (HAP). The causative organisms tend to differ for each classification. The most common causative CAP organism is *Streptococcus pneumoniae* (also called pneumococcal pneumonia), but *Mycoplasma pneumoniae* and *Haemophilus influenzae* are not far behind. Other CAP organisms include *Legionella pneumophila*, *Chlamydia pneumoniae* and *Moraxella catarrhalis*. *Pseudomonas aeruginosa* and *Staphylococcus aureus* are considered the most common, causative organisms for HAP. Other causative HAP organisms include the Gram-negative organisms *Klebsiella pneumoniae* and *Escherichia coli* (*E. coli*).

Viral pneumonia is an acute, self-limiting lung infection most often caused by the influenza virus. Viral pneumonia can exacerbate underlying medical conditions (e.g., pulmonary or cardiac disease) and lead to a bacterial pneumonia. Uncomplicated influenza illness typically resolves after 3–7 days for the majority of persons, although cough and malaise can persist for greater than 2 weeks.

Aspiration, the passage of fluid or solid particles into the lung, can occur in older adults with dysphagia and can lead to aspiration pneumonia (Huether & McCance, 2008). Dysphagia is common in older adults with neurological conditions such as stroke, Parkinson's disease and dementia. It can also occur in individuals with altered level of consciousness caused by sedation, anesthesia, substance abuse, or seizure disorders. Aspiration can be an acute or chronic process with patients who experience acute shortness of breath associated with PO intake or mechanical obstruction of foreign body to the chronic manifestation of dysphagia, GI reflux, vocal cord impairment, and nervous system abnormalities (Palmer & Metheny, 2008). Identifying an impairment in the "normal" swallowing mechanism is paramount as prevention of aspiration is more effective and less costly than treating the known aspiration (d'Escrivan & Guery, 2005).

■ Risk factors

- Advanced age
- Alcoholism
- Altered consciousness
- Co-existing cardiac or liver disease
- Co-existing lung disease such as chronic obstructive pulmonary disease (COPD)

- Dysphagia (common in the elderly patient)
- Endotracheal intubation–ventilator-acquired pneumonia (VAP)
- Immobilization
- Immunocompromise
- Malnutrition
- Neurological disorders that cause paralysis of the diaphragm
- Recent hospitalization
- Residence in group housing such as a nursing home, group home, or dormitory
- Smoking
- Tube feeding

■ Clinical presentation

Most cases of pneumonia are preceded by an upper respiratory infection. This is followed by the onset of cough, dyspnea, and fever. There is usually copious mucus production with bacterial pneumonias but little to no mucus production with viral pneumonias. There may also be malaise, chills, and pleuritic chest pain. Viral pneumonias tend to be milder and self-limiting, but it is not unusual for a secondary bacterial pneumonia to develop as an opportunistic infection in the weakened and damaged lung tissue. Physical exam may reveal inspiratory crackles, with increased tactile fremitus, egophony, and whispered pectoriloquy (McCance & Huether, 2006). There may be dullness on percussion over the affected area of consolidation (Sommers *et al.*, 2007).

Older adults may not present with the typical symptoms of pneumonia. Often, a change in mental (e.g., delirium, increased confusion) or functional status, poor oral intake, or a fall may be the initial sign of pneumonia in an older adult.

Aspiration pneumonia presents radiologically more frequently in the right lung. The right lower lobe (RLL) is more susceptible for aspiration contents due to the straight anatomical angle of the right mainstem.

■ Nursing assessment

Important history includes determining if there is recent history of an upper respiratory infection, recent hospitalization, travel, or illness in other family members or friends. Determining when the illness began and associated symptoms (e.g., headache, anorexia, fever, chills, shortness of breath, or cough) is also necessary. Other critical information includes past medical history, co-existing lung diseases such as COPD and asthma, smoking history, allergies, current medications, and what antibiotics the patient has had in the previous 6 months.

- Physical assessment should include
  - Vital signs
    - Tachycardia, hypotension, tachypnea (respiratory rate >28), and hyperthermia all are significant signs.
    - Obtain baseline oxygen saturation level with patient presentation of symptoms.

- Lung auscultation for adventitious breath sounds (i.e., inspiratory crackles, wheezing, and the decrease or absence of breath sounds).
  - Patients who are dehydrated may not have adventitious breath sounds.
- Ventilations and oxygenation for adequacy
  - Monitor oxygen saturation at rest and with minimal activity.
  - Note presence of cyanosis, tachypnea.
- Color, consistency, odor and amount of sputum
  - Evaluate patient for effective airway clearance (cough) of secretions.
- Observe patient for signs and symptoms of dysphagia and aspiration:
  - Coughing or choking while eating or drinking
  - Hoarse voice following meals
  - Gurgling sounds while speaking
  - Drooling
- Monitor patient for signs and symptoms of sepsis.

■ Diagnostics

- Chest X-ray may be negative in an older adult especially if the patient has a fluid deficit. Common chest X-ray findings include infiltrates that can be patchy, lobar, or diffuse. There is often consolidation in the involved lobe. Consolidation is the solidification of the lung tissue caused by the alveoli filling with exudates.
- Complete blood count: white blood cell count is usually elevated and in the presence of bacterial pneumonia there is usually an increase in polymorphonucleocytes on the differential.
- Serum electrolytes, blood urea nitrogen and creatinine to determine fluid and electrolyte status
- Sputum culture and Gram stain
- Blood cultures, if indicated

■ Differential diagnosis

- CAP vs HAP: Infectious organism
- Congestive heart failure
- Inflammatory lung disease
- Influenza
- Pulmonary emboli
- Pulmonary tumor
- Tuberculosis
- Upper respiratory infection (bronchitis, laryngitis, pharyngitis)

■ Treatment

- Maintain patent airway and provide ventilatory support as needed.
- Provide supplemental oxygen and humidification.
- Nebulized medications (i.e., albuterol and/or itrapropium) will provide humidity and bronchodilation to help patient expel secretions.

- Provide pulmonary hygiene:
  - Teach patient deep breathing and coughing exercises.
  - Consider mild percussion.
  - Consult with physician regarding postural drainage to assist in mobilizing secretions as this can be beneficial in the appropriate patient (cystic fibrosis); however, in older patients, comorbid disease conditions usually prohibit this activity.
  - Nasotracheal suctioning may be needed for patients who cannot raise secretions. Suctioning is effective in removing secretions to improve airway clearance, yet traumatic to mucous membrane and can cause decreased oxygenation and a vasovagal response (decreased heart rate and blood pressure).
    - Consider bedside bronchoscopy for the frail or compromised patient that needs frequent secretion clearance.
- Antibiotics are indicated for bacterial pneumonia and in hospitalized patients are given intravenously.
- Antiviral medications may be a consideration in severe cases of viral pneumonia.
- Administer medications as prescribed:
  - Antibiotics – per causative microorganism
  - Antipyretics
  - Mucolytics
  - Bronchodilators
  - Anti-anxiety
  - Pain medication
- Encourage smoking cessation:
  - Behavioral therapy: individual and/or group
  - Nicotine withdrawal pharmacotherapy options include:
    - Nicotine replacement
    - Bupropion SR
    - Nortriptyline
    - Varenicline (Chantix)
- Reposition immobile patients at least every 2 hours.
- Position "aspiration at risk patients" with HOB >45 degrees.

Monitor "aspiration at risk patients" when eating, drinking, or taking oral medication. Other patients at risk for aspiration include those on enteral feedings, promotility agents, and sedatives or anxiolytics.

- Avoid excessive sedation.
- Anxiety reduction interventions as indicated
- Provide adequate hydration up to 3 liters a day unless contraindicated.
- Provide good oral care at least twice daily (see Box 3.3.4.1).
- Encourage mobilization as much as possible unless there is a specific contraindication.

Box 3.3.4.1 Oral care guidelines

The literature suggests that there is high morbidity and mortality associated with health-care-associated pneumonia. In response, several guidelines for its prevention and control have been published over the last 30 years. The first CDC Guideline for Prevention of Nosocomial Pneumonia was published in 1981 and addressed the main infection-control problems related to hospital-acquired pneumonia. In 1994, the Healthcare Infection Control Practices Advisory Committee (HICPAC) (then known as the Hospital Infection Control Practices Advisory Committee) revised and expanded the CDC Guideline. These guidelines only addressed oral care in the acute care hospital environment, however with the progressive shift in moving healthcare to the outpatient and long term care environment, HICPAC revised it further to cover these settings.

Suggestions for developing an oral care guideline

I. Address standard precautions
- *Hand hygiene* Decontaminate hands by washing them with antimicrobial soap and water and /or by using an alcohol-based waterless antiseptic agent. Visibly soiled hands should be washed with soap & water prior to the alcohol-based agent.
- *Gloving* Wear gloves for handling respiratory and oral secretions or objects contaminated with secretions of any patient.

II. Modify risk for infection
- *Vaccination* (primary prevention): pneumococcal vaccination. Vaccinate patients at high risk for severe pneumococcal infections.

III. Precautions for prevention of aspiration
- *Prevention of aspiration associated with eating and drinking*
  - Sit upright (90 degrees) when possible to consume food /beverages to assist with swallowing.
- *Prevention of aspiration associated with endotracheal intubation*
  - Use noninvasive positive pressure ventilation (NPPV) whenever the option is available.
  - Oral care program for intubated and NPPV patients.
- *Prevention of aspiration associated with enteral feeding*
  - In the absence of medical contraindication(s), elevate at an angle of 30-45 degrees of the head of the bed (if bedridden) of a patient at high risk for aspiration (Wip & Napolitano, 2009; CDC, 2003).
  - Verify appropriate placement of the feeding tube.

- *Prevention or modulation of oropharyngeal colonization*
  - Routinely visually inspect oral mucous membrane, gums and teeth.
  - A soft toothbrush is the most effective mechanical method to control dental plaque.
  - Brush teeth and tongue using toothpaste and toothbrush when possible.
  - Rinse mouth with water.
  - Avoid brushing with a foam swab (unless risk of bleeding or gingivitis) Foam swabs do not provide effective reduction in bacteria.
  - Suction the oral cavity if patient unable to expel oral secretions.
  - Avoid using Lemon glycerin swabs in the mouth. The pH of the oral cavity mouth is normally alkaline @ 6-7. The application of lemon glycerin reduces the oral pH to 2-4 making an acidic environment. An acid environment irritates the mucosa, decalcifies teeth, increases dryness and thus the risk of dental caries (MGH, 2009).
- *Oropharyngeal cleaning and decontamination with an antiseptic agent*
  - Provide a comprehensive oral-hygiene program (that might include the use of an antiseptic agent) for patients in acute-care settings or residents in long-term care facilities who are at high risk for health-care-associated pneumonia.
- *Chlorhexidine oral rinse (non-alcohol rinse)*
  - Oral chlorhexidine gluconate (0.12%) 5 mL BID rinse during the perioperative period on adult patients who undergo cardiac surgery (CDC, 2003). Prophylactic rinsing in other populations can reduce oral bacterial plaque colonization.
  - Apply chlorhexidine to swab and then apply to patient's mouth and tongue if they are unable to apply. Suction excess if patient unable to expel secretions.
  - Do not brush teeth, eat or drink for 30 minutes post chlorhexidine.
  - Oral decontamination with topical antimicrobial agents.
    - If using oral nystatin, do not administer within 2 hours of using chlorhexidine.
- *Prevention of gastric colonization*
  - Preferential use of sucralfate, H_2-antagonists, and/or antacids for stress-bleeding prophylaxis is not recommended by CDC, but offered to some populations with GERD and postoperative reflux issues.
- *Prevention of postoperative pneumonia*
  - Encourage all postoperative patients to take deep breaths, move about the bed, and ambulate unless medically contraindicated.
  - Incentive spirometry on postoperative patients at high risk for pneumonia may be helpful in patients who need reinforcement to take deep breaths.

● Patients at high risk include those who will have abdominal and thoracic surgery, emergency surgery; those who will receive general anesthesia; those ≥60 years; those with totally dependent functional status; those who have had a weight loss >10%; those using steroids for chronic conditions; recent history of alcohol use, COPD or smoking during the preceding year; those with impaired sensorium, a history of cerebrovascular accident (CVA) with residual neurologic deficit, or low (<8 mg/dL) or high (>22 mg/dL) blood urea nitrogen level; and those who will have received >4 units of blood before surgery.

IV. **Staff education with respect to precautions and transmission**

V. **Environmental surveillance and care of medical equipment and devices**
● Changing nebulizer equipment and respiratory equipment per current CDC guidelines.

Oral care is proposed as key to preventing ventilator associated pneumonia, but little work has been done to measure reliably oral care practice (Feider *et al.*, 2009). Despite strong evidence on the role of oral care in the prevention of VAP, it is viewed as a nursing intervention often associated with the hospitalized acute care population. It is often further associated with a specific "type" of patient: the critically ill, neurology, oncology and postoperative groups. There is no definitive evidence to determine the most appropriate method of oral hygiene or oral rinses (Berry & Davidson, 2006; Berry *et al.*, 2007).

Discrepancies exist between reported practices and policies for oral care in the acute care patient (Feider *et al.*, 2010). This may be due to the nursing perception related to the importance of this care. Despite strong evidence on the role of oral care in the prevention of VAP, nursing continues to view oral care as a comfort measure with a low priority and often use foam swabs rather than toothbrushes to provide cleaning of the oral cavity (Ross & Crumpler, 2007; Berry *et al.*, 2007).

The specific guidelines to control discomfort in the oncology population are mostly directly related to treatment of xerostomia or mucositis post chemotherapy or radiation. Caring for this population the healthcare provider must consider the grade of mucositis, potential for further breakdown with immunosuppression, radiation, chemotherapy, medications, and the impact of bone marrow suppression and oral tumors.

This population has more options for medication relief and the application of pain relieving solutions for the oral cavity.

■ Collaborative consultation

- Infectious disease, if indicated
- Physical therapy to help mobilize patient
- Pulmonary consultation, if indicated
- Respiratory therapy to supplement nursing interventions:
  - Bronchodilator therapy
  - Peak flow measurements
- Speech and language pathology (SLP) if aspiration suspected

■ Complications

- Infection can spread via the bloodstream and cause bacteremia, meningitis, and pericarditis.
- Respiratory failure
- Septic shock
- Severe acute respiratory distress syndrome

■ Prevention

- Encourage patients and patient caregivers to receive the influenza vaccine each year.
- Encourage the individual to receive the pneumococcal vaccine as per CDC recommendations.
- Teach susceptible patients the importance of avoiding contact with infected individuals.
- Explain the importance of good Hand hygiene and demonstrate the proper technique.
- Discuss limiting exposure to cigarette smoke.

■ Patient/family education

- Explain all procedures.
- Teach patient coughing and deep breathing exercises including the use of incentive spirometry.
- Teach patient the importance of receiving the flu and pneumococcal vaccines.
- Medication teaching
- Instruct patient to limit excess activity and to take frequent rest periods until the pneumonia is resolved.
- Smoking cessation

References

Berry, A.M. & Davidson, P.M. (2006) Beyond comfort: oral hygiene as a critical nursing activity in the intensive care unit. *Intensive Critical Care Nursing* **22**(6), 318-328.

Berry, A.M., Davidson, P.M., Masters, J. & Rolls, K. (2007) Systematic literature review of oral hygiene practices for Intensive care patients receiving mechanical ventilation *American Journal of Critical Care* **16**(6), 552-562.

CDC (2003) Guidelines for environmental control in health-care facilities. MMWR **52** (No. RR-10). Online. Available from http://www.cdc.gov/mmwr/preview/mmwrhtml/rr5303a1.htm (accessed 14 March 2012).

CDC (2008) Prevention and control of influenza - recommendations of the Advisory Committee on Immunization Practices (ACIP) 2008. MMWR **57**(RR07), 1-60. Online. Available from http://www.cdc.gov/flu/professionals/acip/clinical.htm (accessed 14 March 2012).

d'Escrivan, T. & Guery, B. (2005) Prevention and treatment of aspiration pneumonia in intensive care units. *Treatments in Respiratory Medicine* **4**(5), 317-324.

Feider, L.L., Mitchell, P. & Bridges, E. (2010) Oral care practices for orally intubated critically ill adults. *American Journal of Critical Care* **19**(2), 175-183.

Feider, L.L. & Mitchell, P. (2009) Validity and reliability of an oral care practice survey for the orally intubated adult critically ill patient. *Nursing Research* **58**(5), 374-377.

Huether, S. & McCance, K. (2008) *Understanding Pathophysiology*, 4th edition. Elsevier Mosby, St Louis, MO.

McCance, K. & Huether, S. (2006) *Pathophysiology: The Biologic Basis for Disease in Adults and Children*, 5th edition. Elsevier Mosby, St. Louis, MO.

Massachusetts General Hospital (2009) (General Procedures) Oral Care of the Acutely Ill Guideline (Guanci, M., Goldsmith, T.).

Palmer, J. & Metheny, N. (2008) Preventing aspiration in older adults with dysphagia. *American Journal of Nursing* **108**(2), 40-48.

Rhew, D.C. (2001) Quality indicators for the management of pneumonia in vulnerable elders. *Annalsof Internal Medicine* **135**, 736-743.

Ross, A. & Crumpler, J. (2007) The impact of an evidence-based practice education program on the role of oral care in the prevention of ventilatorassociated pneumonia. *Intensive Critical Care Nursing* **23**(3), 132-136.

Sommers, M., Johnson, S. & Beery, T. (2007) Diseases and Disorders, 3rd edition. F.A. Davis Company, Philadelphia.

Wip, C. & Napolitano, L. (2009) Bundles to prevent ventilator-associated pneumonia: how valuable are they? *Current Opinion Infectious Disease* **22**(2), 159-166.

Web links for further information

All websites correct as of May 2012.

CDC and the Healthcare Infection Control Practices Advisory Committee Guidelines for Preventing Health-Care-Associated Pneumonia, 2003 http://www.cdc.gov/mmwr/preview/mmwrhtml/rr5303a1.htm

Infectious Diseases Society of America/American Thoracic Society Consensus Guidelines on the Management of Community-Acquired Pneumonia http://www.thoracic.org/statements/

Infectious Diseases Society of America Guidelines on Hospital-Acquired Pneumonia American Academy of Family Physicians Guidelines on Diagnosis and Treatment of Community-Acquired Pneumonia http://www.aafp.org/afp/2006/0201/p442.html

Unit 4: Gastrointestinal Disorders

PART 1: APPENDICITIS

Patricia Fitzgerald

Appendicitis is the most common cause of acute abdomen, and the most frequent indication for abdominal surgery worldwide. Although appendicitis usually occurs in the second and third decades of life, it can be seen in patients of all ages (Schmelzer, 2007). It is rarely seen in patients older than age 60, but when present can be easily missed due to its unusual presentation in the older adult. This difficulty in diagnosis leads to a mortality and complication rate in elders that is double that of the general population (Hustey *et al.*, 2005).

The appendix is a small fingerlike appendage that is attached to the cecum below the ileocecal valve. The appendix regularly fills with food and empties into the cecum during digestion. Its small size and inefficient emptying can lead to obstruction and infection. Common sources of obstruction include hard stool, fibrosis or neoplasm. The resulting inflammation and infection are referred to as appendicitis (Smeltzer *et al.*, 2008).

■ Risk factors

There are no known risk factors for appendicitis.

■ Clinical presentation

The classic presentation of appendicitis includes an abrupt onset of epigastric or periumbilical pain that progresses to the right lower quadrant. Patients often complain of a lack of appetite accompanied by nausea and vomiting. Older adults may present with vague, non-specific symptoms (see Box 3.4.1.1). Fever and leukocytosis may not be present. This altered presentation often leads to a delay in diagnosis and treatment resulting in a higher incidence of appendiceal rupture (Smeltzer *et al.*, 2008). Physical exam elicits tenderness on deep palpation. Rebound tenderness may also be present (Wisniewski, 2010).

■ Nursing assessment

- Elicit description of onset of symptoms and location of pain.
- Determine last bowel movement.
- Maintain NPO status preoperatively.
- Monitor vital signs. An increased heart rate and decreasing blood pressure may indicate septicemia. An elevated temperature is often present with appendicitis.

Box 3.4.1.1 Abdominal pain in the older adult

Abdominal pain is a common complaint in the older adult. Proper diagnosis is challenging because patients frequently present with vague non-specific complaints, or display an atypical presentation of many disease states. Pain can be caused by inflammation, mechanical obstruction or trauma and its presentation may provide important clues to the origin. A thorough nursing assessment and examination is crucial, and leads to rapid diagnosis and timely treatment of the underlying disease state. Nurses should carefully obtain the following health data to assist in the care of the older adult.

Health history
- Obtain history of other medical diagnoses and past surgeries.
- Elicit medications patient may be taking.
- Determine history of smoking, drug or alcohol use.
- List any herbal supplements patient may be taking.
- Determine usual bowel pattern and date of last bowel movement.

Pain assessment
- Where is the pain located?
- When did it start?
- Is it constant or intermittent?
- Does anything precipitate the pain?
- Are there any relieving factors?
- Describe the pain. Is it sharp, dull, stabbing, twisting, burning?

Physical exam
- Inspect the abdomen for movement, such as fluid waves.
  - Make note of scars, bruising, distention or bulges.
- Auscultate all four quadrants and note any increase, decrease, or absence of bowel sounds.
- Percuss the borders of the organs to determine the presence of air or solid masses.
- Palpate to assess for tenderness.

Report any findings to the physician. Some common diseases and conditions leading to abdominal pain in the older adult are appendicitis, diverticulitis, ischemic bowel disease, gastroesophageal reflux disease, pancreatitis, constipation, and diarrhea.

- In elders, the abdominal exam may not be abnormal. Tenderness in the right lower quadrant, however, can suggest appendicitis.
- During the abdominal exam note if the abdomen is soft, firm, or distended. Determine if bowel sounds are present in all four quadrants. Note the quality

of bowel sounds (tinkling or diminished). Note any tympany or dullness with percussion. Determine if there is abdominal tenderness and its location. Rebound tenderness or guarding are ominous signs and should be reported to the physician upon discovery.

■ Diagnostics

- Complete blood count with differential. Leukocytosis and elevated neutrophils may be present.
- Serum electrolytes, BUN and creatinine to assess fluid, electrolyte and renal status
- Urinalysis often obtained to exclude a genitourinary problem
- Computed tomography (CT scan) scan with oral and intravenous contrast
- Ultrasonography

■ Differential diagnosis

- Bladder infection
- Crohn's disease
- Diverticulitis
- Pancreatitis
- Pelvic inflammatory disease
- Uterine disease

■ Treatment

Surgical removal of the appendix is the standard treatment for appendicitis.

Preoperative nursing care

- Educate patient and family about the operative procedure and postoperative course.
- Assess vital signs.
- Monitor fluid status and replace fluid and electrolytes as prescribed.
- Assess pain and administer analgesics as ordered.
- Administer antibiotics as ordered.

Postoperative care

- Position patient comfortably in Fowler's position.
- Monitor vital signs and oxygenation.
- Assess lung and bowel sounds.
- Assess intake and output.
- Advance diet as tolerated.
- Encourage coughing and deep breathing exercises every hour to prevent postoperative atelectasis.
- Assess pain level and medicate with analgesics as ordered.
- Administer antibiotics as ordered.

- Assess incision for erythema and drainage.
- If there is a drainage tube present, assess amount of drainage and keep surrounding skin clean and dry.
- Encourage ambulation to maintain mobility and prevent deep vein thrombosis. Patients are usually ambulated on the day of surgery.
- Assess bowel status.

■ Collaborative consultation

Timely communication with the physician is necessary to discuss patient symptoms and any deleterious change in status to prevent serious complications.

■ Complications

- Abscess formation (intra-abdominal)
- Acute respiratory distress syndrome (ARDS)
- Hypovolemia
- Paralytic ileus
- Perforation of the appendix
- Peritonitis
- Sepsis
- Shock

■ Prevention

There are no specific interventions to prevent the occurrence of appendicitis. Timely diagnosis and treatment will prevent appendiceal rupture and peritonitis.

■ Patient/family education

- Teach patient and family to assess incision for erythema or drainage.
- Discuss medications and common side effects.
- Explain the importance of maintaining an adequate fluid intake to avoid constipation.
- Discharge teaching should include information about the importance of contacting the physician if fever, change in mental status, or other change in patient status occurs.

References

Flaser, M.H. & Goldberg, E. (2006) Acute abdominal pain. *Medical Clinics of North America* **90**, 481-503.

Hustey, F.M., Meldon, S.W., Banet, G.E., Gerson, L.W., Blanda, M. & Lewis, L.M. (2005) The use of abdominal computerized tomography in older ED patients with acute abdominal pain. *American Journal of Emergency Medicine* **23**, 259-265.

Schmelzer, M. (2007) Nursing management of lower gastrointestinal problems. In: Lewis, S.L., Heitkemper, M.M., Dirksen, S.R., O'Brien, P.G., & Bucher, L. (eds)

Medical Surgical Nursing: Assessment and Management of Clinical Problems. Mosby, St. Louis.

Wisniewski, A. (2010) Acute abdomen: Shaking down the suspects. *Nursing made Incredibly Easy* **8**(1), 42–52.

Further reading

Ibis, C., Albayrak, D., Hatigpoglu, A.R. & Turan, N. (2010) The amount of comorbidities as a single parameter has no effect in predicting the outcome in appendicitis patients older than 60 years. *Southern Medical Journal* **103**(3), 202–206.

Smeltzer, S.C., Bare, B.G., Hinkle, J.L. & Cheever, K.H. (2006) *Brunner and Suddarth's Textbook of Medical-Surgical Nursing*, 11th edition. Lippincott, Williams & Wilkins, Philadelphia, PA.

PART 2: DIVERTICULAR DISEASE

Patricia Fitzgerald

Diverticula are sacs in the mucosal lining of the gastrointestinal tract that can cause pressure on the surrounding tissues. Although they can occur in any part of the intestine, the most common site is the sigmoid colon, and they are usually found in groups. According to James *et al.* (2006), it is believed that:

> Low dietary fiber decreases the stool bulk and prolongs transit time, causing increased intraluminal pressure. High intraluminal pressure may cause herniation of colonic mucosa through areas of weakness, produced by penetration of vas recta that supply the submucosa and mucosa (p. 271).

Aging contributes to a decrease in the compliance of the colon further contributing to this increased pressure (Camilleri *et al.*, 2000). The presence of diverticula does not always present problems. There are two disorders associated with diverticula: diverticulosis and diverticulitis.

Diverticulosis describes the presence of diverticula, and commonly occurs in the general population "affecting 50% of people by the fifth decade and 67% by the eight decade" (Janes *et al.*, 2006). Patients are usually asymptomatic, although some report a history of constipation. The presence of diverticula is often an incidental finding on a screening colonoscopy or work up of other gastrointestinal disorders.

Diverticulitis occurs when inflammation develops in the diverticula causing further narrowing of the lumen. Stool and bacteria can become trapped in the pouches leading to an overgrowth of bacteria and local tissue ischemia. Complicated diverticulitis occurs when this process progresses to the development of abcesses, fistulas, bowel obstruction, perforation and peritonitis (Jacobs, 2007).

■ Risk factors

- High intake of red meat and fats
- History of constipation
- Low intake of dietary fiber
- NSAID use.
- Obesity
- Physical inactivity
- Smoking

■ Clinical presentation

Diverticulosis

Diverticulosis is usually asymptomatic. Some patients may report alternating episodes of constipation and diarrhea and occasionally abdominal pain, but do not have symptoms suggesting inflammation or infection.

Diverticulitis

Diverticulitis can present as mild or severe. Patients with mild disease frequently describe a loss of appetite, abdominal bloating, constipation, nausea and vomiting, but older patients may stop eating or present with a change in mental status. Abdominal pain is usually located in the left lower quadrant and the onset is gradual and may worsen with movement. This pain is often precipitated by eating, and is relieved when passing flatus or stool. Palpation may reveal tenderness in the area, with or without rebound (Amerine, 2007).

Severe or complicated diverticulitis presents with more acute, constant pain in the left lower quadrant, although location may vary depending upon the diverticula involved. Bowel sounds may be present initially, but can change in frequency and intensity if an obstruction is present (Salzman & Lillie, 2005). Complaints of severe abdominal pain or the presence of blood in the stool may indicate perforation. Urinary frequency may occur if the area of inflammation lies close to the bladder.

Fistula formation between the bowel and the bladder (colovesicular fistula) (Touzios & Dozois, 2009) can lead to the presence of stool in the urine. Passage of stool through the vagina may occur with a colovaginal fistula.

■ Nursing assessment

- Assess patient's regular bowel patterns. Ask patient about a history of constipation or straining with bowel movements.
- Assess description and progression and of pain. Abrupt increase in pain may indicate perforation.
- Monitor vital signs. A temperature elevation more than 2 degrees may indicate infection. Tachycardia may indicate dehydration or the presence of infection. Hypotension may indicate dehydration or worsening infection.

- During the abdominal exam note if the abdomen is soft, firm, or distended. Determine if bowel sounds are present in all four quadrants. Note the quality of bowel sounds (tinkling or diminished). Note any tympany or dullness with percussion. Determine if there is abdominal tenderness and its location. Rebound tenderness or guarding are ominous signs and should be reported to the physician upon discovery.
  - Note frequency and consistency of bowel movements.
  - Assess for the passage of fecal matter in the urine or through the vagina.
  - Examine stool for occult blood.
  - Monitor intake and output.

■ Diagnostics

- Diverticulosis is usually identified through colonoscopy and sigmoidoscopy. These should be avoided during the acute phase of diverticulitis, but are recommended as follow up once the inflammation has resolved to rule out the presence of other disease. This is usually done 6 weeks after the acute episode.
- Computed tomography scan (CT scan) with intravenous contrast is recommended if diverticulitis is suspected. If oral contrast is used it should be water soluble due to the risk of peritonitis.
- Complete blood cell count with differential may reveal leukocytosis.
- Serum electrolytes, BUN, creatinine to assess fluid, electrolyte and renal status.
- Urinalysis

■ Differential diagnosis

- Appendicitis
- Gynecologic problems
- Infectious or ischemic colitis
- Inflammatory bowel disease
- Malignancy
- Nephrolithiasis
- Urinary tract infection

■ Treatment

Asymptomatic diverticulosis

Asymptomatic diverticulosis requires no treatment. A high fiber, low fat diet with adequate fluid intake is recommended to prevent occurrence of diverticulitis.

Symptomatic diverticulitis

- Patients with symptomatic diverticulitis (uncomplicated) are usually treated as outpatients.
  - Administer antibiotics as ordered:

○ Antibiotic coverage for both anaerobic and aerobic bacteria is recommended. The most common recommended antibiotics are metronidazole (Flagyl) and a fluoroquinolone. These should be taken for 7-10 days or longer.
○ Administer analgesics as needed.
● Educate patient to limit intake to clear liquids for 2-4 days gradually increasing to a low residue diet.
● When symptoms completely resolve a high fiber, low fat diet should be initiated to prevent future issues.

If symptoms fail to improve after 24-72 hours of conservative treatment, patients experience increasing pain, or are unable to tolerate fluids, hospitalization is recommended. Inpatient treatment is also recommended for patients older than 85 years of age or those with comorbid conditions (Salzman & Lillie, 2005).

● Administer intravenous antibiotics. Metronidazole and a quinolone are the drugs of choice, although third generation cephalosporins and beta lactams with a beta-lactase inhibitor can also be used. Treatment course is generally 7-10 days.
● Patient should be NPO to facilitate bowel rest.
● Fluid and electrolyte status should be monitored and intravenous fluids administered as ordered.
● If an ileus is present, a nasogastric tube should be placed for drainage.
● Vital signs should be monitored. An acute elevation of temperature could indicate presence of an abcess or increasing inflammation. Tachycardia or hypotension may indicate peritonitis or sepsis.
● Complete blood cell count should be followed. Acute rise in WBC may indicate progressing infection. Decreasing hematocrit could be due to bleeding from perforation.
● Assess for pain and administer analgesics as needed.
● If no improvement occurs within 2-3 days, or if symptoms worsen or new symptoms occur, further imaging is recommended to determine the presence of an abscess, fistula or further obstruction.
● Percutaneous drainage may be required for the presence of an abscess greater than 4 cm in diameter.
● The following occurrences may lead to surgical intervention:
   ○ Generalized peritonitis
   ○ Uncontrolled sepsis
   ○ Uncontained visceral perforation
   ○ Presence of a large, undrainable abscess
   ○ Lack of improvement or deterioration within 3 days of medical management

The surgical procedure most commonly performed is a sigmoid colectomy, with formation of a colostomy. Attempts are often made to reverse the colostomy at a later time if the patient's physical condition and comorbidities suggest that risk for complications is low. Elderly patients rarely have this reversal due to the risk of leakage, small bowel trauma, incisional herniation and the risk presented by additional surgery (Jacobs, 2007).

A resection with primary anastomosis can also be performed, but is often avoided due to the condition of the bowel, amount of bowel contamination present, and nutritional status of the patient (Jacobs, 2007). Elective surgical procedures are often recommended for patients who have frequent reoccurrences of diverticulitis or multiple episodes of abscess formation. The risks versus benefits of elective diverticular surgery in elders must be carefully considered as this surgery in older adults is associated with increased morbidity and mortality, especially in patients with congestive heart failure and chronic obstructive pulmonary disease (Sheer *et al.*, 2011).

■ Collaborative consultation

- Timely communication with the physician concerning patient symptoms and changes in status are necessary to prevent serious complications.
- Collaboration with a nutritionist may be helpful in planning advancement of the patient's diet and patient education around appropriate dietary choices.
- If a colostomy is necessary, collaboration with an enterostomal therapist is essential for successful care and patient teaching.

■ Complications

- Abscess
- Bowel obstruction
- Development of a colovesicular or colovaginal abscess
- Diverticular hemorrhage
- Fistula formation
- Perforation and resulting peritonitis
- Sepsis
- Ureteral obstruction

■ Prevention

- A low-fat high-fiber diet has been shown to decrease the occurrence of diverticulosis and its progression to diverticulitis.
- Adequate intake of fluids will help to prevent constipation and straining with bowel movements.

■ Patient/family education

- Inform patient and families that the presence of diverticula is a common occurrence and usually requires no medical treatment.

- A diet high in fiber and low in fat may decrease the occurrence of diverticulosis, and prevent its progression to diverticulitis.
- Describe to patients and families the fluids included in a clear liquid diet.
- Educate patients and families about the antibiotics ordered, side effects, and the importance of continuing administration for the full number of days prescribed, despite the resolution of symptoms.
- Instruct patients and families to contact their health care provider if symptoms do not resolve within 2-3 days or if more acute pain, fever or nausea and vomiting occur as these may be signs of worsening disease or serious complications.
- For patients requiring surgery, explain the standard course of hospitalization and recovery frequently for the surgical procedure that is planned.
- If a patient is to be discharged with a percutaneous drainage tube, teach patient and family how to care for this tube and the importance of preventing the introduction of bacteria into the system.
- Teach patients and families about the care of a colostomy. Allow patients an opportunity to independently perform care before discharge.
- Discharge teaching should include information about the importance of contacting the physician if fever, change in mental status, or other change in patient status occurs.

References

Amerine, E. (2007) Preventing and managing acute diverticulitis. *Nursing* **37**(9), 56hn1-56hn4.

Camilleri, M., Lee, S.L., Viramontes, B., Bharucha, A.E. & Tangalos, E.G. (2000) Insights into the pathophysiology and mechanisms of constipation, irritable bowel syndrome, and diverticulosis in older people. *Journal of the American Geriatrics Society* **48**(9), 1142-1150.

Jacobs, D. (2007) Diverticulitis. *New England Journal of Medicine* **357**(20), 2057-2066.

Janes, S.E.J., Meagher, A. & Frizelle, F. (2006) Management of diverticulitis. *British Medical Journal.* **332**, 271-275.

Salzman, H. & Lillie, D. (2005) Diverticular disease: Diagnosis and treatment. *American Family Physician* **72**(7), 1229-1234.

Sheer, A.J., Heckman, J.E. Schneider, E.B. *et al.* (2011) Congestive heart failure and chronic obstructive pulmonary disease predict poor surgical outcomes in older adults undergoing elective diverticulitis surgery. *Diseases of the Colon & Rectum* **54**(11), 1430-1437.

Touzios, J.G. & Dozois, E.J. (2009) Diverticulosis and acute diverticulitis. *Gastroenterology Clinics of North America* **38**, 513-525.

Further reading

Mauk, K. (2006) *Gerontological nursing: Core competencies for care.* Jones & Bartlett Learning, Burlington, MA.

PART 3: ISCHEMIC BOWEL

Patricia Fitzgerald

Ischemia is described as a decrease in blood flow to an area that results in tissue damage. Ischemic bowel disease is caused by such a decrease and may have different presentations depending upon the location, degree of ischemia, and duration. It is often divided into three distinct syndromes; acute mesenteric ischemia, chronic mesenteric ischemia and acute colonic ischemia (Flasar & Goldberg, 2006).

Acute mesenteric ischemia is a syndrome where there is diminished blood flow to an area of the intestine and is usually caused by occlusion, vasospasm or hypoperfusion of the mesenteric vasculature. This occlusion often occurs in the parts of the intestine supplied by the celiac, superior mesenteric, and inferior mesenteric arteries. Although the most common cause of arterial occlusion is thromboembolic disease, a mechanical obstruction in the bowel causing decreased blood flow can also lead to intestinal damage. Obstruction of the mesenteric vein can also occur causing edema and decreased perfusion to the tissues. The degree of obstruction and the duration of the hypoperfusion greatly influences the amount of damage incurred. Prolonged or extensive low flow to the mucosa decreases the amount of oxygen being delivered to the area leading to necrosis and perforation of the bowel. This often results in leakage of toxins into the bloodstream. The occlusion is usually sudden, allowing no time for collateral circulation to develop (Dang, 2010; Durston, 2006; Greenwald *et al.*, 2001; McKinsey & Gewertz, 1997).

In chronic mesenteric ischemia there is a gradual decrease in blood supply through the celiac, superior and inferior mesenteric arteries. This is frequently caused by atherosclerosis, and symptoms worsen when an already narrowed lumen becomes occluded. If the occlusion is severe, patients may present with acute mesenteric ischemia.

Acute colonic ischemia is also known as ischemic colitis and is the form of ischemia most usually seen in the older adult. This usually occurs when a section of the intestine does not receive the blood supply it requires, resulting in injury. This decrease is sudden and is usually not associated with a clot, but rather with an acute event where blood is shunted to the brain and other essential organs. Intestinal hypoxia can result in mucosal injury and lead to rectal bleeding. If the injury affects the entire intestinal wall, gangrene can occur and cause septic shock (Green & Tendler, 2005; Pfadt, 2010).

■ Risk factors

Acute ischemia
- Atrial fibrillation
- Congestive heart failure
- History of hypercoagulability

- Hypotension
- Older age
- Peripheral vascular disease
- Valvular disease

Chronic ischemia
- Atherosclerosis
- Diabetes
- Hypertension
- Smoking

▓ Clinical presentation

Patients with acute mesenteric ischemia present with a sudden onset of severe periumbilical pain that is out of proportion with physical findings. This may be accompanied by nausea and vomiting. Sudden pain associated with a forceful bowel movement in a patient with risk factors should heighten suspicion for this condition. Initially, physical exam may be normal or show some distention, but as the disease progresses bowel sounds will be decreased, the abdomen will become more distended, and guarding or rebound tenderness may develop (Durston, 2006; Greenwald *et al.*, 2001; McKinsey & Gewertz, 1997).

Patients with chronic mesenteric ischemia describe episodes of spasmodic pain after eating. This is caused by a decrease in blood flow to the bowel, and is sometimes referred to as intestinal angina (Flasar & Goldberg, 2006). Patients may exhibit weight loss and anorexia due to fear of increased pain. Other symptoms include nausea, vomiting, diarrhea, or constipation (Mukherjee & Tessler, 2010).

Acute colonic ischemia presents as a mild abdominal pain that has a rapid onset and is located over the affected area of the bowel, usually the left side. The patient may also display rectal bleeding or bloody diarrhea within 24 hours after the onset of pain. An urge to defecate is common. Anorexia, nausea, vomiting, or abdominal distension may be present as the result of an associated illeus. Severe ischemia or necrosis may produce leukocytosis, metabolic acidosis, or an elevated lactate (Green & Tendler, 2005).

▓ Nursing assessment

- Patient history should include presenting symptoms, medications, allergies, and past medical history.
  - Assess pain: onset. location, duration, characteristics (e.g., intensity and description (alleviating/aggravating symptoms, treatment).
- Physical assessment:
  - Monitor vital signs.
    - During the abdominal exam note if the abdomen is soft, firm, or distended.

- Determine if bowel sounds are present in all four quadrants. Note the quality of bowel sounds (tinkling or diminished). Note any tympany or dullness with percussion.
- Determine if there is abdominal tenderness and its location. Rebound tenderness or guarding are ominous signs and should be reported to the physician upon discovery.
  ○ Examine stool for occult blood.

Diagnostics

- Complete blood count
- Serum lactate, LDH, CPK amylase, phosphate
- Arterial blood gases to assess for metabolic acidosis, if indicated
- Abdominal X-ray
- Ultrasonography
- Computed tomography scan (CT scan) with contrast – primary test obtained for patients with colonic ischemia
- Mesenteric angiography – primary test for acute mesenteric ischemia
- Magnetic resonance angiography
- Colonoscopy – indicated for colonic ischemia

Differential diagnoses

- Abdominal aortic aneurysm
- Carcinoma
- Diverticulitis
- Infectious colitis
- Inflammatory bowel disease
- Radiation enteritis

Treatment

Acute mesenteric ischemia

- The goal is to restore blood flow to the intestine as quickly as possible.
- Assure hemodynamic stability with careful monitoring and adequate fluid replacement. Use vasopressors cautiously as they may further decrease blood flow to the affected area.
- Patient should have no food or drink (NPO).
- Monitor intake and output.
- Insert a nasogastric tube for decompression, if indicated.
- Correct acidosis and electrolyte imbalances.
- Anticoagulation may be initiated to stop progression of clot if patient is not bleeding.
- Possible procedures:

- Angiography and possible thrombectomy, angioplasty or placement of stent
- Thrombolytic therapy for lysis of clot
- Surgical laparotomy and embolectomy, resection of infarcted bowel if indicated.

Chronic mesenteric ischemia
- Initiate anticoagulation therapy to decrease risk of clot.
- Stents placement may be necessary to increase perfusion.
- Endarterectomy or bypass surgery may be necessary if blood supply is significantly decreased.

Acute colonic ischemia
- Patient should be NPO for bowel rest.
- Administer IV fluids as directed.
- Antibiotics are indicated in severe cases.
- Insert nasogastric tube if ileus is present.
- Monitor for increased pain, fever, and bleeding.
- Surgical intervention is required for colonic infarction. Degree of resection is influenced by the extent of intestinal injury.

■ Collaborative consultation
- Vascular surgeon for pre- and postoperative care
- Dietician for appropriate nutritional support if prolonged NPO status is anticipated
- Pharmacist to discuss potential drug interactions with anticoagulants
- Enterostomal therapist for patients requiring bowel resection

■ Complications
- Anorexia
- Bacteremia
- Death
- Necrotic bowel
- Renal failure
- Respiratory compromise
- Sepsis

■ Prevention
- Adherence to anticoagulant therapy when indicated
- Smoking cessation

■ Patient/family education
- Educate patient and family on importance of adhering to anticoagulation therapy
  - Discuss action of the medication.

- Bleeding precautions
- Desired INR, if patient is started on warfarin and importance of frequent blood tests to determine appropriate dosing.
- Dietary indications
- Educate surgical patients on appropriate wound care and monitoring for increased redness and drainage.

References

Dang, C.V. (2010) Acute mesenteric ischemia. Online. Available from http://emedicine.medscape.com/article/189146-overview (accessed 20 May 2012).

Durston, S. (2006) Puzzled about mesenteric ischemia? *Nursing Made Incredibly Easy!* **4**(3), 58–61.

Flasar, M.H. & Goldberg, E. (2006) Acute abdominal pain. *Medical Clinics of North America* **90**, 481–503.

Green, B.T. & Tendler, D.A. (2005) Ischemic colitis: A clinical review. *Southern Medical Journal* **98** (2), 217–222.

Greenwald, D.A., Brandt, L.J. & Reinus, J.F. (2001) Ischemic bowel disease in the elderly. *Gastroenterology Clinics* **30**(2), 445–473.

McKinsey, J.F. & Gewertz, B.L. (1997) Acute mesenteric ischemia. *Surgical Clinics of North America* **77**(2), 307–318.

Mukherjee, S. & Tesler, D.J. (2010) Chronic mesenteric ischemia. Online. Available from http://emedicine.medscape.com/article/183683-overview (accessed 20 May 2012).

Pfadt, E. (2010) Acute ischemic colitis. *Nursing 2010* **40**(5), 72.

PART 4: PANCREATITIS

Patricia Fitzgerald

Pancreatitis is an inflammatory condition of the pancreas usually associated with alcoholism or gallstones (Andris, 2010). It can be classified as either acute or chronic and its severity can range from mild to life threatening depending on the degree of pancreatic damage sustained.

The pancreas is located in the mid abdomen behind the stomach. It has both exocrine and endocrine functions. The exocrine function of the pancreas involves the acinar cells. These cells synthesize enzymes such as trypsin, amylase, and lipase; enzymes that are secreted into the duodenum to assist with digestion. The pancreas secretes 2–3 liters of pancreatic juices daily (Andris, 2010). The endocrine cells in the pancreas are divided into alpha, beta, and delta cells and release hormones into the bloodstream. Alpha cells are responsible for the production of glucagon, which increases and maintains glucose levels. Beta cells assist with the adjustment of glucose levels through the secretion of insulin. Delta cells inhibit the functions of the acinar, alpha and beta cells, as well as control the secretion of somatostatin. Somatostatin inhibits growth hormone, thyroid-stimulating hormone, insulin, glucagons and other gastrointestinal hormones (Andris, 2010). The inflammatory changes seen in pancreatitis can affect all of these functions.

The most common cause of pancreatitis is ductal obstruction inhibiting the secretion of pancreatic juices into the duodenum. A possible source of this obstruction can be the presence of gallstones which prevent the outflow of pancreatic enzymes or cause reflux of bile into the pancreas (Smeltzer *et al.*, 2008). This leads to the premature activation of the enzymes in the pancreas causing autodigestion, which results in inflammationand possible necrosis. Untreated, this process can lead to fluid shifts, hemorrhage, sepsis, and multiple organ failure. The resulting inflammation can affect both the exocrine and endocrine functions of the pancreas leading to problems with nutrition and glucose control.

Acute pancreatitis is a rapidly occurring inflammatory process in which the pancreas attacks itself. There are two types of acute pancreatitis: interstitial and necrotizing. Interstitial acute pancreatitis can be mild with symptoms lasting on average 3–5 days. The more severe form is acute necrotizing pancreatitis which is associated with a high rate of complications and mortality (Pfrimmer, 2008). The complication rate incidence increases with age, putting the older adult at high risk for multiple organ failure and death.

In chronic pancreatitis, recurrent inflammation destroys the pancreatic cells replacing them with fibrous tissue. Repeated attacks lead to increasing pressure and obstruction within the pancreas. Pancreatic damage occurs over time and the patient is often asymptomatic until the damage becomes severe enough to cause a mechanical obstruction or interfere with the normal function of the pancreas. The presence of these fibrotic changes in the pancreas also increases with age, putting the older adult at risk of developing pancreatic insufficiency. Chronic alcoholism is the most common cause of chronic pancreatitis, and the diagnosis often begins with an episode of acute pancreatitis (Smeltzer *et al.*, 2008).

■ Risk factors

- Alcohol abuse
- Endoscopic retrograde cholangiopancreatography (ERCP)
- Gallstones or biliary sludge
- Hypercalcemia
- Hypertriglyceridemia
- Increasing age
- Infection
- Inflammatory bowel disease
- Malignancy
- Medications
- Parenteral nutrition
- Trauma

■ Clinical presentation

Acute pancreatitis

Patients with acute pancreatitis often describe a sudden onset of sharp, deep twisting abdominal pain located in the mid-epigastrium, which may be associated with nausea and vomiting. Some report biliary colic after meals. Other symptoms include decreased bowel sounds, upper abdominal tenderness with or without rigidity, abdominal distention, and diarrhea. Many patients report a band of pain radiating to the back. The pain often occurs 24-48 hours after a heavy meal or ingestion of alcohol (Smeltzer *et al.*, 2008). Severe cases present with abdominal distention, rebound tenderness and guarding. More diffuse, severe pain may indicate necrotizing pancreatitis (Brenner & Krenzer, 2010).

Other physical findings depend on the severity of the disease. In severe cases patients may display jaundice and fever, progressing to symptoms of septic shock. Extreme fluid shifts result in a decrease in intravascular volume leading to tachycardia and hypotension. Ecchymosis may be present around the umbilicus indicating retroperitoneal bleeding. Respirations may be shallow due to the presence of pleural effusions (Andris, 2010; Pfrimmer, 2008). Serum amylase and lipase levels rise to three times the normal limit.

Chronic pancreatitis

Patients with chronic pancreatitis report similar symptoms, and recurrent attacks are common. Weight loss may occur due to anorexia associated with the severe, chronic pain. Patients also display signs of more extensive pancreatic dysfunction. Fat malabsorption leads to steatorrhea (i.e., loose, greasy, foul smelling stools). Signs of glucose intolerance can also develop (Freedman, 2010).

■ Nursing assessment

- Patient history should determine presenting symptoms, medications, allergies, past medical history and presence of risk factors:
  - Assess onset, location, duration and severity of pain as well as pain characteristics, alleviating/aggravating symptoms, and treatment tried by patient.
- Physical assessment:
  - Vital signs
    - Tachycardia and hypotension may indicate sepsis or hemorrhage.
    - Assess respiratory rate, breath sounds and O$_2$ saturation levels.
  - Monitor mental status.
  - Assess for signs of retroperitoneal hemorrhage noted by Gray Turner's and Cullen's signs, respectively hemorrhagic discoloration of the flanks and umbilicus.
  - During the abdominal exam note if the abdomen is soft, firm, or distended. Determine if bowel sounds are present in all four quadrants. Note the

quality of bowel sounds (tinkling or diminished). Note any tympany or dullness with percussion.

○ Determine if there is abdominal tenderness and its location. Rebound tenderness or guarding are ominous signs and should be reported to the physician upon discovery.

○ Examine stool for occult blood.

■ Diagnostics

- Complete blood cell count:
  - ○ Increasing WBC may be due to inflammation decreasing Hct and HgB may indicate hemorrhage.
- Amylase and lipase levels:
  - ○ Serum amylase rises within 6-12 hours of onset and returns to normal within 48-72 hours. Serum lipase rises within 24 hours but can remain elevated for 5-7 days, making it a more reliable indicator of pancreatitis.
  - ○ Serum amylase and lipase levels are often decreased in the healthy older adult. Caution should be used in interpreting results for diagnosis of pancreatitis.
- Serum electrolytes, BUN, creatinine to monitor fluid and electrolyte status
- Abdominal X-ray to rule out bowel obstruction or perforation
- Chest x-ray to determine the presence of pleural effusion
- Abdominal ultrasound to detect gallstones, examine the biliary tree, and visualize the pancreas
- Computed tomography scan (CT scan) with oral and intravenous contrast
- Magnetic resonance cholangiopancreatography (MRCP)
- Endoscopic retrograde cholangiopancreatogram (ERCP) –Pancreatic surgery

■ Differential diagnoses

- Biliary colic
- Cholecystitis
- Ischemic bowel, though that pain is usually more transient

■ Treatment

Acute pancreatitis

- Monitor vital signs.
  - ○ Monitor O_2 saturation and administer supplemental oxygen as indicated.
- Patient should be NPO until amylase and lipase levels return to normal and pain subsides.
- Administer IV fluids as ordered.
  - ○ Monitor fluid status (careful intake and output).
- Monitor CBC, Serum glucose, serum electrolytes, BUN, creatinine, amylase and lipase levels.

- Insert nasogastric tube for drainage if ileus is present.
- Assess pain and administer analgesics as ordered. Morphine and Dilaudid are preferred.
- Monitor bowel status.
- Administer proton pump inhibitors or H_2 blockers to decrease gastric secretions.
- In patients with prolonged illness, consider jejunal feedings to maintain adequate nutrition. If these are not tolerated parenteral feedings should be initiated.
- Drainage of pancreatic abscesses may be necessary:
  - Record amount of drainage.
  - Keep drain site clean to prevent skin breakdown and infection.

Chronic pancreatitis
- ERCP to remove pancreatic duct stones and release strictures.
- Monitor patient for acute respiratory distress syndrome (ARDS) after ERCP:
  - Dyspnea
  - Tachypnea
  - Decreased oxygen saturation
- Pain management
- Pancreatic enzyme replacement
- Glucose management for diabetes caused by pancreatic destruction
- Counseling on abstinence from alcohol ingestion
- Surgical intervention:
  - Drainage or removal of pseudocyst
  - Pancreaticojejunostomy (Roux-en-Y)
  - Pancreaticoduodenectomy (Whipple procedure)
  - Gallbladder surgery

▨ Collaborative consultation
- Consult nutritionist to determine appropriate methods of feeding.
- Prolonged hospitalization can lead to deconditioning. Consult Physical and Occupational therapy to assist patient's return to baseline level of functioning.
- Consult social services to assist with alcohol counseling and referral to out-patient alcohol rehabilitation programs.

▨ Complications
- Ascites
- Bile duct or intestinal obstruction
- Death
- Hemorrhage
- Pancreatic diabetes
- Pancreatic Insufficiency

- Pancreatic necrosis
- Pleural effusion
- Pseudoaneurysms
- Pseudocyst formation
- Sepsis
- Splenic vein thrombosis

■ Prevention

- Avoid ingestion of high fat foods, heavy meals, and alcohol.

■ Patient/family education

- Reinforce the need for low fat diet.
- Stress the importance of abstaining from alcohol.
- Educate patients on medications and possible side effects.
- Discuss glucose monitoring with patients showing alterations in glucose management.
- Encourage patient to seek medical attention if symptoms recur.
- Discuss use of pancreatic enzymes and other medications.

References

Andris, A. (2010) Pancreatitis: Understanding the disease and implications for care. *AACN Advanced Critical Care* **21**(2), 195-204.

Brenner, Z. & Krenzer, M. (2010) Understanding acute pancreatitis. *Nursing 2010* **40**(1), 32-37.

DiMagno, M.J. & DiMagno, E.P. (2009) Chronic pancreatitis. *Current Opinion in Gastroenterology* **25**, 454-459.

Pfrimmer, M. (2008) Acute pancreatitis. *The Journal of Continuing Education in Nursing* **39**(8), 341-342.

Smeltzer, S.C., Bare, B.G., Hinkle, J.L. & Cheever, K.H. (2006) *Brunner and Suddarth's Textbook of Medical-Surgical Nursing*, 11th edition. Lippincott, Williams & Wilkins, Philadelphia.

PART 5: CONSTIPATION

Patricia Fitzgerald

Constipation is a common complaint in the older adult, but the actual definition of this disorder may vary from patient to patient. The most commonly accepted definition of constipation is a frequency of stools less than three times a week (Crane & Talley, 2007). Many elders who complain of constipation do not base their concern on frequency of stools however, but rather on the need to strain when defecating. Although complaints of constipation increase with age, it is not a normal finding, and the majority of older, active, adults report normal bowel function (Bouras & Tangalos, 2009). The incidence of constipation rises in patients who reside in community dwellings (Crane & Talley, 2007) and is most frequently reported in female patients (Higgins & Johanson, 2004). Chronic constipation has been associated with impairment in quality of life and increased healthcare costs (Gallegos-Orozco et al., 2012).

Constipation can be classified as either primary or secondary. Primary constipation is not related to an existing medical condition or medication. There are three categories of primary chronic constipation: normal transit constipation, slow transit constipation, and defecatory dysfunction.

With normal transit constipation, stool frequency is usually within the normal range, but patients often complain of difficulty passing stool, bloating, and pain. Slow transit constipation occurs when the time it takes for stool to move through the colon is prolonged. Slowing of intestinal peristalsis associated with aging can contribute to this type of constipation (Mauk, 2006). Defecatory dysfunction is the difficulty with the passage of stool. This may be associated with pelvic floor dysfunction. Aging can cause structural changes of the pelvic floor musculature leading to changes in bowel function. This category of dysfunction is commonly seen in older adults, especially in women (Hall et al., 2007).

Secondary constipation is directly related to a medical condition or is caused by medication. Some conditions leading to secondary constipation are:

- Anatomic dysfunction due to surgery or injury to the intestine
- Endocrine or metabolic disorders (hypothyroidism, hypocalcemia, hypokalemia, diabetes)
- Malignancy
- Medications (opiates, anticholinergics, antidepressant, diuretics, antipsychotics)
- Neurologic disorders (Parkinson's, spinal cord injury, dementia, stroke)
- Psychological disorders (depression)
- Rheumatologic disorders (systemic sclerosis)

■ Risk factors

- Decreased fluid intake
- Decreased privacy or inaccessibility of facilities
- Depression
- Female sex
- Impaired mobility or decrease in level of activity
- Low fiber diet
- Low socioeconomic status
- Medications (analgesics anticholinergics, antidepressants, diuretics)
- Pelvic floor dysfunction (PFD)

■ Clinical presentation

Because patients have different perceptions of the term constipation, presenting symptoms may vary. Along with a decreased frequency of bowel movements, patients often describe:

- Excessive straining
- Sensation of incomplete rectal emptying
- Presence of hard stool
- Requirement for manual maneuver to achieve evacuation

In some more severe cases patients may complain of abdominal pain, nausea, or vomiting. Symptoms that have persisted for more than 3 months with an onset of at least 6 months prior to diagnosis lead to a diagnosis of chronic constipation (Hall *et al.*, 2007).

■ Nursing assessment

- Obtain a thorough health history including existing medical conditions and current patient medications including laxatives and stool softeners.
  - Determine patient's present diet and amounts of fiber and liquid intake per day.
  - Elicit information about patient's regular pattern of bowel elimination and any recent changes:
    - What is the frequency and consistency of stools?
    - Is there any particular activity that keeps your bowel pattern regular?
    - Is there any fecal incontinence?
    - Is there any straining with defecation?
    - Identify any lifestyle changes that may have contributed to the change in bowel pattern such as recent immobility, decrease in activity level or surgical procedure.
  - Ask hospitalized or rehabilitation patients daily when the last bowel movement was and document per institutional policy.
  - Ask patients about any changes in urinary pattern as there may be an association with constipation.
- Focused abdominal exam
  - During the abdominal exam note if the abdomen is soft, firm, or distended. Determine if bowel sounds are present in all four quadrants. Note the quality of bowel sounds (tinkling or diminished). Note any tympany or dullness with percussion.
    - Determine if there is abdominal tenderness and its location. Rebound tenderness or guarding are ominous signs and should be reported to the physician upon discovery.
  - Perform a rectal exam to assess for impaction.
  - Stool for occult blood

■ Diagnostics

- Diagnostic testing is not always indicated, but since a change in bowel pattern is an indicator of colon cancer, colonoscopy is recommended when the following conditions occur:
  - Family history of colon cancer
  - Blood in the stool
  - Anemia
  - Unexplained weight loss of greater than 4.5 kg (10 pounds)
- Complete blood count, serum calcium studies, and thyroid function tests to rule out underlying causes of constipation
- Colonic transit studies
- Anorectal manometry

■ Differential diagnosis

- The differential diagnosis is concerned with determining the cause of the constipation. Hypothyroidism, electrolyte disorders, medications, and diet are possible causes. Other disorders to be considered include:
- Colon obstruction
- Ileus
- Irritable bowel syndrome
- Malignancy
- Motility disorder
- Toxic megacolon

■ Treatment

Non-pharmacologic interventions

- Eliminate the causative factor if possible. If this is not possible, a prophylactic medication should be added to the patient's current therapy.
- Gradually increase fiber by 5 g per day at 1 week intervals until goal is met (Hall *et al.*, 2007). A sudden increase in fiber can lead to bloating and flatulence.
- Ensure adequate intake of fluids. This is especially important when increasing fiber in the diet.
- Foods such as prunes and rhubarb have been shown effective in treating and preventing constipation.
- Consumption of beverages containing caffeine are helpful, especially when consumed in the morning when the natural urge to defecate most commonly occurs.
- Increase activity.
- Establish a regular daily routine that will allow the patient to respond to the urge to defecate.
- Pelvic floor rehabilitation and biofeedback have been proven to be effective in strengthening pelvic floor muscles in patients with PFD.

Table 3.4.5.1 Examples of osmotic laxatives.

Medication	Action	Side effects/precautions
Saline laxatives Milk of magnesia Citrate of magnesia Sodium biphosphate	Water is drawn into the intestinal lumen by osmosis.	Use with caution in patients with renal or heart failure as they can cause electrolyte imbalances, fluid overload, and diarrhea
Osmotic laxatives Lactulose Sorbitol Polyethylene glycol (PEG)	Water is drawn into the intestinal lumen by osmosis	PEG may cause excessive stooling, electrolyte imbalance, and abdominal pain

Pharmacologic interventions

- Bulking agents such as Psyllium and methylcellulose may improve symptoms of constipation by adding bulk to the stool. They are sometimes better tolerated by patients than an increase in dietary fiber (Bouras & Tangalos, 2009). These are best tolerated in patients with normal transit constipation.
- Stool softeners such as docusate sodium are sometimes helpful to those complaining of hard stool, though studies have failed to show their effectiveness (Hall *et al.*, 2007).
- Osmotic laxatives work by drawing water into the bowel (Bouras & Tangalos, 2009) (see Table 3.4.5.1).
- Stimulant laxatives such as senna and biscodyl promote increased intestinal motility and draw water into the bowel. Although these drugs have not been shown to cause increased bowel injury, they should be reserved for patients who have not responded to osmotic laxatives and those with constipation related to opiate use. Adverse effects include abdominal distention, electrolyte imbalances and hepatic toxicity (Bouras & Tangalos, 2009).
- Suppositories and enemas can be helpful in patients with obstructive constipation, but should be used cautiously.

Surgical interventions

Patients with slow transit constipation that does not respond to medical management may require surgical intervention such as a subtotal colectomy.

■ Collaborative consultation

- Consult pharmacist to determine role of medications in constipation and discuss possible alternatives with physician.
- Consult nutritionist to compile list of high fiber foods.
- Obtain physical therapy consult for biofeedback and pelvic floor rehabilitation for patients with PFD related constipation.

■ Complications

- Bowel ischemia
- Bowel obstruction
- Diarrhea
- Fecal Impaction
- Fecal Incontinence
- Hemorrhoids
- Megacolon
- Urinary tract infection

■ Prevention

- Increase fiber in the diet.
- Increase activity level as tolerated.
- Assure an adequate fluid intake.
- Provide a time period each day to respond to the urge to defecate, usually after breakfast.

■ Patient/family education

- Educate patient and family about the importance of adequate fiber intake in preventing constipation.
- Reinforce the importance of responding to the urge to defecate.
- Remind patient that sitting in a position with the back leaning backwards somewhat assists in evacuation of stool.
- Explain all medications, actions, and possible side effects.
- Encourage patient to increase fluid intake to 1.5-2 liters/day unless contraindicated by patient's other medical conditions.
- Assist patient in developing a plan to increase physical activity.

References

Bouras, E.P. & Tangalos, E.G. (2009) Chronic constipation in the elderly. *Gastroenterology Clinics* **38**(3), 463-480.

Camilleri, M, Lee, J.S. Viramontes, B., Bharucha, A.E. & Tangalos, E.G. (2000) Insights into the pathophysiology and mechanisms of constipation, irritable bowel syndrome and diverticulosis in older people. *Journal of the American Geriatrics Society* **48**(9), 1142-1150.

Crane, S. & Talley, N.J. (2007) Chronic gastrointestinal symptoms in the elderly. *Clinics in Geriatric Medicine* **23**, 721-773.

Gallegos-Orozco, J.F., Foxx-Orenstein, A.E., Sterler, S. M. & Stoa, J.M. (2012) Chronic constipation in the elderly. *American Journal of Gastroenterology* **107**(1), 18-25.

Hall, K.E., Cash, B.D. & Chang, L. (2007) Managing constipation in the elderly: A CME accredited activity. *Geriatrics*. Online. Available from http://geriatrics.modernmedicine.com/geriatrics/data/articlestandard/geriatrics/332007/449332/article.pdf (accessed 28 May 2012).

Higgins P.D, & Johanson J.F. (2004). Epidemiology of constipation in North America: a systematic review. *American Journal of Gastroenterology* **99**, 750-759.

Mauk, K.L. (2005) Preventing constipation in older adults. *Nursing 2005* **35**(6), 22-23.

Mauk, K. (2006) *Gerontological nursing: Core competencies for care.* Jones and Bartlett Learning, Sudbury, MA.

Tangalos, E.G. (2009) Managing chronic constipation in long term care settings. Online. Available from http://www.annalsoflongtermcare.com/content/managing-chronic-constipation-long-term-care-settings (accessed 21 March 2012).

PART 6: DIARRHEA

Patricia Fitzgerald

Diarrhea is defined as an increase in the frequency and volume of stool. Stools are often described as loose, watery, or fatty. Although many body systems show a decline in function with aging, the absorptive and secretory functions of the bowel do not show any significant changes. There does, however, appear to be some decline in the nervous system of the bowel leading to changes in motility (Schiller, 2009). Despite these changes, the incidence of diarrhea does not increase with aging; but the negative impact of diarrhea is felt more strongly in the older adult. The presence of other medical illnesses or general physiologic decline may make older adults less able to withstand the fluid and electrolyte losses associated with this condition (Schiller, 2009). In addition, physiological compensatory responses to dehydration, such as thirst, may be blunted in older adults (Akhtar, 2003). Older adults who complain of excessive diarrhea often require hospitalization to ensure adequate hydration and monitoring.

Diarrhea can be classified as chronic or acute depending upon the length of time symptoms have been present. The most common cause of acute diarrhea is infection. The number of older adults residing in communal residences and nursing homes may contribute to an increase in the spread of pathogens in this population. Although infections, fecal impaction, or drugs are found to be important causes of acute diarrhea in older patients, in 30 to 50% of all cases of diarrhea precise etiology remains unknown (Akhtar, 2003). Chronic diarrhea is often broken down further into secretory, osmotic, and inflammatory in origin. Secretory diarrhea is caused by a decrease in the absorption of fluid and electrolytes in the bowel, usually caused by an increased transit time. Osmotic diarrhea is generally due to the ingestion of a substance that is poorly absorbed, drawing more water into the bowel. Inflammatory diarrhea is associated with an underlying inflammatory condition. Blood or pus in the stool is characteristic of this type of diarrhea (Schiller, 2009).

■ Risk factors

Acute diarrhea:
● Constipation especially when associated with opioid therapy.

Table 3.4.6.1 Medications associated with diarrhea.

- Acid reducing agents – H$_2$ blockers, proton pump inhibitors
- Antacids
- Antiarrhythmics – quinidine, Pronestyl
- Antibiotics
- Anti-inflammatory agents
- Antihypertensives
- Antineoplastics
- Antiretroviral
- Colchicine
- Heavy metals
- Theophylline
- Misoprostol
- Herbal products
- Vitamins and minerals

Source: Schiller, 2009.

Infection:
- Common pathogens include:
  - *Salmonella*, *Shigella*, *Campylobacter*, *Clostridium difficile*, *Escherichia coli*, norovirus, rotavirus, *Giardia*, *Cryptosporidium*

Medications (see Table 3.4.6.1)
Tube feedings

Chronic diarrhea
Secretory diarrhea

- Bile acid malabsorption
- Endocrine diseases
  - Diabetes, Addison's disease, hyperthyroidism
- Gastrointestinal surgery
- Irritable bowel syndrome
- Medications (see Table 3.4.6.1)
- Microscopic colitis
- Radiation therapy

Osmotic diarrhea

- Lactose intolerance – the ability to break down lactose decreases with age.

Inflammatory diarrhea

- Inflammatory disease
  - Crohn's disease, ulcerative colitis, diverticulitis, ischemic colitis, infection, neoplasm, radiation colitis

Fatty diarrhea

- Malabsorption syndromes
  - Celiac disease
  - Pancreatic insufficiency
  - Short bowel syndrome

■ Clinical presentation

Acute diarrhea

Acute diarrhea is defined as occurring for less than 14 days. Patients complain of a frequent passage of watery stools. They may also describe abdominal cramping, intestinal rumbling, anorexia and thirst (Smeltzer *et al.*, 2008). In severe cases symptoms indicating dehydration may occur. These include weakness, dizziness, tachycardia, and hypotension.

Chronic diarrhea

Patients with chronic diarrhea describe similar symptoms, with onset of symptoms being more than 21 days ago. The length of time symptoms have been present will affect the degree of dehydration as well as the presence of electrolyte imbalances.

■ Nursing assessment

- Obtain thorough health history including weakness, dizziness, fever, chills, nausea, vomiting, abdominal pain, bloody or mucous stools, joint pain, recent constipation, medications, recently ingested foods, and foreign travel:
  - Past medical history is also essential as institutionalized patients may have a nosocomial related diarrhea and patients with acquired immune deficiency syndrome (AIDS) or other immunodeficiency syndrome may be susceptible to particular infectious processes, Older patients with a history of antibiotic use within the past few months may require testing for *C. difficile*.
- Obtain a description of bowel pattern including frequency, consistency, urgency and precipitating factors.
- Assess for signs of dehydration such as loss of skin turgor, thirst, sunken eyes, dry oral mucous membranes, and hypotension.
- Monitor vital signs:
  - Blood pressure and orthostatic vital sign changes: hypotension may indicate dehydration or presence of infection.
  - Tachycardia may indicate dehydration or infection. Electrolyte imbalances can lead to arrhythmia.
  - Monitor temperature for signs of infection.
- During the abdominal exam note if the abdomen is soft, firm, or distended. Determine if bowel sounds are present in all four quadrants. Note the quality of bowel sounds (tinkling or diminished). Note any tympany or dullness with

percussion. Determine if there is abdominal tenderness and its location. Rebound tenderness or guarding are ominous signs and should be reported to the physician upon discovery.

- Examine stool for occult blood.
- Assess perineal area for maceration or fissures due to frequent stool.
- For hospitalized patients an accurate tally of intake and output (including number of diarrheal stools) is essential, as well as daily weights.

■ Diagnostics

Diagnostics depend on the patient history and clinical presentation. Some patients will improve with supportive care while others will require some of the following diagnostic tests.

- Complete blood count/differential
- Serum glucose, electrolytes, magnesium, blood urea nitrogen (BUN), and creatinine
- Thyroid-stimulating hormone (TSH)
- Stool for occult blood, *C. difficile* toxin, fecal leukocytes and culture to determine presence of pathogens, or ova and parasites.
- Abdominal X-ray
- Abdominal CT scan
- Colonoscopy
- Barium enema
- Colon biopsy

■ Differential diagnoses
- Celiac disease
- Diverticulitis
- Infection
- Inflammatory bowel disease
  - Crohn's disease
  - Ulcerative colitis
- Irritable bowel disease
- Ischemic colitis
- Medication side effect
- Mesenteric ischemia
- Neoplasm
- Overflow diarrhea due to obstipation
- Radiation colitis
- Tube feedings

■ Treatment

The goal of treatment is to identify and treat the cause of the diarrhea and treat any associated conditions (e.g., dehydration).

- Administer intravenous or oral fluids as directed.
- Correct electrolyte imbalances.
- Discontinue laxatives or other medications implicated in the cause of the diarrhea.
- Eliminate causative factor if possible.
- Treat underlying conditions.
- Antibiotic therapy is used when bacterial cause is found.
- If no infection is found, and there is no blood in the stool, discuss with physician the administration of antidiarrheals such as loperamide (Imodium) or **diphenoxylate/atropine** (Lomotil). Narcotic medications are usually poorly tolerated in older adults (Schiller, 2009).
- Monitor vital signs including postural vital signs.
- Weigh patient daily and report any weight loss to physician.
- Calculate fluid intake and output daily and discuss with physician fluid replacement strategy for the next 24 hours.
- Provide skin care to prevent breakdown from maceration.

■ Collaborative consultation

- Consult pharmacist for assistance in identifying any medication or drug-drug interaction that may be contributing to diarrhea.
- Collaborate with dietician to determine appropriate tube feeding formula and rate to decrease diarrhea.
- Consult with physican and dietician to determine appropriate advancement of diet, and dietary modifications necessary to assure adequate nutrition.

■ Complications

- Anorexia
- Cardiac arrhythmias
- Dehydration
- Electrolyte imbalances
- Fecal incontinence
- Hypotension
- Paresthesias
- Sepsis
- Skin breakdown
- Weakness

■ Prevention

- Strict hand hygiene after using the bathroom is essential to prevent the spread of pathogens.
- Health care workers should practice hand hygiene before and after interacting with any patient.

- Wash hands well before handling foods.
- Eat only well cooked meats.
- Wash all produce well.
- Tube feeding preparations should be hung for no more than 6-8 hours, and tubing should be changed daily or per institution policy.
- Avoid medications containing sorbitol as they may increase diarrhea.

■ Patient/ family education

- Explain etiology of diarrhea and potential interventions to prevent recurrence.
- Stress the importance of appropriate hand hygiene.
- Describe interventions to prevent skin breakdown.
- Educate patient on proper timing of medication to reduce incidence of diarrhea.

References

Akhtar, A.J. (2003) Acute diarrhea in frail elderly nursing home patients. *Journal of the American Medical Directors Association* **4**(1), 34-9.

Schiller, L.R. (2009) Diarrhea and malabsorption in the elderly. *Gastroenterology Clinics of North America* **38**, 481-502.

Smeltzer, S.C., Bare, B.G., Hinkle, J.L. & Cheever, K.E. (2006) *Brunner and Suddarth's Textbook of Medical-Surgical Nursing*, 11th edition. Lippincott, Williams & Wilkins, Philadelphia.

Further reading

Headstrom, P.D. & Surawicz, C.M. (2005) Chronic diarrhea. *Clinical Gastroenterology and Hepatology* **3**(8), 734-737.

Juckett, G., & Trivedi, R. (2011) Evaluation of chronic diarrhea. *American Family Physician* **84**(10), 1119-1126.

PART 7: GASTROESOPHAGEAL REFLUX DISEASE

Patricia Fitzgerald

The back up of stomach contents into the esophagus is a common complaint among older adults leading to the diagnosis of gastroesophageal reflux disease (GERD). However, the presence of heartburn or regurgitation of stomach contents alone does not define the disease. An international group defined GERD as "a condition which develops when the reflux of stomach contents causes troublesome symptoms or complications" (Richter, 2007, p. 577). Symptoms occurring more than twice a week and the resulting mucosal damage of the esophagus are examples of this. GERD occurs in people of all ages, but in the older adult it can become a chronic problem affecting the quality of life.

GERD may be related to several physiologic changes associated with aging. These include decreased tone of the lower esophageal sphincter, decreased peristalsis, delayed emptying of the stomach, and increased pressure in the stomach and abdomen (Mauk, 2006).

Older adults tend to present with much more severe disease, commonly involving the esophageal mucosa, leading to the development of GERD complications. Therefore, the diagnosis and treatment of GERD should be pursued more aggressively in elder patients (Poh *et al.*, 2010). If left untreated, GERD can lead to erosion of the esophagus and the development of Barrett's esophagus, a precursor to esophageal cancer (Mauk, 2006).

■ Risk factors

- Activities increasing intra-abdominal pressure such as lifting heavy objects
- Advancing age
- Hiatal hernia
- Incompetent sphincter
- Ingestion of large meals before bedtime
- Intake of alcohol, chocolate, carbonated beverages, peppermint, spicy and acidic foods
- Male sex
- Medications:
  - Anticholinergics
  - Narcotics
  - Calcium channel blockers
  - Theophylline
- Obesity
- Smoking

■ Clinical presentation

The most common complaint of patients with GERD is heartburn. This is described as a burning sensation that is located behind the sternum and most commonly occurs after meals. Another symptom often reported is the reflux of stomach contents into the esophagus. Lying down or bending over may make these symptoms worse. Patients who have had symptoms for a long period of time may often report dysphagia (difficulty swallowing) as well. Other less commonly reported symptoms are chest pain, nausea, or the feeling of a lump in the throat. GERD is difficult to diagnose in the older adult because they may have an altered pain perception. Older adults are sometimes asymptomatic or report symptoms not usually associated with GERD such as a hoarse voice, coughing, and respiratory issues such as wheezing and asthma (Crane & Talley, 2007; Poh *et al.*, 2010).

▣ Nursing assessment

- Encourage patient to describe symptoms, as well as precipitating and relieving factors.
- Review medications as well as foods.
  - Medications such as some hormones, anticholinergics, calcium channel blockers and theophylline can increase symptoms.
  - Patients may have different triggers, but, in general, foods associated with GERD include alcohols, coffee, tea, juices, tomatoes, tomato sauce, spicy foods, fried foods, mints, chocolate, high fat foods (e.g., macaroni and cheese), and doughnuts.
- If patient reports chest pain, an electrocardiogram is necessary and vital signs should be monitored to rule out a cardiac origin to symptoms. During the abdominal exam note if the abdomen is soft, firm, or distended. Determine if bowel sounds are present in all – four quadrants. Note the quality of bowel sounds (tinkling or diminished). Note any tympany or dullness with percussion. Determine if there is abdominal tenderness and its location. Rebound tenderness or guarding are ominous signs and should be reported to the physician upon discovery.
- Examine stool for occult blood.

▣ Diagnostics

Diagnosis is primarily based on patient history and symptoms. However, older adults may present with atypical symptoms of GERD which may delay the diagnosis and the start of treatment.

- Proton pump inhibitor (PPI) test is the simplest method of diagnosing GERD. Patients are prescribed a PPI for 1-2 weeks. If symptoms disappear during therapy, and return after discontinuation of the medication, the diagnosis of GERD is established (Richter, 2007).
- Upper endoscopy (esophagoscopy) is recommended for patients who have troublesome dysphagia or who have failed to improve after conservative treatment.
  - Most patients with new onset GERD after age 50 require endoscopy to exclude more serious pathology.
- Ambulatory pH monitoring is helpful in confirming GERD in patients with persistent symptoms who have had a negative upper endoscopy.
- Barium swallow can identify structural defects and alterations in peristalsis especially in patients with dysphagia.

▣ Differential diagnosis

- Angina
- Biliary tract disease
- *Candida*

- Infectious esophagitis
- Peptic ulcer disease
- Pill esophagitis

■ Treatment

- Elimination of risk factors: smoking, alcohol, obesity
- Elevation of the head of the bed on 4 to 6 inch blocks to decrease reflux.
- PPIs are considered the mainstay of treatment for both younger and older patients with GERD.
- Histamine-2 receptor antagonists (H_2RAs) can be used as an adjunctive therapy for breakthrough symptoms in elder patients who have failed PPI therapy taken twice daily. However, if possible H_2RAs (particularly cimetidine) as should be avoided in older adults as they may cause confusion.
- Anti-reflux surgery

■ Collaborative consultation

- Consult dietician to develop a dietary plan to decrease symptoms.
- Consult pharmacist and physician about medications that may increase GERD, and discuss possible alternatives.
- Report any acute increase in symptoms or medication side effects to physician.
- Discuss prescription of medications to aid in smoking cessation.

■ Complications

- Asthma
- Barrett's esophagus
- Chronic pneumonia due to aspiration
- Esophageal cancer
- Esophagitis
- Peptic esophageal strictures

■ Prevention

- Avoid smoking and alcohol.
- Avoid activities that will increase intra-abdominal pressure.
- Avoid eating or drinking 3-4 hours before bedtime.
- Eat small meals to decrease gastric distention and prevent reflux.
- Limit ingestion of foods known to contribute to GERD.

■ Patient/family education

- Educate patient on the contribution of smoking to GERD symptoms. Refer to smoking cessation program or assist in development of smoking cessation plan.

- Provide patients with a list of foods that may contribute to GERD:
  - Chocolate, peppermint, caffeine, coffee, tea, juices, carbonated beverages, alcohol, fried foods, acidic, and spicy foods
- Encourage patient to limit alcohol intake.
- Teach patient to avoid lying down after eating a large meal as this may contribute to reflux. If this can not be avoided encourage elevation of the head of the bed or a side lying position.
- Counsel patient on weight loss.
- Explain to patient the prescribed medications and common side effects.
- Advise patient to report any acute change in symptoms or drug side effects to physician.
- Discuss with patient the need to reconsult physician if symptoms do not resolve at the completion of the course of medication.

References

Crane, S. & Talley, N.J. (2007) Chronic gastrointestinal symptoms in the elderly. *Clinics in Geriatric Medicine* **23**, 721-734.

Mauk, K. (2006) *Gerontological nursing: Core competencies for care*. Jones and Bartlett Learning, Sudbury, MA.

Poh, C.H., Navarro-Rodgriguez, T. & Fass, R. (2010) Review: treatment of gastroesophageal reflux disease in the elderly. *American Journal of Medicine* **123**(6), 496-501.

Richter, J. (2007) The many manifestations of gastroesophageal reflux disease: Presentation, evaluation, and treatment. *Gastroenterology Clinics of North America* **36**, 577-599.

Further reading

Yuhong, Y. & Hunt, R. (2009) Current issues in the management of reflux disease? *Current Opinions in Gastroenterology* **25**, 342-351.

Unit 5: Genitourinary Disorders

PART 1: ACUTE KIDNEY INJURY

Carol A. Tyksienski

Acute kidney injury (AKI) formerly referred to as acute renal failure, accounts for 20-23% of all hospitalizations (USRDS, 2009). AKI is greater with increased age and in older males of African American descent (USRDS, 2009). The Medicare database of 2007 reported an increased incidence of AKI in patients 85 years and older at 27.6% (per 1000 patient years) compared to those 60-69 years of age (8.9%) (USRDS, 2009). These numbers may underestimate the overall incidence of AKI due to the hospital coding of AKI episodes (USRDS, 2009).

Medicare patients age 80 and older have a 41% higher incidence of in-hospital death during an AKI episode than those patients 66-70 years of age (USRDS, 2009). The death rate following discharge for an AKI episode is two times higher for Medicare patients age eighty and older. Elder patients with a history of diabetes and after discharge from an AKI episode are 24% more likely to progress to end stage renal disease (ESRD) (USRDS, 2009).

The kidney undergoes both structural and functional changes as it ages. At 40 years of age the kidney reaches its maximum size and declines thereafter at a rate of 10% for every ten years (Lerma, 2009). This decrease in renal mass is related to "cortical thinning and the loss in number of functioning nephrons" (Lerma, 2009). The number of older adults with glomerulosclerosis (fibrosis of the renal glomeruli), and/or hypertrophy (increase in size of the kidney) increases by the eighth decade of life. Diverticuli may develop in the distal tubule and collecting duct which may lead to urinary tract infections, by harboring bacteria and predisposing the elder to recurrent infections. Vascular changes in the kidney may also occur with the elder population. Thickening of arterioles are common in those with a history of hypertension.

A decrease in renal blood flow (RBF) and a decline in glomerular filtration rate (GFR) occurs at a rate of one milliliter per year after about thirty years of age (Zhou *et al.*, 2009) and with a greater decline noted in males (Lerma, 2009). These changes lead to an increased risk in the development of AKI. It is noted that not all individuals experience a decrease in GFR especially the elder who remains normotensive (Lerma, 2009).

GFR is estimated based on the serum creatinine level. Several factors may influence the creatinine level; these factors include nutritional status, protein intake and muscle mass. Serum creatinine is not a reliable indicator of renal function in elders due to the decrease in muscle mass that occurs in the aging individual. The release of serum creatinine into the bloodstream is variable and therefore abnormal values may not be detected until there is a significant loss in kidney function (Bagshaw & Bellomo, 2007).

Two formulas have been used to calculate the GFR: the Cockcroft-Gault and the Modification of Diet in Renal Disease (MDRD). The accuracy of both of these formulas in estimating the GFR in the older population remains questionable and has not been validated in individuals greater than seventy years of age (Zhou *et al.*, 2009). Utilizing the MDRD formula resulted in higher estimates of GFR than the Cockcroft-Gault (Berman & Hostetter, 2007). This finding is especially important when considering drug dosing in the older adult, as there is an increased risk of drug toxicity when overestimating the GFR. In older patients, the Cockcroft-Gault formula is preferred when estimating the GFR for drug dosing to avoid (Zhou *et al.*, 2009).

Cockcroft-Gault formula for males

$$\frac{(140 - age) \times (body\ weight\ in\ kg)}{(72) \times (serum\ creatinine\ in\ mg/dl)}$$

Cockcroft-Gault formula for females

$$\frac{(140 - age) \times (body\ weight\ in\ kg) \times 0.85}{(72) \times (serum\ creatinine\ in\ mg/dl)}$$

There is an alteration in the tubular function of the aging kidney. Urinary sodium excretion is reduced and increased total body sodium may lead to hypertension in elders. Tubular scarring and atrophy may lead to impaired potassium excretion resulting in hyperkalemia. This occurs more often in elders treated with medications that are potassium sparing, like diuretics (Lerma, 2009).

■ Risk factors

- Advanced age
- Cancer chemotherapy
- Cardiogenic shock
- Chronic diseases: hypertension, diabetes mellitus, cardiovascular, peripheral vascular disease, congestive heart failure, benign prostatic hypertrophy and multiple myeloma
- Contrast media
- Exposure to nephrotoxic medications: angiotensin-converting enzyme inhibitors (e.g., lisinopril, Altace, enalapril, Zestril), aminoglycosides (e.g., amikacin, gentamicin, tobramycin), non-steroidal anti-inflammatory agents, antibiotics (e.g., penicillins, cephalosporins, sulfonamides, ciprofloxacin, rifampin), diuretics (furosemide, and potassium-sparing diuretics), and immunosuppressants
- Hypovolemia

- Multisystem organ failure
- Septic shock
- Trauma with significant blood loss and muscle damage
- Urinary tract obstruction

■ Clinical presentation

There are three major categories of AKI: prerenal, intrinsic and postrenal, identified by the physiological changes assessed in the patient. Older patients may have multiple contributing causes of AKI and these categories may overlap.

Prerenal AKI

Prerenal AKI is related to under perfusion of the kidneys and is frequently associated with intravascular volume depletion which may be seen in elders with congestive heart failure (CHF). Diuretic use in the older adult (elderly) may be related to 40% of prerenal cases of AKI (Abdel-Kader & Palevsky, 2009). Other causes include renal arterial disease resulting in renal artery stenosis and embolic disease (i.e., septic or cholesterol).

The clinical presentation and common causes of volume depletion in prerenal AKI include: diarrhea, vomiting, blood loss related to hemorrhage, increased losses from diuretic use, pancreatitis, and third-spacing after surgery. The treatment of prerenal AKI includes fluid resuscitation and discontinuing the medications that lead to volume depletion with the goal of restoring renal function.

Intrinsic AKI

Intrinsic AKI involves structural damage within the kidney, predominately damage to the tubular epithelium. Causes of intrinsic AKI include: acute tubular necrosis, renovascular obstruction, glomerular disease, glomerulonephritis, collagen disease, vasculitis, interstitial nephritis, or intratubular obstruction.

The hospitalized elder is at an increased risk for the development of intrinsic AKI. ATN may be caused by ischemia (e.g., a severe hypotensive episodes), infection, rhabdomyolysis, or drug toxicity. ATN post surgery may be related to increased gastrointestinal losses or blood loss. The goal of treatment is to correct the primary disorder, provide fluid resuscitation, avoid drug toxicity, and to remove the offending agent.

Postrenal AKI

Postrenal AKI is most often due to obstruction of the upper or lower urinary tract and is common in elders. A frequent cause of urinary obstruction male is benign prostatic hypertrophy (BPH) or rarely prostatic cancer; in older females pelvic and retroperitoneal malignancy is associated with postrenal AKI. Overall, the obstruction may present as partial or complete. The patient with partial obstruction may report symptoms of pain in flank or abdomen, difficulty with voiding and reporting frequency, urgency, hesitancy, hematuria or nocturia. Complete obstruction is characterized by anuria; the patient may report pain in flank or abdomen and suprapubic fullness. The treatment of postrenal AKI is to relieve the obstruction as soon as possible to promote recovery of renal function. A bladder scan or bladder catheterization will confirm urinary retention.

■ Nursing assessment

The patient history is concerned with obtaining information that would identify an event, agent, or an obstruction in the urinary tract that has caused kidney injury. History may be expanded upon as information is gathered in a particular area.

- History of recent surgery, abdominal trauma, falls, cardiac, kidney or liver disease, or infection
- Medical tests that would require nothing by mouth or bowel preparations leading to hypovolemia, dietary fluid restriction, fevers
- Medications that would lead to hypovolemia and decrease in systemic circulation: diuretics and antihypertensives
- Exposure to hot, humid weather for several days and poor fluid intake

Possible physical assessment findings in AKI are listed below, but must be correlated with history and laboratory results.

- Vital signs: is hypotension, tachycardia, tachypnea or fever present?
- Unexplained changes in mental status and/or changes in behavior
- Weakness
- Weight loss
- Poor skin turgor, dry mucous membranes
- Decreased jugular venous pressure
- Decreased urine volume, oliguria, anuria, hematuria, bladder distension
- Nausea, vomiting
- Flank pain, abdominal distension

■ Diagnostics

- The literature describes AKI based on increases in serum creatinine and reduction in urine output. Mehta and colleagues (2007) defined AKI as a rapid "reduction in kidney function (within 48 hours), an absolute increase in serum creatinine of more than or equal to 0.3 mg/dl ($\geq$26.4 µmol/l), a percentage increase in serum creatinine of more than or equal to 50% (1.5-fold from baseline), or a reduction in urine output (documented oliguria of less than 0.5 ml/kg per hour for more than 6 hours)".
- Serum creatinine is currently used to monitor changes in kidney function and measured urine output to gauge kidney function. Urinary chemistry has been used by medical professionals to detect early stages of AKI.

- When diagnosing AKI two serum creatinine values within 48 hours should be evaluated and urine output should be assessed along with the clinical presentation and after fluid resuscitation has been considered (Mehta *et al.*, 2007).
- The increase in creatinine is a late marker in the amount of function lost in AKI, and is influenced by age, body weight, diet and muscle mass and the diagnosis may be delayed up to seventy-two hours (Endre, 2008). Older adults may have other comorbidities that may delay and interfere with the diagnosis of AKI.
- The ADQI or RIFLE criteria may be used to classify AKI (see Box 3.5.1.1). However the AKIN and RIFLE criteria both have flaws that prevent the timely diagnosis and rapid response to failing kidney function.
- There is a need for a marker that would be specific to kidney injury and have the ability to monitor changes and the stage of kidney injury. Bagshaw and Bellomo (2007) reported that there are a number of clinical markers being investigated and validated for the early diagnosis and treatment of AKI including: Cystatin C, neutrophil gelatinase-associated lipocalin (NGAL), kidney injury molecule-1 (KIM-1) and interleukin-18 (IL-18).
- Laboratory and imaging diagnostic testing may include:
  - Urinalysis, microscopic exam of urine, specific gravity and osmolality, myoglobinuria, urinary sodium
  - Serum blood urea nitrogen (BUN), creatinine and electrolytes, albumin, LDH
  - Immunology: serum blood tests antinuclear antibody (ANA), antineutrophil cytoplasmic antibody (ANCA), antiglomerular basement membrane antibodies
  - X-rays of kidney, ureters and bladder (KUB)
  - Intravenous pyelogram (IVP)
  - Ultrasound or magnetic resonance imaging (MRI)
  - Kidney biopsy

■ Differential diagnosis

Differential diagnosis of AKI includes determining the underlying cause of kidney injury. Factors to consider include:

- Advanced cardiac failure
- Changes in mental status
- Consider allergic interstitial nephritis: when presenting patient presentation includes fever, rash, arthralgias and history of exposure to antibiotics nonsteroidal anti-inflammatory and antibiotics.
- Depletion in volume from diarrhea, hemorrhage, vomiting, increased urination or sweating
- Glomerular or tubular injuries
- Gynecologic surgery or abdominopelvic malignancy

Box 3.5.1.1 RIFLE and AKIN Criteria for Acute Kidney Injury

Bellomo *et al.* (2004) and the Acute Dialysis Quality Initiative (ADQI) work group classified AKI according to the stages of renal injury using the acronym RIFLE. The RIFLE criteria identify five stages of worsening renal function from risk to injury to failure to loss to end stage kidney disease. The first three stages: risk, injury, and failure are identified by increasing serum creatinine levels and a decrease in GFR and urine output. The fourth and fifth stages are associated with severe renal dysfunction and correspond to the need for renal replacement therapy. The fourth stage is identified by loss of renal function for more than 4 weeks and the fifth stage denoted by the letter "E" and the loss of function greater than three months.

Mehta *et al.* (2007) and the Acute Kidney Injury Network (AKIN) proposed changes to the RIFLE criteria noting that smaller changes in serum creatinine may influence morbidity and mortality. AKIN criteria were matched to the RIFLE criteria by the following: stage 2 is matched to injury and stage 3 to failure and those patients requiring renal replacement therapy (RRT). The AKIN and RIFLE criteria display common changes in urine output. It is yet to be found if the AKIN and RIFLE criteria will be widely adopted by the medical community in the diagnosis of AKIN.

A comparison of RIFLE and AKIN criteria

RIFLE	AKIN	RIFLE/AKIN
Serum creatinine or GFR	Serum creatinine	Urine output
R increased creatinine × 1.5 or GFR decrease >25%	**Stage 1** increase to ≥150% to 200% from baseline	<0.5 ml/kg hour for more than 6 hours
I increased creatinine × 2 or GFR decrease >50%	**Stage 2** increase to >200% to 300% from baseline	<0.5 ml/kg hour for more than 12 hours
F increased creatinine × 3 or GFR decrease >75%	**Stage 3** increase >300% or creatinine ≥4.0 mg/dl	<0.3 ml/kg hour for 24 hours or anuric for 12 hours
L complete loss of kidney function greater than 4 weeks		
E End stage kidney disease greater than 3 months, renal replacement therapy required		

Adapted from Endre, Z.H. (2008) Acute kidney injury: Definitions and new paradigms. *Advances in Chronic Kidney Disease* **15**(3), 213-221.

- Hyperkalemia
- Hypertensive emergencies
- Hypovolemia
- Interstitial nephritis
- Papillary lesions or necrosis
- Patient presenting with hemolysis or rhabdomyolysis
- Prostate obstruction
- Renal calculi
- Tubular obstruction, necrosis from crystals that form from medications (e.g., acyclovir, methotrexate, triamterene, indinavir or sulfonamides)

■ Treatment

It is essential to identify and treat the underlying cause of AKI. Patients will require management of fluid volume status, correction of electrolyte and acid base imbalances, and nutrition. Fluid and electrolyte disorders can be challenging in the older adult particularly when critically ill. The nurse's role will be to monitor for complications, to treat fluid and electrolyte imbalances, and continually assess the patient's response to collaborative care interventions. Continuous assessment, prompt identification and correction will prevent further renal compromise. Renal replacement therapy (RRT) may be required for those patients who have failed other interventions. The type of RRT will depend of the hemodynamic stability and clinical presentation of the patient. Continuous venovenous hemofiltration (CVVH) may be utilized for those patients hemodynamically unstable and in an intensive care setting and intermittent hemodialysis for those that are hemodynamically stable.

Nurses with specialized training provide CVVH or hemodialysis treatments. A central venous catheter will provide access to the patient's venous blood system. Catheters are the life line for the patient and should only be accessed by the specially trained nurses. Heparin is often used to maintain patency of the catheter when it is not in use. Nursing assessment includes monitoring catheter site for signs of infection.

■ Collaborative consultation

- Nephrologist
- Urologist
- Cardiologist
- Infectious disease
- Radiologist
- Transfer to a hospital that has renal replacement therapy available.

■ Complications

- Anemia related to the reduction in erythropoietin production. Erythropoietin is a hormone produced by the kidneys and responsible for the production of red blood cells.

- Hypocalcemia from the deactivation of vitamin D which results from the decrease in creatinine clearance. There is an increased risk of fractures in the older adult.
- Risk of glucose intolerance due to the aging kidney and decreased GFR insulin clearance
- Progression of AKI to chronic kidney disease which may be related to comorbidities
- Infection
- Death

■ Prevention

- Identify those patients at risk for AKI: older adults, diabetics, and patients with hypertension, cardiac disease, vascular disease and known renal impairment.
- Early identification of AKI is critical to treatment and recovery.
- Prompt consultation with a nephrologist to manage AKI.
- Maintain adequate blood pressure and fluid volume status.
- Avoid nephrotoxic agents.

■ Patient/family education

- Educate the patient and family about the causes of AKI.
- Explain any procedures or tests that may need to be performed.
- Review medications with patient and family for nephrotoxins.
- Encourage patient and family to seek medical consultation before taking any new medications both prescription and over the counter; elders are at risk for AKI due to decreased ability of kidneys to clear drugs.
- Maintain fluid intake especially in hot, humid weather.
- Dietary consultation
- Dialysis nursing staff to explain the purpose and rationale for renal replacement therapy

References

Abdel-Kader, K. & Palevsky, P.M. (2009) Acute kidney injury. *Clinical Geriatric Medicine*, **25**, 331–358.

Bagshaw, S.M. & Bellomo, R. (2007) Early diagnosis of acute kidney injury. *Current Opinion in Critical Care*, **13**, 638–644.

Bellomo, R., Ronco, C., Kellum, J.A., Mehta, R.L., Palevsky, P. & the Second International Consensus Conference of the Acute Dialysis Quality Initiative (ADQI) Group. *Critical Care* **8**, R204–R212.

Berman, N. & Hostetter, T.H. (2007) Comparing the Cockcroft–Gault and MDRD equations for calculation of GFR and drug doses in the elderly. *National Clinical Practice Nephrology* **3**(12), 644–655.

Endre, Z.H. (2008) Acute kidney injury: definitions and new paradigms. *Advances in Chronic Kidney Disease* **15**(3), 213–221.

Lerma, E.V. (2009) Anatomic and physiologic changes of the aging kidney. *Clinical Geriatric Medicine* **25**, 325-329.

Mehta, R.L., Kellum, J.A., Shah, S.V. *et al.* & the Acute Kidney Injury Network (2007) Acute Kidney Injury Network: report of an initiative to improve outcomes in acute kidney injury. *Critical Care* **11**(2). Online. Available from http://ccforum.com/content/11/2/R31 (accessed 28 May 2012).

US Renal Data System, USRDS 2009 Annual Data Report: Atlas of Chronic Kidney Disease and End-Stage Renal Disease in United States National Institutes of Health, National Institute of Diabetes & Digestive & Kidney Diseases, Bethesda, MD, 2009.

Zhou, X.J., Rakheja, D., Yu, X., Saxena, R., Vaziri, N.D. & Silva, F.G. (2008) The aging kidney. *Kidney International* **74**, 710-720.

Further reading

Bellomo, R. (2006) The epidemiology of acute renal failure: 1975 versus 2005. *Current Opinion in Critical Care* **12**, 557-560.

Counts, C.C. (ed.) (2008) *Core Curriculum for Nephrology Nursing*. Jannetti, New Jersey.

PART 2: CHRONIC KIDNEY DISEASE

Carol A. Tyksienski

Chronic kidney disease (CKD) affects approximately 26 million American adults (National Kidney Foundation [NKF], 2010). Advances in medical care and longer life span have lead to an increasing number of older adults with this chronic illness. Since 2000, the prevalent rate of chronic kidney disease patients age 65 and older has increased 24-28% (USRDS, 2009). A closer look at the prevalence of end stage renal disease (ESRD) over the last decade reveals a growth of 42% in individuals' age 65-74 years and 57% growth in those 75 and older (USRDS, 2009). In the year 2007, the ESRD incident rate for those aged 65-74 years increased 1.2% and those age 75 and older an increase of 10% (USRDS, 2009).

The NKF Kidney Disease Outcomes Quality Initiative (KDOQI) (2002) defined CKD as a gradual loss of the kidney's ability to filter the byproducts of protein metabolism. In addition, the loss of other kidney functions leads to an accumulation of fluid and electrolyte imbalance. The following conditions must be met for the diagnosis of CKD:

- Glomerular filtration rate (GFR) <60 ml/min/1.73 m^2 for 3 months or longer; with or without kidney damage
- Structural, functional abnormalities of the kidney, abnormal imaging tests, or abnormalities of blood or urine with or without decreased GFR lasting 3 months or more

The NKF developed guidelines for the clinician to identify the stages of renal failure. There are five stages of renal failure. Each stage is identified by a numerical representation of GFR.

Five stages of CKD

Stage 1: the GFR >90 ml/min/1.73 m² is normal or decreased. CKD is identified by proteinuria, abnormal urinary sediment or abnormal image testing. The patient at this stage is asymptomatic.

Stage 2: the GFR 60–89 ml/min/1.73 m² there is a mild decrease in kidney function. Usually the patient is asymptomatic. Hypertension may develop at this stage.

Stage 3: GFR 30–59 ml/min/1.73 m² the patient may be asymptomatic or laboratory abnormalities may develop identifying anemia and dyslipidemia.

Stage 4: GFR 15–29 ml/min/1.73 m² the patient develops signs and symptoms of CRF such as altered mental status, fatigue, weakness and loss of appetite.

Stage 5: GFR <15 ml/min/1.73 m² the patient will have laboratory abnormalities indicating involvement of many organ systems. Symptoms will vary among patients depending on the severity of loss of renal function. The severity of symptoms and complications will indicate the need for the initiation of renal replacement therapy (RRT).

■ Risk factors

- African-American, American Indian or Asian-American race
- Age 65 years and older
- Bladder or kidney cancer
- Diabetes
- Enlarged prostate
- Family history of kidney disease
- Glomerulonephritis
- Heart disease
- Hypertension
- Kidney infection (pyelonephritis)
- Kidney stones
- Lupus
- Obesity
- Polycystic kidney disease
- Renal artery stenosis
- Scleroderma
- Smoking
- Vasculitis

■ Clinical presentation

Generally, patients in CKD stage 1–3 do not experience any symptoms in fluid and electrolyte imbalances or metabolic abnormalities. In Stages 4–5

(GFR <30 ml/min) disturbances in fluid and electrolyte and metabolic abnormalities usually become apparent. Uremic symptoms in stage 5 are related to the accumulation of toxins. Hyperkalemia may develop when the GFR falls below twenty and the kidneys are unable to excrete potassium. Metabolic acidosis is usually present in the later stages. As the GFR falls to less than 10 ml/min, sodium retention occurs and fluid accumulates leading to peripheral edema, pulmonary edema and hypertension. Anemia develops from the kidneys' inability to synthesize the hormone erythropoietin.

■ Nursing assessment

Nursing assessment for all patients includes determining patient risk factors for CKD. Further patient history should determine the patient's past medical history, allergies, and exposure to nephrotoxic medications (e.g., nonsteroidal anti inflammatory agents (NSAIDs), antibiotics, chemotherapeutic agents or radio contrast agents) which have been identified as causing elevated creatinine levels and renal failure. Useful information also includes a history of hypertension, diabetes, and/or proteinuria and when these disorders were diagnosed. Previous consultation with a nephrologist may also be helpful.

Nursing assessment should determine if the patient has:

- Mental status changes
- Hypertension
- Weight loss: may be related to loss of appetite, nausea or vomiting related to uremia and an increase in weight related to fluid accumulation in the later stage of CKD
- Neck vein distention related to fluid accumulation
- Breath sounds: note any adventitious sounds such as rales, wheezes, and rhonchi.
- Heart sounds: auscultate for extra heart sounds such as S_3 or S_4 or pericardial friction rub. Pericardial friction rub or pleural effusions are signs of uremic pericarditis, a condition that requires urgent initiation of dialysis.
- If RRT has been initiated assess the vascular access. This access is the life line of the patient and only specially trained nurses should use this vascular access device.
- Central venous catheter: Assess site for signs of infection. Heparin may be used to maintain patency of the catheter when not in use.
- Arteriovenous fistula (AVF) and arteriovenous graft (AVG): Auscultate site for bruit (swooshing sound from blood flowing through the access) and palpate for a thrill (the vibration caused by blood flowing). Avoid taking a blood pressure or venipuncture in the extremity with a AVF or AVG.

■ Diagnostics

- Complete blood count to assess for anemia which is common in CKD
- Serum glucose, electrolytes, blood urea nitrogen (BUN), creatinine and calculation of GFR

- Serum calcium, phosphorus, vitamin D, parathyroid hormone level to look for evidence of bone disease
- Albumin, lactate dehydrogenase
- Lipid profile because of the increased risk of cardiovascular disease in CKD
- Hepatitis B and C status
- Calculation of GFR
- Urine microscopic exam aides in identifying the type of renal disease.
- 24 hour urine collection to assess protein excretion
- Renal ultrasound to identify an abscess, cysts, tumors, hydronephrosis, or malformations
- Computed tomography scan to identify obstruction, cysts, stones and tumors.
- Renal biopsy

■ Differential diagnosis

The differential diagnosis is the same as for acute renal failure:

- Advanced cardiac failure
- Changes in mental status
- Consider allergic interstitial nephritis when presenting with fever, rash, arthralgias and exposure to nonsteroidal anti-inflammatory and antibiotics.
- Depletion in volume from diarrhea, hemorrhage, vomiting, increased urination or sweating
- Glomerular or tubular injuries
- Gynecologic surgery or abdominopelvic malignancy
- Hyperkalemia
- Hypertensive emergencies
- Hypovolemia
- Papillary lesions or necrosis
- Patient presenting with hemolysis or rhabdomyolysis
- Prostate obstruction
- Renal calculi
- Tubular obstruction, necrosis from crystals that form from medications (e.g., acyclovir, methotrexate, triamterene, indinavir or sulfonamides)

■ Treatment

- In the early stages of CKD the treatment goal is to slow the progression to ESRD.
- Diagnose and if possible treat the underlying cause.
- Control hypertension: use of angiotensin-converting enzyme inhibitors (ACE inhibitor) or angiotensin-II receptor blockader (ARB) to slow the progression of CKD in patients with proteinuria and diabetic nephropathy.
- Closely monitor patients for hyperkalemia.
- Goal hemoglobin A1C: <7% for healthy elders with diabetes, but for many older adults, the goal HgA1C may need to be higher to prevent hypoglycemia.

- Avoid nephrotoxins, polypharmacy and inappropriate dosing of renally excreted drugs : IV radio contrast, NSAIDs, antibiotics (e.g., gentamicin and vancomycin).
- Symptoms of uremia will indicate the need to initiate renal replacement therapy (hemodialysis, peritoneal dialysis or renal transplantation).
- In stage 5 RRT becomes necessary for patient survival: hemodialysis is achieved by the placement of a venous catheter, AVF, or AVG for access to the bloodstream.
- Hospital nurses should collaborate with the nephrologist and hemodialysis nurse regarding administration of medications before or after the hemodialysis treatment.
- Antihypertensives may lower blood pressure during hemodialysis resulting in inability to remove excess fluid. Water soluble medications (e.g., vitamins) are removed during hemodialysis. Water soluble medications and other medications should be administered towards end of treatment or posttreatment to prevent the need for reloading a dose.
- Monitor laboratory values: serum creatinine, BUN, serum albumin, potassium, glucose, hemoglobin, hematocrit, calcium, phosphorus, white blood count and therapeutic drug monitoring (e.g., antibiotics peak and trough).
- Dietary restrictions for patients undergoing hemodialysis include:
  - fluid restriction to avoid excess fluid weight gain between dialysis treatments
  - sodium restriction
  - avoiding foods high in potassium (e.g., bananas, oranges, potatoes and tomatoes) to control serum potassium
  - avoiding foods high in phosphorus (e.g., milk, chocolate, dried beans) to control serum phosphorus and deter calcium loss from the bones
  - maintain protein (e.g., poultry and seafood) in the diet.
- Peritoneal dialysis is another option for RRT: through a surgically placed peritoneal catheter the dialysate fluid enters the peritoneal cavity, where the peritoneum acts as the semipermeable membrane removing toxins. Several exchanges of the dialysate fluid are completed daily.
- Renal transplantation is not a cure for CKD; it is a treatment for those patients in CKD stage 4 and 5 ESRD. The organ donor may be deceased or a biologically related or biologically unrelated donor.

■ Collaborative consultation

- All patients in Stage 3 or 4 CKD should be referred to a nephrologist. This will lead to better patient outcomes including decreased morbidity and mortality.
- A dietician should be consulted to educate the patient on dietary restrictions.
- In older adults, especially frail elders, the initiation of hemodialysis can become an ethical issue due to poorer outcomes in elders and the number of comorbidities in this age group (Schlanger *et al.*, 2009). Ethical concerns should be discussed with hospital based resources (e.g., pastoral care or optimal care committee) as needed.

- Timely referral to a vascular access surgeon or renal transplant center will result in a smooth transition when the need for RRT occurs.
- Social worker consultation is recommended to review patient/family eligibility requirements for ESRD Medicare benefits.

■ Complications

- Anemia
- Cardiovascular disease and mortality
- Death
- Disturbances in mineral metabolism
- Electrolyte disturbances
- Fluid volume overload
- Hypertension
- Infection
- Inflammation
- Malnutrition
- Sexual dysfunction
- Transplant rejection
- Vascular access/peritoneal catheter problems

■ Prevention

CKD prevention is accomplished with early identification and management of modifiable risk factors. Management of diabetes and hypertension is essential to prevent or delay the onset of CKD. Since elders have a higher incidence of diabetes and hypertension, the goal in this age group is to prevent CKD or delay the progression by treating the comorbidities.

■ Patient/family education

- Education should include information about
  - Progression of CKD
  - Treatment options
  - The importance of weight, blood pressure and glucose control
- Encourage adherence to medication regimen.
- Limit use of nephrotoxic medications.
- Dietary recommendations
- RRT options
- Vascular access for RRT
- Transplantation

References

National Kidney Foundation (NKF) (2002) KDOQI Clinical practice guidelines for chronic kidney disease: Evaluation, classification, and stratification. Online. Available from http://www.kidney.org/professionals/KDOQI/guidelines_ckd/toc.htm (accessed 21 March 2012).

National Kidney Foundation (NKF) (2010) The facts about chronic kidney disease. Online. Available from http://www.kidney.org/kidneyDisease/ckd/index.cfm# facts (accessed 21 March 2012).

Schlanger, L.E., Bailey, J.L. & Sands, J.M. (2009) Geriatric nephrology: Old or new subspecialty. *Clinical Geriatric Medicine* **25**, 311–324.

US Renal Data System, USRDS 2009 Annual Data Report: Atlas of Chronic Kidney Disease and End-Stage Renal Disease in United States National Institutes of Health, National Institute of Diabetes & Digestive & Kidney Diseases, Bethesda, MD, 2009.

Further reading

Counts, C.C. (ed.) (2008) *Core Curriculum for Nephrology Nursing.* Jannetti, New Jersey.

Pagana, K.D. & Pagana, T.J. (2010) *Mosby's Manual of Diagnostic and Laboratory Tests*, 4th edition. Mosby, St. Louis.

PART 3: URINARY TRACT INFECTIONS

Terry Mahan Buttaro

Although urinary tract infections (UTIs) are common infections in all older adults, these infections seem to occur more frequently in women. In the community setting, a urinary tract infection may not require hospitalization unless the infection is considered a complicated one. Uncomplicated UTIs in the community are most often associated with *Escherichia coli* (*E. coli*), *Staphylococcus saprophyticus*, *Enterobacter*, *Proteus*, or *Pseudomonas*. Complicated UTIs can be caused by these same organisms, but usually require hospitalization because they are associated with pyelonephritis, urosepsis, urinary obstruction, strictures, or urinary instrumentation.

Most healthcare-associated UTIs are associated with urinary catheterization, but immunocompetence, incontinence, and abnormalities of the urinary tract such as prostatic hypertrophy, are predisposing factors. Worldwide, nosocomial or hospital acquired urinary tract infections, can also be caused by *E. coli*, but are more frequently associated with *Enterobacter*, *Klebsiella pneumoniae*, *Pseudomonas aeruginosa*, and/or *Proteus mirabilis* (Rosenthal et al., 2006). In the United States, 32% of healthcare associated-infections are UTIs (CDC, 2009a, b). These infections are costly for the health care system and are associated with significant morbidity and mortality for patients, particularly with the increase in drug resistant bacteria.

Younger patients with a UTI are usually symptomatic. In older adults, any infection can cause just subtle changes and the older patient with a UTI or other infection may not be symptomatic. Older women, especially those living in nursing homes, frequently have asymptomatic bacteruria (bacteria in the urine of an asymptomatic person). Asymptomatic bacteruria is common in patients who have a chronic indwelling Foley catheter and these patients can have a UTI and be asymptomatic (Lo *et al.*, 2008). In these patients, a high urinary bacterial count may or may not suggest a UTI as cause of patient's status change complicating diagnosis, treatment and care. Though patients with asymptomatic bacteruria are not always treated, treatment is usually indicated prior to some urologic procedures and for men scheduled for a transureteral resection of the prostate (Nicolle *et al.*, 2006).

■ Risk factors

- Advanced age
- Atonic or neurogenic bladder
- Constipation or fecal impaction
- Immunosuppression (diabetes, cancer, or other chronic illness)
- Inadequate fluid intake
- Incontinence
- Neurologic disorder (e.g., cerebral vascular accident spinal cord injury)
- Urinary instrumentation (Foley catheter or recent urinary instrumentation)
- Urinary obstruction (e.g., benign prostatic hypertrophy [BPH], renal calculi, tumor, etc.)
- Vaginal atrophy, cystocele, or prolapse

■ Clinical presentation

The onset of illness in older patients can be acute or gradual. New or increased confusion or other change in mental or functional status is often the first sign of illness and warrants careful examination. Anorexia, vomiting, fever, or chills are possible, but not necessarily essential clinical components of illness in elders. New or more persistent urinary frequency, dribbling, or incontinence is a subtle change associated with urinary tract infections as is hematuria.

Important patient considerations include patient co-morbid illnesses, recent blood urea nitrogen (BUN) and creatinine, allergies, most recent bowel movement, current medications as well as antibiotic history within the past three months. A recent history of urinary instrumentation or urinary catheterization, as well as previous history of urinary tract abnormalities are important when discussing the change in patient status with the physician. The physician should also be made aware of the patient's history of antibiotic therapy within the past three months, because of potential drug resistance.

■ Nursing assessment

The physical examination findings may be as subtle as the clinical history. Assessment considerations include:

- Mental status changes
- Vital signs:

- Temperature: 0.9°C (2°F) degrees greater than patient baseline or greater than 37.8°C (100°F) suggests illness in an older patient. Many patients will not present with fever or chills despite serious infection or sepsis.
  - Tachycardia: Even a heart rate in the 90s may suggest onset of illness.
  - Blood pressure: Check for hypotension and orthostatic changes.
  - Weight loss, if recent, can indicate dehydration.
- Skin: exclude decubitus ulcer, cellulitis, herpes zoster, or other signs of skin infection.
- Cardiac: auscultate for signs of heart failure or pericarditis which can be associated with UTI or other illness.
- Lungs: auscultate for rales, wheezes, rhonchi to exclude heart failure (commonly associated with UTI in elders) or pneumonia.
- Abdomen: determine presence of bladder distention, abdominal or CVA tenderness. A rectal exam may be indicated to help exclude constipation which is often associated with UTIs.
- Vaginal exam if hematuria is presenting symptom to exclude vaginal bleeding.
- Penile evaluation: determine if edema, lesions, or penile discharge is present.

■ Diagnostics

- Urinalysis
  - Ten or more WBCs in urine requires urine culture and sensitivity.
  - WBC casts suggests upper urinary tract infection.
- Urine culture and sensitivity
- CBC/differential, if indicated to assess degree of leukocytosis
- Chem 8 to determine hydration status, BUN, creatinine*
- Blood cultures, if sepsis is a consideration*
- CT scan, ultrasound, cystoscopy, or intravenous pyelogram may be indicated if urinary obstruction is a consideration.

*If indicated.

■ Differential diagnosis

- Other infectious processes should always be considered particularly in elders.
  - Appendicitis, cholecystitis, cholangitis, diverticulitis, pneumonia
- If hematuria is present, but UTI is excluded, bladder or renal cancer is possible.

■ Treatment

- Obtain urine for urinalysis C&S as soon as possible-preferably before antibiotic therapy is started.

- Obtain urine in a catheterized patient from the appropriate port, not the collection bag. Cleanse port with disinfectant, then aspirate sample with sterile needle and syringe.
- Intravenous antibiotic treatment is usually necessary for patients with fever >37.8°C (100°F) (or 0.9°C (2°F) above baseline), chills, CVA tenderness, delirium, or complicated UTIs.
  - Antibiotic therapy is individualized and based on patient history (e.g., allergies and recent previous antibiotic therapy) and urine culture sensitivities.
  - IV antibiotic therapy is continued until patient is afebrile for 48 hours and able to take oral medications and fluids.
- Encouraging oral fluids is helpful for all patients with subtle mental status changes as these changes are often associated with dehydration.
- Monitor VS carefully, particularly hypotension, tachycardia, increased fever.
- Monitor intake and output, daily weights.
- Monitor for heart failure as any infection can precipitate heart failure in an older adult.
- Notify MD if patient develops diarrhea especially if more than 4 liquid stools a day.

■ Collaborative consultation

- When discussing potential antibiotic treatment with the physician or other health care provider, be certain to review patient allergies and concurrent medications (especially warfarin).

■ Complications

- Hyperkalemia and metabolic acidosis have been associated with trimethoprim and sulfamethoxazole (Bactrim).
- Infections associated with antibiotic therapy (e.g., *Clostridium difficile*, thrush and vaginitis).
- Kidney damage
- Pyelonephritis
- Urosepsis

■ Prevention

- Avoid urinary catheterization whenever possible.
- Encourage adequate oral fluids and place fluids within reach of patients.
- Use the smallest catheter when catheterization is indicated.
- Discuss removing urinary catheters within 24 to 48 hours after surgery and when critically ill patients stabilize to avoid catheter-associated urinary tract infections (CAUTI).
- Discuss with MD obtaining a urinalysis C&S in women 48 hours after a urinary catheter is discontinued, if catheter was placed for 1 week or less (2005 IDSA).

- Anchor all urinary catheters appropriately.
- Maintain closed urinary tract drainage system.
- Cleanse urinary catheter and perineal area daily and as needed with mild soap and water.
- Monitor post-operative patients and other patients with suspected urinary retention by using bladder scans.
- Avoid urinary catheter irrigation unless necessary (e.g., blood clots in the urine).
- Promote bladder and bowel training by encouraging regular toileting on the commode or toilet to prevent incontinence and promote bladder/bowel emptying.
- Check and change incontinent patients frequently.
- Avoid irritating soaps and powders in perineal area.
- Monitor the patient for constipation and discuss bowel protocols with the physician as constipation is a risk factor for UTIs.

■ Patient/family education

- Discuss with patients and families the benefit of drinking adequate fluids daily.
- Encourage patients to toilet frequently.
- Explain the side effects of medications and importance of discussing side effects with the doctor or other health care provider.

References

Centers for Disease Control and Prevention (2009a) Catheter-associated urinary tract infection. Online. available from http://www.cdc.gov/ncidod/dhqp/dpac_uti.html (accessed 21 March 2012).

Centers for Disease Control and Prevention (2009b) Estimates of healthcare-associated infections. Online. available from http://www.cdc.gov/ncidod/dhqp/dpac_uti.html (accessed 21 March 2012).

Lo, E., Lindsay, N., Classen, D. et al. (2008) Strategies to prevent catheter-associated urinary tract infections in acute care hospitals. Online. Available from http://www.journals.uchicago.edu/doi/full/10.1086/591066 (accessed 21 March 2012).

Nicolle, L.E., Bradley, S., Colgan, R., Rice, J.C., Schaeffler, A. & Hooton, T.M. (2006) Infectious Diseases Society of America Guidelines for the diagnosis and treatment of asymptomatic bacteriuria in adults. Online. Available from http://www.journals.uchicago.edu/doi/pdf/10.1086/427507 (accessed 21 March 2012).

Rosenthal, V.D., Maki, D.G., Salomao, R. et al. (2006) Device-associated nosocomial infections in 55 intensive care units of 8 developing countries. Annals of Internal Medicine 145(8), 582-591.

Unit 6: Neurologic Disorders

PART 1: DEMENTIA

Constance Cruz, Sara A. Fisher, Mary Lussier-Cushing and Jennifer Repper-DeLisi

Dementia is a clinical syndrome of neurological impairment affecting an individual's cognitive, neuropsychiatric/behavioral, and functional systems. There are at least 70 pathological conditions (diseases and injuries to the brain) that cause dementia. The most common forms of progressive dementia are Alzheimer's disease, vascular dementia, Lewy body dementia, and frontotemporal dementia. The pathophysiology for each is poorly understood.

In the US, about 4 to 5 million people are affected with dementia (Merck Manual, 2010). The prevalence of this disabling disorder doubles every 5 years after age 60 affecting 40% of people over age 85 and is a leading cause of institutionalization (Merck Manual, 2010). As the population ages, it is expected that incidence and prevalence of dementia are expected to significantly increase in the coming years (Middleton & Yaffe, 2009).

The effects of this disease on both the patient and care giver are well documented, but the financial costs associated with dementia are also staggering at $200 billion a year (Alzheimer's Association, 2012). Community, institutional and internet resources to assist those affected are numerous and growing.

■ Risk factors

- Advanced age
- Alcohol use, excessive (>1 drink/day for women; >2 drinks/day for men)
- Atherosclerosis
- Blood pressure (blood pressure that's that is too high, and also possibly too low)
- Cholesterol
- Depression
- Diabetes
- Family history
- High estrogen levels
- Homocysteine blood levels
- Smoking
- Vascular disease (Mayo Clinic, 2009)

■ Clinical presentation

The clinical presentation of dementia is generally determined by the underlying cause and the severity of the disease. A person with Alzheimer's disease is likely to present with short term memory impairment whereas a patient with

Lewy body dementia may present with new onset visual hallucinations. As dementia is primarily a progressive condition, it is generally described in terms of stage and severity: early, middle and late. Early on, Alzheimer's disease may present with only mild short-term memory impairment or occasional trouble with word finding, with minimal impairment in functioning. In advanced stages of the disease, an individual will experience significant memory loss, disorientation, and disabling functional problems.

Patients with mild dementia may have been functioning at home reasonably well. Illness and hospitalization, however, can cause an "unmasking" of a dementia. The change in cognitive function may be caused by delirium.

▧ Nursing assessment

Assessment starts with a complete physical exam identifying all medications that are being taken as well as past or current use of alcohol or other substances. Assessing for dementia involves identification of cognitive impairment, neuropsychiatric or behavioral symptoms as well as functional impairment. Cognitive impairment includes "perception, imagination, judgment, memory, and language, as well as the processes people use to think, organize, and learn" (Lyketsos, 2009, p. 244). The neuropsychiatric symptoms "include signs and symptoms of disturbed perception, thought, mood, or behavior (Livingston et al., 2005, p. 1996). Functional assessment pertains to physical, social, and economic aspects of daily living (Campbell, 1990).

There are a number of tools used to assess cognitive impairment. The Mini-Mental State Exam (MMSE) is probably the most commonly used measure of cognition in elders. The MMSE takes about 10 minutes to complete; it includes a series of questions assessing orientation, attention, memory, concentration, and two pencil and paper tasks testing language, organization, and constructional ability. The MMSE uses a 30 point scale; a score of 23 or less, in a patient with at least 8 years of education, is indicative of cognitive impairment. Another tool recommended for use by nurses is the Mini-Cog which can uncover cognitive impairment in its earliest stages and can be administered in less than 10 minutes. This test requires the patient to register and recall three unrelated objects and draw the Ten Point Clock Test for determination of visuoconstructional difficulties (Doerflinger, 2007).

Neuropsychiatric symptoms include perceptual disturbances (i.e., delusions and hallucinations), disordered sleep, mood, and anxiety and behaviors such as agitation, aggression, or wandering. These symptoms are common in varying degrees and are often more distressing than the cognitive impairment to both patient and family. It is often these symptoms that lead to nursing home placement. Assessment includes complete mental status exam, careful observation, and patient and care giver report.

Functional ability is impacted by impaired executive function in the brain (i.e., ability to set goals, plan, and multitask), memory, and mental status (Mayo, 2008). Assessment includes evaluating the patient's ability to manage their finances, perform ADLs, navigate their environment, and prepare meals. Two tools that are recommended for functional assessment are The Barthel Activities instrument for measuring ADLs and The Instrumental Activities of Daily Living Scale which measures more complex activities (Graf, 2008).

■ Diagnostics

Recommended diagnostic testing to determine treatable causes of the dementia usually includes:

- Complete blood count, chemistry panel, blood urea nitrogen (BUN), creatinine
- Thyroid-stimulating hormone
- Vitamin B12
- Folate
- FTA-ABS (a test to detect antibodies to the bacteria that causes syphilis)
- Humna immunodeficiency virus (HIV) screening
- Neuroimaging: computed tomography (CT) scan) or magnetic resonance imaging (MRI)

The diagnostic criteria for dementia are identified in the *Diagnostic and Statistical Manual of Mental Disorders IV – Text Revised* (DSM IV-TR; APA, 2000) as:

A. The development of multiple cognitive deficits manifested by both (1) memory impairment…and one (or more) of the following cognitive disturbances:
- aphasia (language disturbance)
- apraxia (impaired ability to carry out motor activities despite intact motor function)
- agnosia (failure to recognize or identify objects despite intact sensory function)
- disturbance in executive function (i.e., planning, organizing, sequencing, abstracting)

B. The cognitive deficits cause significant impairment in social or occupational functioning and represent a significant decline from a previous level of functioning.

C. The course is characterized by gradual onset and continuing cognitive decline.

D. The cognitive deficits are not due to any of the following:
   (1) other central nervous system conditions that cause progressive deficits in memory and cognition (e.g., cerebrovascular disease, Parkinson's disease, Huntington's disease, subdural hematoma, normal-pressure hydrocephalus, brain tumor)
   (2) systemic conditions that are known to cause dementia (e.g., hypothyroidism, vitamin B or folic acid deficiency, niacin deficiency, hypercalcemia, neurosyphilis, HIV infection)
   (3) substance-induced conditions

E. The deficits do not occur exclusively during the course of a delirium.

F. The disturbance is not better accounted for by another Axis I disorder (e.g., major depressive episode, schizophrenia).

With early onset: if onset is at age 65 years or below.

With late onset: if onset is after age 65 years.

■ Differential diagnosis

The initial step in the differential diagnosis is determining whether the changes occurring are a result of normal aging, anatomic abnormality, hydrocephalus, mild cognitive impairment, metabolic disturbance, delirium, dementia, or depression. Making this determination involves carefully obtaining the patient's history, a focused physical examination, laboratory testing, and if indicated neuropsychological testing, brain imaging, obtaining biomarkers, and genetic testing. One aspect of the differential is to determine whether the patient is suffering with a chronic condition or a potentially reversible cause of dementia (Geldmacher, 2004).

■ Treatment

Person-centered care is a key concept in the treatment of a person with dementia. This theory of care considers the individuality of the patient, the presenting symptoms, and the support system to determine the interventions and goals of care. Additionally, in planning care, it is important to recognize that a person suffering with dementia will have a lowered stress threshold; interventions need be provided in a low stress environment. Smith *et al.* (2006) suggest providing unconditional positive regard, supporting all losses both interpersonally as well as environmentally, and using the patient's behaviors to guide activity and stimulation levels. Keeping the stress level to a minimum is a crucial component of care.

Nonpharmacologic nursing care strategies include, but are not limited to the following areas.

Cognitive/environmental

- Provide a quiet and safe environment. Include appropriate sensory stimulation such as calming individualized music, white noise, aromatherapy, visual stimulation (pictures or magazines), and gentle touch/massage.
- To avoid overstimulation, maintain low quiet voice, decrease hall noise, limit multiple visitors or staff, and keep TV off (unless requested by patient).
- Assist the patient with putting on eyeglasses, hearing aids, or dentures to optimize sensory function and speech.
- When interacting with the patient, face the person so they can clearly see and hear you. Present with a smile and calm approach to lead the patient's emotional response.
- Use simple language and short sentences. Guide patient into desired activity with simple one step directions. Provide gentle guidance and cueing for completing activities of daily living.

- Allow for enough time to complete tasks to maximize their functional capacity.
- Allow extra time for cognitive processing; wait for verbal and behavioral responses.
- Use distraction, verbal encouragement, or soothing touch if the patient appears anxious or confused.
- Provide frequent orientation. Tell them your name and role when you enter the room. Remind them they are safe and being cared for at the hospital. Establish a consistent schedule with a core group of nurses. Limit room changes. Provide clock, calendar, and familiar possessions from home to promote orientation, preserve memory and facilitate reminiscing. Provide the family with a poster and encourage them to provide patient information and photos. These can be displayed in the patient's room to help the staff to get to know them. Encourage the patient to talk about old memories.
- Normalize sleep-wake cycle. Keep blinds open during day then close and dim the light at night.
- Maintain a toileting schedule every 2 or 3 hours. Ambulate patient to bathroom or assist with use of bedpan/urinal or bedside commode.
- Ambulate at least one or two times each shift to reduce risks of immobility and to expend psychomotor energy. Allow the patient to wander in safe contained areas to provide exercise, maintain function and promote sleep at night.
- Avoid use of mechanical restraint as it may increase agitation and morbidity. Use least restrictive alternatives.
- Camouflage or hide IV tubes and other lines, which may increase confusion, fear and agitation or be accidentally removed (wrap with gauze, cover with blanket, place lines behind a chair or otherwise out of sight and reach).
- Provide written reminders or notes for the patient to hold or have at the bedside table to help compensate for short term memory deficit.
- Posted signs can also be helpful re: not getting out of bed without calling for assistance.
- Encourage socialization such as daily visits from family, one-to-one interaction with staff and other patients, pet therapy. Presence of family may help to orient and calm patient.

Neuropsychiatric

- *Reminiscence therapy*: A guided, structured therapy used by nurses and other disciplines to promote reflection on life events. Since long-term memory is often preserved in early, middle, and even late stages of dementia, reminiscence allows people to share and value their life experiences. Although results are mixed, some studies have found improved self esteem and decreased depression in patients (Livingston *et al.*, 2005; Remington *et al.*, 2005).
- *Validation therapy*: A method of working with disoriented elders that provides an empathetic listener who does not judge them, but accepts their view of reality (Feil, 1993).

- *Reality orientation therapy*: Frequent reorientation to person, place, time and event through greetings, clocks, calendars, signs, etc. are common strategies that can help diminish maladaptive behaviors.
- *Simulated presence therapy*: Involves use of an audiotape, recorded by friend/family member, containing positive personal memories and anecdotes.
- *Therapeutic activity programs*: Interventions may employ exercise, reading groups, Montessori activities, social activities, and art groups.
- Sensory/multisensory stimulation interventions are individualized. They include the use of music/music therapy, aroma therapy, touch/massage, exposure to various tactile sensations, lights and pleasant images. Numerous studies have found behavioral and affective improvement after exposure to sensory stimulation (Livingston *et al.*, 2005).

Pharmacologic treatments
- Cholinesterase inhibitors are used to temporally improve memory, enhance cognitive function, positively impact sense of well-being and may improve behaviors. Common side effects of cholinesterase inhibitors include head-ache, fatigue, anorexia, diarrhea, and dizziness.
- Antipsychotic medications, both typical and atypical, can be used to treat hallucinations, delusions, and behavioral problems in dementia. These medications, which can have serious side effects, including death, should be considered after nonpharmacological/behavioral interventions have been tried.
- Antidepressant therapy is effective in treating depression, improving quality of life, and targeting maladaptive behaviors of dementia. There are several classes of antidepressants: tricyclic antidepressants (amitriptyline, doxepin, imipramine, desipramine, nortriptyline), monoamime oxidase inhibitors (moclobemide, phenelzine), selective serotonin reuptake inhibitors (SSRI) (citalopram, escitalopram, fluoxetine, fluvoxamine, paroxetine, sertraline), atypical antidepressants (bupropion, trazodone, venlafaxine, nefazodone, duloxetine and mirtazapine). Side effects of antidepressants are class specific.

■ Collaborative consultation
Patients with dementia benefit from a multidisciplinary approach that includes consultation with mental health professionals (psychiatric nurses, social workers, psychologists and psychiatrists), occupational therapists, physical therapists, primary care providers, and the hospital care team to aid in evaluation and treatment.

■ Complications
- Agitation
- Anorexia
- Falls

- Fractures
- Psychosis
- Safety issues
- Sleep disorders

■ Prevention

The prevention of a dementia syndrome is largely dependent on the pathological condition that causes it. Risk factor modification remains the cornerstone for prevention. Researchers recommend regular exercise, cognitive activity including new learning, social engagement, healthy diet, recognition and treatment of depression, and control of chronic diseases.

■ Patient/family education

- Provide education, support and role modeling regarding communication and care of patient with dementia.
- Refer to appropriate support organizations and recommended readings.

References

Alzheimer's Association (2012) Facts and figures. Online. Available from http://www.alz.org/downloads/facts_figures_2012.pdf (accessed 31 May 2012).

American Psychiatric Association (2000) *Diagnostic and Statistical Manual of Mental Disorders*, 4th edition, Text Revision. American Psychiatric Association, Washington DC.

Boustani, M., Callahan, C.M., Unverzagt, F.W. *et al.* (2005) Implementing a screening and diagnosis program for dementia in primary care. *Journal of General Internal Medicine* **20**(7), 572-527.

Campbell, J.M. (1990) Assessment. In: *Geropsychiatric Nursing*, M.O. Hogstel (ed.). CV Mosby, St. Louis.

Doerflinger, D.M.C. (2007) How to try this: The Mini-Cog Simplifies the identification of cognitive impairment with this easy-to-use tool. *American Journal of Nursing* **107**(12), 62-71.

Feil, N. (1993) *The Validation breakthrough: simple techniques for communicating with people with Alzheimer's type dementia*. Health Professions Press, Baltimore, MD.

Geldmacher, D.S. (2004) Differential diagnosis of dementia syndromes. *Clinics in Geriatric Medicine* **20**(1), 27-43.

Graf, C. (2008) The Lawton instrumental activities of daily living scale. *American Journal of Nursing* **108**(4), 52–62.

Lyketsos, C.G. (2009) Dementia and milder cognitive syndromes. In: The American *Psychiatric Publishing Textbook of Geriatric Psychiatry*. Blazer, D.G. & Steffens, D.C. (eds). American Psychiatric Publishing, Inc, Arlington, VA.

Livingston, G., Johnston, K., Katona, C., Paton, J., & Lyketsos, C.G. (2005) Systematic review of psychological approaches to the management of neuropsychiatric symptoms of dementia. *American Journal of Psychiatry* **162**(11), 1996-2021.

Mayo, A.M. (2008) Measuring functional status in older adults with dementia. *Clinical Nurse Specialist* **22**(5), 212-213.

MayoClinic (2009). Risk Factors. Online. Available from http://www.mayoclinic.com/health/dementia/DS01131/DSECTION=risk-factors (accessed 22 March 2012).

The Merck Manual of Diagnosis and Therapy, 18th edition, 2006. Online. Available from http://www.merckmanuals.com/professional/index.html (accessed 22 March 2012).

The Merck Manual of Geriatrics (2000) Online. Available from http://merck.com/mkgr/mmg/sec5/ch40/ch40a.jsp (accessed 22 March 2012).

Middleton, L.E. & Yaffe, K. (2009) Promising strategies for the prevention of dementia. *Archives of Neurology* **66**(10), 1210-1215.

Remington, R., Gerdner, L.A. & Buckwalter, K.C. (2005) Nursing management of clients experiencing dementias of late life: care environments, clients, and caregivers. In: *Geropsychiatric and Mental Health Nursing*, K. Devereaux Melillo & S. Crocker Houde (eds). Jones & Bartlett Publishers, Sudbury, MA.

Smith, M., Hall, G.R., Gerdner, L. & Buckwalter, K.C. (2006) Application of the progressively lowered stress threshold model across the continuum of care. *Nursing Clinics of North America* **41**(1), 57-81.

PART 2: DELIRIUM IN THE OLDER HOSPITALIZED ADULT

Mary Lussier-Cushing, Jennifer Repper-DeLisi, Sara A. Fisher and Constance Cruz

Delirium is a common and serious problem for older adults hospitalized in the acute care setting, and is associated with substantial morbidity and mortality (Inouye *et al.*, 1999, 2001). Delirium is characterized by an acute onset and fluctuating course. Central features include reduced ability to focus, sustain and shift attention, a change in cognitive function (i.e., disorganized thinking and speech, forgetfulness or memory deficit, disorientation, or development of perceptual disturbances), and an altered level of consciousness with reduced awareness of the environment. It is caused by one or more physiologic conditions (DSMIV-TR; APA, 2000). An increase or decrease in psychomotor activity and a disturbance in the sleep wake cycle are also common. The prevalence of delirium at hospital admission is 14-24%, and the incidence of delirium arising during hospitalization ranges from 6-56% among general hospital populations (Inouye, 2006). Though delirium may occur in any age group, it is the most common complication of hospital admission for patients 65 and older (Young & Inouye, 2007), occurring in up to 30% of older patients presenting to the emergency department (Agostini & Inouye, 2003; Inouye, 2006), 53% of older patients post-operatively (Inouye, 2006) and in 70-87% of older ICU patients (Pisani, 2006; Inouye, 2006). Prompt identification of this syndrome and treatment of the underlying cause(s) are essential. Delayed recognition and intervention can result in a more complicated, lengthy and costly hospital stay. Adjusted average annual hospital costs were 2.5 times higher for patients with delirium (Leslie *et al.*, 2008). The problem of delirium in older hospitalized adults is important because patients 65 years and older account for more than 48% of all hospital days of care (Leslie *et al.*, 2008; Inouye, 2006). Confusion, disorientation, forgetfulness, and agitation place this patient group at higher risk for injury. This may include falls, complications associated with restraint use, wandering in the hospital environment, dislodgement of therapeutic or monitoring devices, and hazards associated with prolonged bed rest and immobility.

Nursing care of the delirious patient requires a complicated array of interventions to identify the syndrome, implement effective safety interventions, treat the underlying cause(s) of the syndrome, and sooth the confused and often terrified patient.

■ Risk factors

Delirium develops in a vulnerable patient with superimposed triggers or insults in a stressful and unfamiliar environment. The more predisposing risk factors one has, the more vulnerable one is to developing delirium. For example, an 81-year-old patient with chronic obstructive pulmonary disease (COPD), type 2 diabetes, macular degeneration, and cataracts may be admitted to the hospital with a change in mental status and found to have a urinary tract infection (UTI). However, a UTI is unlikely to cause delirium in a young healthy person.

Predisposing risk factors include:

- Advanced age
- Decreased oral intake, dehydration, or malnutrition
- Drug dependence including alcohol, prescription medications, and illicit drugs
- Frailty (i.e., functional dependence, immobility, or history of falls [Inouye, 2006; Dick & Morency, 2005])
- History of cognitive impairment, dementia, stroke, acquired immune deficiency syndrome (AIDS), or traumatic brain injury (TBI)
- Multiple chronic diseases, especially severe medical illness or terminal illness
- Previous episode(s) of delirium or depression
- Sensory impairment (visual or hearing)
- Treatment with many medications

Precipitating risk factors, also known as contributing or triggering factors, or etiologies are:

- Decreased oral intake, dehydration, poor nutritional status, or low serum albumin
- Environmental: admission to ICU, use of physical restraints, bladder catheters, tubes and lines, multiple procedures, and transfers between care areas and providers (Inouye, 2006; Dick & Morency, 2005)

- Infection, fever, hypothermia, hypoxia, anemia, shock, sepsis, or hypo-perfusion
- Medications – polypharmacy, medication changes, side effects and inter-actions, including withdrawal from alcohol, prescription or illicit drugs
  - Common medications that can impair cognition include:
    - Antibiotics
    - Benzodiazepines (e.g., lorazepam)
    - Cardiac drugs
    - Corticosteroids
    - Digoxin
    - H_2 blockers (e.g., cimetidine)
    - Medications with anticholinergic side effects (e.g., diphenhydramine or scopolamine)
    - Muscle relaxants
    - NSAIDs
    - Opioids (especially meperidine)
    - Psychiatric medications
    - Parkinson medications (e.g., levodopa)
    - Sedatives (e.g., sleep aids)
    - Seizure medications
    - Theophylline
    - Urinary incontinence drugs
- Metabolic derangements (i.e., electrolyte, glucose, or acid-base imbalance)
- Pain, sleep deprivation, or emotional stress
- Primary neurologic disease (e.g., stroke, intracranial bleed, meningitis, encephalitis, tumor, or metastasis)
- Surgery, burns, severe or terminal illness, or iatrogenic complications

Be mindful that delirium, especially the hypoactive presentation often goes unrecognized. Four independent risk factors associated with under-recognition of delirium are:

- Age 80 years or older
- Baseline dementia
- Hypoactive presentation of delirium
- Vision impairment (Inouye, 2006)

Delirium is hypothesized to be the final common pathway of multiple patho-genic mechanisms, including impaired cerebral oxidative metabolism as evidenced by characteristic findings on EEG of generalized slowing, inflamma-tion and activation of cerebral cytokines, a stress reaction with hypercorti-solism, and dysfunction of neurotransmitter systems (Dick & Morency, 2005; Fearing & Inouye, 2009). While the fundamental pathophysiology for delirium is not clearly understood, an imbalance in neurotransmitters is associated with the occurrence of this syndrome, Acetylcholine is a neurotransmitter that plays a central role in mediating consciousness and the ability of an individual to maintain or shift attention (Fearing & Inouye, 2009). Reduced cholinergic activity and excess dopamine are two primary mechanisms believed to be involved in the development of this syndrome (Fearing & Inouye, 2009; Marcantonio et al., 2006; Trzepacz & van der Mast, 2002). This is important to remember for two reasons. First, anticholinergic medications, or those with anticholinergic side effects, often contribute to the development or worsening of delirium. The syndrome may resolve with a dosage reduction or discontinuation when possible. Second, it favors the selection of low-dose antipsychotic medication to treat the symptoms of confusion, fear, and agitation that often accompany delirium (Fearing & Inouye, 2009; Querques et al., 2006).

■ Clinical presentation

Delirium occurs on a spectrum with three presentations.

Hypoactive delirium

A patient with hypoactive delirium may appear lethargic, does not wash, eat or engage verbally and is apt to decline physical therapy (PT) or other treatments and care activities. This presentation is often unrecognized or is mistaken for lack of motivation or depression. The hypoactive form is more common in the older adult and is associated with poorer prognosis (Fearing & Inouye, 2009).

Hyperactive or agitated delirium

This patient gets staff attention as he/she is apt to be yelling, climbing out of bed, pulling at lines or tubes, awake much of the night, uncooperative or even combative with care. When a period of agitation follows shortly after a period of marked orientation and clarity, the period of confused agitation may be mistaken for willful or deliberate behavior.

Mixed delirium

Mixed presentations with fluctuations between hypoactive and hyperactive delirium are common in practice. Sensory perceptual disturbances including hallucinations and illusions may occur at any point along the spectrum as well as paranoid thinking about care providers, and in some instances paranoid thinking may include family.

Brief or intermittent periods of orientation and clarity may contribute to care providers' failure to recognize delirium and also to the experience of fearful uncertainty for concerned family members interacting with patient at the bedside or via telephone.

■ Nursing assessment

Nurses in the acute care setting play a pivotal role in the recognition, prevention and intervention for delirium because of the time spent with patients and the close interactive nature of care. Assessment of cognitive and functional baseline and changes will be directed by the condition of the patient on arrival and over the course of the hospitalization. Some patients are able to provide information on admission, while others may be acutely confused on initial contact. In that case, information from the referring facility, family, primary care provider (PCP) or providers of home services will be helpful to determine cognitive and functional baseline.

A variety of screening tools are available to assess current mental status and cognitive function. The two most commonly used and studied are the Confusion Assessment Method (CAM) and the Folstein Mini Mental State Exam (MMSE). The CAM is a diagnostic algorithm that screens for the presence of the four diagnostic criteria for delirium; acute change or fluctuating course of mental status, inattention, disorganized thinking and altered level of consciousness (Inouye et al., 1990). The CAM is intended to be used in combination with other cognitive screening techniques or tools. The MMSE is a 30-point cognitive screening tool that includes orientation, registration, attention, recall and language (Folstein et al., 1975). Administer the CAM and/or the MMSE and compare results to reported baseline. Repeated administration of these tools can help to track cognitive improvement or decline over time.

Identify the time frame for the acute changes in mental status. Review vital signs, oxygen saturation, respiratory status, urinary and bowel function, hydration (input and output), and sleep pattern, noting any trends. Note any recent medication changes, procedures done, or events that have occurred such as a fall. This information usually yields one or more precipitating factors from the past 2–3 days prior to or coinciding with the onset of delirium symptoms, though the time frame may be more immediate (within 24 hours), or longer (a week or more).

The most common reversible cause of delirium is medications. Therefore the nurse must always perform a thorough medication review whenever delirium is suspected. This review should include close attention to any new medication the patient has received, dosage adjustments, evaluation for any abrupt discontinuation of medications (by plan or inadvertent omission by patient or care provider), especially benzodiazepines, barbiturates, or hypnotics. Monitor for any drug toxicity (e.g., dilantin, digoxin, antibiotic, immunosuppressant, or chemotherapy agents). Discuss taper or discontinuation of any non-essential medications and the identification of possible deliriogenic medications with the prescribing clinician.

■ Diagnostics

There is no definitive laboratory test, X-ray or scan that confirms the diagnosis of delirium. Laboratory tests such as complete blood count (CBC), electrolytes, general chemistries, TSH (thyroid studies), anemia studies (vitamin B12, folate), liver function, urinalysis and chest X-ray are useful for identification of treatable conditions that may be contributing to the clinical presentation. Radiologic diagnostics often are costly and low yield, so their use should be guided by clinical presentation, history and exam. Careful review of medications, both those recently added or discontinued, is essential for the identification of precipitating factors for delirium.

Use the mnemonic "I WATCH DEATH" (**I** = Infection, **W** = Withdrawal from drugs, **A** = Acute metabolic disorders, **T** = Trauma, **C** = CNS pathology, **H** = Hypoxia, **D** = Deficiencies in vitamins, **E** = Endocrinopathies, **A** = Acute vascular insult, **T** = Toxins, **H** = Heavy metals) to identify the underlying physiologic cause(s) or precipitating factors for delirium. Other available mnemonics include DELIRIUM (**D** = Drugs, **E** = Eyes, ears, and other sensory deficits, **L** = Low O_2 states (e.g., heart attack, stroke, and pulmonary embolism), **I** = Infection, **R** = Retention (of urine or stool), **I** = Ictal state, **U** = Underhydration/undernutrition, **M** = Metabolic causes (DM, Post-operative state, Sodium abnormalities), **(S)** = Subdural hematoma or, rule out, the WWHHHHIMPS (**W**ernicke's encephalopathy, **W**ithdrawal, **H**ypertensive crisis, **H**ypoperfusion/hypoxia of the brain, **H**ypoglycemia, **H**yper/hypothermia, **I**ntracranial process/infection, **M**etabolic/meningitis, **P**oisons, **S**tatus epilepticus) for life threatening causes of delirium (Caplan & Stern, 2008).

▪ Differential diagnosis

Dementia, unlike delirium has a more insidious onset and chronic course with stages that often plateau for periods of time. Remember, the patient with dementia is at higher risk for delirium. With any change from baseline mental status assume there is a delirium until proven otherwise, for it can be treated. For the hospitalized older patient in the acute care setting the question may be, is there also an underlying dementia or depression; and if so, has this been clearly diagnosed, suspected or largely unrecognized during or prior to this illness.

Discussion with the family, PCP or outpatient care providers may help to clarify that there has been a cognitive and functional decline over months to a year or longer, or that this is strictly an acute change over hours, days or weeks.

Psychiatric conditions such as depression, mania and nonorganic psychotic orders generally do not develop suddenly in the context of medical illness. Anxiety is a fairly universal experience for both the patient and family during times of acute illness and hospitalization and can usually be reduced with calm education, support, and reassurance. Depression secondary to prolonged medical illness, chronic pain, and other losses of aging is not usually diagnosed and treated until delirium has resolved. See the chapters on anxiety and depression for further discussion of these topics.

▪ Treatment

The goal of treatment is for patient to return to cognitive and functional baseline as quickly as possible. Nursing care interventions include the following:

Physiologic care and monitoring
Identify and treat the underlying physiologic etiologies or precipitating factors (one or more) as specifically as possible. For example correct metabolic

derangements, treat infection with an antibiotic, alcohol withdrawal with a benzodiazepine, hypoxia with oxygen, etc.

- Monitor vital signs, oxygen saturation, and labs.
- Monitor for food and fluid intake, especially adequate hydration. Assist with menu selections, opening meal containers and feeding as needed.
  - The amount of fluid that accompanies meals is not typically enough to maintain adequate hydration.
  - Encourage small frequent amounts of oral fluids throughout the first half of the day, decreasing intake after 7 pm. Ask family to assist with this.
  - It may be helpful to have family visit at mealtime with patient out of bed (OOB) to chair.
- Assess for urinary and bowel function-monitor for signs and symptoms of UTI, urinary retention, constipation.
  - Avoid indwelling urinary catheters unless clinically necessary to reduce risk of infection and trauma from accidental dislodgement.
  - Provide a regular toileting schedule-offer/encourage use of bedpan, urinal or assist to bedside commode or bathroom every 2–3 hours.
- Mobilize patients to reduce hazards of immobility; ideally out of bed to chair for meals, bed linen changes and/or during visits with family/friends.
  - For non-mobile patients reposition, encourage and assist with bed exercise and ROM.
- Assess pain and provide pain management with both pharmacological and non-pharmacological approaches.
- Facilitate a normal sleep–wake cycle with non-pharmacological approaches to sleep and anxiety:
  - Wake up your patients during the day; provide rest periods in morning and afternoon.
  - Offer a small amount of a warm beverage such as milk or decaffeinated or herbal tea (if not contraindicated).
  - Offer/try a back rub, hand or foot massage to facilitate comfort and reduce restlessness.
  - Offer/encourage use of ear plugs, soothing music, use of white noise machine or fan.
  - For patients with sleep apnea, use of continuous positive airways pressure machine may be helpful, especially if used at home.
  - Cluster care and limit night time sleep disruption for non-essential care.

Communication tips

- Approach patient so they see you coming and call them by their preferred name.
- Give a verbal warning before touching them.
- Reorient patient with each encounter to your name and role. Reorient patient also to name of hospital, reason for hospitalization, date and more importantly time of day.

- Provide reassurance and redirect patients by telling them what to do, rather than "don't touch this, don't do that."
- Give a simple explanation for care being provided.
- Guide the patient into desired care activity with simple one step direction.
- Move and talk slowly. Allow ample time for patient to respond.
- Move rounds and discussions out of the room- only one person in a group of staff or visitors should talk at a time. Remember patients with delirium have difficulty maintaining and shifting attention, and can be easily distracted or over stimulated by noise and activity.
- Communication with patient should be short, frequent, orienting, therapeutic and/or meaningful.
  - For example, talk to patient about things that are relevant and of interest to patient- their family, work, hobbies, pets, weather, current events, or TV show.
- TV on for short periods of time only if patient is attending to it
- Quiet or preferred music can be soothing or white noise machines or a fan can help to block out the irritation and distraction of hospital beeps, alarms and noise.
- When a patient becomes over stimulated and agitated by noise, movement and care activities, sometimes a short period of time and space can be helpful to calm them.
- Provide reality testing for the patient with hallucinations or illusions (misinterpretation of an actual stimulus).
  - Acknowledge their experience as being very real to them.
  - "I don't hear or see that," or give simple explanation for what they are actually looking at or hearing.
  - Provide reassurance for their safety and redirect to another topic.

Sensory and environmental support and safety interventions

- Post and update orienting information (hospital name, day, season, physician/nurse names, etc.)
- Presence of family or phone contact may be helpful to calm and reassure patient.
- Encourage and assist with use of sensory aids: glasses, hearing aid, and dentures.
  - Provide magnifier or portable hearing enhancer to facilitate speech with patient who has vision and hearing impairments.
- Room lighting and window shades to avoid glare that may distort vision and to simulate the normal day night sleep-wake cycle
- Provide non-slip footwear and a clear path to the bathroom.
  - Remove unnecessary clutter from room, especially bedside area.
- Careful room selection for ease of monitoring and noise level; limit non-essential room changes.
- Least restrictive alternative to maintain patient and staff safety; bed and chair alarms as needed

Medication management

If the patient shows early signs of escalating agitation and there are safety concerns despite your best efforts with the previous interventions, medication intervention is indicated.

- Treat the symptoms of confusion, fear, agitation and combativeness with a low dose antipsychotic medication such as haloperidol (Fearing & Inouye, 2009; Querques *et al.*, 2006).
  - With the use of haloperidol or other antipsychotic medication, monitor a daily EKG for corrected QT (QTc) due to risk of QTc prolongation.
  - Monitor and maintain serum potassium and magnesium in high normal range.
- Avoid anticholinergic medications such as scopolamine, atropine and diphenhydramine, and benzodiazepines unless their use is essential for a clinical reason, as they may contribute to or worsen delirium.
- One study (Al-Aama *et al.*, 2011) provides evidence that nightly melatonin supplementation, administered early to mid evening, may have a role in decreasing delirium and facilitating sleep in older adults admitted to acute care. Future research studies are required to confirm the potential protective role of melatonin.
- Consultation with psychiatry or geri-psychiatry services for evaluation and medication management is strongly recommended.

■ Collaborative consultation

- Gerontology clinical nurse specialist
- Psychiatric clinical nurse specialist or psychiatry consult for evaluation and treatment recommendations, if possible with geri psych expertise.
- Dietician
- Occupational therapy safety evaluation
- Physical therapy for mobility
- Social worker for patient and family support
- Chaplain

■ Complications

Hazards of immobility include physical deconditioning, pneumonia, aspiration, deep vein thrombosis/pulmonary embolism, injuries from falls, restraints and tubes such as indwelling urinary catheter.

With unrecognized or persistent delirium there is increased risk for cognitive and functional decline, with failure to return to baseline level of functioning and mortality.

■ Prevention

Since delirium is often multifactorial in nature, most prevention strategies are multicomponent. A few of the most well known studies and programs include

The Yale Delirium Prevention Trial (Inouye *et al.*, 1999), the Hospital Elder Life Program (HELP http://www.hospitalelderlifeprogram.org), 10 domains for targeted strategies by Marcantonio *et al.*, 2001), and SPICES: an Overall Assessment Tool for Older Adults (Fulmer, 2007).

Delirium prevention with optimal function and outcomes for the older patient can be facilitated by attention to risk factor assessment, routine systematic screening for delirium and cognitive impairment, and use or targeted delirium prevention and intervention strategies.

- Orienting communication and therapeutic activity
- Early mobilization and walking
- Maintaining hydration and nutrition
- Non-pharmacological approaches to sleep and anxiety
- Adaptive equipment for vision and hearing impairment
- Pain management (Inouye *et al.*, 1999; Young & Inouye, 2007)

■ Patient/family education

Few illness situations are more terrifying and degrading to patients and families than the loss of "personhood," and the ability to reason and understand (Young & Inouye, 2007). The family is often very distressed and frightened when loved ones demonstrate a change in mental status and behavior. They fear that their family member has sustained brain damage or has quickly become demented. They are apt to express this in an angry or frustrated manner, "What have you done to my husband? He was not like this before he came to the hospital!" "This is not my mother. She would be so embarrassed. She never talks or acts like this. She's not making any sense;" or after an episode of combativeness, "He is so easygoing and gentle; he would never hurt anyone." The family may even get upset with the patient for their behavior or try to "talk some sense into them."

- Acknowledge their concerns.
- Reassure them that we understand that this is not how their loved one usually behaves or communicates with others.
- Provide education regarding the acute and fluctuating nature of delirium and how it may be impacting what the patient is saying or doing.
- Role model calm communication with the patient.

It may be therapeutic to give the family useful tasks to help their loved one. This provides a concrete way for them to help and feel useful, while helping to pass time and bind their anxiety. Strategic use of their help may help to prevent delirium. Examples include:

- "She/he needs to rest. It would be helpful if you would sit quietly, or hold his/her hand and encourage rest or a nap."
- A foot or hand massage may be helpful to reduce restlessness.

- Let them know that it would be helpful for their loved ones recovery for him/her to sit up in a chair. "Please encourage him/her to sip/drink a cup of fluid every hour and to use the incentive spirometer during your visit."
- "He/she needs to spend more time awake today. It would be helpful if you can help with completion of menu, watch the news or favorite TV show with him/her, talk to them about things that would be of interest, but preferably nothing that would worry or upset him/her."
- Ask the family to tell you about the patient so care providers can get to know him/her as a person. This may be therapeutic for the family member and helpful to staff.
  - Provide a "Get to Know Me" sheet or poster, to guide this process with the family and to facilitate more meaningful communication with the patient as care is provided (see Figure 3.6.2.1).

Unless the patient initiates conversation or asks questions about the period of time during which they were confused or acted out of character, there is no need to revisit or process this should family inquire about doing so. Some

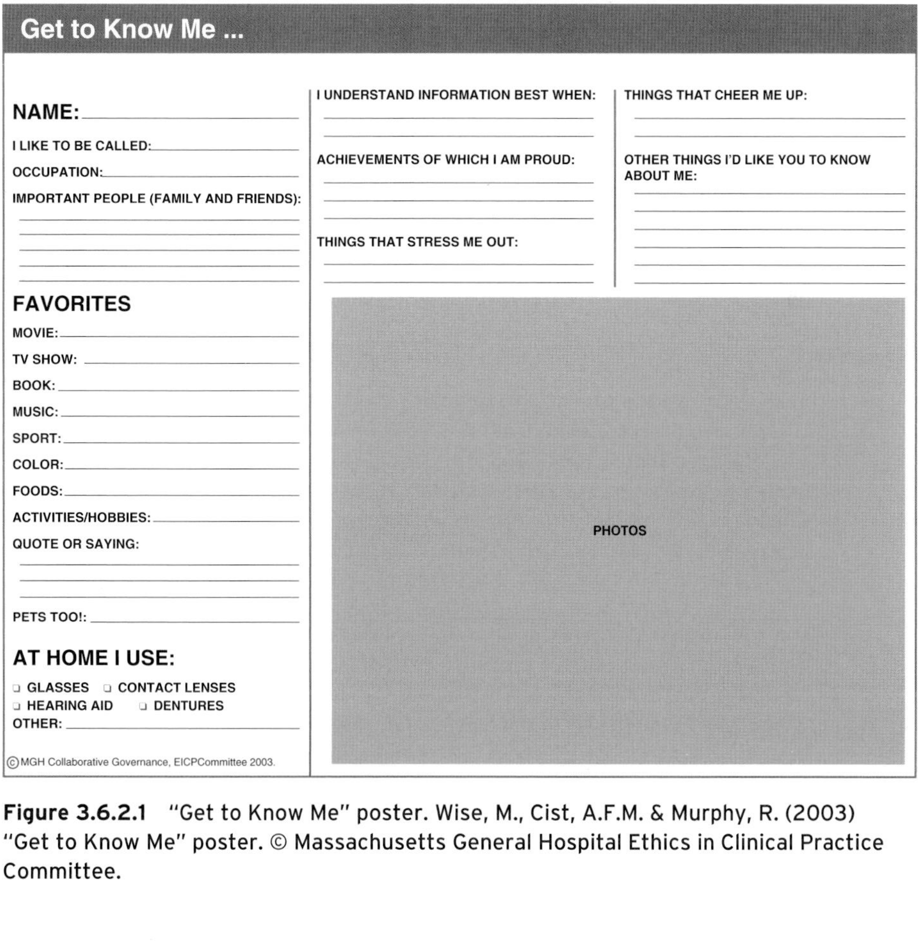

Get to Know Me ...

NAME:_____

I LIKE TO BE CALLED:_____
OCCUPATION:_____
IMPORTANT PEOPLE (FAMILY AND FRIENDS):_____

FAVORITES
MOVIE:_____
TV SHOW:_____
BOOK:_____
MUSIC:_____
SPORT:_____
COLOR:_____
FOODS:_____
ACTIVITIES/HOBBIES:_____
QUOTE OR SAYING:_____
PETS TOO!:_____

AT HOME I USE:
❏ GLASSES ❏ CONTACT LENSES
❏ HEARING AID ❏ DENTURES
OTHER:_____

I UNDERSTAND INFORMATION BEST WHEN:_____
ACHIEVEMENTS OF WHICH I AM PROUD:_____
THINGS THAT STRESS ME OUT:_____

THINGS THAT CHEER ME UP:_____
OTHER THINGS I'D LIKE YOU TO KNOW ABOUT ME:_____

PHOTOS

©MGH Collaborative Governance, EICPCommittee 2003.

Figure 3.6.2.1 "Get to Know Me" poster. Wise, M., Cist, A.F.M. & Murphy, R. (2003) "Get to Know Me" poster. © Massachusetts General Hospital Ethics in Clinical Practice Committee.

patients have no recollection of the delirium experience, while others have vague recollection. On the other hand, during and following recovery from delirium patients may experience recollections of the event as unpleasant and disturbing (Young & Inouye, 2007) (i.e., patient taken to CT scan or MRI during the night has a belief about being taken out of the hospital to a train station and later returned). If the patient has a need to talk about it, listen, acknowledge their experience and provide clarification when possible. Remember, the patient may have a rather fixed belief about this and may not be convinced otherwise refocus on the present infusing realistic hope.

References

Al-Aama, T., Brymer, C., Gutmanis, I., Woolmore-Goodwin, S.M., Esbaugh, J. & Dasgupta, M. (2011) Melatonin decreases delirium in elderly patients: A randomized, placebo-controlled trial. *International Journal of Geriatric Psychiatry* **26**, 687-694.

American Psychiatric Association (2000) *Diagnostic and Statistical Manual IV, Text Revision*. APA, Washington, DC.

Caplan, J.P. & Stern, T.A. (2008) Mnemonics in a nutshell; 32 aids to psychiatric diagnosis. *Current Psychiatry* **7**(10), 27-33.

Dick, K. & Morency, C.R. (2005) Delirium. In: *Geropsychiatric and Mental Health Nursing*. K.D. Melillo & S.C. Houde (eds). Jones and Bartlett Publishers, Sudbury, MA.

Fearing, M.A. & Inouye, S.K. (2009) Delirium. In *Textbook of Geriatric Psychiatry*. D.G. Blazer & D.C. Steffens (eds). American Psychiatric Publishing, APA, Inc., Arlington, VA.

Folstein, M., Fostein, S., & McHugh, P. (1975) Mini-mental....A Practical Guide for grading the cognitive state of patients for the clinician. *Journal of Psychiatric Research* **12**, 189-198.

Fulmer, T. (2007). How to try this: Fulmer SPICES. *American Journal of Nursing* **107**(10), 40-48.

Inouye, S.K. (2006) Delirium in older persons. *New England Journal of Medicine* **354**, 1157-1165.

Inouye, S.K., Bocaardus, S.T., Charpentier, P.A. *et al.* (1999) A multicomponent intervention to prevent delirium in hospitalized older patients. *New England Journal of Medicine* **340**(9), 669-676.

Inouye, S.K., Foreman, M.D., Mion, L.C., Katz, K.H. & Cooney, L.M. (2001) Nurses' recognition of delirium and its symptoms. *Archives of Internal Medicine* **161**, 2476-2473.

Leslie, D.L, Marcantonia, E.R., Zhang, Y., Leo-Summers, L. & Inouye, S.K. (2008) One-year health care costs associated with delirium in the elderly population. *Archives of Internal Medicine* **168**(1), 27-32.

Marcantonio, ER, (2011) In the clinic. Delirium. *Annals of Internal Medicine* **154**(11).

Pisani, M.A., Araujo, K.L.B., Van Ness, P. H. *et al.* (2006) A research algorithm to improve detection of delirium in the intensive care unit. *Critical Care* **10**(4), Online. Available from http://ccforum.com/content/10/4/R121 (accessed 30 May 2012).

Querques, J., Stern, T.A., Tesar, G.E. & Heckers, S. (2006) *Diagnosis and Treatment of Agitation and Delirium in the Intensive Care Unit Patient. Manual of Intensive Care Medicine*, 4th edition. Lippincott, Williams & Wilkins, Philadelphia.

Young, J. & Inouye, S. (2007) Delirium in older people. *British Medical Journal* **334**, 842-846.

Further reading

Breitbart, W., Morotta, R., Platt, M.M., *et al.* (1996) A doubleblind trial of haloperidol, chlorpromazine, and lorazepam in the treatment of delirium in hospitalized AIDS patients. *American Journal of Psychiatry* **153**, 231-237.

Cassem, N.H., Murray, G.B., Lafayette, J.M. *et al.* (2004) Delirious patients, In: *Massachusetts General Hospital Handbook of general hospital psychiatry*, 5th edition, T.A. Stern, G.L. Fricchione, N.H. Cassem *et al.* (eds). Mosby, Philadelphia: pp. 119-134.

Fick, D.M., Cooper, J.W., Wade, W.E. Waller, J.L., Maclean, J.R. & Beers, M.H. (2003) Updating the Beers Criteria for potentially inappropriate medication use in older adults. *Archives of Internal Medicine* **63**, 22.

Inouye, S.K., vanDyck, C.H., Alessi, C.A., Balkin, S., Siegal, A.P. & Horwitz, R.I. (1990) Clarifying confusion: The Confusion Assessment Method. A new method for detection of delirium. *Annals of Internal Medicine* **113**, 941–948.

Inouye, S.K., Studenski, S., Tinetti, M. & Kuchel, G.A. (2007) Geriatric syndromes: clinical research and policy implications of a core geriatric concept. *Journal of American Geriatric Society* **55**(5), 780-791.

Inouye, S.K., Brown, C.J. & Tinetti, M.E. (2009) Medicare nonpayment, hospital falls and unintended consequences. *New England Journal of Medicine* **360**, 2390-2393.

Lakatos, B.E., Capasso, V., Mitchell, M.T. *et al.* (2009) Falls in the general hospital: association with delirium, advanced age and specific surgical procedures. *Psychosomatics* **50**, 218-226.

National Cancer Institute, General Management Approach to Delirium. Online. Available from http://www.cancer.gov/cancertopics/pdq/supportivecare/delirium/HealthProfessional/page5 (accessed 22 March 2012).

Schreier, A.M. (2010) Nursing care, delirium, and pain management for the hospitalized older adult. *Pain Management Nursing* **11**(3), 177-185.

Someya, T., Endo, T., Hara, T. Yagi, G. & Suzuki, J. (2001) A survey on the drug therapy for delirium. *Psychiatry and Clinical Neurosciences* **55**, 397-401.

Warshaw, G. & Mechlin, M. (2009) Prevention and management of postoperative delirium. *International Anesthesiology Clinics* **47**(4), 137-149.

Wei, L.A., Fearing, M., Sternberg, E.J. & Inouye, S.K. (2008) The confusion assessment method: a systematic review of current usage. *Journal of the American Geriatrics Society* **56**, 823-830.

PART 3: ISCHEMIC STROKE

Marion Phipps

A stroke is a clinical syndrome of neurological findings that can occur suddenly or more progressive in nature. The sequence of events results in focal neurological deficits. A stroke is the result of both modifiable and non-modifiable risk factors. Strokes occur because of an impairment of cerebral blood flow resulting in cellular injury and death. The perfusion to the brain may be impaired by one of two mechanisms: a blockage of a blood vessel, defined as an ischemic stroke; or by blood vessel hemorrhage, defined as a hemorrhagic stroke. Symptoms of stroke vary among individuals and are related to the region of the brain deprived of blood supplied by the vessel involved.

In the United States 780,000 individuals sustain a stroke each year: 600,000 being new strokes, and 180,000 recurrent strokes (AHA, 2011). Stroke is the third leading cause of death in the US and the overall yearly mortality rate is approximately 273,000 persons (AHA, 2011). The costs of this disorder are compelling-costing 53.9 billion in 2010 (Heidenreich *et al.*, 2011).

■ Risk factors

Risk factors for stroke may be described as non-modifiable risk factors, modifiable risk factors and cardiac risk factors.

Non-modifiable risk factors
- *Age*: particularly older age
- *Gender*: men are at higher risk, however, after the age of 75, 40,000 more women than men have stroke. Older women are more likely to die than men and women often have more severe strokes.
- *Genetic factors*: there is thought to be a genetic factor for subarachnoid hemorrhage due to ruptured aneurysm.
- *Race*: blacks have higher risk probably due to hypertension.

Modifiable risk factors
- *Carotid stenosis*: consider surgical or radiological intervention.
- *Diabetes mellitus*: tight control especially in presence of hypertension
- *Hypertension*: there is possibly a 30-40% reduction in stroke risk with blood pressure lowering.
- *Lipids* (weaker correlation): treatment with statin medications
- *Prior stroke or transient ischemic attack (TIA)*: risk reduction and behavior modification

Cardiac risk factors
- Atrial fibrillation
- Coronary artery disease
- Congestive heart disease
- Left ventricular dysfunction with mural thrombosis
- Myocardial infarction
- Mitral stenosis

Modifiable behaviors
- Cigarette smoking
- Diet
- Excessive alcohol intake
- Obesity (hypertension, lipids, diabetes): abdominal obesity
- Physical inactivity

■ Clinical presentation

The clinical presentation of a stroke is dependent on the hemisphere of the brain involved as well as the cerebral blood vessels involved and the extent of occlusion within these vessels. The clinical presentations based on vessel involvement include:

- Internal carotid artery symptoms:
  - Aphasia, if the dominant hemisphere is involved
  - Carotid bruit
  - Hemianopsia (blindness in temporal half of one eye, nasal side in other eye), episodes of visual blurring, or amaurosis fugax – temporary blindness in one eye
  - Paralysis of the contralateral (opposite) face, arm, leg
  - Sensory deficits of the opposite face, arm, and leg
- Anterior cerebral artery symptoms:
  - Abulia (inability to make decisions, or perform voluntary acts)
  - Confusion, personality change, judgment, behavior, apathy, flat affect
  - Mental status function may be altered.
  - Opposite side paralysis/ weakness/ of face, arm, leg; greater in leg (foot drop)
  - Sensory loss in the toes, foot, leg
- Middle cerebral artery symptoms:
  - In large volume middle cerebral artery strokes, that can involve almost half of one cerebral hemisphere, there is worry for cerebral swelling and neurological decline. These individuals must be closely monitored and may be considered for hemicranectomy or removal of part of the skull to accommodate the swelling brain.
  - Opposite motor and sensory loss; weakness of arm and face; usually greater loss in leg
  - On same side: hemianopia, gaze preference
- Vertebrobasilar artery symptoms:
  - Ataxic gait and clumsiness
  - Diplopia (double vision), hemianopia, nystagmus, conjugate gaze preference
  - Dysarthria (difficulty manipulating tongue, lips, to produce speech)/ dysphagia (difficulty swallowing)
  - Hemiplegia/hemiparesis; quadriplegia/quadriparesis
  - Locked in syndrome (paralysis from mouth down, involving all four limbs and trunk with intact intellectual function) when basilar artery is occluded.
  - Same side numbness and weakness of the face
  - Vertigo, nausea, dizziness
- Posterior cerebral artery symptoms:
  - Altered mental status
  - Brainstem involvement: pupillary dysfunction, nystagmus, and loss of conjugate gaze

- Cortical blindness
- Diffuse sensory loss from thalamic or subthalamic involvement, intention tremor
- Hemianopsia
- Impaired memory and cognition
- Lack of depth perception
- Perseveration
- Visual agnosia; hallucinations
- Visual deficits
- Posterior-inferior cerebellar artery symptoms:
  - Cerebellar signs including unsteady gait, vertigo, ataxia
  - Contralateral loss of pain and temperature sensation, loss of balance on affected side, and loss of pain and temperature sensation on the ipsilateral face
  - Dysarthria, dysphagia, dysphonia
  - Ipsilateral Horner's syndrome
  - Nausea and vomiting
  - Nystagmus
- Brain stem cerebellar symptoms:
  - Dysarthria
  - Dysconjugate gaze, nystagmus, bilateral visual field deficits
  - Limb or gait ataxia
  - Motor or sensory loss of all four limbs

Handedness determines the dominant hemisphere; but not always.

- In individuals who are right handed:
  - Contralateral motor/ sensory loss
  - Deficit is language; aphasia.
  - Left hemisphere is dominant for language.
  - Memory deficit is language.
  - Slow, cautious behavioral style
  - Visual disturbance in right visual field
- In individuals who are left-handed:
  - Contralateral motor, sensory loss
  - Deficits are visual and sensory neglect; spatial/ perceptual deficits/ denial.
  - Quick, impulsive behavioral style; distractibility; poor insight
  - Right hemisphere is dominant for perception.
  - Visual disturbance in left visual field

It is important to identify those conditions that can mimic stroke. Excluding these conditions is part of the initial care of the stroke patient in the emergency department:

- Acute confusional state/ delirium
- Brain tumor

- Complicated migraine with transient visual changes
- Drug overdose
- Eclampsia
- Head injury: Subdural hematoma or other trauma
- Hypoglycemia/ hyperglycemia
- Hyponatremia
- Infections: brain abscess, encephalitis, or urinary tract infections (UTI) (especially in elders)
- Syncope
- Toxic or metabolic disorders
- Unrecognized seizure: postictal state

■ Nursing assessment

- Neurological assessment and vital sign measurements are needed every 1-2 hours for the first 8 hours after admission to the acute care setting and then every 4 hours while hospitalized.
- Cardiac assessment via cardiac telemetry is needed during the first 24-48 hours or longer to identify cardiac arrhythmias, which are common in the immediate period post stroke.
- Measure orthostatic signs when first when the patient becomes mobile; determine how often to measure after this initial measurement.
- Respiratory assessment: monitor respiratory status and oxygen saturation. Prepare patient for chest X-ray, arterial blood gas levels, and intubation if needed.
- Assessment adequacy of circulation including: presence of peripheral edema, possible deep vein thrombosis (DVT), and potential for pulmonary embolism (PE).
- Assess swallowing ability: patient's responsiveness ability to sit upright, pulmonary function, condition of the mouth, tongue movement, cough, and voice quality.
- Careful glucose measurement during the initial period of hospitalization
- Measurement of intake and output: careful fluid balanceis important to avoid volume overload or depletion.
- Avoid IV dextrose solution in first 24 hours.
- Monitor serum electrolytes, blood urea nitrogen (BUN) and creatinine.
- Maintain IV access.
- Assess possible need for nasogastric tube or gastric tube placement.
- Carefully monitor medication response:
  - Heparin: partial thromboplastin time (PTT) andprothrombin time (PT)
  - Warfarin: International Normalized Ratio (INR)
- Assess language ability.
- Assessment of pain
- Assess bowel and bladder function.
- Assessment of motor function and fall risk
- Assessment of mood to identify possible presence of depression

- Mental status assessment
- Monitoring comorbidities and complications
- Monitoring of all interventions
- Early mobilization
- Patient and family education
- End of life concerns: expressed wishes of the individual; family support needed

■ Diagnostics

- Lab studies:
  - Complete blood count (CBC), electrolytes, glucose level, basic chemistry panel, coagulation studies, BUN, cardiac biomarkers, PT, PTT
- Imaging studies:
  - Computed tomography scan (CT scan):
    - Distinguish ischemia from hemorrhage.
    - Define anatomical distribution of stroke.
    - Normal CT scan first 6 hours
    - After 6–12 hours sufficient edema to produce a regional hypodensity on CT scan
  - Magnetic resonance imaging (MRI) is another important tool in the early care of the stroke patient, which helps to identify the location and extent of the cerebral infarction.
  - Other:
    - Electrocardiogram (EKG), oxygen saturation, Holter monitor
    - Chest film, arterial blood gas (ABG), toxicology screen, liver function tests, electroencephalogram (EEG)
  - Additional testing for stroke and TIA:
    - Carotid duplex scanning: for suspected carotid artery stenosis.
    - Transcranial Doppler: evaluation of proximal vascular anatomyincluding the middle cerebral artery (MCA), intracranial carotid anatomy, and vertibrobasilar artery
    - Echocardiogram: if cardiogenic embolism is suspected and might lead to change in patient's management
    - Transesophogeal echocardiogram: detection of cardio-embolic source, atrial septal defects, or patent foramen ovale
    - Transthoracic echocardiogram: sensitive to ventricular thrombi/evaluation of ventricular function

■ Differential diagnosis

The differential diagnosis includes the type of stroke as well as other potential causes of the patient's symptoms.

- Aneurysm
- Brain tumor
- Complicated migraine with transient visual changes
- Delirium

- Drug overdose
- Eclampsia
- Encephalopathy
- Head injury: Subdural hematoma or other trauma
- Hypoglycemia/hyperglycemia
- Hyponatremia
- Infection
- Infections: brain abscess, encephalitis, UTI
- Metabolic disorder: hypothyroidism or myxedema
- Migraine
- Seizure: post-ictal state
- Subdural or epidural hematoma
- Syncope
- Toxic disorders
- Trauma

■ Treatment

- In the Emergency department:
  - Administration of recombinant tissue plasminogen activator (rtPA) in carefully selected patients with ischemic stroke
- Other interventions/treatments for ischemic stroke:
  - Intra-arterial thrombolysis:
    - Option for treatment of selected patients with major stroke <6 hours duration
    - Large thrombus in the MCA, a life threatening vertebrobasilar stroke and when rtPA is contraindicated
    - Available at centers where studies are being conducted
- Additional interventions:
  - Cerebral stents
  - Removal of clot via a radiological wire placed in the femoral artery – the MERCI Procedure
- Pharmacologic interventions for ischemic stroke include:
  - Heparin, low molecular weight heparin (LMWH), aspirin
  - Agents that inhibit platelet aggregation:
    - Clopidogrel (Plavix), ticlopidine (Ticlid), dipyridamole (Persantine)
    - Research on these drugs in combination with aspirin continues.
- Initiation of rehabilitation strategies as soon as possible.

■ Collaborative consultation

The interdisciplinary team is the cornerstone of stroke care. Members of the team include: nursing, social service, occupational therapy, physical therapy, speech and language therapy, swallowing therapy, physicians, case managers, neuropsychologist, and chaplaincy among others. Stroke rehabilitation can be described as a restorative learning process that seeks to hasten and maximize recovery from stroke by treating the disabilities caused by the stroke, and to prepare the stroke survivor to reintegrate as fully as possible into community life. This requires the coordinated efforts and expertise of members of this team.

■ Complications

- Alteration in motor function causing paralysis, paresis, muscle flaccidity or spasticity
- Alteration in self care activities and altered independence
- Altered bowel and bladder function
- Altered cardiac function: rhythm disturbance, atrial fibrillation, preventricular contractions (PVCs), or congestive heart failure (CHF)
- Altered mental status and cognitive impairments
- Altered neurological function: motor, sensory, visual, auditory
- Depression
- Dysphagia: loss of ability to swallow food or liquids resulting in need for nasogastric or gastric feeding tube.
- Fatigue
- Immobility: possibility of pressure ulcer formation or contracture formation.
- Pain
- Respiratory alterations: pneumonia, aspiration,or pulmonary embolus
- Vascular: DVT
- Visual disturbances

■ Prevention

- Identification of risk factors
- Life style alterations to reduce risk of stroke:
  - Management of blood pressure, diabetes, and cardiac disease
  - Diet to attain and maintain weight reduction
  - Increased activity
  - Moderation in alcohol intake
  - Monitoring of cholesterol and triglyceride levels
  - Smoking cessation
- Careful medication regime management
- Regular follow-up with physician

■ Patient/family education

The goal of public education is early identification of symptoms, rapid transport to a designated stroke center for evaluation, and initiation of treatment. Public education about stroke includes:

- Stroke education about ischemic stroke is focused on identifying the "suddens" as stroke symptoms require immediate hospitalization.

- These include:
  - Sudden numbness in the face, arm, or leg, especially on one side of the body
  - Sudden confusion, or trouble speaking or understanding
  - Sudden difficulty seeing in one or both eyes
  - Sudden trouble walking, dizziness, or loss of balance or coordination

Patient and family education also becomes the work of the team and may address such topics as:

- Description of stroke
- Difference between ischemic or hemorrhagic stroke
- Prevention of recurrent stroke, including:
  - Identification of needed medications
  - Blood pressure management
  - Activity
  - Diet
  - Need for follow-up
- Common complications
- Selection of rehabilitation setting
- Path toward recovery and prognosis for recovery.

Further reading

American Heart Association Statistical Update (2011) Heart Disease and Stroke Statistics–2012 Update. *Circulation* **125**, e2–e220. A Report From the American Heart Association.

American Association of Neuroscience Nurses (2008) Guide to the Care of the Hospitalized Patient with Ischemic Stroke. Clinical Practice Guideline Series. AANN, Glenview, IL.

Bates, B., Choi, J.Y., Duncan, P. *et al.* (2005) Veterans Affairs/Department of Defense clinical practice guideline for management of adult stroke rehabilitation care. *Stroke* **36**, 2049–2056.

Dancer, S., Brown, A. & Yanase, L. (2009) National Institutes of Health stroke scale reliable and valid and in plain English. *Journal of Neuroscience Nursing* **41**(1), 2–5.

Del Zoppo, G., Saver, J.L., Jauch, E.C. & Adams, H.P. Jr. (2009) Expansion of the time window for treatment of acute stroke with intravenous tissue plasminogen activator. AHA/ASA Science Advisory. *Stroke* **40**, 2945.

Garon, B., Seirzant, T. & Ormiston, C. (2009) Silent aspiration: Results of 2000 video fluoroscopic evaluations. *Journal of Neuroscience Nursing* **41**(4), 178–188.

Gross, J. (2003) Urinary incontinence after stroke: Evaluation and behavioral treatment. *Topics in Geriatric Rehabilitation* **19**(1), 60–83.

Harari, D., Norton, C., Lockwood, L. & Swift, C. (2004) Treatment of constipation and fecal incontinence in stroke patients: Ranomized controlled trial. *Stroke* **35**, 2549–2555.

Jauch, E. (2009) Acute stroke management. Emedicine. Online. Available from http://emedicine.medscape.com/article/1159752-overview (acessed 22 March 2012).

Jepson, R., Despain, K. & Keller, D. (2008) Unilateral neglect: Assessment in nursing practice. *Journal of Neuroscience Nursing* **40**(3), 142-150.

Heidenreich, P.A., Trogdon J.G., Khavjou, O.A. *et al.* (2011). Forecasting the future of cardiovascular disease in the United States: a policy statement from the American Heart Association. *Circulation* **123**, 933-944.

Hinkle, J. (2010) Outcome three years after motor stroke. *Rehabilitation Nursing* **35**(1), 23-31.

Hinkle, J. & Guanci, M. (2007) Acute ischemic stroke review. *Journal of Neuroscience Nursing* **39**(5), 285-310.

Ryan, T., Enderby, P. & Rigby, A.S. (2006) A randomized controlled trial to evaluate intensity of community-based rehabilitation provision following stroke or hip fracture in old age. *Clinical Rehabilitation* **20**(2), 123-131.

Sacco, R., Adams, R., Albers, G. *et al.* (2006) Guidelines for prevention of stroke in patients with ischemic stroke or transient ischemic attack: a statement for healthcare professionals from the American Heart Association/American Stroke Association Council on Stroke: co-sponsored by the Council on Cardiovascular Radiology and Intervention: the American Academy of Neurology affirms the value of this guideline. *Stroke* **37**, 577.

Summers, D. & Leonard, A. (2009) Comprehensive overview of nursing and inter-disciplinary care of the acute ischemic stroke patient. AHA Scientific Statement. Stroke **40**, 2911-2944.

Vanhook, P. (2009) The domains of stroke recovery: A synopsis of the literature. *Journal of Neuroscience Nursing* **41**(1), 6-17.

PART 4: DIZZINESS

Jean B. Fahey

Dizziness means different things to different persons. Children love to twirl in circles and ride on the spinning "carousels" at the playground, a testament to the joys that dizziness can bring. Dizziness in elders, conversely, fails to elicit this pleasure and interferes with lifestyle and social behavior. "Dizziness in the elder is more persistent, has more causes, is less often due to a psycho physiologic cause, and seems to be more incapacitating than dizziness in younger patients" (Davis, 1994). The prevalence of dizziness in elders is high and is associated with falls, functional disability, and even death. Assessment of fall risk should be done with all persons who complain of dizziness and strategies to reduce the risk of injury from falls implemented immediately.

Dizziness as described by patients is a non specific term, and is classified into four different categories: syncope or presyncope, disequilibrium, nonspecific dizziness or ill defined light-headedness, and vertigo. Light-headedness or fainting is related to conditions associated with presyncope or syncope, while a spinning sensation is usually related to vertigo.

■ Risk factors

- Anxiety, depression
- Cerebrovascular disease, past myocardial infarction, postural hypotension

- Cognitive dysfunction
- Deconditioning
- Dehydration
- Gait disorders
- Hyponatremia
- Impaired balance
- Medications
- Neck disorders
- Sensory defects, visual, hearing, or tactile impairment

From Tinetti *et al.*, 2000.

■ Clinical presentation

According to Samuels (2010), it is important that the patient describe the dizziness in their own words as this will help the practitioner differentiate the cause. Asking the patient what he or she means by "dizzy", then listening without asking questions is also necessary to determine the sensation the patient is experiencing. Additional information necessary includes the patient's medications (including over-the counter and herbals), a recent history of falls, and associated symptoms (e.g., nausea, vomiting, tinnitus, visual changes, weakness and/or loss of consciousness), what makes it worse or better, when the episodes occur and how long they last.

■ Nursing assessment

- Vital signs, including orthostatics
- Cardiopulmonary evaluation:
  - Heart rate, rhythm, extra heart sounds and carotid bruits
- Neurologic evaluation including cognitive screen, cranial nerves, gait, balance, and Romberg
  - Assess for nystagmus (involuntary oscillation of the eyes).
- Fall risk assessment

■ Diagnostics

Laboratory and imaging studies are guided by patient presentation and are not always indicated. In older adults a cardiac or neurologic etiology is a definite concern requiring physician consultation and diagnostic evaluation that may include an electrocardiogram, echocardiogram, event monitor, computerized tomography (CT) or magnetic resonance imaging (MRI) and laboratory evaluation. Diagnostic testing for patients with vertigo may include audiometry and tests of vestibular function. A blood sugar test is important for patients complaining of lightheadedness.

■ Differential diagnosis

The differential diagnosis is concerned with determining the cause of the patient's dizziness. Symptoms help differentiate the cause and fall into one of the four following categories:

(1) Syncope or presyncope is a sensation of fainting or near fainting and some patients describe this as a feeling of lightheadedness or as if they were going to "pass out". Persons may have other signs and symptoms such as pallor, blurred vision, diaphoresis, nausea and have a feeling of warmth. These signs and symptoms indicate possible diminished cerebral blood flow and usually last a few seconds but sometimes can last longer. Samuels (2010) identifies possible associated conditions below:
 - Cardiac arrhythmias
 - Dehydration
 - Failure of autonomic reflex or a hypersensitive carotid sinus
 - Hyperventilation R/T anxiety
 - Micturition or defecation syncope
 - Neurocardiogenic syncope or vasovagal syncope
 - Orthostatic hypotension
 - Vasovagal syncope
 - Vasodilation or factors that disable vasoconstriction
 - Ventricular outflow obstruction

(2) Disequilibrium is the feeling of imbalance or the feeling like you are about to fall. This sensation can be from problems in two areas:
 - Cerebellar ataxia is related to cerebellar pathology and is characterized by a wide based, uncoordinated unsteady gait (Samuels, 2010).
 - Multiple sensory deficit syndrome frequently affects elders with visual or auditory deficits, peripheral neuropathy and/or muscular disorders or weakness.

(3) Nonspecific dizziness, anxiety, or ill defined lightheadedness is suggested by a patient's inability to explain what they mean by "dizziness". These patients will complain that they are "just dizzy". Potential causes include:
 - Hypoglycemia
 - Medications
 - Psychiatric disorders, panic attacks, depression, personality disorders, alcohol dependence and somatization disorders
 - Nonspecific diseases that may be commonly related to hyperventilation

(4) Vertigo is the cause of about one third of all patient dizzy complaints (Neuhauser et al., 2008). Patients may describe feeling off balance or use a descriptive term like "spinning", or an illusion of movement. Often vertigo is related to a peripheral lesion, though central lesions (e.g., brainstem infarction, cerebellar stroke, demyelinating disease, or tumor) are also possible. Benign positional vertigo, labyrinthitis, Ménière's disease, schwannomas or tumors are common disorders associated with peripheral lesions. Vertigo can occur spontaneously, or with head position change or

middle ear pressure. The sensation is aggravated by head motion and may be worse when the patient's eyes are closed. Patients commonly have difficulty maintaining a steady upright posture when walking, standing or even sitting unsupported. Nystagmus suggests the dizziness is vertigo. Associated hearing loss or tinnitus suggests vertigo from a peripheral origin; other associated brainstem signs are often present and suggest vertigo from a central origin. Because vertigo can have multiple concurrent causes, especially in elders, a specific diagnosis can be elusive (Swartz & Paxton, 2005). Systemic causes of vertigo are rarer; these include diabetes and hypothyroidism. Certain features can aid in the distinction between central and peripheral causes of vertigo. The physical exam should include orthostatic vital signs and an otoscopic exam. The neurological exam should include the Dix-Hallpike maneuver to differentiate peripheral from central vertigo.

- Central vertigo produces other neurologic symptoms, although this generalization has many exceptions. Central vertigo generally does not have hearing loss or tinnitus. Risk factors such as hypertension, atrial fibrillation, history of prior stroke, and advanced age may raise the suspicion of vascular causes. Brainstem signs may be present and include: ataxia, vomiting, headache, diplopia, visual loss, slurred speech, numbness, weakness, or incoordination. Vertical nystagmus is classic from a central cause. The Dix-Hallpike maneuver produces nystagmus that is not fatigable, and not latent. The symptoms are usually mild and last more than 1 minute (Swartz & Paxton, 2005). Potential causes include:
  - All drugs that intoxicate the reticular activating system
  - Demyelinating disorders
  - Brainstem vascular disease (Wallenberg's syndrome, VB insufficiency, cerebellar ischemia)
  - Temporal lobe disorders (seizures) and brain tumors
  - Cerebral hemorrhage
  - Head trauma, concussion
  - Cervical spine muscle ligament injury, stenosis
  - Infection or autoimmune disorder
  - Migraine (10% of all patients with vertigo)
- Peripheral vertigo presents with an abrupt onset of nausea, vomiting, and auditory complaints. Symptoms are usually intense. The majority of causes of vertigo are peripheral. The VIIIth cranial nerves (cochlear and vestibular) are affected. Hearing loss suggests a peripheral cause. Nystagmus is torsional upbeat or horizontal. The Dix-Hallpike maneuver generally shows nystagmus to be latent and fatigable, with symptoms being severe but lasting less than 1 minute (Swartz & Paxton, 2005). Causes include:
  - Foreign body in ear canal
  - The vestibular schwannoma, often incorrectly called an acoustic neuroma. These tumors can become quite dangerous causing cerebellum or cranial nerve compression.

- Ear infections: labyrinthitis, vestibular or cochlear neuritis
- Benign paroxysmal positional vertigo (BPPV), or Barany's vertigo. This benign condition lasts for only seconds. This occurs only in certain positions, and abates when the person stops moving. The Dix-Hallpike maneuver will reproduce the symptoms.
- Ménière's disease is caused by excessive fluid in the endolymphatic system in the ear. It's characterized by a dull ache in the mastoid process or around the ear with severe tinnitus, a cochlear kind of sensory hearing loss and a classic peripheral type of vestibular symptoms with severe spinning vertigo.
- Inner ear fistulas

■ Treatment

Treatment of dizziness depends on the cause:

(1) Presyncopal, or syncopal dizziness may involve reestablishing blood flow. If dizziness occurs during or just following exercise, this may be from a cardiac arrhythmia, aortic stenosis, or asymmetrical septal hypertrophy. If the history suggests a cardiac cause, Holter monitoring is indicated. Discontinuing any precipitating drugs, or addressing any autonomic insufficiency with agents such as midodrine may help. Maneuvers such as leg crossing and constricting the leg muscles or fist clinching can restore cerebral blood flow. Educating elders on avoiding dehydration or rapidly going from a sitting or lying position to a standing position can be very effective.

(2) Disequilibrium from multiple sensory deficit syndrome is treated by correcting/improving sensory deficits. These include surgery for cataracts, hearing aids, and night light use, review of medications, reducing alcohol intake and treatment of peripheral neuropathy.

(3) Anxiety and or depression can be treated with supportive management with or without the use of antidepressants or anxiolytic drugs. Assurance, support and relaxation techniques along with identifying and controlling hyperventilation can reduce episodes of anxiety. Socialization and activity can be helpful for mild depression. Often though, psychiatric care may be indicated.

(4) Treating vertigo will depend on the cause:

Peripheral causes:

- Foreign bodies or fistula repairs
- The Epley, Sermont, or Brantd-Daroff maneuvers for benign paroxysmal positional vertigo
- Supportive measures with Ménière's disease
- Surgical evaluation for the acoustic neuroma (vestibular schwannoma)

- Labyrinthitis, vestibular and cochlear neuritis, generally resolve completely in 3 to 6 weeks.

Central treatment of vertigo:

- Evaluation of all medications
- Reestablishing blood flow and prevention of low flow states
- Surgical intervention may be helpful for spinal stenosis.
- Treatment of infections, autoimmune, or seizure disorder
- Three categories of drugs treat vertigo.
  - Anti-serotonin and antihistamine type drugs: dimenhydrinate, diphenhydramine, meclizine, and cyclizine. All produce major sedation, a significant concern in older adults. Modafinil or methylphenidate can be used in concert with these drugs to reduce side effects.
  - Phenothiazines: promethazine, for nausea can be given rectally. Other phenothiazines are not helpful.
- Belladonna alkaloids: Scopolamine has many cardiovascular and psychiatric side effects. Transdermal scopolamine may help with motion sickness, but transdermal doses will not affect acute vestibular syndromes.

■ Collaborative consultation
- Specialists from neurology, cardiology, otolaryngology and psychiatry may be consulted for patients complaining of dizziness.
- Physical therapy evaluation to determine patient's safety with ambulation and need for assistant devices.

■ Complications
Falls are one of the more serious complications associated with dizziness and vertigo.

■ Prevention
Prevention will depend on the cause of the dizziness or vertigo.

■ Patient /family education
- Explain the cause and prevention of the dizziness. Discuss fall prevention and interventions for both the hospital and home.
- Discuss the importance of a home safety evaluation.
- Evaluate the effectiveness of prescribed drugs.
- Prevention of dehydration and cues to stand up slowly from a sitting or supine position.
- Encourage use of night lights, hearing aids, and eye glasses.

References

Davis, L.E. (1994) Dizziness in elderly men. *Journal of the American Geriatric Society* **42**(11), 1184–1188.

Neuhauser, H.K., Radtke, A., von Brevern, M. *et al.* (2008) Burden of dizziness and vertigo in the community. *Arch Intern Med* **168**, 2118.

Samuels, M. (2010) "The dizzy patient." Entering the mind zone, Brigham and Women's Hospital, Joseph P. Martin Conference Center, Boston, MA, 6 October, 2010.

Swartz, R. & Paxton, L. (2005) Treatment of vertigo. *American Family Physician* **71**(6), 1115–1122.

Tinetti, M.E., Williams, C.S. & Gill, T.M. (2000) Dizziness among older adults: a possible geriatric syndrome. *Annals of Internal Medicine* **132**(5), 337–344.

PART 5: NORMAL PRESSURE HYDROCEPHALUS

Jean B. Fahey

Normal pressure hydrocephalus (NPH) is characterized by ventricular dilation and normal cerebrospinal fluid (CSF) pressure without papilledema (i.e., optic disk swelling). NPH was reported as early as 1956, but Adams and colleagues were the first investigators to categorize and recognize NPH's clinical importance in 1965 (Adams *et al.*, 1965; Osei-Boamah, 2011). Since then, more attention has been focused on the diagnosis and treatment of NPH because it is thought to account for about 5% of all dementias and is a potentially treatable cause of dementia (Osei-Boamah, 2011; Rosenberg, 2008).

NPH can be idiopathic or related to another secondary condition (Vanneste, 2000). When associated with an identified etiology (e.g., head injury), NPH can occur in any age group, but idiopathic NPH usually occurs in adults over the age of 60 years (Osei-Boamah, 2011).

The pathophysiology of idiopathic NPH is not certain. The absence of papilledema with normal CSF pressures at lumbar puncture resulted in the term "normal pressure hydrocephalus", however, the pressure may not always be normal. Intracranial hypertension may begin even before diagnosis (Rowland, 1995) as the cerebral ventricles become enlarged because of the increase in cerebrospinal fluid volume. In theory, the increase in ventricle size allows CSF pressure to normalize, but creates pressure and ischemia in the brain causing the cognition, gait, and urinary incontinence problems. However, numerous studies have not established this or other pathology as the definitive cause of NPH (Bateman, 2007; Osei-Boamah, 2011).

Unfortunately, the changes that occur in NPH are insidious and often attributed to normal aging changes. As a result, the disorder is often not diagnosed and treatment can be delayed because these problems mimic many of the problems commonly seen in older adults: gait difficulty, cognitive decline, and incontinence. To help healthcare providers and physicians recognize NPH, an international team of scientists developed clinical guidelines for diagnosis in 2005 (Graff-Radford, 2007).

■ Risk factors

Risk factors include (Rosenberg, 2008):

- Closed head injury or head trauma
- Craniotomy
- Meningitis or other central nervous system infections
- Subarachnoid hemorrhage

Factors that could aggravate hydrocephalus because they increase jugular venous pressure and decrease CSF flow into the cerebral venous sinuses include (Graff-Radford, 2007; Rowland, 1995):

- Congestive heart failure
- Lung disease
- Obesity
- Recent head injury
- Sleep apnea
- Systemic hypertension

■ Clinical presentation

According to Graff-Radford (2007), patients with normal pressure hydrocephalus may present differently depending on the stage of the disorder. Signs and symptoms include headache, falls, lethargy, malaise, incoordination, weakness and/or urinary incontinence. In early stages, the symptoms and signs may be subtle, but urinary incontinence and the cognitive and gait changes increase over time.

A family member may also notice these signs and symptoms. The patient's history should be verified by a family member, friend, or other collaborator and also include information about recent behavior or cognitive change. A past medical history of secondary causes such as head trauma, intracerebral hemorrhage, meningitis, secondary hydrocephalus, and neurologic or psychiatric disorder should be elicited.

■ Nursing assessment

The initial nursing assessment should include vital signs and full physical assessment. The skin assessment should determine any bruising or lacerations the patient may have incurred in a fall. The neurologic assessment should address the patient's cognitive status, psychomotor skills and ability to ambulate. Important considerations include:

- Is the patient attentive? Alert and oriented?
- Is the patient's short term memory intact? Recall intact?
- Is the speech fluent?
- Is cognition impaired as evidenced by decreased Mini Mental State Examination (MMSE) score?
- Is executive function intact?
- Is the gait apraxic, slowed, shuffling wide based, or magnetic?
- Is fine motor speed diminished?
- Is patient incontinent of urine or stool?
- Does the patient have urinary urgency, urinary frequency, or nocturia?

■ Diagnostics

Diagnostics are based on the patient's clinical presentation. Usual diagnostics include:

- Lumbar puncture (LP)
- Computed tomography (CT) scan
- Magnetic resonance imaging (MRI)

Further diagnostics include tests to determine if the patient will benefit from CSF shunting. These include a large volume spinal tap, temporary external lumbar drainage, and intracranial pressure monitoring B wave presence, a potential indication of NPH and a possible predictor of shunt success (Osei-Boamah, 2011).

■ Differential diagnosis (Graff-Radford, 2007)

- Addison's disease
- Carcinomatous meningitis
- Dementias
  - Alzheimer disease
  - Frontotemporal dementia
  - Parkinson's dementia
  - Parkinsonian syndromes: Lewy body disease, corticobasal ganglionic degeneration, progressive supranuclear palsy, and multiple system atrophy
  - Pick's disease
  - Vascular dementia
- Wilson's disease
- Encephalopathy
- Gait disorders
- Head trauma

- Hypothyroidism
- Intracranial infection
- Intracranial tumor
- Subdural hematoma

■ Treatment

The symptoms of NPH usually increase over time if the condition is not treated, so early diagnosis is important. Varied medications (e.g., acetazolamide, furosemide, and isosorbide) have been tried, but are not effective (Hebb & Cusimano, 2001). Repeated LP drainage has also been used with some patients, but the most effective therapy is ventriculoperitoneal shunting (VP shunt) which decreases cerebral pressures (Osei-Boamah, 2011).

■ Collaborative consultation

Neurology consultation is indicated for patients with suspected NPH. Neuropsychological evaluation assists with diagnosis, determines the patient's baseline function and assists patients and families with information about prognosis and future planning (Graff-Radford, 2007).

Neurosurgical consultation for VP shunt.

■ Complications

VP shunt complications in NPH can be significant. These include:

- Cerebral infarction
- Death
- Hematomas/hemorrhages
- Intracranial infections
- Neurologic disability
- Seizures
- Shunt failures

■ Prevention

NPH is idiopathic. Currently, there is no known prevention.

■ Patient/family education

Safety measures must take a prominent role and must be incorporated with teachings for caregivers. The importance of safety and fall prevention is an important aspect of patient and family education.

Frequent toileting with assistance, ambulatory aids, and frequent nursing assessment can help minimize falls and their associated complications. A safety evaluation of the home environment, and ambulatory and toileting aid use assessment will also be beneficial.

Regular follow up and attention to symptoms are required after surgical treatment because of the risk of infections and shunt failure. Neurologic deterioration should be assessed by the neurologist and possibly imaging to exclude hemorrhage or to check the shunt catheter positioning when necessary.

References

Adams, R.D., Fisher, C.M., Hakim, S., Ojemann R.G., & Sweet, W.H. (1965) Symptomatic occult hydrocephalus with "normal" cerebrospinal fluid pressure (a treatable syndrome). *New England Journal of Meicine* **15**(273), 117-126.

Bateman, G.A. (2007) The pathophysiology of idiopathic normal pressure hydrocephalus: cerebral ischemia or altered venous hemodynamics? *American Journal of Neuroradiology* **29**(1), 198-203.

Graff-Radford, N. (2007) Normal pressure hydrocephalus. *Neurologic Clinics* **25**(3), 809-832.

Osei-Boamah, E. (2011) Normal pressure hydrocephalus in the older patient. *Clinical Geriatrics* **19**(4), 49-4.

Rosenberg, G.A. (2008) Brain edema and disorders of cerebrospinal fluid circulation. In: *Neurology in Clinical Practice*, 5th edition, W.G. Bradley, R.B. Daroff, G.M. Fenichel & J. Jankovic (eds). Butterworth-Heinemann, Philadelphia.

Rowland, L. (1995) *Merritt's Textbook of Neurology*, 9th edition. Williams & Wilkins, New York.

Vanneste, J.A. (2000) Diagnosis and management of normal pressure hydrocephalus. *Journal of Neurology* **247**(5), 5-14.

Further reading

Anger, J.T., & Litwin, C.S. (2006) The prevalence of urinary incontinence among community dwelling adult woman; results from the national health and nutrition examination survey. *Journal of Urology* **175**(2), 601-604.

Hebb, A.O., & Cusimano, M.D. (2001) Idiopathic normal pressure hydrocephalus: a systemic review of diagnosis and outcome. *Neurosurgery* **49**(5), 1166-1184.

Hebert, L.E., Scherr, P.A., Bienias, J.L., Bennett, D.A., & Evans, D.A. (2003) Alzheimer disease in the us population: prevalence estimates using the 2000 census. *Archives of Neurology* **60**(8), 1119-1122.

Jack, Jr. C.R., Shiung, M.M., & Gunter, J.L. (2004) Comparison of different MRI brain atrophy rate measures with clinical disease progression in AD. *Neurology* **62**(4), 591-600.

Ogino, A., Kazui, H., Miyoshi, N. *et al.* (2006) Cognitive impairment in patients with idiopathic normal pressure hydrocephalus. *Dementia, Geriatrics and Cognitive Disorders* **21**(2), 113-119.

Reikin, N., Marmarou, A., Klinge, P., Bergneider, M., & Black, P.M. (2005) Diagnosing idiopathic normal pressure hydrocephalus. *Neurosurgery* **57**(3 suppl), S4-S16.

Stothers, L., Thom, D., & Calhoun, E. (2005). Urologic diseases in America project: urinary incontinence in males-demographics and economic burden. *Journal of Urology* **173**(4), 1302-1308.

Verghese, J., Lipton, R.B., & Hall, C.B. (2002) Abnormality of gait as a predictor of non-Alzheimer dementia. *New England Journal of Medicine* **347**(22), 1761-1768.

PART 6: PARKINSON'S DISEASE

Marion Phipps

Parkinson's disease (PD) is a degenerative disease of the nervous system. It was first described in 1817 by the English physician James Parkinson. In his writings he described this disease as "the shaking palsy" and in an early paper he outlined the initial symptoms of the disease that would bear his name. PD is a chronic and progressive disorder of movement. The disease usually begins insidiously, often unilaterally, with only a few apparent symptoms. Often individuals experience clumsiness in one hand as an initial symptom.

The incidence and prevalence of PD increases with age and it is considered a disease of older adults , but not always, as it can occur in middle age or in younger adults. In the United States it is believed that there are about 500,000 individuals with PD, with 50,000 individuals newly diagnosed each year (National Parkinson Foundation, 2012). Though initial symptoms may occur earlier, Parkinson's disease is usually diagnosed around age 62 (National Parkinson Foundation, 2012). Men are affected more often than women. As the population ages an increased incidence of PD is expected (The National Institute of Neurological Disease and Stroke, 2011).

There are varied types of parkinsonism, but the underlying problem relates to dopaminergic transmission. The basal ganglia are composed of neurons gathered in clusters (ganglia) along the sides of both lateral ventricles, above the thalamus. The basal ganglia are a collective term that includes the sub-cortical motor nuclei of the cerebrum. The structures of the basal ganglia include: the striatum, globus pallidus, subthalamic nuclei, substantia nigra, and the red nucleus. PD is thought to be caused by the destruction of the substantia nigra, the area where the brain chemical dopamine is created. Dopamine is a chemical transmitter responsible for the coordination of smooth, purposeful movement. It is possible that individuals with PD have lost 60-80% of their dopamine-producing cells before symptoms appear. The pathophysiology of PD is thought to include the following changes. Pigmented cells in the substantia nigra are lost because of degenerative changes and are replaced by Lewy (protein) bodies. With this change, dopamine, normally stored in these cells is depleted. This results in impairment of extrapyramidal motor tracts, semiautomatic motor function, and coordinated movements.

■ Risk factors

One of the diagnostic problems of PD is that early symptoms may be disregarded as normal consequence of aging. Researchers believe PD is caused by a combination of genetic susceptibility and exposure to environmental factors that may trigger the disease. Other causative factors continue to be investigated, but concerns include:

- Exposure to neurotoxins
- Family history Parkinson's Disease
- History of head injury
- Male gender

■ Clinical presentation

Symptoms of PD usually begin gradually and worsen over time. As symptoms become more pronounced functional ability may be altered with increased difficulty walking, in self care activities, and in speaking.

The four main symptoms and motor manifestations of PD include:

- *Resting tremors*: tremors of the hands, arms, jaw, or head. The tremor may have a characteristic PD appearance: 4–6 beats/second, with "pill rolling" tremor of the thumb and forefinger.
- *Bradykinesia*: slowness of movement and loss of spontaneous, automatic movements making activities of daily living (ADLs) difficult.
- *Muscle rigidity*: resistance to movement through muscle tension leading to stiffness and aching of the limbs and trunk.
- *Postural instability*: the individual with PD develops a stooped and bowed posture causing postural instability and an increase in falls.

Secondary manifestations

- *Depression*: May be an early symptom of PD; depression needs to be identified and treated with appropriate pharmacologic or therapeutic interventions.
- *Emotional changes*: Individuals may become fearful, insecure, irritable, and/or sad. These changes may be accompanied by mask-like face from muscular rigidity that may make emotional state difficult to interpret through facial expression.
- *Monotone voice*: speech may be soft and hesitant. It may be difficult to understand the patient when they speak.
- *Cognitive problems*: Seen in some but not all patients; dementia may develop in some patients.
- General weakness and muscle fatigue with chewing and swallowing, leading to dysphagia, malnutrition and weight loss. These changes place the individual at risk of aspiration pneumonia.
- General weakness and muscle fatigue leading to pain and muscle cramps of the extremities and trunk, but particularly in the legs and toes
- Edema of the feet and legs due to immobility
- *Problems with sleep*: insomnia, wakefulness, fatigue from lack of sleep

Autonomic manifestations

- Drooling: may lead to maceration of the lips, face, and chin.
- Seborrhea: oily, greasy skin, excessive perspiration
- Constipation and potential urinary incontinence; urinary hesitancy and frequency
- Orthostatic hypotension: increasing the risk of falls

The classification of Parkinson's disease

Stage I: One side of the body involvement only

Stage II: Both sides of the body involvement; balance intact

Stage III: Impaired postural and righting reflexes, balance affected; mild to moderate disease; remains physically independent

Stage IV: Fully developed, severe disease, marked disability, may be unable to walk or stand unassisted

Stage V: Confinement to bed or wheelchair.

■ Nursing assessment

The nursing assessment of an individual with PD may change as the symptoms of the disease increase.

In the initial stages the nurse carefully monitors:

- Motor function
- Balance
- Blood pressure changes with standing that would indicate orthostatic hypotension
- Self care ability
- Changes in bladder and bowel function

As the disease progresses the nurse continues to assess the above areas but additional assessment includes:

- Risk of falls
- Swallowing ability
- Nutritional balance
- Skin integrity
- Range of joint motion
- Presence of depression, delusions, or altered mental status
- Need for adaptive equipment and consultation with interdisciplinary team

As the individual becomes more debilitated the nurse may assess:

- End of life questions
- The need for additional supports in the home or transfer to another more appropriate setting of care

■ Diagnostics

There is no diagnostic blood or laboratory test that can diagnose PD. The diagnosis of PD is based on the description by the individual of their symptoms over time and by physical examination. Brain computerized tomography scan (CT scan) or magnetic resonance imaging (MRI) usually appear normal, but may be completed to rule out other conditions. However, it is important to diagnose this disease as early as possible so that appropriate interventions can be initialed. Progression of symptoms occurs over time. There is great individual variation in this process, but symptoms may progress over 20 years or longer.

■ Differential diagnosis

Parkinson's disease is a fairly prevalent neurodegenerative disorder, but other conditions may have a similar presentation. The differential can be extensive and may include the following:

- Hallervorden–Spatz disease
- Hemiatrophy-hemiparkinsonism
- Huntington's disease
- Infection
- Lewy body dementia
- Medication induced tremor
- Movement disorder
- Multisystem atrophy
- Normal pressure hydrocephalus
- Progressive supranuclear palsy
- Shy–Drager syndrome
- Striatonigral degeneration
- Toxicity (carbon dioxide, cyanide, ethanol, manganese, 1-methyl-4-phenyl-1,2,3,6-tetrahydropyridine)
- Trauma
- Tumor
- Wilson's disease

■ Treatment

Treatment of PD includes multiple modalities. Control of disease symptoms is managed with carefully regulated and monitored drug therapy and potential surgical interventions. Supportive therapy and maintenance is needed for the management of additional symptoms. Participation in physical therapy and continued physical activity and mobility is essential as is referral for psychotherapy, if necessary. Depression may be treated with psychotherapy and/or antidepressant medication.

Drug therapy for PD generally falls into one of three categories. These include: drugs that increase the level of dopamine; drugs that impact the symptoms of the disease, such as tremors and muscle stiffness; and drugs that treat non-motor problems: depression, etc.

Drugs that increase levels of dopamine (dopamine replacement therapy) are the cornerstone of the symptomatic treatment of PD. These include:

- Levodopa:
  - Metabolic precursor to dopamine
  - L-dopa crosses the blood–brain barrier; converts to dopamine in basal ganglia.
  - When administered alone induces a high incidence of nausea and vomiting
  - Best given in combination levodopa/peripheral decarboxylase inhibitor (PDI)
- Levodopa with decarboxylase inhibitor (PDI):
  - Standard of symptomatic treatment for PD; given with the onset of functional disability
  - Provides the greatest anti-parkisonian benefit with fewest adverse effects: bradykinesia and rigidity
  - Lacks efficacy in later disease
  - Started at low dose, increased slowly, and titrated to control symptoms:
    (1) Levodopa and carbidopa (Sinemet)
      - Immediate release: 25/100 milligrams 1/2 tablet daily initially and increased every 1-2 days to 1 tablet po TID
      - CR form: 25/100 milligrams. 1 tab po qd, increased to TID or 50/200 milligrams po BID
- Dopamine agonists:
  - Mimic the role of dopamine in the brain.
  - Directly stimulate postsynaptic dopamine receptors to provide anti-parkinsonian benefit.
  - Can be used as monotherapy to improve symptoms in early disease or as an adjunct to levodopa in patients whose response to levodopa is deteriorating and those experiencing fluctuations in response to L-dopa.
  - After 6 months to a few years these medications may not be as effective as levodopa/PDI.
  - Drugs include: bromocriptine, pergolide, pramipexole, and ropinirole.
  - Dosed according to symptoms
- Monoamine oxidase-inhibitors
  - Inhibit the enzyme that breaks down dopamine in the brain.
  - Reduces symptoms of PD:
    - Drug: selegiline – can delay need for levodopa for up to a year.
    - Given with levodopa can prolong response to drug.
- Catechol-O-methyl transferase inhibitors:
  - An enzyme that helps to break down dopamine.
  - Helps to reduce needed level of dopamine or when a drug holiday is needed for levodopa.
  - Side effects: diarrhea, nausea, and sleep disturbance
  - Drugs: tolcapone and entacapone

Drugs that impact the symptoms of PD include:

- Amantadine
  - An antiviral drug that can reduce symptoms of PD. This drug is often used alone in early stages of disease. May be given with an anticholinergic medication and levodopa.
  - Effect wears away after about 1 year.
  - Side effects: insomnia, mottled skin, edema, and agitation
  - May in rare cases cause liver disease; liver function must be monitored.
- Anticholinergic drugs
  - Decrease activity of neurotransmitter acetycholine; reduces resting tremor, cramps, and rigidity.
  - Not effective in treating bradykinesia, gait disturbance, or other features of advanced PD:
    - Artane: 2-5 milligrams tid or qid
    - Pagitane: 1.25-5 milligrams tid or qid
    - Kemardrin: 5-10 milligrams tid or qid
    - Akineton: 1-2 milligrams tid or qid
    - Cogentin: 0.5-6.0 milligrams daily

Additional pharmacologic interventions include: antidepressants, anti-anxiety agents, and antipsychotics if psychosis is caused by Parkinsonian drugs or neurological involvement.

Surgical interventions for the treatment of PD have been developed and studied in surgical trials. Surgeries for PD include the following.

Steriotactic surgery

- Pallidotomy: the surgeon selectively destroys part of the basal ganglia, the globus pallidus, via surgical implementation.
  - Used to eliminate tremors, bradykinesia, and rigidity
  - May improve gait and imbalance and decrease need for levodopa
  - Only one side of the brain at a time; if symptoms are bilateral 6 month lapse between surgeries.
- Thalamotomy: surgically destroying part of the thalamus, the collection of nuclei responsible for sensory integration
  - Primarily to reduce tremor

Deep brain stimulation (DBS)

- High frequency stimulation through electrodes placed in parts of the brain (usually the subthalamic nucleus, the globus pallidus, or the thalamus, a cluster of nuclei responsible for the integration of sensation). An implantable pulse generator is connected to the electrodes and is tunneled down under the skin to beneath the collarbone.
- Stimulates the brain to decrease symptoms of PD
- Approved by the Food and Drug Administration (FDA)

- Can be applied to both sides of the brain
- Reduces need for medications
- Patient needs to return to hospital to have pulse generator adjusted to needs.
- Not effective with all PD patients

■ Collaborative consultation

The entire interdisciplinary team is involved in the care of the individual with worsening symptoms of PD. These team members include: nurses, neurologist, neurosurgeon, physiatrist, physical therapy, occupational therapy, speech and language pathologists, nutritionist, social worker, psychologist, and clergy.

■ Complications

The possible complications of advancing PD include:

- Adverse response to medications
- Alteration in sleep; insomnia
- Alterations in bowel function
- Altered mental status
- Constipation
- Contracture formation
- Depression
- Fatigue and exhaustion
- Immobility
- Impaired balance with the possibility of injury from falls
- Inability to swallow and possible aspiration pneumonia
- Pain from limited movement
- Pressure ulcer formation
- Urinary tract dysfunction and possible infection

■ Prevention

The goal of interdisciplinary care of the individual with PD is prevention of the complications listed above. Involvement of the team and frequent follow-up is an essential aspect of care.

■ Patient/family education

- Patient and family education regarding the course of the disease:
  - National Parkinson's Foundation: http://www.parkinson.org
- Medication education:
  - Review of all prescribed medications and potential side effects
  - Encourage patient to carry drug information at all times.
  - Encourage adherence to drug regime.

- Describe signs and symptoms in need of medical consultation.
- Accident prevention:
  - Muscle strengthening through prescribed exercise regime
  - Physical therapy: maintenance of range of joint motion and increased muscle strength and tone
  - Prevention of orthostatic hypotension leading to falls and potential injury
- Nutritional consultation/ weight loss/ swallowing problems:
  - Diet: normal, well balanced diet essential; rich in fiber and fluids to prevent constipation
- Evaluation of bowel and urinary problems:
  - Prevent constipation
  - Evaluation with urologist for possible pharmacologic or surgical management of urinary problems
- Interventions to combat impact of immobility:
  - Skin care: bathing and frequent repositioning
  - Range of joint motion to prevent contracture formation.
  - Positioning equipment
  - Appropriately fit wheelchair; wheelchair cushion
  - Prevention of pneumonia, deep vein thrombosis (DVT), and pulmonary emboli (PE)

References

The National Institute of Neurological Disease and Stroke (2011) Parkinson's Disease: Hope through Research. Online. Available from http://www.ninds.nih.gov/disorders/parkinsons_disease/detail_parkinsons_disease.htm (accessed 22 March 2012)

National Parkinson Foundation (2012) Parkinson's Disease Overview. Available @ http://www.parkinson.org/parkinson-s-disease.aspx (accessed May 30, 2012).

Further reading

Hagell, P. (2007) Nursing and multidisciplinary interventions for Parkinson's disease. What is the evidence? *Parkinsonism and Related Disorders* **13** (Supplement 3), S501-508.

Krack, P., Batir, A. & Van Blercom, N. (2003) Five-year follow-up of bilateral stimulation of the subthalamic nucleus in advanced Parkinson's disease. *New England Journal of Medicine* **349**, 1925-1933.

MacMahon, D. & Thomas, S. (1998) Practical approach to quality of life in Parkinson's disease. *Journal of Neurology* **245**, S19-S22.

Pagonabarraga, J. (2010) Parkinson's disease: Definition, diagnosis, and management. *Encyclopedia of Movement Disorders*. Elsevier, Oxford, pp. 405-412.

Reynold, H. Wilson-Barnett, J. & Richardon, G. (2000) Evaluation of the role of the Parkinson's disease nurse specialist. *International Journal of Nursing* 337-349.

Sadowski, C., Jones, C., Gordon, B. & Feeny, D. (2007) Knowledge of risk factors for falling reported by patients with Parkinson's disease. *Journal of Neuroscience Nursing* **39**(6), 336-342.

PART 7: SEIZURES

Susan R. Gavaghan

Seizures often occur as a consequence of disease and conditions that are prominent in older adults. Cerebrovascular disease is the most common condition that results in a seizure, but trauma and dementia are other risk factors in this population. The incidence of new seizures is highest in individuals over the age of 60 and it is anticipated that elders will constitute half of all new-onset epilepsy patients by 2020 (Pugh *et al.*, 2009). Some studies suggest the incidence is actually higher since seizures are often unrecognized in elders. Seizure activity is not as readily recognized in this age group because seizure activity in elders may be atypical or may not be witnessed in the elder who lives alone and has limited social interactions (Pugh *et al.*, 2009; Sutton, 2007). Although an isolated seizure is a possibility, 80% of older adults who have had a single seizure are likely to have another (Ramsey, 2004).

A seizure is a hyperexcitation and disorderly discharge of neurons in the brain leading to a sudden, violent, involuntary series of muscle contractions (Gilbert, 2012). Seizures can be classified as acute symptomatic seizures or epilepsy. Acute symptomatic seizures are provoked by a particular trigger (e.g., hypoglycemia, alcohol withdrawal, and medication; Gilbert, 2012). Epilepsy involves recurrent unprovoked seizure activity that occurs in the absence of treatment. After a seizure, an older adult may present with confusion, memory loss or delirium (Waterhouse & Towne, 2005). Caregivers may report periods of staring or disorientation (Sutton, 2007).

There are many types of seizures, but seizures are usually categorized as focal (i.e., simple partial or complex partial) or generalized (i.e., tonic–clonic) (Herman, 2007). Initially, a partial seizure starts in one part of the brain, but a partial seizure can develop into a generalized seizure. Consciousness is not affected in a simple partial seizure, but is in complex partial and generalized seizure. Further categorization of seizures includes the following:

- *Partial (focal) seizures* arise from localized area of brain and cause specific symptoms
  - *Simple partial seizures* involve muscle twitching or sensory changes without change in memory or level of consciousness.
  - *Complex partial seizures* are the most common seizure type in older adults. The seizure may be preceded by antecedent symptoms (e.g., paresthesias, dizziness and muscle cramps), an aura or sense of *déjà vu*, but many patients do not experience an aura. Automatisms (e.g., lip smacking, or repeating phrases over and over again) are common.
  - Simple or complex seizure progressing to generalized seizure.

Generalized seizures cause a generalized electrical abnormality in the brain

- *Convulsive*
  - Clonic: fast repetitive motor activity
  - Myoclonic: brief jerking or stiffening of extremities lasting only a few seconds
  - Tonic: sudden episodes of increased muscle rigidity/stiffness without loss of consciousness
  - Tonic-clonic: generalized seizures that usually last two minutes, but no longer than five minutes. These seizures are characterized by stiff muscles and immediate loss of consciousness. The patient may bite the tongue and be incontinent.
  - Status epilepticus: continuous seizures that lasts 15 minutes or a series of seizures that occur over a 20-30 minute period in which patient does not regain consciousness (Gilbert, 2012). In the older adult these seizures occur in the setting of hypoxia, hyperglycemia, intracranial infection, brain tumor, or withdrawal (Velez & Selwa, 2003).
    - Postictal states are frequently more prolonged in the older patient.
    - Convulsive and nonconvulsive status epilepticus is not infrequent in elders , almost twice as prevalent as in the general population.
- *Nonconvulsive*
  - Atonic: sudden loss of muscle tone in most cases causing the patient to fall
  - Absence (petit mal): seizure that usually involves staring
- *Unclassified or idiopathic seizures* occur in about half of all seizures. These occur for no known reason and do not fit into any classification (Ignatavicius *et al.*, 1999).

■ Risk factors

Acute symptomatic seizures:

- Acute stroke or transient ischemic attack
- Alcohol, benzodiazepine or barbiturate withdrawal
- Head trauma
- Infection
- Metabolic encephalopathy (e.g., hyperglycemia/hypoglycemia, nonketotic hyperglycemia, hyponatremia, hypocalcemia, uremia and hepatic encephalopathy)
- Medications (e.g., beta-lactam antibiotics, isoniazid, quinolones, opioid analgesics, bupropion, opioid analgesics, and antipsychotics)
  - Medication induced seizure due to polypharmacy or impaired drug clearance

Epilepsy:

- Age related brain changes
- Cerebrovascular disease (leading cause in elders [Velez, 2003])
- Cryptogenic
- Dementia

- Head trauma (second leading cause [Velez, 2003])
- Intracranial tumors

■ Clinical presentation

A reliable first hand account by a witness is critical to describe the events leading up to the seizure, as well as what occurred during and following the seizure (Gilbert, 2012; Sutton, 2007). Most seizures in elders are partial onset seizures with or without a tonic clonic seizure, a secondary generalization (Hiyoshi & Yagi, 2000). In elders the presentation is often atypical and classic descriptions are uncommon. Older adults may report localized parasthesias, dizziness and muscle cramps, while observers often note confusion, sleepiness or clumsiness rather than motor manifestations (Kellinghaus et al., 2004).

If a seizure is observed or suspected, obtain an accurate history of events leading up to, during and after seizure, onset sudden or gradual, any systemic illness, current medications and medication changes, recent stress or illness, and history of head trauma (Gilbert, 2012).

■ Nursing assessment

- Actions taken by nurse should be appropriate for type of seizure.
- Observe, document and time length of seizure.
- Turn patient on side to prevent aspiration.
- Remove objects in area that may injure patient.
- Do not restrain patient.
- Do not force anything into patient's mouth.

Post seizure assessment:

- Elders are more likely to suffer debilitating fractures, subdural hematomas and prolonged postictal states than younger people (Kutluay et al., 2003):
  - Assess vital signs.
  - Perform a neurological assessment.
  - Document seizure description and timing.

■ Diagnostics

- CBC/differential
- Glucose
- Serum electrolytes
- Blood urea nitrogen, creatinine
- Alcohol and/or drug toxicology
- Neuroimaging:
  - Magnetic resonance imaging (MRI)
  - Cerebral angiography
- Lumbar puncture to exclude cerebral infection
- Electroencephalography (EEG)

■ Differential diagnosis

- Delirium
- Drop attacks
- Psychogenic factors
- Sleep disorders
- Syncope
- Transient global ischemia
- Transischemic attacks

■ Treatment

- Remove or treat underlying condition or cause of seizure.
- Primary epilepsy is routinely treated with antiseizure medication.
  - Antiepileptic drug treatment is an option but seizure type, pharmokinectic profile, expected adverse effect and cost should be considered. Monotherapy is desirable in this population as polypharmacy tends to increase incidence of side effects.
  - In an emergency, generalized seizure activity is often treated with an intravenous (IV) benzodiazepine (e.g., lorazepam or diazepam).
  - Status epilepticus is treated with oxygen and IV benzodiazepine (e.g., lorazepam or diazepam). Discuss consideration of IV glucose, thiamine, fosphenytoin, or phenobarbital with physician if SE does not abate (Gilbert, 2012). Intubation and anesthesia consultation for induced coma may be necessary (Gilbert, 2012).
  - Common antiseizure medications for generalized tonic-clonic seizures include carbamazepine (Tegretol), divalproex (Depakote), lamotrigine (Lamictal), levetiracetam (Keppra), and phenytoin (Dilantin).

    In older adults, normal physiologic changes of aging alter the pharmacodynamic and pharmacokinetic profiles of medications prescribed. Additionally, older adults have lower circulating protein concentrations, decreased renal elimination, altered distribution volumes, impaired hepatic metabolism, and potential alterations in gastrointestinal (GI) absorption (Sutton, 2007).
- Seizure precautions and nursing interventions to protect patient from traumatic injury:
  - Protect patient during a seizure.
  - DO NOT insert objects into patient's mouth, as this intervention may break teeth and lead to aspiration.
  - DO NOT restrain patient as limbs can be fractured.
  - Turn patient on side to prevent aspiration.
  - Have oxygen and suction available.
  - Assure IV access.
  - Keep bed in lowest position.
- Post-seizure care:
  - Note signs present prior to seizure and time of onset.
  - Document body parts involved, types of movement, time seizure started and stopped and any postictal response.

- Monitor respiratory pattern , heart rate.
- Check patient for bowel incontinence, bitten tongue, injuries.
- Document eye deviation and papillary response.

■ Collaborative consultation

- Obtaining information from patient and family regarding seizure description, events surrounding seizure and whether aura was present is helpful
- Once seizure occurs, call physician and consult pharmacist for appropriate medications.
- Consultation with neurology is also beneficial.

■ Complications

- Untreated status epilepticus can lead to death. Other complications include:
  - Aspiration
  - Brain damage that may be irreversible
  - Cardiac dysrhythmias
  - Hypoxia
  - Lactic acidosis
  - Traumatic injury

■ Prevention

- Antiseizure medications should not be stopped even if the seizures have stopped as this can lead to a recurrence of seizures.
- Avoid alcohol and nicotine as these stimulants can precipitate seizure activity.

■ Patient/family education

- Older adults are already vulnerable to loss of independence. Seizure activity imposes driving restrictions, impaired self confidence, and risk for falls.
- Do not take any medication without asking the doctor. Always discuss the impact of new medications on seizure threshold.
- Explain importance of medical alert bracelet.
- Advise patient to carry identification stating he has seizures, name and phone number of care provider.
- Carry medication information: name, dosage, and time of medication administration.
- Discuss with patient and family the therapeutic and adverse effects of prescribed anticonvulsant(s) as well as need to discuss side effects with physician.
- Emphasize importance of taking medication.
- Discuss need to return for lab work to monitor serum drug levels.

References

Gilbert, K. (2012) Seizures. In: *Primary Care: A Collaborative Practice*, 4th edition, T.M. Buttaro, Trybulski, Bailey, & Sandberg-Cook (eds). Mosby, St. Louis.

Herman, S. (2007) Classification of epileptic seizures. Continnum. *Epilepsy* **13**(4), 13–47.

Hiyoshi, T. & Yagi, K. (2000) Epilepsy in the elderly. *Epilepsia* **41**(Suppl 9), 31.

Kellinghaus, C., Loddenkemper, T., Dinner, D.S., *et al.* (2004) Seizure semiology in the elderly. *Epilepsia* **45**, 263.

Kutluay, E., McCaque, K. & Beydoun, A. (2003) Safety and tolerability of oxcarbazepine in elderly patients with epilepsy. *Epilepsy Behavior* **4**(2), 175–180.

Pugh, M.J.V., Knoefel, J.E., Mortensen, E.M., Amuan, M.E. *et al.* (2009) New-onset epilepsy risk factors in older veterans. *Journal of the American Geriatric Society* **57**(2), 237–242.

Ramsay, R.E., Rowan, A.J. & Pryor, F.M. (2004) Special considerations in treating the elderly patient with epilepsy. *Neurology* **62**(5), S24–S29.

Sutton K.A. (2007) New onset seizures in the elderly patient, JAAPA. Online. Available from www.jaapa.com.

Velez L. & Selwa L.M. (2003) Seizure disorders in the elderly. *American Family Physician* **67**(2), 325–332.

Waterhouse, E. & Towne, A. (2005) Seizures in the elderly: Nuances in presentation and treatment. *Cleveland Clinic* **72**(3), S26–S37.

Unit 7: Endocrine

PART 1: DIABETES

Susan L. Wood

In 2010, 10.9 million adults over age 65 were known to have diabetes (CDC, 2011). The prevalence of diabetes in this cohort is more than 26% compared with an 11.3% prevalence in younger adults (CDC, 2011). Functional impairment, reduced health status, and problems with activities of daily living are all associated with diabetes (Sinclair *et al.*, 2008).

Diabetes mellitus is a group of disorders associated with relative or an absolute lack of circulating insulin. The end result of this decrease or lack of insulin is hyperglycemia. Type 1 diabetes, usually diagnosed in young children or young adults, is characterized by little or no insulin. Type 1 diabetes develops when pancreatic beta cells are destroyed, often by an autoimmune process (NIDDK, 2011). Type 2 diabetes can develop in children as well as adults. The cause may be both genetic and environmental. In adults, type 2 diabetes accounts for the majority of diabetes diagnoses. Type 2 diabetes begins as insulin resistance. Diminished responsiveness of insulin receptors rather than lack of insulin is the cause of this type of diabetes. However, the pancreas also loses its ability to produce insulin as the disorder progresses (NIDDK, 2011).

Other causes of diabetes include steroid-induced diabetes and gestational diabetes, Older adults receiving glucocorticoids require careful monitoring because of the risk of developing hyperglycemia.

■ Risk factors
- Type 1 diabetes mellitus
  - Autoimmune, genetic, and environmental
  - Pancreatectomy
  - Whipple's procedure
- Type 2 diabetes mellitus
  - Age greater than 45
  - Central obesity
  - Family history of diabetes
  - History of gestational diabetes or high birthweight baby (>4 kg (9 lbs) or more at birth (NIDDK, 2011)
  - Hypertension (>140/90 mmHg)
  - Low HDL cholesterol (<35 mg/dl) or high triglycerides (>250 mg/dl)
  - Medications
    - Current history of steroid therapy causing steroid induced hyperglycemia
    - Atypical antipsychotics
  - Over weight

● Racial/ethnic risk: (non-Hispanic blacks, Hispanic/latinoLatino Americans, Asian Americans, and Pacific Islanders, American Indians, and Alaskan natives)
● Sedentary lifestyle

■ Clinical presentation

Older adults present unique challenges in diabetes care. The prevalence of diabetes increases with age, as aging is associated with a reduction in beta-cell function, decreased insulin sensitivity, and altered carbohydrate metabolism. Some symptoms of diabetes such as frequent urination, cognitive impairment, weight loss, depression and incontinence, often go unnoticed because they are thought to be related to medications or the aging process. Additionally, evidence suggests that poor glycemic management may synergistically interact with other age related pathology to accelerate disease progression (Gregg & Narayan, 2002). Thus individualizing nursing care to the older adult is essential to achieve the overall goal of improving quality and quantity of life.

■ Nursing assessment

Essential subjective and objective data to elicit includes:

Subjective data
Because many elders have diabetes and the disorder is undiagnosed, it is important that nurses carefully assess patient data to aid in identifying those patients with undiagnosed diabetes.

● History of present illness
● Cardiovascular risk factors: age, sex, hypertension, hyperlipidemia, weight/body mass index, smoker, physical inactivity, and family history
● Past health history should determine:
  ● Recent history of mumps, rubella, coxsackievirus or other recent viral infections
  ● Recent trauma, infection or stress
  ● Pregnancy history (birth to infant >4 kg)
  ● History of chronic pancreatitis, Cushing syndrome, acromegaly, or frequent fungal infections
  ● Habits: smoking history; alcohol, drugs, and illicit substances use
  ● Lifestyle
    ○ Diet
      ■ 24 hour dietary review
    ○ Exercise
● Sleep patterns
● Allergies
● Current medication
  ● Current medications including possible recent corticosteroid therapy
  ● Over the counter and herbal supplements

- Family history
  - Age, sex, health or cause of death: grandparents, parents, siblings, spouse, and children
- Social history: home situation and patient support systems
- Review of systems
  - General: recent weight loss or gain, weakness, fatigue, or presence of blurry vision
  - Skin: rashes, pruritus, or poor healing
  - Head: headache or dizziness
  - Eyes: blurred vision, glasses/contacts, and last eye exam
  - Nutritional assessment: recent weight loss or gain
  - Nose: recent upper respiratory infection
  - Ears: hearing aids or ear pain
  - Mouth: dentures, bleeding gums, toothache, difficulty swallowing, and last dental exam
  - Neck: swollen glands or neck pain
  - Respiratory: cough, shortness of breath or wheezing
  - Cardiac: heart problems, chest pain, or paroxysmal nocturnal dyspnea
  - Gastrointestinal: heartburn, change in appetite, nausea, vomiting, constipation, diarrhea, abdominal pain, or food allergies
  - Urinary: burning, frequency, polyuria, nocturia (how often), or incontinence
  - Genital: rashes, discharge, or frequent vaginal infections
  - Peripheral vascular: leg cramps, numbness/tingling, or previous history deep vein thrombosis
  - Musculoskeletal: gout, weakness, or stiffness
  - Endocrine: thyroid history, polydipsia, or polyphagia
  - Psychiatric: depression, anxiety, irritability, or apathy

Objective data

Many patients with diabetes will not exhibit signs of the disorder. Concerning signs of illness in patients with diabetes may include the following:

- Weight loss
- Eyes: soft, sunken, vitreal hemorrhage, and cataracts
- Integumentary: dry, warm, inelastic skin, rashes, poor wound healing, and loss of hair on toes
- Respiratory: rapid, deep respirations
- Cardiovascular: hypotension and a weak, rapid pulse
- Gastrointestinal: dry mouth, vomiting, and fruity breath
- Neurological: altered reflexes, restlessness, confusion, stupor, and coma

■ Diagnostics

- Screening of people without risk factors should begin at 45 years of age and then every 3 years (Executive Summary, Standards of Medical Care in Diabetes, 2012).

- A diagnosis of diabetes is based on any of the following test results, confirmed by testing on a second day.
  - a blood glucose of 126 mg/dl or higher after an 8 hour fast
  - a blood glucose level of 200 mg/dl or higher 2 hours after drinking a beverage containing 75 grams of glucose dissolved in water (OGTT)
  - a random blood glucose of 200 mg/dl or higher, along with presence of diabetes symptoms
  - a HgB A1C >6.5% (Executive Summary, Standards of Medical Care in Diabetes, 2012)
- Serum electrolytes, blood urea nitrogen (BUN), creatinine
- Lipid panel
- Thyroid stimulating hormone (TSH)
- Urine for glucose, ketones, urea, albumin

■ Differential diagnosis

Stress, medications, sleep deprivation, and infection can all affect blood glucose. The differential diagnosis includes insulin resistance, Type 1 or Type 2 diabetes.

■ Treatment

The hospitalized patient with diabetes can present unique challenges. Important nursing interventions include:

- Monitor blood glucose closely as stress, medications, infection and inadequate insulin can all affect blood glucose. Acute illness, injury and surgery are situations that may evoke a counterregulatory hormone response resulting in hyperglycemia.
- Monitor patients closely for signs of hypoglycemia as patients may eat less, antibiotics can affect blood sugar levels, and patients may be NPO for diagnostic testing.
- Monitor anion gap (AG), normal value AG=16. Increased anion gap is associated with an increase in metabolic acid which can be life threatening

$$AG = (Na+K) - (Cl+CO_2).$$

- Monitor serum electrolytes, BUN, creatinine.
- Electrocardiogram (EKG) is indicated if electrolyte changes occur or if patient complains of chest heaviness or discomfort.
- Monitor fluid balance.
  - Monitor amount patient eats at meals as a decrease in food intake may result in hypoglycemia.
- Administer insulin as ordered.
- Administer intravenous fluid (IVF) as ordered.
- Observe patient carefully for signs of hypoglycemia.

■ Collaborative consultation

- Coordination of care may be complex as hospitalized patients may have multiple health care providers. Changes in drug therapy may occur when patients see specialty providers or during acute illness or hospitalization. When a patient's history includes multiple disease states and numerous medications that include over the counter drugs, herbal products, and other supplements, diligent nursing management is required to ensure continuity of care that is well coordinated.
- When discussing potential treatments with the physician or other health care provider, be certain to review patient allergies and concurrent medications as certain medications may increase blood glucose (e.g., steroids).
- Dietician: Nutritional therapy is the cornerstone of care for the person with diabetes. Achieving nutritional goals requires a coordinated team effort that considers the behavioral, cognitive, socioeconomic, cultural and religious aspects of the patient.
- Annual ophthalmology consultation: Diabetic retinopathy is a common complication of diabetes. Elevated blood sugar damages the retinal blood vessels, causing them to break down, leak, or become blocked. Over time, this causes retinal hemorrhage and impaired oxygen delivery to the retina that can lead to the growth of abnormal vessels. These new vessels are fragile and can break easily, causing permanent vision loss. Annual dilated eye examinations are recommended for early detection and prevention of diabetic retinopathy. Refer patients to dilated eye exam at least every 2 years, and yearly when diabetes-related eye problems or other eye problems exist, or if risk factors are present (high blood pressure or poor glucose control).
- Annual dental examination: Poor glycemic control is associated with gingivitis and more severe periodontal diseases. Oral signs and symptoms of diabetes can also include a neurosensory disorder known as burning mouth syndrome, taste disorders, abnormal wound healing, and fungal infections (candidiasis). Individuals with diabetes may notice a fruity (acetone) breath, frequent xerostomia (dry mouth), or a change in saliva thickness. Dry mouth can also lead to a marked increase in dental decay. Oral findings in people with diabetes are associated with other systemic findings such as excessive loss of fluids through frequent urination, altered response to infection, altered connective tissue metabolism, neurosensory dysfunction, microvascular changes, medications causing dry mouth, and possible increased glucose concentration in saliva.
- Podiatry: A comprehensive foot examination for abnormalities, including evaluation of pulses, sensation, foot biomechanics (general foot structure and function), and nails helps determine the person's category of risk for developing foot complications. Persons with diabetes who are at high risk have one or more of the following characteristics: (1) loss of protective sensation, (2) absent pedal pulses, (3) foot deformity, (4) history of foot ulcers, or (5) prior amputation. Low-risk individuals have none of these characteristics.

■ Complications

- Hypoglycemia
- Diabetic ketoacidosis (DKA)
- Hyperglycemic hyperosmolar state (HHS). Chronic complications of diabetes are generally divided into two categories: macrovascular complications and microvascular complications. Macrovascular complications are diseases of the large and medium sized vessels which include cerebrovascular, cardiovascular and peripheral vascular disease.
- Microvascular complications result from thickening of the vessel membranes in the capillaries and arterioles. Most notably affected are the eyes (retinopathy), the kidneys (nephropathy) and the skin (dermopathy).

■ Prevention

- Increase level of exercise because physical activity reduces the risk of diabetes.
- Maintain a healthy weight because obesity increases the risk of developing type 2 diabetes.
- If overweight, weight loss and physical activity should be reinforced.
- Encourage a diet that is low in fat, total calories, and processed foods, but high in fruits and vegetables.
- If overweight and over age 45, a periodic glucose screening test is recommended.
- Teach patients and families signs and symptoms of hypoglycemia and management of hypoglycemic episodes. Discuss skin care, foot care, blood glucose monitoring, and medication management.

■ Patient/family education

The goals of diabetes self management are to enable the patient to become the most active participant in his or her care. The patient education issues for the older adult include those related to vision, mobility, skin care, medication management and effects of multiple medications, mental status, and functional ability. Discussing the patient's financial and social situation, eating habits, quality of life issues and the potential for undetected hypoglycemic episodes are important.

Hypoglycemia

Hypoglycemia is often defined as blood glucose below 50 mg/dl. However, hypoglycemia cannot be defined numerically as patients may experience a hypoglycemic reaction with varied serum blood sugar concentrations. Hypoglycemia is usually caused by medications used to treat diabetes and is the most common endocrine emergency (NIDDK, 2011). Unfortunately, some patients, particularly elders, may not exhibit the common signs and symptoms associated with hypoglycemia.

■ Risk factors

- Critical illness: especially hepatic or renal failure, and sepsis
- Excessive alcohol ingestion
- Hormonal deficiencies
- Meals or snacks that are delayed or missed
- Medication (e.g., salicylates, pentamidine, fluoroquinolones, and sulfon-amides)
- Oral hypoglycemic agent and insulin
- Postprandial hypoglycemia
- Strenuous activity without adjusting insulin or food intake
- Tumors
- Weight loss

■ Clinical presentation

- Change in mental status, confusion
- Hunger
- Irritability
- Shakiness/anxiety/nervousness
- Diaphoresis
- Difficulty speaking
- Palpitations
- Seizures
- Death

■ Nursing assessment

- Mild hypoglycemia:
  - Diaphoresis, hunger, impaired concentration, irritability, paresthesias, pallor, tachycardia, or tremulous
- Moderate hypoglycemia:
  - Some degree of mental status changes, anger, or irritability
- Severe hypoglycemia:
  - Confusion, fatigue/drowsiness, seizure, or loss of consciousness
  - *Patient would be unable to recognize symptoms or treat self.*

■ Diagnostics

An immediate blood glucose is indicated for any patient with change in level of behavior/level of consciousness or other signs and symptoms associated with hypoglycemia.

■ Differential diagnosis

Initial differential diagnosis is concerned with determining the cause of the patient's symptoms. An immediate point of care blood sugar is necessary.

If the blood sugar is below normal, the degree of hypoglycemia (i.e., mild, moderate, severe) is determined. After the hypoglycemia is identified and treated, the underlying cause of the hypoglycemia must be learned to prevent further episodes of low blood sugar. In hospitalized patients common causes of low blood sugars include:

- Incorrect insulin or dose
- Delayed or missed meals
- False readings:
  - Possible lab error or related to leukocytosis or thrombocytosis
- Heart failure
- Hepatic failure
- Medications associated with lowered blood glucose:
  - Levofloxacin, moxifloxacin, pentamidine, quinine, salicylates, sulfon-amides, sulfonylureas
- Postprandial (reactive) hypoglycemia
- Prolonged fast
- Renal failure
- Sepsis

Other causes of hypoglycemia include:

- Addison's disease
- Alcohol
- Chronic heart failure associated with liver engorgement
- Insulinoma
- Leukemia
- Liver disease
- Past history of bariatric or gastric surgery
- Non-islet cell tumor of pancreas
- Strenuous exercise

■ Treatment

Treatment is based on the classification of hypoglycemia. Usually a patient with mild hypoglycemia could be expected to treat themselves safely, but that might not be true for an older adult with cognitive or physical impairment.

Mild hypoglycemia
- 15 to 20 grams of a simple carbohydrate (i.e., 4 to 6 oz. orange juice or a glucose gel) by mouth.
  - *Patients who are taking acarbose or α-glucosidase inhibitors must be given pure glucose to treat hypoglycemia.*
    Repeat blood sugar in 10-15 minutes. If blood sugar is less than 60 mg/dl, give an additional 10-15 grams carbohydrate by mouth. Recheck blood sugar every 15 minutes until blood sugar >70 mg/dl or above (NIDDK, 2011).

- In 30 minutes, patient should eat a snack with both protein and carbohydrate.

Moderate hypoglycemia

- Give patient 15-30 grams of a simple carbohydrate and follow protocol above.

Severe hypoglycemia

- If patient is alert and can swallow safely, give 30-45 grams of a simple carbohydrate (i.e., 8-12 oz. orange juice or glucose gels).
- If patient is unresponsive give 25-50 grams of 50% dextrose intravenous solution. May repeat, if no improvement in 15 minutes and blood sugar is still low. Intravenous D5W is frequently infused after patients receive 50% IV dextrose.
- An alternative treatment is 0.5 to 1 milligram glucagon IM or SQ.
- Patients with hypoglycemia should respond to these treatments in 10-15 minutes, but cognition can remain somewhat impaired for 30-45 minutes longer.
- Repeat blood glucose every 15 minutes until blood sugar is >70 mg/dl (NIDDK, 2011), then every one to two hours or more frequently if necessary (Buttaro et al., 2006).

Quick fix foods to treat hypoglycemia

- 3 or 4 glucose tablets
- 1 serving of glucose gel—the amount equal to 15 grams of carbohydrate
- 1/2 cup, or 4 ounces, of any fruit juice
- 1/2 cup, or 4 ounces, of a regular - not diet - soft drink
- 1 cup, or 8 ounces, of milk
- 5 or 6 pieces of hard candy
- 1 tablespoon of sugar or honey (NIDDK, 2011)

■ Collaborative consultation

- Notify the physician of hypoglycemic event and treatment.
- Further consultation regarding current medications and comorbidities may also be indicated.

■ Complications

- Patient safety is a primary concern.
- Other complications can include falls, seizures, coma, and death.

■ Prevention

- Patients, friends and families should be able to recognize the signs and symptoms of hypoglycemia (e.g., agitation, confusion, difficulty concentrating, shakiness, sweating).

- Check your blood sugar before meals, at bedtime, before and after exercise, and if you wake up in the middle of the night. Keep a record of your blood sugars to determine if your blood sugar is trending too low or too high.*
- Record your blood sugars to discuss with your doctor.
- If signs of hypoglycemia occur, drink orange juice, eat graham crackers, pretzels, or take a glucose tablet or glucose packet. Check your blood sugar within 15 minutes and repeat snack if blood sugar is still below.
- Eat your meals and snacks on a regular time schedule.
- Don't skip meals. If you are sick and cannot eat or drink fluids, call the doctor.
- Call your doctor if you are having frequent low blood sugar symptoms as your medicine might need to be decreased or changed.
- Keep snacks close by at all times: in your pocket, purse, car, and by the bedside table.
- Monitor your blood sugar before and after exercise as exercise can cause low blood sugar.*
- Discuss drinking alcohol with your doctor as alcohol can cause low blood sugar.
- Do not drive or operate heavy equipment if you think your blood sugar is low.

*Note. Older adults may not be able to check blood sugars because of functional impediments. For these patients, the goal blood sugar goals may be higher than for other adults.

■ Patient/family education

Educate patient and family regarding prompt recognition and treatment (NIDDK, 2011).

Hyperglycemic crises

DKA and HHS are acute complications of hyperglycemic crisis that may occur with diabetes. If untreated, either crisis may result in coma or death. DKA occurs most often with Type 1 diabetes and is associated with the biochemical triad of hyperglycemia, ketosis, and acidosis.

HHS occurs most often in Type 2 diabetes. This medical emergency is characterized by severe hyperglycemia and dehydration, the absence of ketosis, marked hyperosmolarity, renal function impairment and central nervous system (CNS) manifestations. A concurrent illness usually accompanies the disorder (e.g., pneumonia, burns, trauma, or sepsis). Iatrogenic causes also have been associated with HHS; among these are hypertonic enteral feedings, dialysis, and medications (e.g., thiazide diuretics, steroids, mannitol, or phenytoin). Persons most at risk for the disorder are older adults, institutionalized patients, the mentally impaired, and those who cannot recognize signs of dehydration (Kitabchi et al., 2001).

Although the pathophysiology of DKA is better understood than that of HHS, the basic underlying mechanisms of both disorders is a reduction in circulating insulin, coupled with an elevation of counterregulatory stress hormones (glucagon, catecholamines, cortisol and growth hormone). The main difference is that the patient with HHS typically has some circulating insulin, so fat breakdown and ketoacidosis do not occur. Both disorders result in electrolyte disorders and significant fluid loss, dehydration and potentially shock and death.

■ Risk factors

- Accidental or deliberate omission of insulin
- Acute illness
- Diabetes mellitus (mainly type 1)
- Infection
- Physiological or psychological stress

■ Clinical presentation

An acute illness or infection can unmask or precipitate hyperglycemia. DKA or HHS should be suspected in elders with an illness accompanied by a change in mental status, nausea, vomiting, dehydration and infection. Pertinent history should determine the onset of symptoms, illness course, allergies, medications, previous history of diabetes or hyperglycemia, polyuria, polydipsia, malaise, recent surgery or other physiologic stress, or non healing wounds.

■ Nursing assessment

The physical exam findings may be subtle. Assessment considerations include:

- Mental status changes: aphasia, confusion, visual hallucinations, seizure activity, stupor and coma
- Vitals signs: hypotension, tachycardia, temperature (may be elevated, normal or subnormal) and diminished pulmonary wedge pressure which reflects reduced circulating volume
- Skin: pronounced tissue dehydration, dry mucous membranes, poor turgor, and possible skin infection
- Cardiac: tachycardia is often present initially. Dysrhythmias are associated with potassium and magnesium imbalance. Monitor heart sounds for signs of fluid overload in elders receiving IV fluid repletion.
- Lungs: evaluate for Kussmaul respirations (i.e., deep, labored, and fruity smelling breaths associated with acidosis) that suggest DKA. Shallow breaths may suggest HSS. Lungs sounds may be initially clear, particularly in dehydrated older adults, but continuous monitoring for cough, egophony, percussion, dullness and adventitious breath sounds is important to determine if pneumonia is a precipitant. Monitoring lung sounds for fluid overload with IV replacement is necessary.

- Abdomen: assess for abdominal pain, distention, bowel sounds and tenderness. Gastric stasis can lead to acute abdominal distension with copious vomiting.
- Peripheral vascular: monitor for diminished peripheral pulses and leg cramps
- Neurologic: monitor for mental status changes, focal deficits, seizures, and unresponsiveness.

■ Diagnostics

HHS
- Serum glucose >600 mg/dl
- Serum or urine ketones absent
- Serum osmolality elevated >330 mOsm/l
- Serum electrolytes normal or high sodium
- BUN and creatinine elevated
- Complete blood count (CBC): elevated hematocrit and leukocyte levels

DKA
- Serum glucose >250 mg/dl
- Serum ketones present
- Urine ketones present
- Serum osmolality variable
- Decreased serum sodium
- Increased serum potassium level initially, then decreased because of increased diuresis and reversal of acidosis.
- BUN and creatinine elevated
- CBC: elevated hematocrit and leukocyte levels because of diuresis and dehydration
- Arterial blood gas: metabolic acidosis.
- Anion gap >10

■ Differential diagnosis
- DKA
- HHS

■ Treatment
- Management includes treating the underlying cause, insulin therapy to decrease serum glucose (initially an insulin bolus, then IV insulin drip), and replacing fluids and electrolytes.
- Institute aspiration precautions if your patient has neurologic signs and symptoms.
- Replace fluids. Patients can lose 8-12 L. While repleting intravascular fluid, monitor for evidence of fluid overload.
  - Monitor intake and output.

- Monitor blood glucose hourly. Inform physician when blood glucose is 250 mg/dl.
- Monitor and replete serum electrolytes (potassium, magnesium, calcium and phosphate initially, then check serum potassium every 2 hours and discuss results with physician).
  - As DKA progresses, diuresis triggers potassium loss. Once the patient is rehydrated and the acidosis resolves, potassium moves into the cells, causing plasma levels to drops. Insulin therapy causes more potassium to enter the cells, causing levels to fall even further. In HHS, potassium problems aren't as common or significant. However diuresis may cause potassium, magnesium, and calcium losses and patients may need replacement.
  - Combat acidosis. Metabolic acidosis in DKA should resolve with fluid replacement and insulin therapy. Discuss the physician if serum pH $\ll$ 7.
- Discuss with physician need for anti-emetic therapy if patient is vomiting.

Collaborative consultation

- Continuous consultation with the physician is necessary for patients with HHS or DKA.
- Further consultation with specialists (e.g., endocrinology) may also be necessary.

Complications

- Acute renal failure
- Dehydration
- Electrolyte abnormalities
- Infection
- Shock
- Death

Prevention

Patients and families need to understand the risks of hyperglycemia and the need to notify the physician if illness occurs.

Patient/family education

The key to the prevention of DKA and HHS and related complications is adequate patient and family education regarding diabetes management (Boord *et al.*, 2001; Kitabchi *et al.*, 2001; Moore, 2004). Understanding the importance of monitoring blood sugars, adherence to the medication regimen, and management of blood sugar during illness is essential.

References

American Diabetes Association (2012) Standards of Medical Care in Diabetes. Online. Available from in http://care.diabetesjournals.org/content/35/Supplement_1/S11/T2.expansion.html (accessed 28 May 2012).

American Geriatrics Society (2003) Guidelines for improving the care of older adults with diabetes mellitus. JAGS51:S265–S280. Online. Available from www.americangeriatrics.org/files/documents/JAGSfinal05.pdf (accessed 7 June 2012).

Boord, J., Graber, A., Christman, J. & Powers, A. (2001) Practical management of diabetes in critically ill patients. *American Journal of Respiratory Critical Care Medicine* **164**(10), 1763–1767.

Buttaro, T.M., Aznavorian, S. & Dick, K. (2006) *Clinical management of patients in subacute and long-term care settings*. Mosby, St. Louis.

Centers for Disease Control (2011) National Diabetes Fact Sheet, 2011. Available from http://www.cdc.gov/diabetes/pubs/pdf/ndfs_2011.pdf (accessed 28 May 2012).

Executive Summary: Position Statement: Standards of Medical Care in Diabetes – 2010 *Diabetes Care* **33**, S4–S10; doi:10.2337/dc10-S004.

Gregg, E.W. & Narayan, V. (2002) Complications of diabetes in elderly people: underappreciated problems include cognitive decline and physical disability. *British Medical Journal* **325**, 916–917.

Kitabchi, A.E., Umppierrez, G.E., Murphy, M. *et al.* (2001) Management of hyperglycemic crises in patients with diabetes. *Diabetes Care* **24**(1), 131–153.

Moore, T. (2004) Diabetic emergencies in adults. *Nursing Standard* **3**(18), 45–52.

National Institute of Diabetes and Digestive and Kidney Diseases (NIDDK) Online. Available from http://diabetes.niddk.nih.gov/dm/pubs/overview/index.htm (accessed 21 March 2012).

National Institute of Diabetes and Digestive and Kidney Diseases (NIDDK) Online. Available from http://diabetes.niddk.nih.gov/dm/pubs/hypoglycemia/ (accessed 21 March 2012).

Sinclair, A., Conroy, S. & Bayer, A. (2008) Impact of diabetes on physical function in older people. *Diabetes Care* **31**, 233–235.

Further reading

California Healthcare Foundation/American Geriatrics Society Panel on Improving Care for Elders with Diabetes. Mangione, C.M., Brown, A.F., *et al.* (2003) Guidelines for improving the care of the older person with diabetes mellitus. *Journal of the American Geriatrics Society* **51**, S265–S280.

Olson, D.E. & Norris, S.L. (2004). Diabetes in older adults: overview of of AGS Guidelines for the treatment of diabetes mellitus in geriatric populations. *Geriatrics* **59**(4), 20.

Selected websites

American Diabetes Association: http:diabetes.org

Centers for Disease Control and Prevention's National Center for Chronic Disease Prevention and Health Promotion Division of Diabetes Translation http:www.cdc.gov/diabetes

National Institute of Diabetes and Digestive and Kidney Diseases of the National Institutes of Health: http//www.niddk.nih.org

PART 2: HYPO/HYPERTHYROIDISM

Susan L. Wood

Thyroid disorders are characterized by either thyroid hormone overproduction (i.e., hyperthyroidism) or deficiency (i.e., hypothyroidism), as well as gland inflammation and enlargement. In most cases thyroid disorders are easily treated. The difficulty, especially in elders, is that because symptoms of a thyroid problem are often subtle, thyroid disorders are frequently undiagnosed resulting in potentially serious consequences (American Thyroid Association, 2011).

The thyroid gland, located below the larynx, is regulated by thyroid-stimulating hormone (TSH), secreted from the anterior pituitary gland. TSH causes conversion of thyroglobulin, produced by the thyroid follicles, into the thyroid hormones: T3, T4, and calcitonin. If thyroid hormone production is below normal, the endocrine negative feedback system causes the hypothalamus to secrete thyrotropin-releasing hormone (TRH). TRH in turn stimulates the pituitary to release TSH (Braimon & Hislop-Chestnut, 2012). T3 and T4 affect cellular metabolism and calcitonin regulates body calcium (Braimon & Hislop-Chestnut, 2012).

Hypothyroidism

The causes of thyroid dysfunction are varied. Decreased thyroid hormone synthesis or thyroid tissue destruction is the cause of primary hypothyroidism, most often caused by an autoimmune process (e.g., Graves' disease or Hashimoto's thyroiditis (Camera, 2010). Pituitary dysfunction is usually the cause of secondary hypothyroidism. Other causes of hypothyroidism include congenital disorders (e.g., cretinism), iodine deficiency, thyroidectomy, radiation therapy, and medications such as amiodarone, interferon alpha, lithium, methimazole, and propylthiouracil. Older adults taking amiodarone are at risk for amiodarone-induced thyrotoxicosis (AIT) or amiodarone-induced hypothyroidism (AIH) (Bogazzi et al., 2001). The risk of developing either AIT or AIH is 14-18% for patients taking this medication (Gopalan & Burks, 2009).

Thyroid screening occasionally reveals an elevated TSH, but normal T4 in patients who are asymptomatic. Known as subclinical hypothyroidism, this type of hypothyroidism requires follow-up. If the TSH is less than 10 mU/l and the patient is not having symptoms, treatment may not be necessary, though monitoring of the TSH is indicated. If the TSH is greater than 10 mU/l, patients are usually treated with exogenous thyroid hormone.

Older adults with untreated or under treated hypothyroidism are at risk of developing myxedema coma, a life threatening endocrine emergency. In years past the mortality rate for patients with myxedema coma was 60-70% (Rodríguez et al., 2004). More recently, the estimated mortality rate for mIxedema coma approached 40% (Kim & Ladenson, 2007).

■ Risk factors

- Age
- Autoimmune disorder
- Family history
- Female gender
- Medications
- Radiation to head/neck
- Thyroidectomy

■ Clinical presentation

Older patients developing hypothyroidism may complain of cold intolerance, constipation, dry skin, fatigue, hair loss, lethargy, memory problems, and weight gain. Often, however, an elder may not notice the symptoms or attribute them to aging. Healthcare providers also may attribute patient complaints to aging or comorbid disorders (Kim & Ladenson, 2007).

■ Nursing assessment

The physical findings may be difficult to interpret because the findings may be subtle or associated with other disorders.

A careful physical assessment looking for the following abnormalities is important.

- Vital signs: possible weight gain, hypertension (particularly diastolic), possible subnormal temperature, or bradycardia
- Skin: dry or yellow carotene tone
- HEENT: puffy facial appearance, alopecia, brittle, thinning hair, diminished visual acuity or hearing, small or enlarged thyroid (goiter), slow, deep voice, or enlarged tongue
- Extremities: edema fingers, toes, peripheral edema (non pitting), or delayed relaxation phase tendons-especially Achilles' tendon (Kim & Ladenson, 2007; Braimon & Hislop-Chestnut, 2012)

■ Diagnostics

- TSH: elevated
- T4: below normal
- Thyroid autoantibodies (if indicated)

Other possible laboratory abnormalities:

- Decreased hemoglobin and hematocrit
- Possible low vitamin B12 level
- Low serum sodium
- Hyperlipidemia
- Hypoglycemia (in myxedema coma) (Camera, 2011)

■ Differential diagnosis

The differential diagnosis is concerned with the underlying cause of the hypothyroidism.

■ Treatment

Treatment for hypothyroidism requires T4 replacement with daily oral levo-thyroxine sodium. In older adults, the initial prescribed amount of levothyrox-ine ordered is a lower dose than is usually prescribed for younger adults. The TSH and T4 are repeated in 4-6 weeks and the medication is increased by small increments until the TSH and T4 values are within normal limits. After stabilization of the TSH, the TSH is usually monitored once a year and as necessary depending on the patient's symptoms.

■ Collaborative consultation

- Consider endocrinology consultation

■ Complications

- Untreated hypothyroidism can cause myxedema coma and death.
- Overtreated hypothyroidism can cause a medication-induced hyperthy-roidism. Symptoms associated with hyperthyroidism can cause anxiety, sleep difficulties, tachycardia, palpitations, angina, ischemia, and weight loss.

■ Prevention

- There is no known prevention for hypothyroidism. For patients taking medications that can cause hypothyroidism, it is important to review the symptoms of hypothyroidism so that the patient can discuss the symp-toms with their doctor.
- Infants are screened at birth for congenital hypothyroidism. There is no way to prevent acquired hypothyroidism and not all organizations recommend regular screening, but the American Thyroid Association does recommend screening female adults over age 35 with TSH every 5 years (Ladenson et al., 2000). If the TSH is below or above normal, a free T4 is recommended.

■ Patient/family education

- Discuss with patients and families the effects of thyroid hormones on the body when thyroid hormone levels are low.
- Explain the importance of taking the medication each morning ½ hour before eating or taking other medications.
- Patients should understand the importance of not stopping the medication without discussing it with the doctor and call the physician if any adverse symptoms occur (e.g., palpitations, shortness of breath, or chest discomfort).

Hyperthyroidism

The causes of hyperthyroidism in elders frequently differs from the causes of hyperthyroidism in younger patients. Grave's disease is the most common cause of an overactive thyroid in younger patients, but multinodular and uninodular toxic goiter (Plummer's disease) are usually the cause of hyperthyroidism in elders. Other potential causes of hyperthyroidism include thyroiditis, exogenous iodine excess, pituitary tumors, and thyroid cancer. Patients with hyperthyroidism have high levels of circulating thyroid hormones. The excess thyroid hormones can be related to a problem with the thyroid gland itself (primary hyperthyroidism) or caused by excess TSH stimulating the thyroid to produce thyroid hormones. Thyrotoxicosis refers to the physiologic effects or clinical syndrome of hypermetabolism that result from excess circulating levels of T3, T4, or both.

■ Risk factors

- Age
- Female gender
- Past medical history
  - Autoimmune disorder
  - Excessive iodine intake
  - Family history
  - Head or neck radiation therapy
  - Medications (e.g., amiodarone, antiretroviral treatment for acquired immune deficiency syndrome, Campath-1H, interferon beta-1b and interleukin-4, immunosuppressant therapy, levothyroxine supplements, and lithium)
  - Neck trauma
  - Stress

■ Clinical presentation

When the thyroid is overactive, common complaints may include anorexia or polyphagia, diarrhea or constipation, weight loss, emotional lability, insomnia, palpitations and heat intolerance. Elders may complain of feeling edgy, weak, fatigued, or notice chest heaviness, shortness of breath (due to heart failure) or discomfort. Many elders have hyperthyroidism but have unexpected signs and symptoms appearing depressed and lethargic. A good history is important to determine subtle changes as well as medication history, family history, past medical history of head or neck radiation, recent illness, or failure to thrive (Golden et al., 2011).

■ Nursing assessment

In elders, the most common physical findings may be a depressed appearance, atrial fibrillation, and myopathy. The physical assessment should be focused to determine presence or absence of the following findings associated with hyperthyroidism.

- Vital signs:
  - Possible weight loss
  - Blood pressure: possible increased blood pressure or increased pulse pressure
  - Heart rate: tachycardia or possible irregular rhythm (e.g., atrial fibrillation)
  - Respiratory rate may be normal.
  - Temperature: fever is possible in thyroiditis.
- HEENT:
  - Check for exophthalmus, conjunctival erythema, lid lag, and/or ophthalmopathy.
  - Neck: palpate thyroid for enlargement, tenderness, and nodules.
  - Cardiac: auscultate for rhythm changes and murmurs. Note heart rate.
  - Lungs: in heart failure, rales or crackles are possible.
  - Extremities: possible edema
  - Neurologic: possible tremor, extremity weakness, or hyperactive reflexes (Golden *et al.*, 2011)

■ Diagnostics

- Laboratory:
  - Decreased serum TSH with elevated free T4 levels
  - Free T3 (if indicated)
- Imaging:
  - Radioadsorbed iodine uptake scan
  - Thyroid ultrasound (if indicated)
- Pituitary magnetic resonance imaging (MRI), if secondary hyperthyroidism
- Other:
  - Electrocardiogram (ECG) is recommended for angina symptoms, tachycardia, or irregular rhythm.

■ Differential diagnosis

The differential diagnosis is concerned with the underlying cause of the hyperthyroidism.

■ Treatment

The goal in treating hyperthyroidism is to first determine the cause and promote patient comfort. Depending on the underlying pathology, treatments will differ. If the hyperthyroidism is related to exogenous thyroid medication (i.e., levothyroxine), the medication dose should be decreased. If the hyperthyroidism is related to a medication, can the medication be stopped or dose decreased? Beta adrenergic blockers can help alleviate symptoms and require careful monitoring because of potential adverse effects with certain comorbid disorders. Antithyroid medications (e.g., methimazole or propylthiouracil) given daily can return the patient to the euthyroid state, but require monitoring for agranulocytosis, drug induced hepatitis, and potential drug-drug interactions. Antithyroid drugs inhibit the synthesis of thyroid hormones, but the drugs are not curative and compliance issues can impact successful control of the thyroid hormones.

Other therapies include radioactive iodine, to destroy the thyroid gland, for a single autonomous nodule or Grave's disease. For multinodular goiter, surgery may be preferred.

■ Collaborative consultation

- Consider endocrinology consultation.
- Consult ophthalmologist for patients with Graves ophthalmopathy.

■ Complications

Untreated hyperthyroidism can result in thyrotoxic crisis (thyroid storm), an unusual, but potentially life threatening exacerbation of hyperthyroidism. Most often the result of illness or injury, thyroid storm is an overproduction of T2 and T4, causing an increase in adrenergic activity. Cardiac, gastrointestinal, and sympathetic nervous system decompensation occurs as a result of epinephrine over production.

Symptoms of thyrotoxic crisis include: tachycardia, vomiting, stupor, irritability, restlessness, tremor, weakness, angina, warm, flushed skin, and temperature elevation. If suspected, treatment to inhibit thyroid hormone synthesis and secretion is started immediately as there is no specific diagnostic test for thyrotoxic crisis. Management will include cardiac monitoring, oxygen, intravenous fluid and electrolyte replacement (American Thyroid Association, 2011).

■ Patient/family education

Patients and families need to understand the cause of the patient's symptoms and potential treatments.

Hyperthyroidism may run in families, so families need to be aware of the signs and symptoms of the disorder.

References

American Thyroid Association. Treatment Guide for Hypothyroidism. Online. Available from http://www.thyroidguidelines.net/hypothyroidism_1995/guidelines/hypothyroidism (accessed 26 March 2012).

Bogazzi, F., Bratalena, L., Gasperi, M., Braverman, L. & Martino, E. (2001) The various effects of amiodaorone on thyroid function. *Thyroid* **11**(5), 511–519.

Braimon J.C. & Hislop-Chestnut, D. (2012) Thyroid disorders. In: Buttaro, T.M., Trybulski, J, Bailey, P.P. & Sandberg-Cook, J (eds) *Primary Care: A Collaborative Practice*, 4th edn. Elsevier, St. Louis.

Camera, I.A. (2010) Endocrine problems. In: Lewis, S., Heitkemper, M., Dirksen, S., Bucher, L. & Camera, I.A. (eds) *Medical Surgical Nursing Assessment and Management of Clinical Problems*, 8th edition. Mosby, St. Louis.

Gopalan, M. & Burks, J. Thyroid dysfunction induced by amiodarone therapy. Online. Available from http:emedicine.medscape.com/article/129033 (accessed 26 March 2012).

Golden, A.K., Thomas, D.J. & Porter, B.O. (2011) Endocrine and metabolic problems. In: Dunphy, L.M., Winland-Brown Porter, B.O. & Thomas, D.J. (eds). *Primary Care: the Art and Science of Advanced Practice Nursing*, 3rd edn. FA Davis, Philadelphia.

Kim, M.I. & Ladenson, P.W. (2007) Hypothyroidism in the elderly. In Online. Available from http://www.endotext.org/aging/aging9/agingframe9.htm (accessed 26 March 2012).

Ladenson, P., Singer, P., Ain, K., *et al.* (2000) American Thyroid Association Guideline for detection of thyroid dysfunction. *Archives of Internal Medicine* **160**, 1573-1575.

Rodríguez, I., Fluiters, E., Pérez-Méndez, L.F., Luna, R. Páramo, C. & García-Mayor, R.V. (2004) Factors associated with mortality of patients with myxoedema coma: prospective study in 11 cases treated in a single institution. *Journal of Endocrinology* **180**, 347-335.

The American Thyroid Association and American Association of Clinical Endocrinologists Taskforce on Hyperthyroidism and Other Causes of Thyrotoxicosis (2011) Hyperthyroidism and Other Causes of Thyrotoxicosis: Management Guidelines of the American Thyroid Association and American Association of Clinical Endocrinologist. Online. Available from http://thyroid-guidelines.net/sites/thyroidguidelines.net/files/file/THY_2010_0417.pdf (accessed 26 March 2012).

PART 3: HYPERPARATHYROIDISM/ HYPOPARATHYROIDISM

Susan L. Wood

Understanding parathyroid disorders in older adults requires appreciating parathyroid function. There are four parathyroid glands located behind the thyroid. These glands secrete parathyroid hormone (PTH), the primary determinant of calcium and phosphorous homeostasis. In response to low serum calcium levels, the parathyroid glands secrete PTH to (1) release bone calcium into extracellular fluid, (2) stimulate calcitriol production to increase intestinal absorption of calcium, and (3) decrease urinary calcium excretion in the kidneys (Owens, 2009; Malabanan, 2012).

Calcium is involved in numerous body functions: cell structure, cell membrane permeability, muscle contraction, bone and teeth formation and structure, and impulse transmission. Additionally, calcium is instrumental in hormone secretion and normal coagulation and (Owens, 2009). An overactive or underactive parathyroid can seriously impact elder health and wellness.

Hyperparathyroidism

In 2005, Coker *et al.* proposed that more than 3.9 million people in the US age 65 or older have primary hyperparathyroidism (PHPT). For postmenopausal women the prevalence of PHPT is increased (Coker *et al.*, 2005; Owens, 2009).

Primary hyperparathyroidism results in calcium, phosphate and bone metabolism disorders and is related to increased PTH secretion causing an elevated serum PTH and high normal or elevated serum calcium levels (Coker *et al.*, 2005). A benign tumor in the parathyroid (adenoma) is the most common cause of this inappropriate hypersecretion of PTH, but familial hypocalciuric hypercalcemia (FHH)is another cause (Malabanan, 2012).

Secondary hyperparathyroidism also results in inappropriately elevated PTH and is related to renal failure or vitamin D deficiency (Malabanan, 2012). Other causes of secondary hyperparathyroidism include inadequate dietary calcium, malabsorption, urinary calcium loss, lithium therapy, and hyperphosphatemia. Tertiary hyperparathyroidism occurs when there is hyperplasia of the parathyroid glands usually related to prolonged hypocalcemia.

■ Risk factors

- Age
- Chronic kidney disease
- Family history: Familial hypocalciuric hypercalcemia
- Medications (e.g., anticonvulsants, lithium, and rifampin)
- Menopause
- Multiple endocrine neoplasia, Type 1
- Neck irradiation history
- Sunscreen (heavy usage)
- Vitamin D deficiency:
  - Gastric bypass surgery
  - Lack of adequate sun exposure
  - Malabsorption

■ Clinical presentation

Most patients with hypercalcemia associated with hyperparathyroidism are asymptomatic. Some patients may have vague symptoms that include:

- Abdominal discomfort
- Anxiety
- Bone pain
- Cognitive impairment
- Constipation
- Depression
- Fatigue
- Hypertension
- Insomnia
- Irritability
- Paresthesia
- Polydipsia
- Proximal muscle weakness
- Urinary symptoms: hematuria, nocturia, polyuria (Malabanan, 2012)

■ Nursing assessment

Vigilance and attentiveness can suggest hypercalcemia though the signs of hypercalcemia are as vague as the symptoms and are easily attributed to other disorders. The clinical signs associated with hypercalcemia include:

- Band keratopathy, a white cloudiness at the cornea border
- Cardiac changes: coronary artery disease (CAD), calcifications on cardiac valves, hypertension, or left ventricular hypertrophy
- Fracture
- Kidney stones

■ Diagnostics

Laboratory

Laboratories may have different normal ranges.

Normal adult serum calcium is usually 8.4-10.2 mEq/dl

- High or low serum calcium levels must always first be correlated with the serum albumin level. The corrected calcium formula is:

4 - albumin (0.8) + serum calcium level

- Serum calcium: can be normal if serum albumin is low, otherwise elevated.
- Serum Albumin
- Fasting serum phosphorus will be decreased or normal.
- Serum magnesium: possibly increased in FHH
- PTH, measured by radioimmunoassay may be elevated.
- Fractional excretion of calcium (FECa): used to exclude FHH
- Ionic calcium >5.6 mg/dl
- Vitamin D 25OH below normal
- Serum 25 - hydroxyvitamin D creatinine clearance
- 24 hour urinary calcium

Electrocardiogram (EKG)

- Shortened QT interval
- Ventricular arrhythmias
- Hypertension (Owens, 2009)

Imaging

- Bone density
- Technetium sestamibi scan if surgery is anticipated
- Parathyroid biopsy if indicated

■ Differential diagnosis

- Primary hyperparathyroidism vs. Secondary hyperparathyroidism
- Hyperparathyroidism related to medications (e.g., lithium) or radiation therapy

- Excessive exogenous calcium
- FHH
- Hyperthyroidism
- Malignancy
- Medications (e.g., thiazide-induced hypercalcemia)
- Multiple endocrine neoplasia syndrome
- Vitamin D deficiency
- Chronic kidney disease

■ Treatment

Treatment depends on the cause of the hyperparathyroidism, but many patients are managed medically. The treatment goals are (1) to relieve patient symptoms and (2) prevent complications associated with hyperparathyroidism. Potential treatments include:

Surgical therapy – parathyroidectomy

- The treatment for primary hyperparathyroidism is surgical removal of the parathyroid adenoma (s). Indications for surgery may include hypercalcemia, hypercalciuria, and reduced bone mineral density (Rodgers et al., 2008). Postoperative care includes:
- Monitor patient for bleeding.
- Monitor intake and output.
- Monitor serum electrolytes (calcium, potassium, phosphate and magnesium levels).
- Monitor for signs of hypocalcemia (Chvostek's sign and Trousseau's sign)
  - Chvostek sign: An abnormal reaction to the stimulation of the facial nerve. When the facial nerve is tapped at the angle of the jaw, the facial muscles on the same side of the face will contract momentarily (typically a twitch of the nose or lips) because of hypocalcemia with resultant hyperexcitability of nerves.
  - Trousseau's sign: A blood pressure cuff is placed around the arm and inflated to a pressure greater than the systolic blood pressure and held in place for 3 minutes. This occludes the brachial artery. In the absence of blood flow, the patient's hypocalcemia and subsequent neuromuscular irritability will induce spasm of the muscles of the hand and forearm. The wrist and metacarpophalangeal joints flex, the distal and proximal interphalangeal joints extend, and the fingers adduct.
  - Mild tetany manifestations include unpleasant tingling of the hands and mouth.
  - Severe tetany manifestations include muscle spasms and laryngospasms.
  - Low serum calcium can be repleted with intravenous calcium gluconate or oral calcium supplements.

Nonsurgical therapy
Medications
Bisphosphonates given intravenously (IV) can be used to lower serum calcium levels in patients with critically elevated calcium levels. Additionally,

bisphosphonates can be used to control the osteopenia associated with hyperparathyroidism.

- Vitamin D deficiency requires correction to achieve a serum 25 hydroxy-vitamin D level greater than 30 ng/dl.
- Hyperphosphatemia may be controlled with diet or if necessary with phosphate binders.
- Patients with chronic kidney disease (stage 3-5) may require calcitriol, cinacalcet, and/or vitamin D.

■ Collaborative consultation

- Referral to a parathyroid surgeon if surgery necessary
- Consider endocrinology consultation.
- Consultation with a dietician to help patients address calcium elevation or deficiency

■ Complications

- Cardiac
  - CAD
  - calcifications on cardiac valves
  - hypertension
  - left ventricular hypertrophy
- Fractures
- Kidney stones
- Osteoporosis
- Excision of parathyroid adenomas may cause hypocalcemia.

■ Prevention

- Monitor patients taking medications that may raise calcium levels (e.g., lithium and thiazide diuretics).
- Monitor renal status of older adults as those with chronic kidney disease will require evaluation for hypocalcemia, hyperphosphatemia, vitamin D deficiency and hyperparathyroidism.

■ Patient/family education

Instruct patient to avoid immobility and prolonged bedrest.Encourage patients to engage in physical activity to minimize bone resorption. Walking 20 minutes, three to four times a week has been demonstrated to minimize bone decalcification in postmenopausal women.

Explain the importance of adequate hydration: at least 6 glasses of water per dayDiscuss the importance of medication therapy when indicated.

Hypoparathyroidism

Hypoparathyroidism is associated with decreased levels of parathyroid hormone (PTH) and hypocalcemia, Most often, trauma or neck surgery causes removal or injury to the hypothyroid glands and this is the cause of the hypoparathyroidism. Other causes are possible and include hereditary hypothyroidism, radioactive iodine treatment for hyperthyroidism, irradiation of the head or neck, low or elevated serum magnesium, or autoimmune disease. Low calcium levels can also be related to a low albumin level.

■ Risk factors

- Surgery for hyperparathyroidism
- Thyroid surgery

■ Clinical presentation

The clinical features of hypoparathyroidism are caused by the low serum calcium level. Most patients with hypocalcemia complain of numbness and tingling in the toes, fingertips, or around the lips, but dysphagia, abdominal cramping, muscle cramps, fatigue, weakness, headaches, memory problems, and anxiety and depression are also possible symptoms (Shoback, 2008).

■ Nursing assessment

When patients complain of symptoms it is important to address their concerns and assess for signs of the disorder.

- Patients with hypocalcemia can be anxious and apprehensive and may complain of perioral or digital numbness and tingling.
- Monitor patients for laryngospasm, seizures and arrhythmias
  - Check Chvostek's sign by tapping the facial nerve. Observe for facial muscle contraction.
  - Check Trousseau's signs by using a blood pressure cuff to occlude the brachial artery. Observe for carpal spasm.
  - Respiratory function may be compromised.
- Monitor ECG for prolonged QT interval.

■ Diagnostics

Laboratory

Normal adult serum calcium is usually 8.4-10.2 mEq/dl. High or low serum calcium levels must always first be correlated with the serum albumin level. The corrected calcium formula is:

$$4 - albumin (0.8) + serum calcium level$$

- Serum calcium
- Serum albumin
- Other important laboratory diagnostics include:

- Ionized calcium: normal is 4.0-<4.5 mg/dl is consistent with hypocalcemia.
- Fasting serum phosphorus: normally 2.5-4.5 mg/dl; >4.5 mg/dl suggests hyperphosphatemia.
- Magnesium
- Serum 25 OH-hydroxyvitamin D
- Serum 1,25-dihydroxyvitamin D
- PTH_i.
- 24 hour urine for urinary calcium
- Urinary cyclic AMP, if indicated

■ Differential diagnosis

- Acquired hypoparathyroidism
- Acute pancreatitis
- Chronic kidney disease
- Hereditary hypoparathyroidism
- Hyper/hypomagnesemia
- Hypoalbuminemia
- Metabolic alkalosis
- Metastatic disease
- Pseudohypocalcemia
- Transient hypocalcemia (may be related to burns, sepsis, transfusion with citrated blood, or medication induced)

■ Treatment

The goal of treatment is to replete the calcium and provide comfort to the patient during a hypocalcemic episode.

- Mild hypocalcemia is treated with oral calcium supplementation 1 to 3 grams PO in divided doses.
- Immediate treatment for severe hypocalcemia includes:
  - IV calcium gluconate 1 mg/ml in D5W to be infused per hospital policy (usually 30-100 ml/hour). Infuse slowly as IV calcium may cause hypotension, dysrhythmias.
  - Calcium infusions require ECG monitoring.
    - Monitor patient for IV patency as extravasation could lead to cellulitis and/or tissue necrosis.
- Long-term treatment includes:
  - Oral calcium supplements
  - Vitamin D preparations (e.g., calcitriol) will raise calcium levels rapidly by enhancing intestinal calcium absorption and bone resorption.

■ Collaborative consultation

Consider consultation with an endocrinologist.

■ Complications

- Arrhythmias
- Bronchospasm
- Heart failure
- Increased intracranial pressure
- Laryngospasm
- Lenticular cataracts
- Papilledema
- Respiratory arrest
- Seizures

■ Prevention

There are no lifestyle changes that can help prevent hypoparathyroidism. During thyroid and other neck surgeries, surgeons take great care to avoid excising or damaging these glands.

■ Patient/family education

Patients and families should understand the cause of the disorder and that hypoparathyroidism can be a chronic condition requiring treatment and continued follow-up. Additional information should include:

- The importance of a high calcium diet as well as available sources of dietary calcium
- Avoidance of long-term laxative use
- Importance of exercise
- Importance of monitoring calcium levels three to four times a year and life-long care (Camera, 2011)

References

Camera, I.A. (2011) In: Lewis, S., Heitkemper, M., Dirksen, S., O'Brien, P., Bucher, L. & Camera, I.A. (eds) (2007). *Medical Surgical Nursing. Assessment and Management of Clinical Problems*, 8th edition. Mosby, St. Louis, pp. 1308-1311.

Coker, L.H., Rorie, K., Cantly, I. & Kirkland, K. (2005) Primary hyperparathyroidism, cognition, and health-related quality of life. *Annals of Surgery* **242**(5), 64226-64650.

Goodman, W. (2002) Calcimimetic agents and secondary hyperparathyroidism: Treatment and prevention. *Nephrology, Dialysis and Transplantation* **17**(2), 204-207.

Malabanan, A. (2012) Parathyroid gland disorders. In: Buttaro, T.M., Trybulski, J.J., Bailey, P.B. & Sandberg-Cook, J. (eds) *Primary Care: A Collaborative Practice. Mosby*, St. Louis.

Owens, B. (2009) A Review of primary hyperparathyroidism. *The Art and Science of Infusion Nursing* **32**(2), 8779-8792.

Rodgers, S., Lew, J. & Solorzano, C. (2008) Primary hyperparathyroidism. *Current Opinion in Oncology* **20**, 52–58.

Shoback, D. (2008) Hypoparthyroidism. *New England Journal of Medicine* **359**, 391–404.

Sloand, J. (2007) Treating hyperparathyroidism with Cincalet HCl. *Nephrology Nursing Journal* **34**(3), 341–342.

PART 4: SYNDROME OF INAPPROPRIATE ANTIDIURETIC HORMONE SECRETION

Susan L. Wood

Syndrome of inappropriate antidiuretic hormone secretion (SIADH) is the most common cause of hyponatremia in older persons both in the hospital and in the community (Miller, 2009). Older adults are at greater risk for disease-induced SIADH than younger patients, partly because of age-related physiologic changes in fluid, body mass, and electrolyte balance and also because they receive treatment with many medications that cause SIADH.

The hyponatremia of SIADH is associated with normal extracellular volume. Caused by excess antidiuretic hormone (ADH) production, in SIADH there is an increase in water reabsorption resulting in excess body water, not a serum sodium deficiency. The excess free water absorbed results in dilutional hyponatremia (Rottman, 2007).

SIADH is most frequently related to malignancy, especially small cell lung cancer. Other causes include malignant tumors (e.g., pancreatic, lymphoid, thymus, prostate, and colorectal cancers); central nervous system disorders (e.g., head injury, cerebrovascular injury, and brain tumors), infection, Guillain-Barré syndrome, systemic lupus erythematosus, drug therapy (e.g., carbamazepine, chlorpropamide, opioids, general anesthesia agents, thiazide diuretics, selective serotonin reuptake inhibitors, tricyclic antidepressants and antineoplastics), and other miscellaneous conditions (e.g., hypothyroidism, lung infection, chronic obstructive pulmonary disease, HIV, and adrenal insufficiency) (Robertson, 2006; Camera, 2011).

■ Risk factors

- Central nervous system disorders
- Head trauma
- Medications
- Neoplasms
- Older age
- Pulmonary disease

■ Clinical presentation

Signs and symptoms of SIADH are variable and depend on the extent of the osmotic fluid shift that results in cerebral edema. In elders, signs and symptoms are often attributed to other causes. Patients with a rapid fall in serum sodium levels will usually have more pronounced signs and symptoms. Dark concentrated urine, anorexia, nausea, malaise, dyspnea, and falls can be early symptoms. Headache, vomiting, irritability, confusion, lethargy, muscle cramps or twitching, weakness, obtundation, seizures and coma occur as the serum sodium continues to decrease (Holm *et al.*, 2009; Camera, 2011).

■ Nursing assessment

The physical examination findings may be subtle as patients with mild to moderate hyponatremia may be asymptomatic and physical examination findings may not occur until the serum sodium level decreases to <120 mEq/l. Assessment considerations include:

- Evaluation of volume status:
  - Vital signs including postural vital sign changes
  - Check skin for signs of dehydration or edema.
  - Monitor intake and output carefully.
  - Daily weights
- Neurologic: Monitor for any alteration in level of consciousness: personality change, confusion, anorexia, or weakness.
- Cardiopulmonary: Monitor heart and lung sounds (Holm *et al.*, 2009; Camera, 2011).
- GI: Assess for bowel sounds.

■ Diagnostics

Initial diagnostics are concerned with identifying hyponatremia:

- Laboratory
  - Serum glucose, serum electrolytes, blood urea nitrogen (BUN), and creatinine
    - SIADH is associated with hyponatremia (sodium <135 mEq/l) and low serum osmolality (<280 mOsm/kg).

$$\text{Serum osmolality} = 2(\text{Na [in mEq/l]}) + \text{K (in mEq/l)} + (\text{BUN [in mg/dl]}/2.8) + (\text{glucose [in mg/dl]}/18)$$

  - Urine specific gravity >1.005
  - Elevated urinary sodium level (>20 mmol/l)
  - Elevated urine osmolality (>100 mOsm/l)
  - Normal thyroid stimulating hormone (TSH)
  - Normal or low uric acid
- Imaging
  - Chest radiographs may reveal underlying cause (e.g., pulmonary disease or lung carcinoma).
  - Computed tomography (CT) scan may show cerebral edema or may identify a central nervous system disorder (e.g., brain tumor) responsible for SIADH (Fitzgerald, 2008).

■ Differential diagnosis

SIADH is a diagnosis of exclusion and can usually be made with routine history, physical examination, and laboratory information (Robertson, 2006).

Other disorders commonly associated with hyponatremia should be excluded including:

- Hyponatremia associated with hypervolemia (e.g., generalized edema due to severe congestive heart failure, cirrhosis or nephrosis)
- Hyponatremia associated with hypovolemia (e.g., renal or non renal disorders)
  - Renal disorders: chronic renal disease, osmotic diabetic diuresis, mineralocorticoid deficiency, angiotensin-converting enzyme [ACE] inhibitors, and diuretics
  - Non renal disorders: dehydration, diarrhea, vomiting, burns, extreme exercise, diaphoresis, and third-space fluid loss (Buttaro, 2012)
- Pseudohyponatremia associated with elevated serum glucose, hyperlipidemia or hyperproteinemia
- Psychogenic polydipsia
- Beer potomania (the association of severe hyponatremia with ingestion of large quantities of beer)
- Reset osmostat
- Adrenal insufficiency and adrenal crisis
- Hyperkalemia and metabolic acidosis coexisting with hyponatremia suggest adrenal insufficiency
- Plasma cortisol levels should be obtained to rule out adrenal insufficiency.
- Cerebral salt wasting (rare syndrome described in patients with cerebral disease that mimics SIADH)
- Pulmonary infection
- Chronic obstructive pulmonary disease
- HIV
- CNS disorders
- Medications

■ Treatment

- Discontinue offending medications whenever possible.
- Intravenous therapy with 0.9% or 3% normal saline. *Serum sodium must be monitored carefully to prevent too rapid an increase in serum sodium.*
- Fluid restriction:
  - The goal is to establish a negative fluid balance and slowly increase in serum sodium levels.
  - May be no more than 1000 ml/day, though the degree of fluid restriction can be variable and should be discussed with the physician.
  - Provide distractions to decrease discomfort of thirst related to fluid restrictions.
- Protect from injury because of potential mental status changes:
  - Bed alarm
  - Assist with ambulation.
  - Seizure precautions

- Pharmacologic agents are sometimes, but not always indicated. These include:
  - Vasopressin receptor antagonists
  - Diuretics (e.g., furosemide)
  - Demeclocycline
- Provide support for patient and family regarding diagnosis and mental status changes (Fitzgerald, 2008; Holm *et al.*, 2009).

■ Collaborative consultation

- When discussing treatment for SIADH with the physician or other health care provider, be certain to review the treatment orders carefully to avoid too rapid a rise in sodium.
- Dietician consultation may be indicated to manage supplements and teach the patient symptoms of fluid and electrolyte imbalances, especially those involving sodium and potassium.

■ Complications

- Initial complications of hyponatremia include nausea, loss of appetite, fatigue, headache, thirst, dyspnea on exertion, decreased urine output and increased body weight.
- As the serum sodium levels continue to decrease, symptoms become more severe causing muscle cramps, muscle twitching, vomiting, seizures, coma and death.

■ Prevention

Prevention is directed at the underlying cause. Medications that stimulate the release of ADH should be avoided or discontinued. Therapy is then directed at restoring the normal fluid volume osmolarity as described above. When SIADH is chronic, the patient must learn to self manage treatment regimens and recognize symptoms of fluid and electrolyte imbalances. The patient's ability to observe severe restriction of fluid intake may determine the degree of ongoing symptoms. SIADH usually improves after stopping a drug or curing an infection when that is the cause. When cancer is the direct cause of SIADH, one hopes for similar improvement of SIADH from treatments that reduce the amount of cancer in the body.

■ Patient/family education

- Emphasize the importance of compliance with fluid restriction.
- Ice chips or sugarless gum can help decrease thirst.
- Patient and family should be taught the symptoms of fluid and electrolyte imbalances and when to seek medical attention.

References

Buttaro, T.M. (2012) Hypernatremia and hyponatremia. In: Buttaro, T.M., Trybulski, J., Bailey, P.B. & Sandberg-Cook, J. (eds) *Primary Care: A Collaborative Practice*, 4th edition. Mosby, St. Louis.

Camera, I.M. (2011) Endocrine problems. In: Lewis, S., Heitkemper, M., Dirksen, S., O'Brien, P. & Bucher, L. (eds). *Medical Surgical Nursing Assessment and Management of Clinical Problems*, 8th edition. Mosby, St. Louis.

Fitzgerald, M. (2008) Hyponatremia associated with SSRI use in a 65 year old woman. *The Nurse Practitioner* **February**, 11-12.

Holm, A., Bie, P., Otteson, M., Odum, L. & Jesperson, B. (2009) Diagnosis of the syndrome of inappropriate secretion of antidiuretic hormone. *Southern Medical Journal* **102**(4), 380-383.

Miller, M. (2009). Hyponatremia in the elderly: risk factors, clinical consequences, and management. *Clinical Geriatrics* **17**(9), 34-39.

Robertson, G. (2006) Regulation of arginine vasopressin in the syndrome of inappropriate antidiuresis. *The American Journal of Medicine* **119**, S36-S42.

Rose, B.D. & Post, T.W. (2001) *Clinical Physiology of Acid-Base and Electrolyte Disorders*, 5th edition. McGraw-Hill, New York, pp. 703-711.

Rottmann, C. (2007) SSRI's and the syndrome of antidiuretic hormone secretion. *AJN* **107**(1), 51-58.

Further reading

Bourgeois, J., Babine, S. & Bahadur, N. (2002) A case of SIADH and hyponatremia associated with citalopram. *Psychosomatics* **43**(3), 241-242.

Miller M. (1998) Hyponatremia: age-related risk factors and therapy decisions. *Geriatrics* **53**, 32-48.

Unit 8: Musculoskeletal

PART 1: SEPTIC ARTHRITIS

Susan Bardzik

Septic arthritis, also known as infectious arthritis, is a bacterial infection of the joint. The bacteria may enter through the skin or travel from a distant location through the blood to invade the joint and cause damage. More than one joint may be involved. The bacteria may invade any joint of the body, large or small. The joints usually affected include the knee, hip, shoulder, elbow, wrist, and joints of the fingers.

Organisms most commonly causing septic arthritis include *Staphylococcus aureus*, streptococci, *Escherichia coli*, and *Niesseria gonorrheae*. Other causes may include *Borrelia burgdorferi* (Lyme disease) and *Mycobacterium tuberculosis*. Fungal, parasitic, and some viral infections such as rubella, mumps, and hepatitis, have also been implicated (Madoff, 2012).

Septic arthritis occurs in 2 cases per 10,000 persons in the general population (Smith *et al.*, 2006). Young children and elders are most commonly affected. Older adults are particularly vulnerable since they often have more risk factors and co-morbid conditions.

■ Risk factors

- Age
- Alcoholics
- Animal bites or other penetrating injury
- Central line placement
- Hemodialysis
- History of arthritis
- Immunocompromised patients, especially those with HIV, diabetes, liver or kidney problems, and cancer, or post organ transplantation
- Immunosuppressant medications
- Infection – local or systemic
- Intravenous drug abuse
- Open skin wounds (that allow bacteria to access the body)
- Previous intra-articular (joint) steroid injection
- Prosthetic joints
- Psoriasis
- Sexually transmitted diseases
- Sickle cell disease
- Surgery to the joint, especially joint replacements
- Tick bite
- Trauma to the joint (Langford & Mandell, 2012)

■ Clinical presentation

- Pain in the affected joint that is worse with movement
- Edema in the affected joint
- Decreased mobility
- Erythema and warmth of the affected joint
- Fever (chills are not always present)
- Malaise

■ Nursing assessment

- A thorough patient history including the history of present illness, allergies, current medications, past medical history, and pain assessment will give clues to the sources of infection and help guide treatment.
- Review all current medications. Remember that immunosuppressant medications can mask signs of infection.
- Vital signs: although older adults and immunocompromised patients may not develop a fever, an elevated temperature usually indicates infection. Tachycardia may occur in response to fever. Hypotension may occur with sepsis.
- Musculoskeletal: assess joints for erythema, edema, warmth, tenderness and decreased mobility. Nearby tendons and muscles may be painful.
- Skin: examine for trauma, bites, open or ulcerated areas, and cellulitis –this may be a portal of entry for bacteria to enter the body. A rash may suggest gonococcal infection (Madoff, 2012).
- Assess lungs for any signs of a respiratory infection. Tuberculosis is sometimes implicated.
- Assess any intravenous or invasive lines or catheters for signs of infection.
- Inspect genitalia for signs of ulcers or drainage that may indicate a sexually transmitted disease.

■ Diagnostics

- Arthrocentesis/synovial fluid analysis (aspiration of synovial fluid or joint fluid to check for white blood cells (WBC) and bacteria) is necessary for accurate diagnosis. Purulent synovial fluid indicates inflammation and infection.
- Complete blood count (CBC) with differential and blood cultures
- Erythrocyte sedimentation rate (ESR) and C-reactive protein (CRP) are increased in response to inflammation.
- X-ray
- Ultrasound
- Computed tomography scan (CT scan) and magnetic resonance imaging (MRI) may be ordered to assess joint damage.
- Throat, sputum, spinal fluid, urine, and skin lesions are cultured if suspected as an infectious source.

■ Differential diagnoses

- The differential diagnosis is concerned with determining the cause of the infected joint so that appropriate therapy is administered. Examination of the synovial fluid with culture and sensitivity will aid diagnosis, but other considerations in the differential include:

- Bursitis
- Cellulitis
- Flares of other forms of arthritis
- Gout
- Joint injury, such as fracture, meniscal tear, osteonecrosis
- Lyme disease
- Osteoarthritis
- Osteomyelitis
- Other infections
- Parasitic arthritis
- Pseudogout
- Reactive arthritis
- Reiter's syndrome
- Systemic lupus erythematosus
- Tumors (Madoff, 2012; Margaretten et al., 2007)

■ Treatment

- Synovial fluid, CBC with differential, and blood cultures are an essential component of therapy and should be obtained prior to beginning antibiotic therapy (Madoff, 2012).
- Antibiotic therapy – a prolonged course of intravenous antibiotics may be necessary depending upon the extent of the infection.
  - Monitor for associated side effects of antibiotic therapy.
- Drainage of infectious material in the joint is an essential treatment.
- Arthrocentesis (needle aspiration), arthroscopy (viewing of a joint space through an endoscope), or open surgical drainage are also typically performed. Surgical lavage (washing out of the joint) and debridement (removal of infected tissue) can be done during arthroscopy or open surgical procedures.

Preprocedure

- Inform the patient that needle aspirations are painful. Premedicate the patient with pain medication prior to the procedure.
- Inform the patient that aspirations may need to be done serially for several days or until the infection has cleared.
- Provide emotional support and reassurance to the patient to decrease anxiety.

Post-procedure

- Monitor the aspiration site for erythema and drainage.
- Apply a sterile dressing to the aspiration site if draining.
  - Monitor elders for signs of discomfort and administer analgesics to decrease pain (Mandell, 2009).

- Maintain affected joint in its natural position. Splints can be used temporarily in the acute phase to maintain correct positioning of the joint and decrease pain.
- Avoid weight bearing initially until pain and inflammation resolve (Madoff, 2012; Smith *et al.*, 2006).
- Assist the patient with passive and active range of motion (ROM) exercises. Physical therapy and ROM are important to avoid joint immobility and muscle atrophy (Drees & Ross, 2005).
- Apply heat or ice to the affected areas to decrease inflammation and pain.
- Monitor for fevers, increasing pain, erythema , edema at the joint site and increases in WBC which can indicate progressing infection that can lead to complications.

■ Collaborative consultation

A rheumatologist is an essential team member in diagnosing and prescribing appropriate treatment. An infectious disease physician and pharmacist may also guide treatment in regards to appropriate antibiotic coverage. The physical therapist will help preserve joint mobility and function. An orthopedic surgeon is consulted for reconstruction.

■ Complications

Loss of joint function and mobility is common. Septic arthritis destroys tissue quickly and may lead to permanent bone and cartilage damage and destruction. Joint replacement may be necessary. In severe cases, amputation and prosthetic surgery may occur. Septic arthritis may also cause septicemia. Mortality rates vary depending upon age, speed and appropriateness of treatment and co-morbid conditions.

■ Prevention

- Identify at risk patients.
- Use sterile technique with all procedures.
- Treat any open skin area immediately to avoid infection.
- Discuss prophylactic antibiotics with physician for at risk populations undergoing invasive procedures.
- Patients may wish to weigh the risk versus benefits to receiving intra-articular steroid injections for previous joint problems.
- Avoidance of at risk sexual behaviors and intravenous drug abuse.

■ Patient/family education

- Teach patient and family to report signs of redness, swelling, or pain in a joint.
- Explain all treatments and procedures to patients and families.
- Discuss with both patient and family the expected treatment regimen (i.e., the long course of antibiotics and possible antibiotic side effects).

- Discuss importance of physical therapy to maintain joint mobility and avoid muscle atrophy.
- Discuss safety precautions with the patient and family since pain and the medications used to treat pain and joint instability may increase the patient's risk for falls or other injury.

References

Drees, M., & Ross, J. (2005) Septic arthritis: treat early to minimize morbidity: treatment stats with empiric antibiotic therapy, includes joint drainage. *Journal of Musculoskeletal Medicine* **22**(4), 161-166.

Madoff, L.C. (2012) Chapter 334. Infectious arthritis. In Longo, D.L., Fauci, A.S. Kasper, D.L., Hauser, S.L., Jameson, J.L. & Loscalzo, J. (eds), *Harrison's Principles of Internal Medicine*, 18th edn. Online. Available from from http://0-www.access-medicine.com.library.simmons.edu/content.aspx?aID=9139388 (accessed 5 June 2012).

Langford C.A. & Mandell B.F. (2012) Chapter 336. Arthritis associated with systemic disease, and other arthritides. In Longo, D.L., Fauci, A.S., Kasper, D.L., Hauser, S.L., Jameson, J.L. & Loscalzo, J. (eds), *Harrison's Principles of Internal Medicine*, 18th edn. Online. Available from http://0-www.accessmedicine.com.library.sim-mons.edu/content.aspx?aID=9139559 (accessed 5 June 2012).

Mandell, B.F. (2009) Septic arthritis. ACP Medicine, Decker Intellectual Properties.

Margaretten, M., Kohlwes, J., Moore, D., & Bent, S. (2007) Does this adult patient have septic arthritis? *Journal of the American Medical Association* **297**(13), 1478-1488.

Smith, J.W., Chalupa, P., & Hasan, M. (2006) Infectious arthritis: clinical features, laboratory findings and treatment. *Clinical Microbiology and Infectious Diseases* **12**, 309-314.

Further reading

Garcia-De La Torre, I. (2006) Advances in the management of septic arthritis. *Infectious Disease Clinics of North America* **20**, 773-788.

Matthews, C., & Coakley, G. (2008) Septic arthritis: current diagnostic and therapeutic algorithm. *Current Opinion in Rheumatology* **20**(4), 457-462.

Zeller, J. (2007) Septic arthritis. *Journal of the American Medical Association* **297**(13), 1510.

PART 2: GOUT

Sharon R. Smart

Gout is an arthritic disorder that commonly affects older adults. However, it can also occur in adults as young as 30. More common among men than women, gout is caused by a build-up of monosodium uric acid crystals in one or more joints, causing painful joint inflammation. Uric acid crystals are formed with the breakdown of purines, a substance which naturally occurs in protein. The body produces uric acid naturally during cellular regeneration, and as food containing protein is broken down for use. If the kidneys are unable to excrete excess uric acid, crystals form in one or more joints, causing an acute inflammatory reaction known as gout. Patients can have elevated levels of uric acid, but be asymptomatic. However, the elevated uric acid levels increase the risk of nephrolithiasis, hypertension, and renal disease (Schlesinger, 2012).

Gout is considered the most common form of inflammatory arthritis with an increasing worldwide prevalence. Between 1990 and 1999, the prevalence of gout increased by nearly 60%. In those 75 years and older, the prevalence has doubled. A greater risk of gout has been contributed to certain comorbid conditions including cardiovascular disease, hypertension, renal disease, diabetes, metabolic syndrome, obesity, hyperlipidemia and certain medication use. Lifestyle choices, such as alcohol use and red meat consumption, also play a role. The increased risk of gout in elders is thought to be related to the increase in comorbid conditions that occur with aging (Zychowicz et al., 2010; Zychowicz, 2011).

Gout symptoms can be mistaken for pseudogout (inflammation with crystals other than uric acid, such as calcium), septic arthritis, or rheumatoid arthritis. These conditions may also cause joint pain and inflammation and should be excluded prior to gout treatment.

Intercritical gout is the asymptomatic period between acute gout attacks. When these periods of latency become shorter or the acute attacks last longer, prophylactic treatment for gout is usually initiated with a uric-acid lowering medication such as allopurinol or probenecid.

■ Risk factors

- Age
- Alcohol consumption (beer and spirits)
- Cardiovascular disease
- Diabetes
- Dehydration
- Diet high in red meat and seafood
- Drugs which affect serum urate, such as thiazide diuretics and aspirin
- Glucocorticoid withdrawal
- Hyperlipidemia
- Hypertension
- Hyperuricemia
- Injury
- Malnutrition/starvation
- Metabolic syndrome
- Obesity
- Post-menopausal female
- Renal disease
- Trauma or surgery

▓ Clinical presentation

Gout is diagnosed by both clinical presentation and diagnostic testing. Patient presentation usually includes an acute, severe, onset of monoarticular pain. The patient often notices the pain during the night. Though gout may occur in any joint, most often it is the first metatarsophalangeal joint (big toe joint) that is affected. Gouty pain in this joint is known as podagra. Gout can occur in multiple joints, though this presentation is less common.

▓ Nursing assessment

The history of the present illness as well as allergies, medication, past medical and family history should be obtained.

- Vital signs may be normal, but the patient may have fever or chills.
- The patient often appears uncomfortable. Gout in the knee, foot, or toe will cause so much pain that the patient will have difficulty walking or limp. The affected joint will have low grade inflammation - erythema, edema, warmth, and usually exquisite tenderness. Tophi (urate deposits) in soft tissue may also be present on bony prominences, extensor surfaces and ear helices. In elders, gout can affect joints not commonly affected (i.e., Heberden's nodes) (Schlesinger, 2012).

▓ Diagnostics

Treatment for gout is generally initiated based on clinical presentation. However, diagnostic testing can include:

- Serum uric acid level may be elevated or normal.
- Joint aspiration of synovial fluid to assess presence of uric crystals on microscopic evaluation
- Complete blood count (CBC) with differential if septic joint suspected
- Imaging studies: X-ray, computed tomography (CT) scan) or magnetic resonance imaging (MRI) if indication of crystal formation in the joint

▓ Differential diagnosis

- Bursitis
- Nodular rheumatoid arthritis
- Pseudogout - calcium pyrophosphate dihydrate (CPPD) disease or other mineral deposit in a joint
- Septic arthritis
- Trauma

▓ Treatment

Untreated an acute attack of gout will resolve, but the pain can be immobilizing, so patients are treated during the acute attack for pain. Administering ordered medications and monitoring for symptom relief and side effects are important.

Commonly used medications for acute gout include:

- Corticosteroids – given with food to decrease gastric upset may be the safest treatment for older adults because of side effects associated with other therapies.
- Nonsteroidal anti-inflammatory drugs (NSAIDs) such as ibuprofen and Indocin (use cautiously in elders)
  - Frequent side effects of NSAIDs include nausea, GI bleeding, rash, and/or fluid retention.
- Colchicine – 0.6 milligrams up to five times daily, titrated for diarrhea
  - Rarely used in elders because side effects of colchicine that include diarrhea, gastrointestinal upset, and vomiting.

For patients who are having frequent gout attacks, preventive medications include:

- Uric-acid lowering agents such as allopurinol, febuxostat, or and probenecid. In older patients, the dose of allopurinol is lower (100 to 200 milligrams PO daily), depending on renal status. When allopurinol is started, the treatment can precipitate attacks of gout for several weeks.
- For patients on allopurinol or probenecid, it is important to monitor renal status carefully.

Additional nursing considerations include:

- Monitor affected joint for skin breakdown due to edema of the area.
- Limit diet intake of red meat, shellfish, and purine-rich foods such as wine, beer, cheese and other aged products.
- Monitor CBC and serum electrolytes for any abnormalities that may be associated with medication used for treatment. Monitor uric acid levels (goal serum uric acid <6.0).
- Discuss with physician possible precipitant medications.

■ Collaborative consultation

Be sure to inform the physician or health care provider of any allergies to medications, history of GI bleed or renal disease.

Notify the physician or other health care provider if the patient experiences side effects or medications, especially abdominal pain or diarrhea, or if there is no improvement in symptoms within 24 hours.

■ Complications

- Gouty tophi
- Recurrent or chronic symptoms which require long-term use of allopurinol or other antigout medication

- Complications related to medications for gout include:
  - GI bleed associated with NSAID or steroid use
  - Renal insufficiency with use of allopurinol or NSAIDs
  - Diarrhea or abdominal pain with use of colchicines, NSAIDs, steroids or allopurinol

■ Prevention

- Limiting foods high in purines and nitrates such as aged meats, shellfish, beer, and wine
- Weight reduction
- Adequate hydration
- Adequate nutrition – avoidance of malnutrition

■ Patient/family education

- Teach patient and family how to use pain medications appropriately and monitor for side effects of treatment medications.
- Explain the importance of monitoring the affected joint site for skin breakdown and superimposed cellulitis. Patient/family needs to understand the importance of calling the doctor if signs of infection are present.
- Encourage adequate fluid intake, and minimal dietary nitrates and purines.
- Notify provider if no symptom improvement within 24 hours of initiation of treatment for acute exacerbation.

References

Schlesinger, N. (2012) Gout. In: Buttaro, T.M., Trybulski, J., Polgar-Bailey, P. & Sandberg-Cook, J. (eds) *Primary Care: A Collaborative Practice*. Mosby, St. Louis.

Zychowicz, M.E. (2011) Gout: no longer the disease of kings. *Orthopaedic Nursing* **30**(5), 322-330.

Zychowicz, M., Pope, R. & Graser, E. (2010) The current state of care in gout: Addressing the need for better understanding of an ancient disease. *Journal of American Academy of Nurse Practitioners* **22**(11), Supplement 1, 628-629.

PART 3: JOINT REPLACEMENT

Nichole Spencer

Total joint replacement is medically referred to as total joint arthroplasty. Individuals with osteoarthritis, osteonecrosis, or connective tissue disorders, such as rheumatoid arthritis, may elect to have an affected joint replaced to manage pain or to improve mobility if all other attempted measures have been unsuccessful. The replacement of hip and knee joints is the most common

(Lucas, 2007a). Other joints such as shoulders, elbows, wrists, fingers, ankles or feet can be replaced as well. Osteoarthritis or degenerative joint disease is characterized by the deterioration and loss of cartilage in the joint. In the United States, osteoarthritis is the most common cause of pain and decreased mobility in a joint which could lead to an elective joint replacement (Lucas, 2007a). Osteoarthritis usually occurs in the weight bearing joints such as the hip and knee, posing particular problems for older adults in terms of mobility and ability to perform activities of daily living (ADLs).

■ Risk factors

- Advanced age
- Increased wear and tear on joint secondary to occupation, activity, or injury (e.g., carpet lying, and sports such as football, soccer, and gymnastics).
- Muscle loss can lead to joint deterioration if the muscle is not supporting the joint and leads to wearing down of cartilage.
- Obesity
- Smoking
- Trauma

■ Clinical presentation

Joint replacement is selected when all other conservative measures have failed. It is usually uncontrollable pain and/or an inability to perform those activities associated with daily functioning that result in a patient choosing a joint replacement.

The criteria used for determining the need for a joint replacement includes the inability of the patient to sleep secondary to the joint pain or that the joint pain interferes with daily activities and functioning (e.g., the patient may not be able to use stairs, may not be able to walk as far as needed, or cannot provide self care). Usually, the patient will have tried medical treatment for greater than three months, but when pain is uncontrollable and the patient is unable to participate in therapy to assist with functioning, joint replacement is an option to improve quality of life (Agency for Healthcare Research and Quality, 2002).

■ Nursing assessment
Preoperative

Preoperatively a detailed history must be established. This includes allergies or untoward reactions to medications or anesthesia as well as all medications including over-the counter medications and herbals. Medications are also reviewed to determine if the patient has been taking agents that may interfere with clotting such as nonsteroidal anti-inflammatory drugs (NSAIDs), warfarin (Coumadin), or aspirin.

All previous medical conditions and surgeries must be elicited and the patient's previous functional capabilities determined. Any possible infections, but especially urinary tract infections, should be excluded. The patient's primary care physician and pertinent specialists (e.g., cardiology) will be involved to provide clearance for surgery.

Evaluating the psychological status of the patient is also helpful as is assessment of the home environment (e.g., how many stairs into the home and the location of the bedroom and bathroom) since the patient will likely have some mobility limitations after surgery. Evaluation of the patient's support system is important for post operative success (Lucas, 2007a, b).

The preoperative nursing assessment should be thorough and focused. Document the extremity baseline neurovascular assessments prior to surgery.

Postoperative

Vital signs:

- Monitor for fever or 0.8°C (2°F) increase in baseline temperature.
- Monitor heart rate and blood pressure (increased heart rate and decreased blood pressure may suggest bleeding).
- Assess respiratory rate and oxygen saturation. Increased respiratory rate and/or decreased oxygen saturation could suggest pneumonia, heart failure, or pulmonary emboli.

Neurological status:

- Observe for any mental status changes from baseline. An acute change in mental status suggests delirium and should be further evaluated.

Skin:

- Monitor surgical incision dressings for blood and drainage:
  - Check wound daily and as needed for signs of infection including edema, erythema, exudates and increased pain. Document characteristics of wound exudate: color, clarity, odor, and consistency.
- Observe approximated edges of surgical incision.
- Prevent skin breakdown with skin protectants especially over the sacral area and other bony prominences. Heels should be kept OFF the bed and patient repositioned according to surgeon's instructions and hospital policy.

Respiratory:

- Assess lung sounds for rales, wheezes, rhonchi, and respiratory rate each shift and as needed.
- Monitor oxygen saturation level and the need for oxygen.
- Instruct patient to take deep breaths frequently and encourage use of incentive spirometer.

Cardiac:

- Monitor heart rate and rhythm and for extra heart sounds and murmurs.
- Check pulses distal to joint replacement and bilateral peripheral pulses each shift and as needed.
  - Assess capillary refill bilaterally.
- Assess extremity edema and color of skin bilaterally.
- Apply compression stockings or sequential compression stockings as ordered.
- Provide anticoagulation therapy as ordered.

Gastrointestinal:

- Assess bowel function daily and monitor for constipation. Patients receiving narcotics for pain should have a daily bowel movement and need a bowel protocol.
  - Monitor for bowel sounds/paralytic ileus.
- Patient should be nothing by mouth (NPO) until a diet change is ordered by the surgeon.
  - Patient should have bowel sounds and be passing flatus.
  - Document and report presence of bowel sounds which will indicate the likelihood for diet increase.
- Monitor all stools for occult blood.

Genitourinary:

- Assess for adequate urinary output, at least 30 ml/hour.
- Monitor patient for urinary retention (e.g., small frequent voiding, restlessness, and bladder distention) and symptoms of urinary tract infection.

Musculoskeletal:

- Monitor extremity position and use ordered devices to prevent dislocation (i.e., abduction device such as foam wedge used with hip replacement)
  - knee should remain in a neutral position; immobilizer used with shoulder replacements.
- Assess for possible dislocation (i.e., increased pain to the joint orrotation of the extremity).
- Clarify and follow surgical orders regarding extremity weight bearing status after joint replacement.
- Follow postoperative precautions to range of joint.
  - Hip replacement: Hip should not be bent more than 90 degrees.
  - Knee replacement: Goal is to increase flexion of knee. Continuous passive motion (CPM) machine can assist if ordered by surgeon.
- Evaluate patient's mobility (e.g., ability to transfer from bed to chair and bed mobility). Determine possible needs for assistive devices to assure safe transfers and ambulation.

Neurovascular:

- Monitor for distal pulses and color of extremity with joint replacement.
- Monitor for circulation, movement, and sensation (CSM). Assess for numbness and pressure.
- Compare the extremity with the joint replacement with the other extremity.
  - Always note and document the baseline of extremity assessments prior to surgery.

Pain control:

- Provide analgesics as ordered and assess the need for scheduled versus upon patient request dosing.
- Follow surgeon's orders regarding ice, elevation, and positioning.

■ Diagnostics

Preoperative

- Preoperative diagnostics usually include X-ray and/or magnetic resonance imaging (MRI), complete blood count (CBC), comprehensive metabolic profile (CMP), prothrombin time (PT), partial thromboplastin time (PTT), type and cross match, and a urinalysis. A nasal swab for methicillin-resistant *Staphylococcus aureus* (MRSA) may also be ordered (per hospital policy).

Postoperative

- CBC/differential
- Serum electrolytes, BUN, creatinine
- PT and PTT
- International normalized ratio (INR) if patient is on warfarin (Coumadin)
- Other serologies are dependent on patient co-morbidities.
- Doppler ultrasound to exclude deep venous thrombosis (DVT) if patient has lower extremity unilateral edema, erythema, and pain or discomfort.

■ Differential diagnosis

There is no differential diagnosis for a joint replacement.

■ Treatment

- Assess and document patient's pain level.
- Administer pain medications and assess and document patient response to pain medication.
  - If patient has patient-controlled anesthesia explain use to patient.
- Continuous postoperative assessments as indicated above.
- Administer antibiotics and/or anticoagulants therapies as ordered.
- Monitor intake and output carefully. For patients who are able to eat, monitor meal intake as eating less than 50% of two meals in 24 hours can suggest change of status in older patients.

- Begin discharge teaching with patient and family prior to or immediately after surgery:
  - Is patient home safe for discharge?
  - Will home be accessible for assistive devices?
  - Is bedroom/bathroom accessible for patient?
  - Does patient live alone?
  - Who will help patient with food shopping, transportation to physician appointments?
  - Is caregiver readily available? Will patient need homemaker? Short-term rehabilitation?
  - Does patient/caregiver understand mobility concerns (e.g., weight bearing), exercise regimen, medications, signs of infection, joint prosthesis dislocation, or other important reasons to call surgeon?
- If patient will be discharged home arrange for a visiting nurse, physical therapy, and a home safety evaluation.
- Physical therapy and occupation therapy evaluation

■ Collaborative consultation

- Joint care protocols are specific to the joint replaced and the particular prosthesis type. Each surgeon may also have particular concerns about joint positioning, assistive devices, and pain management. To promote maximum collaborative care, careful discussion about each surgeon's postoperative protocols should be discussed and documented.
- Anticoagulation therapy: if patient is started on warfarin, discuss goal PT/INR and anticoagulation therapy with surgeon daily or as indicated.
- Consult dietician for all patients discharged on warfarin for a review of dietary recommendations.

■ Complications

- Anemia
- Bleeding and clotting problems
- Constipation
- Dislocation or loosening of the hardware or prosthesis
- Infection to incision or hardware
- Neurological injury
- Pneumonia
- Respiratory depression
- Thromboembolism or pulmonary embolism
- Uncontrollable pain

■ Prevention

- Primary goal of therapy after joint replacement is to return patient to optimum state of health and mobility. Other essential goals are to ensure patient safety and prevent infection, dislocation, falls, adverse reaction to a medication, or drug-drug interactions.

■ Patient/family education

Preoperative instruction

- Education about medications to avoid (e.g., aspirin or NSAIDs) is essential. The patient should understand how many days prior to surgery the medications need to be discontinued.
- Pain should be controlled prior to surgery to assist with pain control postoperatively. Patients should be educated on pain control and to be able to rate pain accurately to not let pain become uncontrolled.
- Instruction should be provided on exercises that will be expected postoperatively. Physical and occupational therapists can be helpful preoperatively to provide instruction on how transfers, positioning, and exercises will be performed after surgery. Continued strengthening of muscles surrounding the joint to be replaced is indicated for potential improved recovery with pain and time (Hohler, 2007).
- Instruction should be provided on what to expect postoperatively (e.g., pain, limited mobility, surgical drains, compression stockings, surgical incision, and respiratory exercises).
- Risk for thromboembolism postoperatively requires instruction on the use of anticoagulants status post surgery.
- Since joint replacement, or joint arthroplasty, is elective it is possible that the patient will be able to donate blood for this procedure prior to the surgery (i.e., autologous blood donation).

Postoperative instruction

- Patients should understand the life span of a joint prosthesis is variable.

References

Agency for Healthcare Research and Quality (2002) Managing osteoarthritis: Helping the elderly to maintain function and mobility. Online. Available from http://www.ahrq.gov/research/osteoria/osteoria.htm (accessed 26 March 2012).

Hohler, S.E. (2004) Minimally invasive total hip arthroplasty. *AORN Journal* **79**(6), 1244-1258.

Howell, B. (2007) Joint surgery: Paving the way to hip and knee replacements can relieve pain, allowing people live more active lives. *RN* **70**(1), 32-37.

Lucas, B. (2008a) Total hip and total knee replacement: preoperative nursing management. *British Journal of Nursing* **17**(21), 1346-1351.

Lucas, B. (2008b) Total hip and total knee replacement: postoperative nursing management. *British Journal of Nursing* **17**(22), 1410-1414.

PART 4: OSTEOMYELITIS

Lesley Caracci

Osteomyelitis is an infection of the bone. The root words *osteon* (bone) and *myelo* (marrow) and *itis* (inflammation) define the state of the bone infected with microorganisms. Osteomyelitis was first defined in 1844 by Auguste Nelaton, a surgeon from Paris, (Chen & Balloch, 2010).

Osteomyelitis can be classified as acute, subacute, or chronic. Acute osteomyelitis develops 2 weeks after disease onset. Subacute osteomyelitis develops one to several months after onset and chronic osteomyelitis develops after a few months of disease onset. Acute osteomyelitis can develop into chronic osteomyelitis if left untreated.

Osteomyelitis can also be classified by the source of the infection. Hematogenous osteomyelitis, more common in children, originates from bacteremia. Contiguous osteomyelitis is caused from an infection in nearby tissue and is associated with surgery, trauma, or open wounds. Vascular insufficiency osteomyelitis results from soft tissue necrosis leading to decreased healing of wounds, placing the nearby bone at risk for infection. Other sources of bone infection include endocarditis, urinary tract infections, orthopedic joint implants, or stabilizing devices (e.g., screws andplates) and direct penetration of microorganisms into the bone which may occur with traumatic injury or surgery.

Vertebral osteomyelitis, an infection in the spine is estimated to occur in 2.4 cases per 100,000 with incidence increasing with age. Frequently associated with bacterial infections of the urinary tract, vertebral osteomyelitis often affects elders (Tice, 2012). In patients over age 70 the incidence is 6.5 per 100,000 (Zimmerli, 2010).

Patients with diabetes are at increased risk for developing osteomyelitis due to vascular insufficiency and neuropathy. Osteomyelitis in the foot is usually preceded by a nonhealing soft tissue wound. Patients who develop heel or decubitus ulcers are also at increased risk for developing osteomyelitis.

Staphylococcus aureus is the most common organism present with osteomyelitis. Other organisms include *Staphylococcus epidermidis, Pseudomonas aeruginosa, Serratia marcescens* and *Escherichia coli*. Fungal infections and *Mycobacterium tuberculosis* are other potential causes (Tice, 2012).

■ Risk factors

- Cancer
- Diabetes mellitus
- Extremes of age
- Immunosuppression or immunosuppressant therapy
- Intravenous drug abuse
- Lymphedema

- Male gender
- Malnutrition
- Neuropathy
- Prosthetic joint
- Renal or hepatic disease
- Skin and soft tissue infections
- Tobacco use
- Venous stasis or vascular insufficiency

■ Clinical presentation

- Clinical manifestations of osteomyelitis vary depending on the stage of the disease, site affected and type of infection. Exposed bone is concerning because of the high correlation with underlying osteomyelitis (Carek *et al.*, 2001). Obtaining a detailed history of the patient's complaint as well as the patient's orthopedic history, recent illnesses, pertinent past medical surgical, and family history is essential. Reviewing patient allergies, current medications and antibiotic treatment within the past 3 to 6 months for other illnesses is also important.

Acute osteomyelitis:

- Symptoms have a sudden onset that include:
  - Localized bone pain
  - Fever, malaise
  - Decreased range of motion at site of infection

Chronic osteomyelitis:

- If acute osteomyelitis is not treated or if treatment fails, chronic osteomyelitis may develop. Assessment may reveal:
  - Localized bone pain
  - Erythema and edema
  - A draining sinus tract may be present
  - Decreased range of motion at site of infection

Hematogenous osteomyelitis:

- Symptoms are usually systemic
  - Pain may be non-specific, but accompanied by fever, chills, malaise and other systemic signs and symptoms.
  - Edema and erythema of affected area may be present.

Contiguous osteomyelitis:

- Often associated with a soft tissue infection preceding osteomyelitis
- Symptoms are more localized than those associated with hematogenous osteomyelitis.

- Often:
  - Localized joint and bone pain
  - Erythema and edema
  - Exudate at the site of surgery, trauma or wound infection - a sinus tract or abscess may be present.
  - Fever, chills may be present in the acute phase but may be absent in the chronic phase.

Vertebral osteomyelitis:

- Back pain
- Fever is not always present
- Neurologic impairment - sensory loss, weakness, or radiculopathy

Osteomyelitis of the diabetic foot:

- Usually asymptomatic secondary to neuropathy
- Should be suspected for deep, chronic nonhealing ulcers

▓ Nursing assessment
- Obtain history
- Monitor vital signs
- Assess and document all wounds: location, size, drainage, surrounding tissue, and determine if bone is exposed.
- Pain assessment: location, severity, and duration
- Assess range of motion if joint involvement is present.

▓ Diagnostics
Diagnostic testing is based on the patient's clinical presentation, history, and physical exam.
- Laboratory
  - Complete blood count (CBC) with differential
  - White blood cells (WBC) may be elevated in the acute phase, but may be normal in the chronic phase.
  - Erythrocyte sedimentation (ESR) and C-reactive protein (CRP) are frequently elevated, but are not specific indicators of osteomyelitis.
  - Blood cultures may be positive, especially in hematogenous osteomyelitis. Blood cultures should always be collected prior to initiation of antibiotic therapy.
- **Imaging**
  - Plain radiography - X-ray changes may not be present for up to 2 weeks after onset of infection.
  - Magnetic resonance imaging (MRI) - useful for soft tissue assessment and detects early infection.

- Computed tomography (CT) scan – determines the extent of bone destruction and severity of soft tissue damage.
- Bone biopsy for microbiology and histology is considered the gold standard for identifying the causative organism, although this is completed infrequently. Cultures from sinus tract are not reliable.

■ Differential diagnosis

- Acute leukemia
- Avascular necrosis
- Bone fracture
- Cellulitis
- Degenerative disk disease
- Degenerative joint disease
- Gout
- Malignant bone tumors
- Metastatic malignancy
- Multiple myeloma
- Osteoporosis
- Osteoporotic fracture
- Pyelonephritis
- Spinal stenosis
- Spondylarthritis
- Tumor
- Vertebral osteomyelitis

■ Treatment

- Antimicrobial therapy – usually 4-6 weeks of intravenous therapy
- Surgical debridement may be necessary for chronic osteomyelitis.
  - After debridement, dead space (space created by removing necrotic bone) needs to be managed – this can be done by completing a bone graft. Also, antibiotic-impregnated beads may be temporarily used to fill dead space.
- The bone must be stabilized using plates, screws, rods, or external fixator.
- Muscle and skin flaps can be used to restore open wounds.
- Removal of prosthetic joint if the joint is the cause of the osteomyelitis
- Lower extremity wounds associated with peripheral vascular disease may require vascular stents or grafts for improved circulation and healing.
- Pain management

■ Collaborative consultation

- Infectious disease
- Surgery
- Endocrinologist for diabetic management
- Pain service

- Nutrition
- Physical/occupational therapy
- Wound specialist

■ Complications
- Amputation of affected limb
- Bone abscess
- Draining sinus
- Fracture
- Immobility
- Sepsis
- Skeletal or joint deformities

■ Prevention
- Antibiotic prophylaxis can be used to prevent wound infection after surgery.
- Proactive skin care to prevent decubiti and heel ulcers
- Early wound management to prevent infection

■ Patient/family education
- Discuss with patient and family the importance of completing the full course of antibiotic therapy.
- Review the signs and symptoms of a worsening infection: fever, erythema, should be erythema, swelling, warmth, increased pain, and any change in wound appearance
- Diabetic management

References

Carek, P.J., Dickerson, L.M. & Sack, J.L. (2001) Diagnosis and management of osteomyelitis. *American Family Physician* **63**(12), 2413-2420.

Chen, K. & Balloch, R. (2010) Management of calcaneal osteomyelitis. *Clinics in Podiatric Medicine and Surgery* **27**, 417-429.

Tice A.D. (2012) Chapter 126. Osteomyelitis. In Longo, D.L., Fauci, A.S., Kasper, D.L., Hauser, S.L., Jameson, J.L. & Loscalzo, J. (eds), *Harrison's Principles of Internal Medicine*, 18th edn. Online. Availalable from http://0-www.accessmedicine.com.library.simmons.edu/content.aspx?aID=9119589 (accessed 5 June 2012).

Zimmerli, W. (2010) Vertebral osteomyelitis. *The New England Journal of Medicine* **362**, 1022-1029.

Further reading

Game, F.L. & Jeffcoate, W.J. (2008) Primarily non-surgical management of osteomyelitis of the foot in diabetes. *Diabetologia* **51**, 962-967.

Gelfand, M.S., Cleveland, K.O., Heck, R.K. & Goswami, R. (2006) Pathological fracture in acute osteomyelitis of long bones secondary to community-acquired methicillin-resistant *Staphylococcus aureus*: Two cases and review of the literature. *The American Journal of the Medical Sciences* **332**(6), 357-360.

Lazzarini, L., Mader, J.T. & Calhoun, J.H. (2004) Osteomyelitis in long bones. *The Journal of Bone and Joint Surgery* **86-A**(10), 2305-2318.

Lew, D.P. & Waldvogel, F.A. (2004) Osteomyelitis. *Lancet* **364**, 369-379.

McCance, K.L. & Huether, S.E. (2010) *Pathophysiology: The Biologic Basis for Disease in Adults and Children*, 6th edition. Elsevier Mosby, MO.

PART 5: METABOLIC BONE DISEASE: OSTEOPOROSIS AND PAGET'S DISEASE

Nichole Spencer

Osteoporosis and Paget's disease are the two primary metabolic bone diseases. Paget's Disease is the less common metabolic bone disorder and many patients are asymptomatic. Paget's disease is hereditary and usually affects people over age 40. Also known as osteitis deformans, Paget's involves rapid bone resorption and abnormal bone formation throughout the skeleton causing osteoarthritis, bone pain, fractures, and if involvement of the cranial skull, deafness, headaches, tinnitus and headaches (National Institutes of Health, 2009).

It is estimated that 10 million Americans have osteoporosis (National Institutes of Health, 2010). The risk of developing osteoporosis is greatest in females and 80% of people with osteoporosis are women, but men are also affected (National Osteoporosis Foundation, 2010). This bone disorder, which is asymptomatic until a fracture occurs, is related to a reduction in bone mass, which decreases bone density. As a result, the bone weakens increasing the risk for injury and fracture. Osteoporosis is the most common cause of bone fractures, and a frequent reason elders are hospitalized. Unfortunately, when bone fractures occur in older adults a cascade of events may occur which can lead to death (Bone Health and Osteoporosis, 2004a).

Age-related osteoporosis is the most common form of osteoporosis. In women, there are generally two phases of bone loss. The first phase is usually during menopause when the speed of bone loss is greatest and related to estrogen deficiency. The second phase is after menopause when the rate of the loss of bone mass does decrease but will continue throughout the remainder of the individual's life. The slower periods of bone loss are thought to be related to multiple factors: the inability to absorb calcium and vitamin D as well as limited or decreased weight bearing activities (Bone Health and Osteoporosis, 2004a).

Secondary osteoporosis results in bone loss from another physical disease process or the use of a particular medication. Secondary causes of osteoporosis include:

- Adrenal insufficiency
- Alcoholism
- Anorexia nervosa
- Athletic amenorrhea
- Diabetes mellitus type i
- Emphysema
- End stage renal disease
- Inflammatory bowel disease
- Leukemia
- Lymphoma
- Malabsorption celiac disease
- Rheumatoid arthritis
- Multiple sclerosis

Medications that cause osteoporosis include:

- Anticoagulants such as heparin
- Anticonvulsants
- Glucocorticoids
- Lithium
- Methotrexate
- Thyroxine (Bone Health and Osteoporosis, 2004a)

■ Risk factors

- Advanced age
- Anorexia
- Family history
- Female gender
- History of bone fractures
- Low levels of testosterone and estrogen in men
- Menopausal
- Modifiable factors include:
  - Alcohol abuse
  - Low body weight
  - Low calcium and vitamin D intake
  - Sedimentary lifestyle
  - Smoking
  - Steroid therapy
  - Thyrotoxicosis

- Race ethnicities: Caucasian, Asian, and Hispanic/Latino
- Small body frame

■ Clinical presentation

Paget's disease is often asymptomatic, but with skull involvement, the patient may complain of headache, tinnitus, or hearing loss. Bone pain or fracture is also a common presentation.

Osteoporosis is typically asymptomatic and may go undiagnosed until an injury or fracture occurs. Obvious signs include vertebral column curvature, or kyphosis of the dorsal spine. It is also common for an individual to state that he or she has become shorter, or the patient's medical records may indicate a height decrease.

Patients may present with impaired mobility such as difficulty with bending or walking. A decrease or change of daily functioning such as dressing, bed and transfer mobility, using stairs, or household chores may also be reported.

Symptoms of severe back pain may suggest vertebral compression fractures (Bone Health & Osteoporosis, 2004b). This pain may increase with activity and decrease with rest. When palpated, the spinal column or area of pain may be tender to touch.

■ Nursing assessment

It is important to determine if there is a family history of osteoporosis or other metabolic bone disease. In women, a menstrual and perimenstrual history is important. For all patients a nutritional history to learn about daily calcium intake and supplemental intake is essential. Eliciting information about any pain should include the description of the pain as well as onset, relieving and aggravating factors. Additional helpful information includes a fall risk assessment including concerning factors such as delirium, dementia, debility, impaired mobility, incontinence, pain, psychotropic medications and sensory impairments.

- *Height and weight*: Assess height or weight loss.
- *Lungs*: Assess for lung expansion symmetry secondary to spinal column changes.
- *Cardiac*: Blood pressure and heart rate to be monitored for elevation secondary to pain. Assess for orthostatic changes which increase fall risk.
- *Genitourinary*: Evaluate mobility safety for toileting and incontinence. Monitor for intake of calcium and history of or risk for renal calculi.
- *Musculoskeletal*: Observe ambulation and the ability to get up out and into of chair/bed safely. Evaluate for spinal column changes, joint changes, pain with range of motion, and pain that may impact functional mobility.

■ Diagnostics

Paget's disease

- Alkaline phosphatase
- X-ray

Osteoporosis
- Monitor serum calcium, 25-hydroxy-vitamin D, and phosphorus.
- Biochemical markers can be used to monitor effectiveness of treatment.
  - Conventional X-ray of spine and long bones can indicate decreased bone density
- Dual X-ray absorptiometry (DXA) most commonly used for measuring bone mineral density.
- Quantitative computed tomography (QCT) measures bone density is more costly than the DXA and has more radiation exposure.

■ Differential diagnosis

Primary osteoporosis is associated with age or estrogen related bone loss while secondary osteoporosis is associated with potentially reversible causes of bone loss (Malabanan, 2012). Secondary causes of osteoporosis include connective tissue diseases and medications as well as endocrine, gastrointestinal, hematologic, and rheumatologic disorders (Malabanan, 2012). In older adults, undiagnosed Paget's disease, metastatic disease, and end-stage renal disease should be considered (Malabanan, 2012).

■ Treatment

Paget's disease
There is no known prevention for Paget's disease. However, treatment is similar to that for osteoporosis. Adequate calcium and Vitamin D are necessary. Bisphosphonates are indicated to decrease bone pain and delay disease progression.

Osteoporosis
- Education for prevention or to slow progression of osteoporosis is important for everyone.
- Nutrition teaching should include simple, understandable information about adequate protein, calcium, and vitamin D intake. Avoiding alcohol smoking, and excessive caffeine is highly recommended.
- Exercise is encouraged. Instruct patients to perform weight bearing activities such as ambulating for 30 minutes three to five times per week. Teach patients with osteoporosis to avoid activities such as running, jogging, and skiing which could cause injury to bone structure (e.g., vertebral spine).
- Fall prevention instructions need to be provided to all patients with osteoporosis.
- Home safety evaluation to reduce environmental hazards such as loose rugs and poor lighting. Evaluate need of supportive devices in the home (e.g., bath tub or shower rails, stair rails, and if indicated for ramps over outdoor steps).
- External hip protectors are currently being researched for effectiveness. Medication review to determine what agents might increase fall risk (e.g., psychotropics including antidepressants, hypnotics and anxiolytics) (Cumming, 1998).

- Medications and supplements to improve bone mineral density (calcium and vitamin D) should be taken at the recommended daily amount per gender and individual situation.
  - Recommended doses:
    - Women under age 50: Total dietary and supplemental calcium should be 1000 milligrams each day and Vitamin D3, 400 to 1000 international units PO daily.*
      *Patients with hypercalcemia cannot take calcium supplements.
      Patients should be encouraged to consume dietary sources of calcium rather than use calcium supplements.
    - Women over age 50: Total dietary and supplemental calcium should be 1000 milligrams each day and vitamin D3, 800 to 1000 international units PO daily.†
      †Patients who live in the Northern hemisphere may need additional Vitamin D while those living in sunnier climates may need less Vitamin D.

- Bisphosphonates (i.e., Actonel, Boniva, Fosamax, and Reclast) are slow bone resorption medications that are considered first line treatment for prevention and treatment of osteoporosis.
  - An oral bisphosphonate must be taken with 250 milliliters (8 ounces) of water before eating food or drinking other fluid. The patient then needs to remain upright and without food for one hour to avoid gastric/esophageal irritation (esophageal reflux or esophagitis) (Bone Health and Osteoporosis, 2004c; National Osteoporosis Foundation, 2010).
  - Zoledronic acid (Reclast), a 5 milligram intravenous infusion is also available for patients with osteoporosis once a year. Caution is indicated for patients with impaired renal function.
- Raloxifene (Evista, a selective estrogen receptor modulator (SERM), raloxifene is another treatment option if a bisphosphonate is contraindicated. A venous thromboembolism is a potential risk with this medication (Bone Health and Osteoporosis, 2004c; Honkanen, 2004; Malabanan, 2012; National Institutes of Health, 2008).
- Teriparatide (Forteo), a parathyroid hormone (PTH) analog is the only anabolic medication for treatment of osteoporosis. Forteo stimulates osteoblastic activity and high-quality bone formation and is used for patients with severe osteoporosis who are unable to use the antiresorptive treatment or at high risk for fractures. This medication is a daily subcutaneous injection but is not recommended for long-term use due to the risk of osteosarcoma (Bone Health and Osteoporosis, 2004c; Honkanen, 2004).
- Denosumab (Prolia), a monoclonal antibody and RANK ligand inhibitor, is also approved to decrease fractures in postmenopausal women diagnosed with osteoporosis.
- Kyphoplasty (bone cement injected into the vertebral body increasing bone height and stabilizing bone fracture) or vertebroplasty (bone cement injected into vertebral body) stabilizes fracture but does not increase bone

height) are minimally invasive procedures used to fix acute compression fractures of vertebrae, which sometimes will occur secondary to osteoporosis of the vertebral spine.

■ Collaborative consultation

- Nutritionist for adequate intake of necessary nutrients such as fruits, vegetables, low-fat dairy and protein sources, fiber, and assistance with meal planning.
- Physical therapy to provide exercises for strengthening the abdominal core of the body, back, and legs.
- Physical therapy evaluation to determine if an assistive device such as a cane or walker will help decrease fall risk.
- Surgical consultation for fractures, Paget's disease, or bony abnormalities (Bone Health and Osteoporosis, 2004b).

■ Complications

Paget's disease

- Fractures
- Hearing loss
- Heart failure
- Hypercalcemia
- Kidney stones
- Osteoarthritis
- Pain
- Tinnitus

Osteoporosis

- Uncontrolled pain may indicate fracture, could lead to impaired mobility and decreased daily function.
- Risk for falls secondary to the weakness and fragility of the bone and skeletal structure.
- Risk for fractures secondary to bone fragility.
- Skeletal deformities related to spinal compression fractures.

■ Prevention

Paget's disease

There is no known prevention.

Osteoporosis

Prevention should start by age 9 and include

- Calcium 1300 milligrams daily in divided doses until age 19 when 1000 milligrams a day will be enough until age 50 (National Institutes of Health, 2011)

- Daily vitamin D
- A well balanced daily diet that includes skim milk, leafy green vegetables, and low fat dairy products
- Weight bearing exercise (e.g., walking 30 minutes a day)
- Muscle strengthening exercises for upper and lower body
- Avoid smoking.
- Avoid too much alcohol.

For patients with osteoporosis the focus is on adjusting modifiable factors:

- Teach the recommended daily doses of calcium and vitamin D.
  - After age 60 most women require 1200 milligrams of calcium daily in divided doses.
- Weight bearing activities such as walking 30 minutes three to five times per week. Muscle strengthening exercises such as leg lifts and core abdominal strength
- Smoking cessation
- Decrease or avoid alcohol use.

Screening for bone mass density at the age of 65 years or younger postmenopausal women with risk factors that include smoking, familial history of osteoporosis, history of fractures, or weight loss.
Monitor for effectiveness of osteoporosis treatment.

■ Patient/family education

- Osteoporosis prevention strategies:
  - Eat a diet rich in calcium and vitamin D.
  - Exercise.
  - Do not drink alcohol in excess or smoke.
- Fall prevention interventions for both the hospital and home:
  - Vitamin D supplementation as indicated (USPSTF, 2012)
  - Physical therapy and regular exercise (USPSTF, 2012).

References

Bone health and osteoporosis: A report of the Surgeon General. (2004a) Online. Available from http://www.surgeongeneral.gov/library/bonehealth/chapter_3.html (accessed 26 March 2012).
Bone health and osteoporosis: A report of the Surgeon General. (2004b) Online. Available from http://www.surgeongeneral.gov/library/bonehealth/chapter_8.html (accessed 26 March 2012).
Bone health and osteoporosis: A report of the Surgeon General. (2004c) Online. Available from http://www.surgeongeneral.gov/library/bonehealth/chapter_9.html (accessed 26 March 2012).
Cumming, R.G. (1998) Epidemiology of medication - related falls and fractures in the elderly. *Drugs and Aging* **12**(1), 43-53.

Honkanen, L. (2004) An overview of hip fracture prevention. *Topics in Geriatric Rehabilitation* **20**(4), 285-296.

National Institutes of Health (2008) Raloxifene. Online. Available from http://www.ncbi.nlm.nih.gov/pubmedhealth/PMH0001022 (accessed 26 March 2012).

Malabanan, A.O. (2012) Metabolic bone disease: osteoporosis and Paget's disease of the bone. In Buttaro, T.M., Trybulski, J., Bailey, P.P., & Sandberg-Cook, J. (Eds). *Primary Care: A Collaborative Practice*, 4th edn. Elsevier, St. Louis.

National Institutes of Health (2009) Osteoporosis and related bone diseases resource center. Fast facts about Paget's disease. Online. Available from http://www.niams.nih.gov/Health_Info/Bone/Pagets/pagets_disease_ff.asp#who (accessed 26 March 2012).

National Institutes of Health (2010) Osteoporosis and related bone diseases resource center. Fast facts about Osteoporosis. Online. Available from http://www.niams.nih.gov/Health_Info/Bone/Osteoporosis/osteoporosis_ff.asp (accessed 26 March 2012).

National Institutes of Health (2011) Dietary Supplement Fact Sheet: Calcium. Online. Available from http://ods.od.nih.gov/factsheets/calcium/ (accessed 26 March 2012).

National Osteoporosis Foundation (2010) Fast facts. Online. Available from http://www.nof.org/node/40 (accessed 26 March 2012).

United States Preventive Services Task Force (2012) Online. Available from http://www.uspreventiveservicestaskforce.org/uspstf11/fallsprevention/fallsprevfact.pdf (accessed 3 June 2012).

Unit 9: Hematology/Oncology

PART 1: THE ONCOLOGY PATIENT

Kristina N. Wickman

The term *oncology* refers to the medical specialty that deals with the diagnosis, treatment, and study of cancer. Cancer is a disease of the cell in which the normal mechanisms of the control of growth and proliferation have been altered. Cancer can be benign or malignant. A benign cancer is usually a harmless growth that does not spread or invade other tissues. A malignant cancer is a harmful growth, capable of invading other tissues and spreading (metastasis) to vital organs. Uncontrolled, cancer can result in death (American Cancer Society, 2012). The risk of being diagnosed with cancer increases as individuals age, and most cases occur in adults 55 years and older (American Cancer Society, 2012). The increase in life expectancy over the past few decades has caused an increase in the elder population, which has important implications in the nursing care of the older oncology patient.

According to the National Cancer Institute, people 65 years or older are at the highest risk for cancer. For all cancers combined, those over age 65 years have an incidence rate 10 times greater than the rate for younger people (National Cancer Institute, 2010). The mortality rate for older cancer patients is also greater than that of younger adults (National Cancer Institute, 2010).

The need for highly-trained, knowledgeable oncology nurses is evident. It is also important that nurses feel competent caring for aged patients. The oncology nurse must be an advocate for older patients, especially for issues dealing with quality of life and ethical dilemmas, which may be more apparent when caring for older adults with cancer. One of the major ethical issues in caring for older adults with cancer focuses on treatment decisions and financial resources. The decision to treat these patients is complex and must be evaluated on an individual basis with consideration of multiple factors including cancer stage, comorbidities, risks versus benefits, and available social and financial supports. Older adults may have limited incomes, and some cancer treatments are costly and require alternative financial support resources. Elders require a multifaceted approach to nursing care, including diagnosis, treatment, assessment, in-patient and out-patient care and education, and most importantly, the utmost emotional support.

Cancer development begins at the molecular level. Mutations or genetic changes cause pathology affecting cellular appearance, growth, and function that occur over time (American Cancer Society, 2010).

There are two types of cancer classifications, including solid tumors and hematological cancers. Solid tumors are associated with the organs from which they develop, such as breast or lung cancer. Hematological cancers originate from blood cell-forming tissues, such as leukemia or lymphoma.

Grading and staging are methods used to describe the extent of the cancer, including the extent to which the malignancy has increased in size, the involvement of regional nodes, and metastatic development (American Cancer Society, 2010).

■ Risk factors

- Advanced age
- Dietary factors: high-fat and low-fiber diets, high animal fat intake, preservatives, and high alcohol consumption
- Environmental factors:
  - Chemical carcinogen: Factors include industrial chemicals, drugs, and tobacco.
  - Physical carcinogen: Factors include ionizing radiation (diagnostic and therapeutic X-rays), UV radiation (sun and tanning beds), chronic irradiation, and tissue trauma.
  - Viral carcinogen: Viruses that are capable of causing cancer are known as oncoviruses (Epstein–Barr virus, hepatitis-B virus, and human papillomavirus).
- Genetic predisposition
- Immune function
- Obesity

■ Clinical presentation

Clinical manifestations usually appear once the cancer has grown sufficiently large enough to affect organ function. Presenting symptoms depend on the type of cancer and may not occur until the cancer is well advanced. Anorexia, weight loss, weakness and fatigue are related to the oncology patient's inability to use nutrients appropriately. The oncology patient with central nervous system (CNS) difficulties may complain of partial or total loss of vision. A patient with a hearing or speech disorder may be experiencing metastatic CNS disease. Pain that is not adequately treated and is constant and severe could be a sign of an obstruction or damage of an organ or pressure on tissue, bone or nerves caused by a cancerous process in the body. Pain could also be a sign of a pathological fracture. Most of these signs and symptoms can be ambiguous and an older adult patient might relate these symptoms to the aging process or other comorbidities. The presenting picture is further complicated by an atypical or altered presentation of disease (such as failure to thrive or fatigue).

■ Nursing assessment

The critical first step in diagnosing an older adult with cancer is to obtain a complete history and physical examination. A thorough nursing assessment is essential. Although some patients will not have obvious clinical signs of cancer, typical physical assessment indicators in the older patient with cancer may include:

Vital signs

- Fever – related to immunosuppression
- Hypotension – related to weight loss, dehydration or hypovolemia
- Hypoxia – if pulmonary involvement is indicated
- Tachycardia – related to dehydration, malnutrition, or weight loss
- Tachypnea – related to anxiety or pulmonary involvement

Neurologic:

- Mental status changes, confusion, headache, extremity weakness, or gait changes. Alterations in neurological function could be indicative of a cancer with CNS involvement.
  - Additional neurological deficits include vision or hearing loss which could indicate a malignancy.

Head, eyes, ears, nose, and throat (HEENT):

- Eyes: determine visual changes and/or papilledema.
- Nose: nosebleeds or bleeding gums could be indicative of a hematological disorder such as leukemia.
- Mouth: dysphagia, oral lesions, a change in voice quality, or a burning sensation could be related to a malignant tumor in the mouth, larynx or trachea.
- Neck: determine presence of neck masses or lymphadenopathy.

Cardiac:

- Palpitations, tachycardia, and orthostatic hypotension could be related to weight loss, dehydration, and failure to thrive.
- Assess for chest pain that is constant rather than intermittent or associated with movement.

Respiratory:

- Cough, dyspnea, shortness of breath, hoarseness, and hemoptysis may suggest a lung malignancy.

Gastrointestinal:

- Weight loss, loss of appetite, abdominal discomfort and gastrointestinal (GI) disturbances such as diarrhea or constipation are sometimes associated with a GI malignancy.
  - Physical assessment requires looking for abdominal discomfort, abdominal masses, nausea, vomiting, gastroesophageal reflux disease (GERD) symptoms, or ascites which could be indicative of a gastric cancer or ovarian cancer.

Genitourinary:

- Dysuria, hematuria or pelvic/lower back pain which could be indicative of a kidney or bladder cancer
- Testicular swelling, palpable lymphadenopathy, or abnormal masses in the testicles and scrotum, which could be indicative of testicular cancer
- Vulva pruritus or vaginal bleeding/discharge could be indicative of gynecologic cancer.

Skin:

- Petechiae can be associated with a hematological disease such as leukemia.
- Palpate for masses under the skin.
- Specialized assessment includes a breast examination: observe for skin dimpling, retraction, erythema, lymphadenopathy, nipple discharge or asymmetry of the breast tissue suggesting presence of breast cancer.

Musculoskeletal:

- Joint or bone pain could indicate bony metastasis.
- A new onset abnormal gait may be associated with a CNS disturbance and is a risk for falls.

■ Diagnostics

Accurate diagnosis is essential to effective cancer treatment. A cancer diagnosis is a complex process that requires laboratory evaluation, imaging studies, and pathology results before the cause of the patient's symptoms is identified. Laboratory and imaging studies provide data to support or refute a cancer diagnosis. There are numerous lab diagnostics used in determining if a cancer is the cause of the patient's symptoms. The more common blood tests performed to help diagnose cancer include:

- Complete blood count (CBC) with differential. Unexplained leukopenia, anemia, and/or thrombocytopenia could be indicative of a hematologic cancer.
- Metabolic panel. Liver enzyme abnormalities or metabolic changes such as hypercalcemia or hypocalcemia can suggest the possibility of cancer.
- Tumor marker measurements such as prostate-specific antigen (PSA) in prostate cancer

Other diagnostic tests for cancer include imaging studies such as:

- Basic X-ray
- Computed tomography scan (CT scan)

- Magnetic resonance imaging (MRI)
- Ultrasound

Biopsy provides a definitive diagnosis of cancer, aids in cancer grading and staging and provides healthcare providers with information to determine the best treatment options for the patient.

■ Differential diagnosis

The differential diagnosis is dependent on the type of cancer suspected as the differential is often concerned with the specific system affected. Other conditions should always be considered in older adults. Some conditions to consider include the following:

- Arthritis (bone and joint pain)
- Depression (fatigue, lethargy)
- Hyperthyroidism (weight loss, anorexia)
- Hypothyroidism (weight gain, fatigue, lethargy)
- Influenza (altered immune function, fatigue, bone pain)
- Malnutrition (weight loss, anorexia, fatigue)
- Pneumonia (altered immune function, productive cough)
- TIA/stroke (alteration in CNS, hearing or vision loss)
- Virus (altered immune function)

■ Treatment

The primary goal of cancer therapy in an older adult is to control the cancer and preserve the elder's quality of life and function. Decisions made at the time of initial diagnosis are crucial because early intervention usually offers the best hope of a cure. If a cure is not possible, many elders with cancer will benefit from an extended life span and improved quality of life as a result of cancer treatment. The different types of cancer treatment include: surgery, radiation, chemotherapy, biotherapy, and bone marrow transplantation. The treatment depends on the type of cancer, disease extent, and the patient's other comorbidities.

Important nursing considerations in caring for elder patients with cancer include:

- Surgery in the older patient is typically more risky than surgery in the younger patient.
- Older adults are more at risk for infection, deep vein thrombosis, pneumonia, and skin breakdown: all common complications of surgery.
- Radiation can cause severe skin reactions and fatigue. The response of normal skin to radiation varies from mild redness to a second-degree burn. Older patients typically have more delicate and fragile skin in comparison with a younger patient with normal skin.

- Chemotherapy should be tailored to hepatic and renal function for older patients.
- Assessing cardiac and pulmonary functions are important factors in determining if chemotherapy is safe in the older patient. The side effects of chemotherapy also vary from patient to patient, but are typically more severe in elders. Some side effects include fatigue, infection, imbalanced nutrition, anorexia, nausea, vomiting, mouth sores, and hair loss.
- Biotherapy includes hematopoietic growth factors, interferons, and biologic response modifiers. Side effects of biotherapy include flu-like symptoms, bone pain, fatigue and headache. Side effects in the older patient are typically more exacerbated as a result of the aging process. Bone marrow transplantation (BMT) is used as the primary treatment in hematologic cancers, such as leukemia, lymphoma and multiple myeloma. BMT involves receiving high-dose chemotherapy, and then replacing damaged bone marrow with healthy bone marrow. There are two types of BMTs (autologous and allogenic). An autologous BMT refers to one in which the patient's own marrow can be harvested before treatment and then receives their own marrow after chemotherapy. An allogenic BMT refers to one in which the patient uses the marrow from a matching donor. Side effects of a BMT are similar to those of chemotherapy, with an increasing concern on immunosuppression. Typically, older patients will receive a "mini-BMT," referring to a less intense course of chemotherapy prior to their transplant. Due to the aging process, the older patient's immune system is already weakening. It would not be beneficial to completely wipe out an already weakened immune system in an older patient.

■ Collaborative consultation

Collaborating with multidisciplinary teams is a critical component in the care of an older patient with cancer. Consultation with members of different medical and surgical specialties is necessary when discussing the plan for treatment because of the increased risks associated with an elder's co-morbidities.

In addition to cancer treatment, rehabilitation therapy is important to the older patient's quality of life. Many of the side effects of cancer are debilitating and affect the functional status of an older patient, including ambulation and their ability to perform ADLs. Physical and occupational therapy assists older patients in maintaining functional status in the outpatient and inpatient settings.

Because cancer is not just a physical disease, it is necessary to consult with social work to assist with the emotional and financial side effects of cancer. Cancer care can place a financial burden on the older patient with cancer. Collaboration with a social worker can assist in this burden. A social worker can also assist the older patient and their family in coping with the cancer diagnosis. Social workers can offer other services such as chaplaincy and support groups in the community for patients and their families. Fellow patients with cancer can have a significant impact on the morale and drive of another cancer patient.

■ Complications

Cancer produces serious health problems in the older patient such as:

- Impaired immune system: bacterial, fungal, viral infections
- Impaired hematopoietic system: anemia, thrombocytopenia, or leukopenia
- Altered gastrointestinal tract function: nausea, vomiting, diarrhea, constipation, anorexia
- Sensory deficits: impaired taste buds, hearing loss, visual changes
- Motor changes: weakness, fatigue, or falls
- Decreased respiratory function
- Diminished renal function
- Impaired liver function
- Chronic pain
- Depression
- Sepsis
- Disseminated intravascular coagulation (DIC)
- Spinal cord compression

■ Prevention

- *Primary prevention*
  - Avoidance of known or potential carcinogens, including tobacco, UV radiation, and X-rays
  - Adopting a healthy and physically active lifestyle, in conjunction with limiting sun exposure and other sources of UV radiation, modifying sexual practices, and decreasing exposure to occupation and environmental carcinogens would lead to further reduction in cancer incidence.
- *Secondary prevention*
  - Early detection including mammogram, Pap smear, colonoscopy, sigmoidoscopy, breast self-examination, testicular self-examinations, and skin inspection. As a result of early detection, premalignant lesions may be removed or cancer treatment can be started earlier.
- *Tertiary prevention*
  - For older patients with cancer, it is important to maintain optimal wellness for treatment outcome and quality of life. Reinforce healthy lifestyles and to reinforce rest, relaxation, and therapeutic coping techniques.

■ Patient/family education

The first step in educating an older patient with cancer is to assess their readiness for learning. The initial diagnosis of cancer is overwhelming for patients and their families. Regardless of the stage and severity of the disease, the diagnosis of cancer is devastating for patients. There is a negative stigma surrounding a cancer diagnosis, with a lot of emphasis on the futile nature of its prognosis and cure-rate. Older adults need emotional support to deal with initial diagnosis and treatment options. Education should focus on:

- Infection control – frequent hand-washing, wearing gloves and mask when in crowded places, using aseptic technique when using central line (if applicable), eating cooked foods, avoiding contact with children or sick people
- Medications – side effects, schedules, dosages
- Stress management – relaxation techniques, rest periods when feeling fatigued, coping support, social work
- Daily hygiene and skin care – preventing infection, wound care (if applicable)
- Signs or symptoms of any complications – when to call MD office, what to watch out for that could indicate a complication of the disease, including spinal cord compression, electrolyte disturbances, sepsis

References

American Cancer Society (2012) Cancer Facts and Figures. Online. Available from http://www.cancer.org/acs/groups/content/@epidemiologysurveilance/documents/document/acspc-031941.pdf (accessed 5 June 2012).

National Cancer Institute (2010) Cancer Statistics. Online. Available from http://www.cancer.gov/statistics (accessed 26 March 2012).

Unit 10: Infectious Disease

PART 1: HIV/AIDS

Caroline Sturm-Reganato

Human immunodeficiency virus (HIV) and acquired immune deficiency syndrome (AIDS) tend to be thought of as illnesses affecting mostly young adults. Health care providers may not even consider older adults at risk of contracting HIV because of the misconception that older adults do not engage in sexual activity nor use intravenous (IV) drugs (Vance *et al.*, 2009). However, recent statistics from the Centers for Disease Control (CDC) make evident that older adults are significantly affected by HIV/AIDS. The CDC's HIV/AIDS Surveillance Reports for 2007 found that the percentage of older adults living with HIV/AIDS increased annually by 14% between 2004 and 2007 (Justice, 2010). Moreover, the proportion of older adults living with HIV/AIDS is expected to grow considering that in 2007, over 65% of all people living with HIV/AIDS were over 40 or older, according to the CDC's statistics from 2007 (Gay Men's Health Crisis, 2010). Also, the United States Senate Special Committee on Age forecasts that half of the HIV/AIDS population will be over 50 by 2015 (Luther & Wilkin, 2007).

The aging of the HIV/AIDS population in the US can be explained by two phenomena: longer life expectancy in patients on antiretroviral therapy and new HIV infections in older adults (Vance *et al.*, 2009). Highly active antiretroviral therapy (HAART), introduced in the mid 1990s, has turned a deadly disease into a chronic and manageable one (Vance, 2010). HAART has significantly increased the life expectancy of HIV patients who are living well into their 50s, 60s and 70s (Gay Men's Health Crisis, 2010). Second, new HIV infections in older adults are attributed to the increasing prevalence of older adults living with HIV/AIDS. Older adults who are sexually active and use intravenous (IV) drugs are at a higher risk of infection because of the increased potential exposure to HIV (Justice, 2010). As in the overall HIV/AIDS statistics, African-Americans and men who have sex with men age 50 and older are disproportionately affected by HIV (Gay Men's Health Crisis, 2010).

The aging of the HIV population has significant implications for nursing care (Halloran, 2006). First, nurses must acknowledge that older adults are at risk for HIV and other sexually transmitted infections (STI) and must facilitate discussion on at-risk behaviors with older patients to promote HIV education and prevention (Wooten-Bielski, 1999). Counter to popular belief, older adults engage in at-risk behaviors (Bhavan *et al.*, 2008). Halloran (2006) and Vance *et al.* (2009) explain that nurses must be aware of the specific clinical presentation of HIV/AIDS in older adults as well as the side effects of antiretroviral therapy and potential drug–drug interactions.

HIV is a retrovirus; it contains its genetic information in RNA rather than DNA (Fauci & Lane, 2012; Sweeney, 2005). Once in the host cell, HIV transcribes its RNA into DNA by using the enzyme reverse transcriptase, and then integrates its DNA into the host cell DNA by using the enzyme integrase (Janeway *et al.*, 2001). The host cell will spread the virus by producing new copies of HIV and releasing them in the blood (Janeway *et al.*, 2001).

HIV travels throughout the body as free virus in the blood, semen, vaginal fluid and breast milk (Janeway *et al.*, 2001). This explains its route of infection via sexual contact, blood-to-blood contact, and from mother-to-child. HIV also infects different cells, part of the immune system. It targets a subset of lymphocytes, CD4 T cells, which regulate the immune response by activating antibody producing B cells and CD8 cytotoxic T cells to eliminate foreign antigens (Sommer, 2005; Sweeney, 2005). Activated HIV-infected CD4 T cells spread HIV by producing new copies of the virus. Infected CD4 T cells are destroyed once the virus replication process is over. HIV also infects to a lesser extent, macrophages and dendritic cells without killing them, which enables the virus to establish a reservoir of infection and spread to other tissues, such as the brain (Fauci & Lane, 2012; Janeway *et al.*, 2001).

The immune system controls HIV levels for a period of time, but ultimately HIV successfully evades the response of the immune system via the following two mechanisms. First, CD8 cytotoxic T cells and neutralizing antibodies do not keep up with the high rate of virus replication and the continuous genetic mutation of the virus (Fauci & Lane, 2008). Second, HIV establishes a reservoir of infection, particularly in lymphoid tissue, by hiding in resting CD4 T cells and by infecting macrophages and dendritic cells without killing them (Fauci & Lane, 2012; Janeway *et al.*, 2001).

By targeting CD4 T-cells and by successfully invading the immune system, HIV gradually leads to the depletion of CD4 T cells, which causes immune deficiency and the development of AIDS (Fauci & Lane, 2012). AIDS is characterized by a CD4 cell count below 200 or a CD4 percentage below 14% and the presence of an AIDS-defining illness; the most common ones are esophageal candidiasis, bacterial pneumonia, tuberculosis, and herpes simplex and zoster (Justice, 2009). AIDS-defining illness are caused by pathogens (bacteria, virus, fungus and parasites) that would normally be controlled by a healthy immune system. Another significant characteristic in HIV is that its chronic presence within the body results in the constant activation of the immune system, which leads to a persistent state of inflammation (Appay & Sauce, 2008). Over a long period of time, this chronic inflammatory state is believed to accelerate the aging process and the deterioration of the immune system (Appay & Sauce, 2008).

■ Risk factors

- Age-associated declines in immunity
- Blood transfusions (screening of blood for HIV was not widely practiced before 1985)
- Denial of HIV status
- IV drug use
- Knowledge deficit about HIV and other sexually transmitted diseases

- Multiple sexual partners
- Thinning of the vaginal membranes and vaginal dryness, which increases the risk of vaginal tear
- Unknown HIV status
- Unprotected sex (includes oral, anal, and vaginal sex)

■ Clinical presentation

The clinical presentation of HIV in older adults can follow the same course as that of younger individuals. In the first stage of the illness, 2 to 6 weeks after infection, the patient can experience flu-like symptoms including fever, fatigue, rash, sore throat, gastrointestinal problems, headache, night sweats, and oral and genital ulcers (Fauci & Lane, 2012; Sweeney, 2005). In the second stage, clinical latency, the patient can be clinically asymptomatic for a period of 5 to 10 years (Fauci & Lane, 2012; Sweeney, 2005). In the third stage, the immune system is so compromised that it can no longer fight off infections and opportunistic infections ensue. Justice (2009) clarifies that the most prevalent HIV-related conditions have changed. *Pneumocystis carinii* pneumonia (PCP), Kaposi sarcoma and atypical mycobacterial infections have been replaced by conditions commonly seen in HIV-negative people such as esophageal candidiasis, bacterial pneumonia, tuberculosis, herpes simplex and zoster (Justice, 2009).

Several important considerations should be taken into account regarding the clinical presentation of HIV/AIDs in older adults. First, older adults can develop symptoms less specific to HIV such as fatigue, weight loss, chest infection, cognitive decline (e.g., confusion and memory loss), malignancies, and dermatological abnormalities (e.g., shingles), which can be difficult to distinguish from normal aging and/or age-related illnesses (Luther & Wilkin, 2007). Second, there is a higher incidence of HIV dementia and HIV wasting syndrome in HIV positive older adults compared to their younger counterparts (Luther and Wilkin, 2007). Wasting syndrome is characterized by a weight loss greater than 10% of body weight, 30 days or more of diarrhea or weakness and fever (Sweeney, 2005). HIV dementia in older adults has a rapid onset, unlike Alzheimer's and Parkinson's disease, for which it is often mistaken (Wooten-Bielski, 1999). Patients can experience the following symptoms: first withdrawal and social isolation, then difficulty concentrating, apathy and confusion, followed by neuromuscular tremors, peripheral neuropathy, progressing to weakness and ataxia (Wooten-Bielski, 1999). Older adults with HIV/AIDS dementia do not experience aphasia seen in Alzheimer's disease nor the bradykinesia, rigidity, and tremors seen in Parkinson's disease (Wooten-Bielski, 1999). Third, studies have found that older adults report fewer symptoms to their doctors than younger HIV positive adults (Luther and Wilkin, 2007; Myers, 2009). According to the studies, older adults tend to omit reporting the following symptoms: diarrhea, headache, fever, chills, nausea, vomiting, feeling down, white oral patches, and sinus trouble (Luther and Wilkin, 2007; Myers, 2009). On the other hand, older adults were more likely to report neuropathic symptoms and weight loss, according to the HIV Cost and Service Utilization Study (Luther & Wilkin, 2007).

Considering the similarities in clinical presentation among HIV, normal aging and age-related illness, and the lack of symptoms reported from older adults, a thorough and complete medical and social history, including recent and past sex and drug use history, is of critical importance for the clinician to assess the patient's risk of HIV exposure and to evaluate whether an HIV test is warranted. Linsk (cited in Justice, 2009) suggests the following questions to obtain sex and drug history with older patients:

- Do you have sexual or intimate contact with another man or woman? If yes, with men, women or both?
- Do you take disease precautions? If yes, explain your precautions? If no, why not?
- Do you take any recreational drugs that involve the use of needles? If yes, do you share needles? If yes, how do you clean them?
- Do you drink alcohol before sex? Do you use any illicit drugs or other substances before sex?

Patients presenting with unexplained anemia, severe fatigue and weight loss, peripheral neuropathy, oral candidiasis, widespread herpes zoster, recurrent bacterial pneumonia, or other more traditional AIDS-related disorders such as Kaposi's sarcoma and *Pneumocystis carinii* pneumonia should be tested for HIV (Justice, 2009).

■ Nursing assessment

Adapted from the primary care guidelines for the management of persons infected with human immunodeficiency virus (Aberg *et al.*, 2009).

- *Vital signs*:
  - Temperature: abnormal in the presence of infection
  - Tachycardia may be present in the case of infection.
  - Blood pressure: check for hypertension and hypotension.
  - Weight loss can indicate sarcopenia.
- *Eyes*: note visual disturbances (e.g., blurriness, seeing double, or blindness). Notewhite or yellow retinal discoloration, infiltrate, or hemorrhage which are indicators of ocular opportunistic infections.
- *Mouth*: assess for thrush on tongue, lesions, ulcers and warts on lips, buccal mucosa and gums.
- *Lymph nodes*: palpate for lymphadenopathy.
- *Skin*: examine the entire body including scalp, axillae, palms of hand, pubic and peri-anal area and soles of feet. Look for abnormal lesions and rashes.
- *Cardiac*: note rate and rhythm, heart sounds, murmurs, and extra heart sounds.
- *Lungs*: auscultate for any abnormal sounds including crackles or wheezes.

- *Musculoskeletal*: note muscle wasting, pedal and peripheral edema, and peripheral fat atrophy.
- *Vaginal, penile and rectal exam*: assess for signs of pruritus, note lesions, warts and discharges. Examine for sexual diseases common in HIV positive patients including genital herpes, genital and rectal warts and vaginal candidiasis. Exclude sexually transmitted diseases such as *Chlamydia* and gonorrhea.
- *Neurologic*: assess for cognitive ability including speed of information processing, executive functioning and reasoning, memory and attention, and psychomotor functioning which could indicate HIV dementia or opportunistic infections affecting the central nervous system. Note specificity of cognitive decline to distinguish between age-related cognitive disorders (age related dementia and Alzheimer's) and HIV-related neurological disorders.
- *Psychiatric*: assess patient's general mood. Screen for depression, suicidal ideation, and recreational drug use. Note inappropriate or unusual behavior (e.g., denial, hostility, compulsiveness, carelessness, emotional lability or apathy).

■ Diagnostics

Adapted from the primary care guidelines for the management of persons infected with human immunodeficiency virus (Aberg *et al.*, 2009).

- To diagnose HIV:
  - Rapid HIV test or enzyme-linked immunosorbent assay (ELISA): uses saliva or blood specimen, results are read visually after a waiting period of 20 minutes.
  - Western Blot (detects proteins specific to HIV) or indirect immune-fluorescence assay (detects antibodies to HIV).
    - If the ELISA is positive, the Western Blot test is necessary to confirm the presence of HIV antibodies (Marsh & Martin, 2012).
- Baseline HIV laboratory evaluation: to determine illness progression, the need for antiretroviral therapy and prophylactic treatment for opportunistic infections, and optimal treatment regimen:
  - Lymphocytes count with percentages
  - Plasma HIV RNA (viral load): increase in viral load despite medication adherence suggests resistance to therapy.
  - Resistance testing: done prior to treatment to choose optimal therapy and when patients are showing signs of virologic failure. The most commonly used resistance test is the genotype; it identifies mutations on the virus'genetic code that are linked to antiretroviral therapy resistance.
  - Coreceptor tropism assay: used to determine which patients are eligible candidates for the new class of antiretroviral therapy: CCR5 entry inhibitors.
- Laboratory tests to monitor for adverse effects of medication and complications of HIV.
  - Complete blood count (CBC) and chemistry panel including fasting glucose, liver function, and blood urea nitrogen and creatinine:

- To screen patient for anemia, leucopenia and thrombocytopenia; common in HIV positive patients
- To obtain baseline and monitor renal and hepatic function and nutritional status. Antiretroviral therapy can have myelosuppressive, nephrotoxic and hepatotoxic effects.
- CD4$^+$ T-lymphocyte count
- HIV RNA-PCR
- Fasting lipids: HIV infection and antiretroviral therapy can increase cholesterol and triglycerides.
- Urinalysis and calculated creatinine clearance: used to evaluate and monitor kidney function, to be done especially with African-Americans and patients with advanced HIV or co-morbid conditions (e.g., hypertension and diabetes), because of an increased risk of nephropathy.
- Glucose-6-phosphate dehydrogenase (G6PD): G6PD is a genetic condition that may lead to hemolysis with exposure to oxidant drugs. Dapsone, primaquine, and sulfonamides are antiretroviral drug that can cause hemolysis in HIV positive patients with G6PD deficiency. G6PD deficiency is seen in 10–15% of African-American men and women.
- HLA-B*5701: used to determine whether a patient is allergic to Abacavir. A positive result indicates a higher risk for hypersensitivity reactions to Abacavir.
- Serum testosterone level: in male patients with signs of reduced bone density and who complained of fatigue, weight loss, loss of libido or erectile dysfunction
- Laboratory testing of comorbidities
  - Tuberculosis (TB) skin test: an induration >5 mm is positive in a HIV positive patient and needs to be followed up with a chest X-ray to rule out active TB.
  - Anti-*Toxoplasma* IgG: test for prior exposure to *Toxoplasma gondii*.
  - Hepatitis A
  - Hepatitis B: HBsAg (if positive indicates acute or chronic infection), HBsAb (marker for immunity), and HBcAb (nonspecific marker for acute and resolved infection)
  - Hepatitis C: HCV antibody, if positive HCV RNA is required.
  - Herpes viruses
  - Syphilis: if rapid plasma regain (RPR) test result is positive, lumbar puncture for suspected late latent disease is required.
  - Human papillomavirus infection, chlamydia, and gonorrhea
  - Pap smear: to screen for cervical cancer, vaginal candidiasis and genital warts

■ Differential diagnosis

Fauci and Lane (2012) describe idiopathic CD4 lymphocytopenia (ICL) as a very rare disease, which is characterized with the following diagnostic criteria:

- Two CD4$^+$ T cell counts below 300/microliter or CD4$^+$ T cell percentage <20% at least 6 weeks apart

- No laboratory evidence of HIV infection
- Absence of any other illness (e.g., blood cancer) or therapy (e.g., immuno-suppressive medication or chemotherapy) explaining the decrease in $CD4^+$ T cell count

Patients with ICL have a better prognosis than HIV-positive patients: they remain clinically stable and may even recover spontaneously with their CD4+ T cell count returning to normal values (Fauci & Lane, 2012). Because of the immunodeficiency, ICL patients are also at risk of developing opportunistic infections, particularly cryptococcosis (Fauci & Lane, 2012).

■ Treatment

HAART is the recommended treatment option for patients with clinical AIDS infection, co-infection with HBV requiring treatment, HIV-associated nephrop-athy, or with a CD4 count less than $500/mm^3$ (Marsh & Martin, 2012). However, the decision to initiate therapy, particularly in elders, is based on the individual patient's risk/benefit ratio (Marsh & Martin, 2012). Specific treatment options are an individualized combination of antiretroviral agents based on patient's history (naïve or experienced patient) and blood work (cholesterol, liver and kidney function tests, phenotype, G6PD, HLA-B*5701). HIV medications are organized into different classes based on their mechanism of action:

- Non-nucleoside reverse transcriptase inhibitors (NNRTIs): bind to the enzyme reverse transcriptase, which prevents HIV from converting its RNA into DNA.
- Nucleoside reverse transcriptase inhibitor (NRTIs): they imitate natural nucleosides which the virus uses to incorporate in its DNA, consequently breaking the DNA chain.
- Protease inhibitors (PIs): interfere with the enzyme protease, needed by HIV to cut up long chains of its enzymes and proteins that would infect other cells.
- Entry/fusion inhibitors: block HIV from entering into the cell.
- Integrase inhibitors: disable the enzyme integrase which HIV uses to incor-porate its genetic material into the DNA of the host cell.
- Fixed dose combination: tablets that contain two or more antiretroviral medi-cation from one or more drug classes. The most common one is Atripla, which contains Sustiva (a NNRTI), emtricitabine (a NRTI) and tenofovir (a NRTI).

According to the *Guidelines for the Use of Antiretroviral Agents in HIV-1-infected Adults and Adolescents* (Department of Health and Human Services, 2012) the recommended treatments for first time patients on antiretroviral are:

(1) Atripla: combination tablet with Sustiva, emtricitabine and tenofovir
(2) Ritonavir-boosted atazanavir and Truvada
(3) Ritonavir-boosted darunavir + Truvada
(4) Raltegravir + Truvada

- Antibiotics and antifungal therapy for treatment or prevention of opportunistic infections
- Maintain the number of total medications (HIV and non-HIV medication) to a minimum to reduce the risk of drug-drug interactions (Justice, 2009).
- Monitor for signs and symptoms of allergic reactions to antiretroviral medication and antibiotics (e.g., fever or rash throughout the body).
- Monitor adverse effects of HIV medication: pancreatitis, lactic acidosis, hyperglycemia, gastrointestinal upset, nephrotoxicity, hepatotoxicity, hyperlipidemia and lipodystrophy (Greene, 2003; Marsh & Martin, 2012; McLennon *et al.*, 2003). It is common for HIV positive adults to have sarcopenia and muscle wasting (Vance, 2009). According to Roach (as cited in Vance, 2009) older adults with HIV have an increased risk for adverse effects from HIV therapy, because they lack the adequate muscle mass and fat tissue needed for drug metabolism and elimination.
- Monitor for skin integrity.
- Monitor for signs and symptoms of immune reconstitution inflammatory syndrome (IRIS): fever, swollen lymph nodes, skin lesions and rashes, changes in breathing, pneumonia, hepatitis, abscesses and eye inflammation. IRIS is an accentuated response of the immune system to a pre-existing opportunistic infection that can occur after patients start antiretroviral therapy.

■ Collaborative consultation

- When discussing the patient's condition make sure that signs and symptoms are not interpreted as part of normal aging or as an indicator of an age-related illness, and that an HIV test has been considered.
- Review patient's medications and be aware for potential harmful interactions between HAART and other medications commonly used with older patients such as: lipid lowering agents, antidepressants, cardiac medications, benzodiazepines, acid reducers, and anticoagulants (McLennon *et al.*, 2003).
- Review kidney and liver function tests.

■ Complications

- Allergic reaction to antiretroviral medication
- Depression
- HIV medication adverse effects
  - Table 3.10.1.1 lists HIV medication adverse effects and their respective signs and symptoms.
  - Table 3.10.1.2 illustrates interactions between HIV medications and concomitant drugs used in older patients.
- All NRTIs, except for abacavir, are eliminated by the kidneys unlike the PIs and NRTIs that are metabolized via the CYP3A4 system (McLennon *et al.*, 2003). Consequently, NRTIs are not associated with as many drug-drug interactions as PIs and NNRTIs.

Table 3.10.1.1 HIV medication adverse effects and their respective signs and symptoms.

Adverse effect	Signs and symptoms	HIV medication associated with adverse effect
Central nervous system	Vivid dreams, dizziness, somnolence, impaired concentration, nervousness, anxiety	NNRTI: Sustiva (efavirenz) >50% of patients can experience adverse effect from Sustiva
GI upset	Nausea, vomiting, diarrhea, abdominal pain	All PIs NRTI: zidovudine (ZDV), Videx (didanosine)
Hepatotoxicity:	Abnormal liver function test Jaundice Weight loss	All NNRTIs and PIs Most NRTIs Entry/ fusion inhibitors: Selzentry (maraviroc)
Hyperglycemia	Increased urination, increased thirst, unexplained weight loss	Associated with some PIs; unclear if class effect
Hyperlipidemia	Elevated lipid profile	All PIs except unboosted Reyataz NNRTI: Sustiva (efavirenz)
Lactic acidosis: lactate level greater than 5 mmol/l	Severe lactic acidosis: • persistent nausea, vomiting • abdominal pain • unexplained tiredness • shortness of breath • rapid breathing • enlarged or tender liver • cold or blue hands and feet • abnormal heart beat • weight loss	NRTIs: especially Zerit (stavudine) and Retrovir (zidovudine)
Lipodystrophy		NRTIs especially combined with Sustiva (efavirenz)
Nephrotoxicity	Proteinuria Hypophosphatemia Hypokalemia Increased serum creatinine	NRTI: Viread (tenofovir) PI: Crixivan (indinavir)
Stevens–Johnson syndrome	Skin eruption with mucosal ulcerations Blisters or bullae formation	NNRTIs: Viramune (nevirapine), Rescriptor (delavirdine), Sustiva (efavirenz), Intelence (etravirine) PIs: Agenerase (amprenavir), Lexiva (fosamprenavir) NRTIs: Ziagen (abacavir), Retrovir (zidovudine)

Adapted from *Antiretroviral Therapy-Associated Adverse Effects and Management Recommendations*, by the US Department of Health and Human Services panel on Antiretroviral Guidelines for Adults and Adolescents, 2009, *Guidelines for the use of antiretroviral agents in HIV-1-infected adults and adolescents*, p.116.

Table 3.10.1.2 Interactions between HIV medications and concomitant drugs used in older patients.

Concomitant drug Class/name	Interaction between HIV medication and concomitant drug	Clinical comments and management
Anticoagulant		
Warfarin	NNRTIs: • Viramune and Sustiva can increase or decrease effect of Warfarin. • Intelence increases effect of Warfarin.	Increased risk of bleeding. Monitor INR and adjust Warfarin level.
Acid reducers		
Antacids	PIs: Effects of Reyataz, Lexiva and Aptivus boosted with Norvir are decreased.	Take PIs 2 hrs before or 1 hr after antacid.
Proton pump inhibitors (PPIs)	PIs: Effects of boosted and unboosted Reyataz are decreased. Effect of Viracept is significantly decreased.	Take PPIs 12 hrs prior to Reyataz boosted with Norvir. Coadministration of unboosted PIs with PPIs not recommended. **Do not coadminister PPIs and Viracept.**
Antidepressants		
St John's Wort	Decreases levels of all PIs and NNRTIs.	**Do not coadminister St John's wort with PIs and NNRTIs.**
Selective serotonin uptake inhibitors: Zoloft and Paxil	Sustiva(NNRTI) decreases blood concentration of Zoloft Prezista (PI) boosted with Norvir (PI) decreases blood concentration of Zoloft and Paxil.	Monitor for antidepressant effect. Monitor for antidepressant effect.
Wellbutrin	Sustiva (NNRTI) and Kaletra boosted with Norvir (PI) decrease blood concentration of Wellbutrin.	Adjust Wellbutrin dose based on clinical response.
Benzodiazepines		
Alprazolam (Xanax) Diazepam (Valium)	All PIs increase effects of alprazolam and diazepam.	Consider other benzodiazepines such as lorazepam (Ativan), oxazepam (Serax) and temazepam (Restoril).
Triazolam	All PIs increase level of triazolam. Sustiva increases level of triazolam.	Do not coadminister PIs and triazolam. Do not coadminister Sustiva with triazolam.

(Continued)

Table 3.10.1.2 *(Continued)*

Concomitant drug Class/name	Interaction between HIV medication and concomitant drug	Clinical comments and management
Cardiac medications		
Calcium channel blockers (CCBs)	All PIs can increase levels of CCBs.	Use CCB and PIs with caution. ECG monitoring recommended.
	Sustiva and Viramune (NNRTIs) can decrease levels of CCBs.	Adjust CCBs dose based on clinical response.
Grapefruit juice		
	Level of indinavir decreases when taken with grapefruit juice.	Monitor virologic response. Avoid large consumption of grapefruit juice.
Methadone		
	PIs boosted with Norvir decrease methadone effect.	Risk of methadone withdrawal. Monitor for signs and symptoms of withdrawal. Adjust methadone dose if clinically indicated.
Lipid lowering agents		
Simvastatin Lovastatin	All PIs significantly increase level of simvastatin and lovastatin.	Risk of rhabdomyolysis **Do not coadminister simvastatin and lovastatin with PIs.** Use low dose atorvastatin or pravastatin.
	NNRTIs Sustiva, Viramune, Intelence decrease levels of simvastatin and lovastatin.	Adjust dose level based on lipid response when administered with NNRTIs.
Phosphodiesterase type 5 inhibitors		
Sildenafil (Viagra)	All PIs increase concentration of sildenafil.	For treatment of erectile dysfunction start with lowest dose and monitor for adverse effects of sildenafil. Contraindicated for treatment of pulmonary arterial hypertension.

Adapted from *Drug interactions between protease inhibitors (PIs) and other drugs* and *Drug interactions between NNRTIs and other drugs*, by the US Department of Health and Human Services panel on Antiretroviral Guidelines for Adults and Adolescents, 2009, *Guidelines for the Use of Antiretroviral Agents in HIV-1-Infected Adults and Adolescents*, p. 130 and 136.

- Immune reconstitution inflammatory syndrome
- Progression to AIDS: development of opportunistic infections
- Social isolation
- Suicidal ideation

■ Prevention

- Include questions about past and recent sexual and drug use in health assessment.
- Safe sex education at each routine medical visit: teach or review correct condom use.
- Refer patients to clean needle exchange program.
- Provide at-risk patients with a message tailored to their need and circumstances.

■ Patient/family education

- Emphasize that aging with HIV is possible.
- Discuss the importance of safe sexual practices to prevent HIV transmission.
- Explain the importance of medication adherence: antiretroviral therapy must be taken at the same time every day. Failure to do so increases the risk of the virus becoming resistant to therapy. Patient must take a forgotten dose as soon as it is remembered.
- Encourage immunization updates.
- Discuss the need for careful and routine follow-up with the primary care provider and infectious disease specialist to monitor patient health.
- Review side effects and potential adverse effects of antiretroviral therapy.
- Promote physical activity to maintain and improve muscle mass and strength.
- Promote mental exercises to maintain and improve cognitive abilities.
- Emphasize the importance of a balanced nutrition to prevent sarcopenia.
- Encourage socializing to prevent social isolation and depression.
- Provide patient with information on organizations for older adults living with HIV.

References

Aberg, J.A., Kaplan, J.E., Libman, H. *et al.* (2009) Primary care guidelines for the management of persons infected with human immunodeficiency virus: 2009 update by the HIV Medicine Association of the Infectious Diseases Society of America. *Clinical Infectious Diseases* **49**(5), 651–681.

Appay, V. & Sauce, D. (2008) Immune activation and inflammation in the HIV-1 infection: causes and consequences. *Journal of Pathology* **214**(2), 231–241.

Bhavan, K.P., Kampalath, V.N., & Overton, E.T. (2008) The aging of the HIV epidemic. *Current HIV/AIDS Reports* **5**(3), 150–158.

Fauci A.S., & Lane H.C. (2012) Human immunodeficiency virus disease: AIDS and related disorders. In Longo, D.L. Fauci, A.S. Kasper, D.L. Hauser, S.L. Jameson, J.L. and Loscalzo, J. (eds) *Harrison's Principles of Internal Medicine*, 18th edition. Chapter 189. Online. Available from http://0-www.accessmedicine.com.library.simmons.edu/content.aspx?aID=9123335 (accessed 6 June 2012).

Gay Men's Health Crisis (2010) *Growing older with the epidemic: HIV and aging*. Online. Available from http://www.gmhc.org/files/editor/file/a_pa_aging10_emb2.pdf (accessed 27 March 2012).

Greene, M.D. (2003) Older HIV patients face metabolic complications. *The Nurse Practitioner* **28**(6), 17-25.

Halloran, J. (2006) Increasing survival with HIV: impact on nursing care. *AACN Clinical Issues:Advanced Practice in Acute & Critical Care* **17**(1), 8-17.

Janeway, C.A., Travers, P., Walport, M. & Shlomchik, M. (2001) Failure of the host defense mechanisms. In: P. Austin and E. Lawrence (eds) *Immunobiology: the Immune System in Health and Disease*. Garland, New York, pp. 425-469.

Justice, A.C. (2009) Human immunodeficiency virus infection. In: J.B. Halter, J.G. Ouslander, M.E. Tinetti, S. Studenski, K.P. High and A. Asthana (eds) *Hazzard's Geriatric Medicine and Gerontology*. Online. Available from http://www.accessmedicine.com.ezproxy.med.nyu.edu/content.aspx?aid=5138130 (accessed 27 March 2012).

Justice, A.C. (2010) HIV and aging: Time for a new paradigm. *Current HIV/AIDS Reports* **7**(2), 69-76.

Luther, V.P. & Wilkin, A.M. (2007) HIV Infection in older adults. *Clinics in Geriatric Medicine* **23**(3), 567-583.

Marsh, B.J. & Martin, C.F. (2012). In Buttaro, T.M., Trybulski, J, Bailey, P.P., and Sandeberg-Cook, J. (eds). *Primary Care: A Collaborative Practice*, 4th edn. Elsevier, St. Louis.

McLennon, S.M., Smith, R. & Orrick, J.J. (2003) Recognizing and preventing drug interactions in older adults with HIV: Older adults face the added challenge of drug interactions among HIV and AIDS medications and those used to treat conditions associated with aging. *Journal of Gerontological Nursing* **29**(4), 5-12.

Myers, J.D. (2009) Growing old with HIV: The AIDS epidemic and an aging population. *Journal of the American Academy of Physician Assistants (Jan)*. Online. Available from http://jaapa.com/growing-old-with-hiv-the-aids-epidemic-and-an-aging-population/article/123907/ (accessed 27 March 2012).

Sommer, C. (2005) The immune response. In: C.M Porth (ed) *Pathophysiology: Concepts of Altered Health States*. Lippincott Williams & Wilkins, Philadelphia, pp. 365-385.

Sweeney, K.A. (2005) Acquired immunodeficiency syndrome. In: C.M. Porth (ed) *Pathophysiology: Concepts of Altered Health States*. Lippincott Williams & Wilkins, Philadelphia, pp. 427-445.

US Department of Health and Human Services Panel on Antiretroviral Guidelines for Adults and Adolescents. (2012) *Guidelines for the Use of Antiretroviral Agents in HIV-1-Infected Adults and Adolescents*. Online. Available from http://aidsinfo.nih.gov/contentfiles/lvguidelines/adultandadolescentgl.pdf (accessed 6 June 2012).

Vance, D.E. (2010) Aging with HIV: Clinical consideration for an emerging population. *American Journal of Nursing* **110**(3), 43-47.

Vance, D.E., Childs, G., Moneyham, L. & McKie-Bell, P. (2009) Successful aging with HIV: a brief overview for nursing. *Journal of Gerontology Nursing* **35**(9), 19-25.

Wooten-Bielski, K. (1999) HIV & AIDs in older adults. *Geriatric Nursing* **20**(5), 268-272.

PART 2: SEPSIS AND ARDS

Vince M. Vacca, Jr.

Sepsis can occur at any age; however, individuals with sepsis are typically in their sixth or seventh decade. The average age and costs associated with treating septic patients has consistently increased over time. The incidence of sepsis is predicted to reach a million cases in the next decade with costs estimated at 16 billion dollars annually. Factors such as aging of the population, invasive procedures, and antibiotic resistant organisms are contributing reasons for this predicted increase of sepsis (Linderman & Janssen, 2008).

When bacteria from a focal infection enter the lymphatic and bloodstreams, the inflammatory response becomes systemic causing systemic inflammatory response syndrome (SIRS). SIRS is a physiologic compensatory action intended to protect and maintain homeostasis in response to a threatening infection. SIRS can be recognized by the presence of two or more of these signs and symptoms:

- Core temperature below 36°C (96.8°F) or above 38°C (100.4°F)
- Heart rate above 90 beats/minute
- Respiratory rate greater than 20 breaths/minute
- $PaCO_2$ less than 32 mmHg (normal is 35–45 mmHg)
- White blood cell count (WBC) less than 4000/mm³ or greater than 12,000/mm³ (normal; 5000 to 10,000/mm³) (Martin & Wheeler, 2009)

The presence of SIRS responding to an active infection meets the criteria for sepsis. Sepsis is a clinical syndrome characterized by inflammation, enhanced coagulation, and impaired fibrinolysis, in response to a focal infection. Sepsis as a syndrome can range from mild to severe septic shock with associated multisystem organ failure (see Table 3.10.2.1) (Dellinger *et al.*, 2008; Funk *et al.*, 2009).

For example, a pulmonary infection causing a lobar or focal pneumonia can lead to a localized inflammatory response. White blood cells, primarily neutrophils and macrophages migrate and accumulate in the area of infection to combat the bacterial invaders. Phagocytes engulf the bacteria, then die and create an exudate that accumulates between alveoli. Capillary membranes deteriorate and become more permeable as a result of the effect of bacterial endotoxin present in the exudate. These changes lead to impaired gas exchange across the alveolar-capillary interface. Bacterial endotoxins alter vasomotor and smooth muscle tone resulting in vasodilation. Inadequate tissue perfusion and ischemia result from vascular occlusion by leukocytes and erythrocytes caused by effects of endotoxic and inflammatory mediators (Casserly *et al.*, 2009; Linderman & Janssen, 2008; Martin & Wheeler, 2009).

Table 3.10.2.1 Organ systems affected by sepsis.

- Gastrointestinal (GI) tract – decreased blood flow and perfusion can lead to disruption of the normal protective mucosal barrier, predisposing the intestines to erosive ulceration and bleeding. Deterioration of the protective gastrointestinal mucosal barrier can also lead to translocation of bacteria from the GI tract into the bloodstream, worsening sepsis.
- Hepatic system – hypoperfusion of the liver will lead to impaired utilization of cellular oxygen causing accumulation of ammonia and lactate in the blood. Progression of hepatic hypoperfusion-ischemia leading to infarction causes liver cells to die and serum liver enzymes to rise. Hyperammonemia can contribute to encephalopathy and result in coma.
- Renal system – Decreased blood flow to the kidneys activates the rennin-angiotensin-aldosterone system, leading to production of angiotensin II, a powerful vasoconstrictor. Angiotensin II also stimulates release of aldosterone from the adrenal cortex resulting in sodium and water reabsorption in an attempt to restore effective circulating blood volume. Prolonged kidney hypoperfusion in sepsis can cause acute tubular necrosis (ATN) and possibly acute renal failure.
- Cardiac system – decreased coronary artery blood flow impairs cardiac function resulting in hypotension, decline in cardiac output and significant hypotension.
- Central nervous system – cerebral hypoperfusion and ischemia results in impairment and failure of the brain's vasomotor center leading to inability to vasoconstrict blood vessels, reducing tissue perfusion and worsening hypotension.
- Coagulation system – sepsis results in release of pro-inflammatory cytokines causing an imbalance between normal coagulation and clot lysis leading to formation of thrombi that can occlude micro-vasculature, worsening cellular perfusion.
- Buffer system – Impaired cellular respiration and anaerobic metabolism results in reduction of pyruvate, accumulation of lactate and worsening lactic acidosis.
- Pulmonary system - Activation of neutrophils and macrophages are accompanied by a marked increase in cellular oxygen consumption which leads to generation of toxic oxygen inflammatory intermediates.

From Martin & Wheeler (2009) and Dellinger *et al.* (2008).

Signs and symptoms associated with lobar pneumonia, such as fever, tachycardia, tachypnea, hypocapnia and leukocytosis, meet the criteria for both SIRS and sepsis (Dellinger *et al.*, 2008; DiMarco *et al.*, 2010).

As sepsis worsens, hypotension and hypovolemia occur because of decreased cellular perfusion and widespread increase in capillary permeability. Fluid and proteins leak from the vascular space into surrounding tissues, leading to edema and hypovolemia. This is known as third spacing of fluids, which will intensify the existing hypovolemia and hypotension. Unchecked, this can lead to multi-system organ failure (MSOF) from ischemia and infarction causing septic shock.

■ Treatment

Guidelines from the Surviving Sepsis Campaign 2008 (Nichols & Nielsen, 2010):

- Initiation of antibiotic therapy as early as possible
- Specific anatomical diagnosis with source control
- Fluid therapy – central venous pressure (CVP) >8 mmHg, 12 mmHg if mechanically ventilated
- Maintain mean arterial pressure (MAP) ≥65 mmHg, using vasopressor support if indicated
- Increase cardiac index (CI) to goal using inotropic support
- Steroid administration for adults with hypotension despite fluid and vasopressor support
- Consider administration of recombinant human activated protein C for severe septic shock with organ dysfunction.

Conditions that activate SIRS also have the potential to cause acute respiratory distress syndrome (ARDS). Pro-inflammatory cytokines activated through sepsis travel to the lungs through the bloodstream and cause alveolar inflammation and tissue damage, leading to pulmonary edema and ARDS (Dellinger *et al.*, 2008; Martin & Wheeler, 2009).

ARDS is defined by the American-European Consensus Conference as having:

- Acute onset
- Presence of a pre-disposing condition
- Bilateral infiltrates on chest X-ray
- Pulmonary artery wedge pressure (PAWP) <18 mmHg or no clinical evidence of left atrial hypertension
- PaO_2/F_iO_2 ratio ≤200 mmHg

ARDS can be divided into three phases:

- Acute exudative phase – associated with damage to the alveolar capillary endothelial cells and the alveolar epithelial cells. Proteinaceous fluid leaks and floods the alveoli impairing gas exchange and inactivates surfactant triggering diffuse alveolar collapse. This initial phase can last up to a week.
- Proliferative phase – This phase can last up to 3 weeks and with positive response to treatment, recovery is possible, if not, then the individual will progress to the third phase.
- Fibrotic phase – Fibrotic tissue replaces normal lung tissue causing a progressive vascular occlusion and permanent pulmonary hypertension (Levy & Choi, 2012).

ARDS can result from pneumonia, can coexist with pneumonia, can occur without pneumonia and will often cause pneumonia (see Table 3.10.2.2). Approximately half of all patients with SIRS and sepsis develop acute lung injury leading to ARDS (Martin & Wheeler, 2009).

Table 3.10.2.2 Signs and symptoms associated with ARDS.

- Adventitious breath sounds such as rhonchi, wheezes and crackles
- Arterial blood gases reveal initial hypoxemia and respiratory alkalosis followed by respiratory acidosis.
- Bilateral fluffy infiltrates on chest X-ray
- Cardiac dysfunction such as arrhythmias
- Decreased breath sounds
- Diaphoresis
- Dyspnea
- Hypotension
- Hypoxemia
- Oliguria
- Pallor
- Respiratory/metabolic acidosis
- Tachypnea
- Use of accessory muscles

Risk factors for ARDS include individuals who have experienced direct lung injury such as aspiration.

Diagnostics

Bronchoalveolar lavage is a reliable method to either confirm or exclude ARDS. A high protein concentration in lung lavage fluid compared to protein level in serum is evidence of lung inflammation. An elevated neutrophil count in the lung lavage fluid is considered evidence for ARDS (The National Heart, Lung, and Blood Institute, 2006).

Treatment

The main therapeutic intervention for ARDS is mechanical ventilation utilizing lung-protective strategies to improve oxygenation and eventually restore normal lung function and ventilation. Mechanical ventilator strategies in ARDS are designed to maintain a safe level of pressure in the alveoli to prevent over-stretch injury and to prevent alveolar collapse on exhalation. Mechanical ventilators in ARDS are set using a low tidal volume strategy to deliver adequate amounts of oxygen without causing alveolar damage from pressure or stretch to vulnerable lung tissue. Either volume or pressure modes can be applied to achieve the goals of mechanical ventilation in ARDS. Positive end expiratory pressure (PEEP) helps to prevent collapse of alveoli on exhalation, maintaining functional residual capacity (FRC). PEEP can improve oxygenation independent of increasing the delivered oxygen concentration (F_iO_2). Alveolar damage from oxygen toxicity associated with $F_iO_2 > 50\%$ is possible. Persistent, high levels of oxygen replace nitrogen in airways, causing nitrogen washout. This leads to alveoli containing only oxygen, carbon dioxide and water vapor. Oxygen diffuses out and secretions occlude the airways, which then cause alveolar collapse (ARDS Clinical Trials Network, 2000, 2004; Briel *et al.*, 2010).

In addition to mechanical ventilation support, treatments for ARDS include:

- Pulmonary vasodilators such as inhaled prostacyclin and nitric oxide.
- Anti-inflammatory agents:
  - Ibuprofen
  - Drotrecogin alfa – recombinant form of the natural anticoagulant – activated protein C (anti-inflammatory, anticoagulant, fibrinolytic)
- Glucocorticoids – suppress fibrotic lung tissue changes, may increase immune system suppression and increase incidence of infections. Current recommendations from the Surviving Sepsis Campaign advocate that steroids should only be used in the setting of septic shock if a patient's blood pressure is poorly responsive to both adequate fluid resuscitation and vasopressor support.
- Positioning therapy:
  - Prone – helps mobilize pulmonary secretions and may improve ventilation/perfusion matching by preventing atelectasis.
- Maintain euvolemia.
- Prevent deep venous thrombosis, venous thromboembolism with a combination of mechanical and pharmacological agents as appropriate.
- Prevent gastrointestinal bleeding with prophylactic agents as appropriate.
- Maintain sleep-wake cycles.
- Provide appropriate nutritional support.
- Keep head of bed elevated 30-45° if possible.
- Provide appropriate oral care to prevent translocation of oral bacteria to pulmonary system.
- Monitor vital signs.
- Provide adequate sedation and analgesia as appropriate.
- Provide range of motion for extremities.
- Turn and reposition every 2 hours and prn.
- Prevent skin breakdown.
- Provide patient and family education and support (Dellinger *et al.*, 2008; Martin & Wheeler, 2009).

Caring for patients with SIRS, sepsis, and ARDS is challenging and complex. The nursing plan of care must recognize and address a range of clinical signs, interventions and responses all designed to provide comfort, support tissue perfusion and maximize oxygenation. A thorough understanding of the pathophysiology of SIRS, sepsis, and ARDS, will lead the nurse to develop an effective plan of care.

References

The Acute Respiratory Distress Syndrome Network (2000) Ventilation with lower tidal volumes as compared with traditional tidal volumes for acute lung injury and the acute respiratory distress syndrome. *New England Journal of Medicine* **342**(18), 1301-1308.

Briel, M., Meade, M., Mercat, A. *et al*. (2010) Higher vs lower positive end-expiratory pressure in patients with acute lung injury and acute respiratory distress syndrome. Systematic review and meta-analysis. *JAMA* **303**(9), 865-873.

Casserly, B., Read, R. & Levy, M.M. (2009) Hemodynamic monitoring in sepsis. *Critical Care Clinics* **25**, 803-823.

Dellinger, R.P., Levy, M.M., Carlet, J.M. *et al*. (2008) Surviving Sepsis Campaign: International guidelines for management of severe sepsis and septic shock. *Critical Care Medicine* **36**(1), 296-327.

Di Marco, F., Devaquet, J., Lyazidi, A. *et al*. (2010) Positive end-expiratory pressure-induced functional recruitment in patients with acute respiratory distress syndrome. *Critical Care Medicine* **38**(1), 127-132.

Funk, D.J., Parrillo, J.E. & Kumar, A. (2009) Septis and septic shock: a history. *Critical Care Clinics* **25**, 83-101.

Linderman, D.J. & Janssen, W.J. (2008) Critical care medicine for the hospitalist. *Medical Clinics of North America* **92**, 467-479.

Levy, B.D., & Choi A.M. (2012) Acute respiratory distress syndrome. In Longo, D.L. Fauci, A.S. Kasper, D.L. Hauser, S.L. Jameson, J.L., Loscalzo, J. (eds) *Harrison's Principles of Internal Medicine*, 18th edn. Chapter 268. Online. Available from http://0-www.accessmedicine.com.library.simmons.edu/content.aspx?aID=9105737 (accessed 7 June 2012).

Martin, J.B. & Wheeler, A.P. (2009) Approach to the patient with sepsis. *Clinics in Chest Medicine* **30**, 1-16.

The National Heart, Lung, and Blood Institute ARDS Clinical Trials Network (2004) Higher versus lower positive end-expiratory pressures in patients with the acute respiratory distress syndrome . *New England Journal of Medicine* **351**(4), 327-336.

The National Heart, Lung, and Blood Institute Acute Respiratory Distress Syndrome (ARDS) Clinical Trials Network (2006) Efficacy and safety of corticosteroids for persistent acute respiratory distress syndrome. *New England Journal of Medicine* **354**(16), 1671-1684.

Nichols, D. & Nielsen, N.D. (2010) Oxygen delivery and consumption: a macrocirculatory perspective. *Critical Care Clinics* **26**, 239-253.

Further reading

Bernard, G.R., Margolis, B.D., Shanies, H.M., *et al*. (2004) Extended evaluation of recombinant human activated protein C United States trial (ENHANCE US) - a single-arm, phase 313, multicenter study of drotrecogin alfa (activated) in severe sepsis. *Chest* **125**(6), 2206-2216.

Bridges, E.J. & Dukes, S. (2005) Cardiovascular aspects of septic shock: physiology monitoring and treatment. *Critical Care Nurse* **25**(2), 14-16, 18-20, 22-24.

Hollenberg, S.M. (2009) Inotrope and vasopressor therapy of septic shock. *Critical Care Clinics* **25**, 781-802.

Schorr, C. (2009) Performance improvement in the management of sepsis. *Critical Care Clinics* **25**, 857-867.

PART 3: TUBERCULOSIS

Melissa Donovan

Tuberculosis (TB) is an airborne infectious disease that is preventable and in most cases, curable. As a result of recent global initiatives to reduce the burden of TB and ultimately eliminate the disease, the incidence rate for TB worldwide is in gradual decline and overall prevalence and death rates are falling (WHO, Global plan to stop TB 2011–2015, p. 6). However, despite these achievements, it is estimated that nine million people still develop active TB each year and nearly two million people die from the disease (WHO, Global plan to stop TB 2011–2015). Global initiatives focus on the identification and elimination of two TB-related conditions: latent TB-*infection* and active TB *disease*.

TB is caused by the acid-fast bacterium *Mycobacterium tuberculosis* . These bacilli are carried in particles called droplet nuclei and are only viable when airborne. *M. tuberculosis* is transferred when a patient with active TB disease coughs, sneezes, shouts, or sings. If a susceptible patient inhales the droplet nuclei containing *M. tuberculosis*, there is a 25% chance he will become infected with the pathogen (Fay & Narajan, 2006). When infection is present, most patients' immune systems will mount a response and limit the multiplication of the bacilli, preventing the patient from developing TB disease. This immunologic response to *M. tuberculosis* is identified by a positive purified protein derivative (PPD) skin tuberculin test within 2–12 weeks of initial infection.

Although the patient's immune response may have prevented the progression to TB disease, certain bacilli remain in the body and are viable for many years. A patient with a positive PPD but no signs of TB disease noted on chest X-ray, is considered to have latent TB infection (LTBI). Patients with LTBI are asymptomatic and non-infectious, however if left untreated, approximately 10% of patients with LTBI will develop TB disease during their lifetimes (Surana & Kasper, 2012). In the past, 6–9 months of treatment was indicated for LTBI to decrease the likelihood of developing TB disease (CDC, 2005). More recently, rifapentine plus INH given once a week for 12 weeks as directly observed therapy was recommended for treatment of latent TB (Centers for Disease Prevention and Control, 2012).

TB infection is a prerequisite to TB disease. TB disease occurs when the patient's immune system fails to mount an adequate response to the infection allowing *M. tuberculosis* bacilli to multiply and progress to active disease. It is defined as either pulmonary TB (occurs within the lungs) or extrapulmonary TB (occurs in other organs such as the brain, kidneys, or spine). Patients with extrapulmonary disease are usually noninfectious unless they have concomitant pulmonary, oral cavity, or larynx disease, or extrapulmonary disease that includes abscesses or lesions with extensive drainage (CDC, 2005).

Even though TB disease affects all age groups, it has become a serious health issue among older adults (Mori & Leung, 2010). In the United States in 2005, 74% of subjects with LTBI were over 60 years old and 35% of subjects with active TB disease were over 65 years old (Mori & Leung, 2010). This striking statistic highlights the importance of gathering information regarding previously treated LTBI or TB disease and assessing for risk factors, which may indicate the need for additional TB screening. The diagnosis of TB disease in the older adult may be delayed or overlooked entirely due to differences in clinical presentation. Understanding the unique presentation of TB disease among older adults allows a nurse to identify risk factors, institute precautionary measures to prevent transmission, advocate for early diagnosis and treatment, and educate patient and family members regarding management of the disease.

■ Risk factors

Risk factors of LTBI

- Patients in close contact to others with active TB disease
- Foreign-born patients, especially moving within the past 5 years from areas with a high incidence of TB (Africa, Asia, Eastern Europe, Latin America, and Russia)
- Patients who visit areas with a high incidence of TB
- Residents or employees within high risk congregate settings (e.g., correctional institutions, long-term care facilities, and homeless shelters)
- Healthcare workers who care for high risk patients
- Healthcare workers with unprotected exposure to a patient before TB disease was identified

Risk factors for developing TB disease if infected with LTBI

- Age *itself* is generally not a risk factor for disease. However, associated medical conditions often present in elders may weaken the immune system and increases risk of disease (Mori & Leung, 2010).
- Patients infected with *M. tuberculosis* within the previous 2 years
- Patients with HIV infection
- Patients with conditions affecting the immune system such as: diabetes mellitus, silicosis, chronic renal failure, end-stage renal disease, leukemias, lymphomas, cancer of the head, neck or lung, low body weight (>10% below ideal body weight), prolonged corticosteroid use, other immunosuppressive treatments, organ transplant, intestinal bypass or gastrectomy (CDC, 2005).
- Patients with a history of untreated or inadequately treated TB disease

■ Clinical presentation

The identification of TB infection is often overlooked because patients with LTBI are asymptomatic and symptoms only arise when LTBI progresses to TB disease. However, healthcare providers may also overlook TB disease in elders since the older adult may not exhibit classic signs of TB, and instead present with only subtle changes in physical exam.

Classic symptoms for both pulmonary and extrapulmonary TB include fevers, chills, night sweats, anorexia, weight loss, and fatigue. In addition to these, symptoms associated with pulmonary TB may include chest pain, hemoptysis, and a productive cough for greater than 3 weeks duration. For the older adult, symptoms such as fever, night sweats, and weight loss may not be present. Instead, the older adult may present with a low-grade fever, fatigue, loss of appetite, and a decrease in his/her ability to perform daily activities (Mitty, 2009).

■ Nursing assessment

- Gather a thorough history to determine patient risk factors for TB (especially due to the limited changes noted on physical exam).
- Ask about recent night sweats, weight loss, fever (may not be present in elders).
- Evaluate nutritional status for loss of appetite or unintentional weight loss.
- Physical exam considerations:
  - Changes in mental status
    - May include decreased ability to perform activities of daily living (ADLs)
    - General fatigue
  - Vital sign abnormalities
    - Older patients may or may not exhibit low-grade fever
    - Decreased oxygen saturation and/or increased respiratory rate related to pulmonary TB
    - Heart rate: may be elevated due to infection/fever
    - Blood pressure: monitor for hypotension associated with septicemia.
  - Cardiopulmonary abnormalities (often associated with pulmonary TB but may or may not be present in older adults):
    - Productive cough
    - Chest pain
    - Hemoptysis
    - Crackles or diminished breath sounds noted on lung exam
- Monitor for symptoms associated with TB-drug related hepatoxicity:
  - Liver tenderness
  - Vision changes
  - Dark-colored urine
  - Clay-colored stools
  - Ascites and/or lower extremity edema
  - Jaundice
  - Nausea/vomiting
  - Prolonged bleeding time
- Monitor liver function tests (LFTs).

■ Diagnostics

Screening for TB is necessary to identify patients who require treatment or preventive therapy (Bailey, 2012). Most often the tuberculin skin test is used (See Table 3.10.3.1). If a person has had TB in the past or had a previous positive tuberculin skin test, tuberculin skin tests should not be administered to that patient again. In older adults, the tuberculin skin test can be negative because

Table 3.10.3.1　Diagnostics for LTBI and TB disease.

LTBI	TB disease
Positive TST • Intradermal injection of 5 tuberculin units of PPD • Induration (hard, red, raised area) ≥10 mm after 48–72 h of PPD injection considered positive. For patients with HIV or other immunocompromising conditions, induration ≥5 mm considered positive. • Older adults may not mount an appropriate immune response and therefore TST result may be falsely negative. Recommend a second TST two weeks later to monitor for increased induration of >6 mm from previous test.	*Medical history* that includes exposure to TB or the presence of risk factors *Physical exam* and patient *report of symptoms* related to TB (see clinical manifestation section) *Chest X-ray:* • Abnormalities consistent with pulmonary TB disease include upper-lobe infiltration, cavitation, and effusion (CDC, 2005). • Prior to initiating treatment for LTBI, *all patients with positive TST results must have a chest X-ray to rule out TB disease.* *Positive TST result:* • Elders may or may not test positive (see above). *Sputum culture* • A sputum for AFB culture that is positive for *M. tuberculosis* is considered the current gold standard for diagnosing TB disease. However, it may take up to 12 weeks for culture to grow *M. tuberculosis.* • A positive smear of AFB can be identified within 24 hrs of sputum collection. An AFB-positive smear is predictive of TB disease, and an AFB-negative smear does not exclude the diagnosis of disease if clinical suspicion is high (CDC, 2005). • *A presumptive TB diagnosis is made,* and treatment is often initiated, based upon an AFB-positive smear, abnormal chest X-ray, and suggestive history (Fay & Narajan, 2006).

AFB, acid-fast bacilli; PPD, purified protein derivative; TST, tuberculin skin test.

of the patient's weakened immune system. A repeat tuberculin skin test (the two step) in 2–3 weeks is necessary. Interferon gamma release assays (IGRAs) can also be used to screen for TB (Bailey, 2012). The IGRA laboratory test is a blood test to measure the patient's immune system reaction to mycobacterial antigens (Bailey, 2012).

- Chest X-ray is indicated for patients with a positive tuberculin skin test or positive IGRA.
- Three first morning sputum samples for acid-fast bacilli if laryngeal or pulmonary TB is suspected (Bailey, 2012)
- All suspected or confirmed cases of TB disease must be reported to the local or state health department (CDC, 2005, p. 55).

■ Differential diagnosis

Differential diagnosis' for pulmonary TB may include:

- Pneumonia, bronchitis, influenza, pleural effusion, lung cancer, fungal infection, Wegener's granulomatosis, sarcoidosis, or other pulmonary processes

Differential diagnosis' for extrapulmonary TB may include:

- Lymph nodes: lymphadenitis
- Heart/pericardium: pericardial effusion, or pericarditis
- Gastrointestinal: Crohn's disease, gastrointestinal infection, or colon cancer
- Genitourinary: bladder infection, or pyelonephritis
- Peritoneum: other causes of peritonitis and ascites
- Skeletal: septic arthritis, or osteomyelitis
- Meninges: Lyme disease, neurosyphillis, or other forms of meningitis
- Miliary TB (disseminated): deep fungal infections or metastatic disease

■ Treatment
LTBI
- If a patient has a positive TST and chest X-ray is negative for TB disease, a 9-month course of isoniazid (INH) or 12 weeks of rifapentine plus INH given once a week as directly observed is recommended (Surana & Kasper, 2012).
- Due to the risk of treatment-induced hepatotoxicity, patients with a history of liver injury or excessive alcohol use may not be appropriate candidates for treatment with INH. Active hepatitis and end-stage liver disease are relative contraindications for therapy (CDC, 2005; Bailey, 2012).
- Despite positive TST results, if a patient has been treated for LTBI in the past, additional treatment is not indicated. Therefore, documentation of treatment for LTBI is essential.

TB disease (CDC, 2005)
- Standard treatment regime:
  - 2-month intensive phase of four drugs: Isoniazid (INH) therapy, rifampin, pyrazinamide, and ethambutol
  - Additional 4-month continuation phase of INH and rifampin (total treatment at least 6 months)
- If a patient with cavitary pulmonary TB continues with positive sputum cultures after 2-months of the intensive treatment regime:
  - Requires additional 7-month continuation phase of INH and rifampin (total treatment requires at least 9 months).
- Medication adherence is the key to successful treatment. To ensure that patients adhere to the scheduled treatment regime, directly observed therapy (DOT) by a healthcare provider is required, both in the inpatient and outpatient setting.
- Patients usually report improvement in symptoms after a several weeks of effective treatment.
- The patient is considered noninfectious and no longer requires isolation precautions when he/she has 3 negative AFB smears (taken daily for 3 days in a row), is tolerating the medication regime, and appears clinically improved (Fay & Narajan, 2006).

▮ Collaborative consultation
- Local or state health department: to ensure that the DOT program is continued upon discharge from the inpatient setting
- Medical team: to identify patients at risk for TB disease and initiate TB screening and isolation precautions as soon as possible
- Respiratory therapists: to assist with inducing sputum production for sputum culture
- Infectious disease RN or MD: to ensure that appropriate isolation precautions and prevention measures are in place
- Nutritionist: to optimize nutritional status

▮ Complications
- TB disease can be fatal if left untreated.
- Hepatotoxicity related to TB-medications
- Extrapulmonary involvement in the cardiovascular, genitourinary, gastrointestinal, skeletal, and central nervous systems
- Multi-drug resistant TB (MDR-TB):
  - Definition: strains of *M. tuberculosis* that are resistant to both isoniazid and rifampicin *with or without* resistance to other drugs (Sharma & Mohan, 2006)
  - Potential causes of MDR-TB include:
    - Previous incomplete or inadequate treatment of TB/LTBI
    - Poor diagnostic measures; inability to identify culture susceptibilities due to limited laboratory resources

- ○ Nonadherence to treatment
- ○ Virulence of organism itself
- ○ Host genetic factors
- Second-line drugs are necessary to treat patients with MDR-TB however these drugs are often less effective and cause more side effects than first-line TB therapy.

■ Prevention

- Infection control programs incorporate (Jarvis, 2010):
  - ○ Administration controls
    - ○ Early identification of TB and initiation of treatment
    - ○ Ensure that patients are rapidly triaged and isolated appropriately, sputum samples sent and treatment initiated.
  - ○ Environmental controls
    - ○ Aim is to reduce the concentration of infectious airborne particles.
    - ○ Place patient in a negative pressure isolation room or a single room with the door closed and air vented to the outside.
  - ○ Personal respiratory protection
    - ○ Healthcare workers and staff must wear a filter respirator mask such as a N95 Mask when working with a patient with known or suspected TB.
    - ○ Patients wear ordinary surgical mask whenever they leave the room until two weeks of drug adherence completed.
- Adequate treatment of LTBI
- Management of underlying medical conditions
- Maximize nutritional status.

■ Patient/family education

- Educate patients that TB can be prevented, treated, and cured.
- Understand that older patients may be at greater risk due to other medical conditions that weaken their immune system.
- Explain to patients that TB is *not* spread by: sharing drinks, utensils, toilet seat, or shaking hands.
- Reinforce that medication adherence is essential to TB treatment (make sure that the patient is set up with an outpatient DOT program upon discharge).
- Explain the importance of regular follow-up to monitor hepatic and renal status while taking TB medications.
- Tell patients to inform future healthcare providers about treatment for LTBI or TB disease.

References

Bailey, P.P. (2012) Tuberculosis. In Buttaro, T.M., Trybulski, J. Bailey, P.P. & Sandberg-Cook, J (Eds). *Primary Care: A Collaborative Practice*, 4th edn. Elsevier, St. Louis.

Centers for Disease Control and Prevention (2005) Guidelines for preventing the transmission of Mycobacterium tuberculosis in health-care settings. *Morbidity and Mortality Weekly Report*; 54 (No. RR-17). Online. Available from http://www.cdc.gov/mmwr/preview/mmwrhtml/rr5417a1.htm?s_cid=rr5417a1_e (accessed 5 June 2012).

Centers for Disease Control and Prevention (2012) Tuberculosis Fact Sheet. Online. Available from http://www.cdc.gov/tb/publications/factsheets/treatment/LTBItreatmentoptions.htm (accessed 5 June 2012).

Fay, S., & Narajan, M.C. (2006) Diagnosis: tuberculosis. *Home Healthcare Nurse* **24**(4), 236–246.

Jarvis, M. (2010) Tuberculosis: infection control in hospital and at home. *Nursing Standard* **25**(2), 41–47.

Mitty, E. (2009) Infection control practices in assisted living communities. *Geriatric Nursing* **30**(6), 417–423.

Mori, T., & Leung, C. (2010) Tuberculosis in the global aging population. *Infectious Disease Clinics of North America* **24**, 751–768.

Sharma, S., & Mohan, A. (2006) Multi-drug resistant tuberculosis: A menace that threatens to destabilize tuberculosis control. *Chest* **130**(1), 261–272.

Surana, N.K., & Kasper, D.L. (2012) Short-course isoniazid-rifapentine is effective for latent tuberculosis (update). In Longo, D.L. Fauci, A.S. Kasper, D.L. Hauser, S.L. Jameson, J.L. & Loscalzo, J. (eds) *Harrison's Principles of Internal Medicine*, 18th edn. Online. Available from http://0-www.accessmedicine.com.library.simmons.edu/updatesContent.aspx?aid=1001850 (accessed 5 June 2012).

World Health Organization (2010) The global plan to stop TB 2011-2015: transforming the fight towards elimination of tuberculosis. Online. Available from http://www.stoptb.org/global/plan (accessed 27 March 2012).

Unit 11: Multisystem Disorders

PART 1: FEVER

Monica G. Staples

A fever is part of the body's normal inflammatory response. In the presence of inflammation, cytokines are released and cause metabolic changes affecting an increase in body temperature. The increase in body temperature and cytokines are an important component of the body's defense system resulting in increased phagocytosis and other mechanisms to fight infection or inflammation. Fevers can be acute or chronic and there are innumerable causes of fever. These range from a central nervous system trauma or hemorrhage, simple cold or viral infection, life-threatening infectious process, autoimmune process, or malignancy. Usually a core body temperature over 38°C (100.4°F) is considered a fever, but in older adults and immunocompromised patients a temperature rise 0.8°C (2°F) above the patient's normal body temperature can suggest an infection or other inflammatory response. Often, however, in elders, a change in status may be the first sign of illness and fever may not present until the patient is seriously ill (Dinarello & Porat, 2012; Norman, 2000).

Fever of unknown origin (FUO) is defined as a temperature higher than 38.3°C (101°F) on several occasions, lasting 3 or more weeks, or uncertain diagnosis after 1 week of hospital study (see Table 3.11.1.1 and Gelfand & Callahan, 2012; Petersdorf & Beeson, 1961). The original definition was later modified to distinguish between classical FUO and three other types: nosocomial FUO, neutropenic FUO, and HIV-associated FUO. The clinical approach to the latter three types of FUO, are different from classical FUO (Gelfand & Callahan, 2012).

There are other causes of elevated body temperature (i.e., hyperthermia) in all age cohorts. These include medications, heat stroke, and malignant hyperthermia (Dinarello & Porat, 2012).

■ Risk factors

- Age
- Chronic disease
- Failure to avoid pathogens (exposure)
- Inadequate acquired immunity
- Inadequate primary defenses: broken skin, injured tissue, body fluid stasis
- Inadequate secondary defenses: immunosuppression, leukopenia
- Indwelling catheters, drains
- Intravenous (IV) devices
- Intubation

Table 3.11.1.1 Classification of fever of unknown origin (FUO).

Category of FUO	Definition	Common etiologies
Classic	Temperature >38.3°C (100.9°F) Duration of >3 weeks Evaluation of at least 3 outpatient visits or 3 days in hospital	Infection, malignancy, collagen vascular disease
Nosocomial	Temperature >38.3°C Patient hospitalized ≥24 hours but no fever or incubating on admission Evaluation of at least 3 days	*Clostridium difficile* enterocolitis, drug-induced, pulmonary embolism, septic thrombophlebitis, sinusitis
Immune deficient (neutropenic)	Temperature >38.3°C Neutrophil count ≤500 per mm^3 Evaluation of at least 3 days	Opportunistic bacterial infections, aspergillosis, candidiasis, herpes virus
HIV-associated	Temperature >38.3°C Duration of >4 weeks for outpatients, >3 days for inpatients HIV infection confirmed	Cytomegalovirus, *Mycobacterium avium-intracellulare* complex, *Pneumocystis carinii* pneumonia, drug-induced, Kaposi's sarcoma, lymphoma

HIV, human immunodeficiency virus.
Reprinted from Durack, D.T. & Street, A.C. (1991) Fever of unknown origin-reexamined and redefined. *Current Clinical Topics in Infectious Disease* **11**, 37.

- Invasive procedures
- Malnutrition
- Prosthetic devices
- Rupture of amniotic membranes

■ Clinical presentation

Fever can be accompanied by back pain, generalized myalgias, anorexia, malaise and fatigue. Rigors (episodes of profound chill with piloerection) may occur with septicemia. Sweating may be accompanied by drop of high temperature due to cooling effect of evaporation of perspiration.

Fever reduces mental acuity and may cause delirium and stupor. In infants and children under the age of 5 years, fever is associated with febrile seizures, particularly if there is a previous history of seizure disorder. Older patients, particularly those with dementia or hepatic or renal failure are also susceptible to febrile seizures. Dehydration and weight loss occurs with prolonged fever. Cardiovascular collapse and cardiac arrest may occur with extremely high temperatures.

■ Nursing assessment

Obtain a health history that includes:

- Onset of fever and accompanying symptoms
- Recent travel, exposure to pets and other animals, the work environment, and recent contact with persons exhibiting similar symptoms
- Family history that examines possible hereditary causes of fever, such as familial Mediterranean fever
- Medical history that illustrates conditions such as lymphoma, rheumatic fever, prosthetic device, or a previous abdominal disorder (e.g., inflammatory bowel disease), the reactivation of which might account for the fever
- Allergy review including the type of reaction associated with the offending medication
- Medication review to determine if patient is taking an antipyretic such as acetaminophen or a nonsteroidal anti-inflammatory drug (NSAID), a gluco-corticoids-an anticytokine which will potentially diminish the fever response, or a medication associated with drug-induced fever (Dinarello & Porat, 2012)

Physical examination that assesses:

- Skin, mucous membranes and lymphatic system
- HEENT
- Cardiac:
  - Heart rate, rhythm, and presence of murmur or rub
- Lungs:
  - Respiratory rate, presence of rales, wheezes, rhonchi, or rubs
- Abdominal:
  - Assess any surgical site.
  - Presence and quality of bowel sounds/percussion
  - Palpitation for masses, organomegaly, tenderness, guarding, and rebound tenderness
- Monitor vital signs including orthostatic blood pressure changes.
- Monitor temperature using the same method consistently (i.e., oral, temporal, or rectal):
  - Sustained fever implies that the temperature elevation is persistent.
  - Intermittent fever pattern has wide fluctuations in temperature, indicating a deep-seated septic focus, malignancy, or drug fever.
  - Remittent fever is one where the temperature falls every day but not to normal level and fever recurs. It is typical of some diseases such as tuberculosis.
  - In relapsing fevers, febrile episodes are separated by intervals of normal temperature, which may stretch into days.
- Monitoring daily weights is especially important in older patients as weight loss helps determine fluid replacement needs.
- Monitor intake and output daily to help determine fluid replacement needs.

- Monitor white blood cell (WBC) count: Rising WBC indicates body's efforts to combat pathogens; normal values: 4000 to 11,000/mm^3. Very low WBC (neutropenia <1000/mm^3) indicates severe risk for infection because patient does not have sufficient WBCs to fight infection.
- Monitor serum electrolytes, blood urea nitrogen (BUN), and creatinine for fluid and electrolyte repletion.
- Monitor for the following signs of infection:
  - Change in mental status may be the first sign of infection in older adults.
  - Monitor intake and output. Decreased intake <50% for two meals suggest change in status and may indicate impending infection.
  - Erythema (redness), edema (swelling), increased pain, or purulent drainage at incisions, injured sites, and exit sites of tubes, drains, or catheters
    - Any suspicious drainage should be cultured; antibiotic therapy is determined by pathogens identified at culture.
  - Elevated temperature. Fever of up to 38°C (100.4°F) for 48 hours after surgery is related to surgical stress; after 48 hours, fever above 37.7°C (99.8°F) suggests possible impending infection. Fever spikes that occur and subside are indicative of wound infection. A very high fever accompanied by sweating and chills may indicate septicemia.
  - Color of respiratory secretions: yellow or yellow-green sputum is indicative of respiratory infection.
  - Appearance of urine: blood tinged or cloudy, foul-smelling urine with visible sediment may indicate urinary tract or bladder infection.
- Assess nutritional status, including weight, history of weight loss, and serum albumin. Patients with poor nutritional status may be anergic, or unable to muster a cellular immune response to pathogens and are therefore more susceptible to infection.

■ Diagnostics

Diagnostic evaluation for the patient with fever is dependent on patient presentation and physical assessment findings, but may include:

- Laboratory studies
  - Hematology/inflammatory markers
    - Complete blood count (CBC) with differential
    - Blood smear
      - Thick blood smears should be examined for *Plasmodium*.
      - Thin blood smears should be used to speciate *Plasmodium* and to identify *Babesia*, *Trypanosoma*, *Leishmania*, *Rickettsia*, and *Borrelia*.
    - Erythrocyte sedimentation rate (ESR): striking ESR elevation and anemia of chronic disease are frequently seen in association with giant cell arteritis or polymyalgia rheumatica, common causes of FUO in patients >50 years of age.
    - C-reactive protein: Useful cross-reference for ESR, more sensitive and specific indicator of acute-phase inflammatory metabolic response
  - Chemistries

- Liver function tests
- Muscle enzymes
- BUN/creatinine
- Electrolytes
- Calcium
- Iron
- Transferrin
- Total iron-binding capacity
- Vitamin B$_{12}$
- Urinalysis
- Serum protein electrophoresis
- Specific testing for infection
- Cultures
  - Blood, at least 3 samples, cultured for 2 weeks to rule out HACEK organisms
    - A HACEK organism refers to a group of slow-growing gram negative bacteria that can cause endocarditis: *Haemophilus* species (*Haemophilus parainfluenzae*, *Haemophilus aphrophilus*, *Haemophilus paraphrophilus*), *Actinobacillus actinomycetemcomitans*, *Cardiobacterium hominis*, *Eikenella corrodens*, and *Kingella* species.
  - Urine: bacteria with or without mycobacteria, fungi
  - Sputum
  - Fluids and biopsy specimens, as appropriate
  - Stool for fecal leukocytes and culture
- Cytomegalovirus (CMV) serology
- Monospot with or without Epstein–Barr virus (EBV) serology
- Acute-/convalescent-phase serum samples set aside
- Collagen vascular disease and vasculitis evaluation
  - Antinuclear antibody (ANA)
  - Antineutrophil cytoplasmic antibody
  - Rheumatoid factor
  - Serum cryoglobulins
- Sarcoid-related testing
  - Serum angiotensin-converting enzyme levels may be elevated.
- Purified protein derivative (PPD) to rule out tuberculosis (TB)
- Biopsy
  - Temporal artery biopsy if temporal arteritis is a consideration
- Imaging may include:
  - X-rays, ultrasonography, computed tomography (CT), magnetic resonance imaging (MRI), radionuclide scanning, and positive emission tomography (PET)
    - Chest: all patients with FUO should undergo chest radiography. Repeat chest radiography with or without chest CT: indicated if new symptoms develop
    - Heart: echocardiography may be helpful in evaluating for: bacterial endocarditis, pericarditis, and nonbacterial thrombotic endocarditis.

    ○ Respiratory tract signs/symptoms should prompt consideration of bronchoscopy with bronchoalveolar lavage to obtain fluid for cultures or cytology.

    ○ Abdomen: abdominal signs/symptoms may be evaluated by ultrasound, CT, or MRI. Ultrasonography of the abdomen is useful for investigation of the: Hepatobiliary tract, kidneys, spleen and pelvis and in the absence of localizing signs, symptoms, or initial laboratory testing, patients should undergo abdominal imaging. CT of abdomen, pelvis with intravenous and oral contrast unless MRI is specifically indicated (e.g., in patients with intravenous-contrast allergy, or if spinal or paraspinal abscess is suspected).

    ○ Prosthetic devices require imaging to assess device and possible inflammation around prosthesis.

    ○ Spine: MRI preferred if spinal or paraspinal lesion is suspected.

■ Differential diagnosis

The differential diagnosis for fever is wide and can vary regionally as well. The diagnosis can be divided into four subgroups that differentiate by infection, malignancy, autoimmune conditions, and miscellaneous.

■ Treatment

Pharmacologic treatment

Antipyretics: Endogenous pyrogens released by leukocytes in response to infection, drugs, blood products, or other stimuli cause fever by stimulating cerebral prostaglandin-E synthesis and as a result raise the hypothalamic temperature set point (Mackowiak, 1998). Antipyretic agents, including acetaminophen, aspirin, and other NSAIDs, are believed to block this process by inhibiting cyclo-oxygenase-mediated prostaglandin synthesis in the brain, resulting in a lowering of the hypothalamic set point. This activates the body's two principal mechanisms for heat dissipation: vasodilatation and sweating (Mackowiak, 1998). The effectiveness of antipyretic agents is tightly linked to conditions in which thermoregulation is intact. Antipyretic medications are helpful to alleviate patient discomfort and to treat fever over 38.3°C (101°F), but it is important to assess the patient's hepatic and renal status to determine adequate daily dosing. Acetaminophen can cause liver damage and NSAIDs are concerning in older patients because of the risk of gastrointestinal bleeding and their impact on the renal system (i.e., fluid overload).

Antibiotics: Initiation of therapy may be necessary for unstable or high-risk patients while the diagnostic evaluation is ongoing, and certainly before the results of cultures are available. Usually, this entails antimicrobial therapy, but treatment may also have to be considered for noninfectious causes of fever as well. If an infectious cause of fever is suspected, empirical antimicrobial therapy may be urgent. Delay of effective antimicrobial therapy has been associated with increased mortality from infection and sepsis (Garnacho-Montero *et al.*, 2003). However, cultures should usually be obtained before antibiotic therapy is started. Patients with severe leukopenia may require antibiotic treatment before cultures are obtained.

The choice of regimen depends on the suspected infectious etiology, whether the infection is community-, healthcare-, or hospital-related, and whether the patient is immunocompromised. If drug-resistant pathogens are suspected, initial broad-spectrum empirical antimicrobial therapy directed against both resistant Gram-positive cocci (including methicillin-resistant *Staphylococcus aureus*) and Gram-negative bacilli is indicated. This may require several agents to ensure that resistant pathogens are covered. In addition, empirical antifungal coverage may be appropriate in selected patients. The antibiotic regimen is changed when the culture and sensitivities reveal the offending microbe and appropriate therapy.

Nonpharmacologic methods

Though controversial and not routinely recommended due to limited efficacy, external cooling modalities are sometimes used to decrease body temperature when other measures fail (Chan & Chen, 2010; Kiekkas *et al.*, 2008). External cooling reduces body temperature by promoting heat loss without affecting the hypothalamic set point. Four modes of heat transfer constitute the basis of interventions to promote heat loss: (1) evaporation (e.g., water sprays or sponge baths), (2) conduction (e.g., ice packs, water-circulating cooling blankets, or immersion), (3) convection (e.g., fans or air-circulating cooling blankets), and (4) radiation (i.e., exposure of skin) (Polderman, 2004). In patients with temperature elevations caused by impaired thermoregulation (e.g., occurring after brain injury), antipyretic agents are usually ineffective, and temperature reduction may only be achieved by external cooling. External cooling can result in reflex shivering, vasoconstriction, and patient discomfort as the body attempts to generate heat and counteract the cooling process.

■ Collaborative consultation

- Infectious disease specialists may provide assistance with diagnosis and treatment planning.

■ Complications

Complications can vary based on the underlying cause of fever. However, serious morbidity and mortality is a consideration in all patients, but particularly older adults.

■ Prevention

- Limit exposure to infection.
- Proper hand hygiene

■ Patient/family education

- Teach patient or caregiver to wash hands often, especially after toileting, before meals, and before and after administering self-care.
- Instruct patient to take medications as prescribed and complete course of antibiotics.
- Teach patient and family signs and symptoms of infection and when to report to nurse or physician.
- Instruct patient on all care instructions for discharge including dressing changes, peripheral or central IV site care, peritoneal dialysis, and self-catheterization (may use clean technique).
- Explain the side effects of medications and importance of discussing side effects with the doctor or other health care provider.

References

Chan, E.Y. & Chen, W.T. (2010) External cooling methods for treatment of fever in adults: a systematic review. *Journal of Advanced Nursing* **67**(2).

Dinarello, C.A., & Porat, R. (2012) Chapter 16. Fever and Hyperthermia. In: *Harrison's Principles of Internal Medicine*, 18th edition (Longo, D.L., Fauci, A.S., Kasper, D.L., Hauser, S.L., Jameson, J.L., Loscalzo, J. eds). Online. Available from http://0-www.accessmedicine.com.library.simmons.edu/content.aspx?aID=9095580 (accessed 9 June 2012).

Gelfand, J.A., & Callahan, M.V. (2012) Chapter 18. Fever of unknown origin. In: *Harrison's Principles of Internal Medicine*, 18th edition (Longo, D.L., Fauci, A.S., Kasper, D.L., Hauser, S.L., Jameson, J.L., Loscalzo, J. eds). Online. Available from http://www.accessmedicine.com.library.simmons.edu/content.aspx?aID=9095700 (accessed 9 June 2012).

Gaeta, G.B., Fusco, F.M. & Nardiello, S. (2006) Fever of unknown origin: a systematic review of the literature for 1995-2004. *Nuclear Medicine Communications* **27**, 205-211.

Garnacho-Montero, J., Garcia-Garmendia, J.L., Barrero-Almodovar, A. *et al.* (2003) Impact of adequate empirical antibiotic therapy on the outcome of patients admitted to the intensive care unit with sepsis. *Critical Care Medicine* **31**, 2742-2751.

Kiekkas, P., Brokalaki, H., Theodorakopoulou, G. & Baltopoulos, G.I. (2008) Physical antipyresis in critically ill adults. *American Journal of Nursing* **108**(7), 40-49.

Mackowiak, P.A. (1998) Concepts of fever. *Archives of Internal Medicine* **158**(17), 1870-1881.

The Merck Manual for Healthcare Professionals. Manifestations of infection. Online. Available from http://www.merck.com/mmpe/print/sec14/ch167/ch167d.html (accessed 27 March 2012).

Norman, D.C. (2000) Fever in the elderly. In: *Clinical Infectious Disease* **31**. Online. Available from http://www.jstor.org/pss/4482277 (accessed 27 March 2012).

O'Grady N., *et al.* (2008) Guidelines for evaluation of new fever in critically ill adult patients: 2008 update from the American College of Critical Care Medicine and the Infectious Diseases Society of America. *Critical Care Medicine* **36**, 1330.

Petersdorf, R.G. & Beeson, P.B. (1961) Fever of unexplained origin: report on 100 cases. *Medicine (Baltimore)* **40**, 1-30.

Polderman, K.H. (2004) Application of therapeutic hypothermia in the ICU: opportunities and pitfalls of a promising treatment modality: part 1: indications and evidence. *Intensive Care Medicine* **30**(4), 556-575.

Further reading

De Kleijn, E.M., Vandenbroucke, J.P. & van der Meer, J.W. (1997) Fever of unknown origin (FUO). I. A prospective multicenter study of 167 patients with FUO, using fixed epidemiologic entry criteria. The Netherlands FUO Study Group. *Medicine (Baltimore)* **76**, 392–400.

Knockaert, D.C., Vanneste, L.J. & Bobbaers, H.J. (1993) Recurrent or episodic fever of unknown origin. Review of 45 cases and survey of the literature. *Medicine (Baltimore)* **72**, 184–96.

Leggett, J. (2007) Approach to fever or suspected infection in the normal host. In *Cecil Textbook of Medicine*, 23rd edition (Goldman, L. & Ausiello, D, eds). WB Saunders Company, New York, Chapter 302. Read more at http://www.umm.edu/ency/article/003090.htm#ixzz1xL88IjwA

National Cancer Institute. Fever. Online. Available from http://www.cancer.gov/cancertopics/pdq/supportivecare/fever/healthprofessional (accessed 3 August 2010).

National Institute of Neurological Disorders and Stroke. Febrile seizures fact sheet. Online. Available from http://www.ninds.nih.gov/disorders/febrile_seizures/detail_febrile_seizures.htm (accessed 27 March 2012).

Roth, A.R. & Basello, G.M. (2003) Approach to the adult patient with fever of unknown origin. *American Family Physician* **68**(11), 2223–2229.

PART 2: POLYMYALGIA RHEUMATICA

Monica G. Staples

Polymyalgia rheumatica (PMR) is one of the most common inflammatory rheumatic diseases of older adults, affecting twice as many women as men. Predominantly found in adults 50 years and older, PMR is characterized by severe bilateral pain and stiffness, usually of sudden onset, affecting the limb girdle areas (shoulder and hip), neck, and torso (Dasgupta & Kalke, 2004). It has many non-specific features and a wide differential diagnosis.

The cause of PMR is not known, but it may be due to an abnormal response of the immune system. In an autoimmune disorder, the body's immune system mistakes healthy tissues as foreign and potentially dangerous invaders into the body and attacks them. This results in inflammation and may lead to the painful symptoms of PMR.

The disorder may occur alone, or with or before temporal or giant cell arteritis (GCA) (Langford & Fauci, 2012), GCA is an inflammatory disorder that affects the arterial blood vessels of the head.

■ Risk factors

- Advanced age: the average onset of the disease is 70.
- Ethnicity: people of northern European origin and Scandinavian descent in particular are more susceptible.
- Gender: women are two times more likely to develop this disorder.

■ Clinical presentation

Typically, PMR has an abrupt or rapid onset that begins with a severe, deep, aching rheumatic pain in the shoulder and pelvic area. The pattern of pain is usually symmetric and may be aggravated by the motion of joints in the vicinity. However, pain may occur at rest, and frequently awakens the patient during the night.

Patients have trouble combing their hair, putting on a coat, or getting up out of a chair. A few patients have joint swelling, usually of the knees, wrists and sternoclavicular (mid and upper chest) joints. A number of systemic complaints may occur including fever (usually low-grade), malaise, fatigue, morning stiffness, and weight loss.

Findings on physical examination are typically nonspecific. On examination, limitation of active and, often, passive movements of the shoulders due to pain is present. Shoulder pain is the presenting finding in the majority of patients. The hips and neck are less frequently involved. In both the shoulder and pelvic girdles the pain usually radiates distally toward the elbows and knees. The discomfort may begin on one side, but it soon becomes bilateral. The diagnosis is usually made within two to three months after the onset of symptoms.

■ Nursing assessment

Daily nursing assessment should include:

- Range of motion
- Monitor for pain; specifically worsening headache or jaw pain.
- Monitor for headache and change in visual acuity.

■ Diagnostics

The diagnosis of PMR is based on a thorough medical history, symptom analysis, and physical examination. There is no precise test to diagnose PMR. Medical tests generally include a variety of blood tests that are nonspecific, but their results may increase the suspicion of a diagnosis of PMR.

- Creatine kinase (CPK) is normal.
- Hemoglobin or hematocrit may be normal or low.
- Erythrocyte sedimentation rate (ESR) is usually elevated, but may be normal.
- C-reactive protein (CRP)
- Liver function tests may be abnormal.
- Alkaline phosphatase may be elevated.

Diagnosis is based on the presence of the following criteria:

- The patient is >50 years of age.
- Duration of symptoms is longer than 2 weeks.
- Presence of bilateral shoulder or pelvic girdle aching

- Morning stiffness lasting longer than 45 minutes
- Evidence of an acute phase response

■ Differential diagnosis

A wide variety of conditions may mimic PMR (Gonzalez-Gay *et al.*, 2000). When present, distal-limb symptoms may initially make it difficult to differentiate PMR from rheumatoid arthritis or other, similar syndromes. Pronounced symmetric involvement of peripheral joints, seropositivity for rheumatoid factor, and the development of joint erosions and extra-articular manifestations clearly differentiate rheumatoid arthritis from PMR. It may be difficult to differentiate PMR with swelling and edema of the hands and feet from the uncommon syndrome of remitting seronegative, symmetric synovitis (RS3PE) with pitting edema. The latter condition is characterized by the acute onset of bilateral, diffuse, symmetric swelling of the wrists and hands associated with marked, pitting edema of the dorsum of the hands and, less frequently, of the feet. Affected patients are persistently seronegative for rheumatoid factor and do not have rheumatoid arthritis. Articular symptoms of RS3PE respond rapidly to small doses of corticosteroid.

In the older adult, systemic lupus erythematosus may sometimes present as PMR. The presence of pleuritis or pericarditis (which are common in late-onset systemic lupus erythematosus), leukopenia or thrombocytopenia, and antinuclear antibodies should raise the clinical suspicion of systemic lupus erythematosus. The predominant proximal muscular weakness demonstrated with movement, rather than pain and an increase in muscular enzyme levels, differentiate polymyositis from PMR.

The presence of peripheral enthesitis, dactylitis, anterior uveitis, and radiologic evidence of sacroiliitis differentiate late-onset spondyloarthropathy from PMR. The younger age at the onset of symptoms, the presence of other, related conditions, such as irritable bowel syndrome, the presence of multiple, small, localized areas of muscle tenderness ("trigger points"), and a normal erythrocyte sedimentation rate clearly differentiate fibromyalgia from PMR.

Bacterial endocarditis and solid-organ cancers (of the kidneys, ovaries, or stomach) or hematologic (myeloma) cancers may also cause conditions mimicking PMR (Gonzalez-Gay *et al.*, 2000). The lack of an adequate response to prednisone and the presence of atypical features (the absence of the accentuation of symptoms with motion, the absence of morning stiffness or the presence of minimal stiffness, and a diffuse pattern of aches) should suggest the need for further investigations.

■ Treatment

PMR may resolve without treatment. However, this may take several years. In the meantime, treatment can be very effective in relieving symptoms and helping people to live normal, active lives. Treatment varies depending on the severity of symptoms, the presence of complications, a person's age and medical history, and other factors. Treatment can include a combination of medication, regular exercise, and eating a healthy diet.

PMR treatment is based on low-dose glucocorticoid therapy. The response to corticosteroids is rapid, with the resolution of many symptoms after a few days of therapy. A lack of improvement should alert physicians to question the diagnosis. The initial dose of corticosteroids is usually given for 2–4 weeks; then, it can be gradually reduced each week or every 2 weeks by a maximum of 10% of the total daily dose. Steroid dose reduction is usually based on maintaining a normal ESR. If the corticosteroid dose is reduced or withdrawn too quickly, a relapse or recurrence of symptoms usually occurs.

Recently, glucocorticoid-sparing agents have been tested with conflicting results. (Hernández-Rodríguez et al., 2009). Oral corticosteroids continue to be the standard medication for treatment with higher doses initially necessary if GCS is suspected (Langford & Fauci, 2012). Therapy may continue for 1–2 years while the prednisone dose is slowly tapered..

Other treatment options for patients with PMR may also be indicated. Calcium supplements and vitamin D are recommended to help prevent bone loss. Additionally, a bisphosphonate (e.g., alendronate or risedronate) may be recommended to prevent bone loss associated with glucocorticoid therapy.

■ Collaborative consultation

- Immediate consultation with the physician is indicated for new onset headache, scalp tenderness, or visual changes as any of these symptoms could suggest GCA in an adult older than age 60.
- Consultation with ophthalmologist should be considered for suspicion if temporal arteritis or CGS is suspected. Surgical consultation is necessary for temporal artery biopsy in suspected GCA.
- Physical therapy consultation can be helpful to promote mobility and maintain range of motion.
- Nutrition consult may be helpful for patients with anorexia.

■ Complications

Temporal arteritis or GCA, the most common primary vasculitis in older adults, is found in approximately 10% to 30% of people who have PMR (Langford & Fauci, 2012). GCA is characterized by temporal pain, headache, jaw pain, scalp tenderness, fatigue, and sometimes fever and can result in permanent loss of vision if not treated promptly (Langford & Fauci, 2012).

Other complications are related to treatment. Steroid therapy is associated with gastrointestinal bleeding, hypokalemia, steroid induced hyperglycemia, and bone loss.

■ Prevention

There is no known means of prevention for PMR or GCA.

■ Patient/family education

- Discuss with patients and families pain management.
- Explain the risk of GCA associated with PMR and discuss the importance of contacting the healthcare provider if GCA symptoms occur (e.g., headache, visual changes, or scalp tenderness).
- Explain the side effects of long-term corticosteroid use and emphasize the importance of not stopping steroid therapy abruptly.
- Discuss the importance of adequate vitamin D and calcium to help prevent bone loss.

References

Dasgupta, B. & Kalke, S. (2004) Polymyalgia rheumatica. In: *Oxford Textbook of Rhematology*, 3rd edition. Oxford University Press, Oxford, pp. 977–982.

Gonzalez-Gay, M.A., Garcia-Porrua, C., Salvarani, C., Olivieri, I. & Hunder, G.G. (2000) The spectrum of conditions mimicking polymyalgia rheumatica in northwestern Spain. *Journal of Rheumatology* **27**, 2179–2184.

Hernandez-Rodriguez, J., Cid, M.C., Lopez-Soto, A., Espigol-Frigole, G. & Bosch, X. (2009) Treatment of polymyalgia rheumatica; a systemic review. *Archives of Internal Medicine* **169**(20), 1839–1850.

Langford, C.A. & Fauci, A.S. (2012) Chapter 326. The vasculitis syndromes. In *Harrison's Principles of Internal Medicine*, 18th edition (Longo, D.L., Fauci, A.S., Kasper, D.L., Hauser, S.L., Jameson, J.L., Loscalzo, J. eds). Online. Available from http://0-www.accessmedicine.com.library.simmons.edu/content.aspx?aID=9138083 (accessed 9 June 2012).

Further reading

Ntatsaki, E. & Watts, R.A. (2010) Management of polymyalgia rheumatica. *British Medical Journal* **340**, c620.

Polymyalgia rheumatica. American College of Rheumatology. http://www.rheumatology.org/practice/clinical/patients/diseases_and_conditions/polymyalgiarheumatica.asp (accessed July 14, 2010).

Roane, D. & Griger, D. (1999) An approach to diagnosis and management of initial management of systemic vasculitis. *American Family Physician* **60**, 1421–1430.

Unwin, B., Williams, C.M. & Gilliland, W. (2006) Polymyalgia rheumatica and giant cell arteritis. *American Family Physician* **74**(9), 1547–1554.

PART 3: RHEUMATOID ARTHRITIS

Monica G. Staples

Classified as an autoimmune disease, rheumatoid arthritis (RA) is character-ized by recurrent inflammation of connective tissue, primarily diarthroidal joints and their related structures. A painful and disabling disease, RA affects approximately 1% of the population and children as well as adults and elders (Grosser & Smyth, 2011). While RA can affect any joint, the small joints in the hands and feet tend be involved more frequently than others. The cause of RA remains unknown, but the primary focus of the inflammation is in the synovium, which is the tissue that lines the joint. Inflammatory chemicals released by the immune cells cause swelling and damage to cartilage and bone.

Rheumatoid factors (RFs) usually consist of two classes of immunoglobulin antibodies – antibodies for IgM and IgG (occasionally IgA). Their main targets are portions of the immunoglobulin molecule. RFs bind with their target self-antigens in the blood and synovial membrane, forming immune complexes (antigen-antibody). Synovial inflammation (synovitis) occurs when the immune complexes in blood and synovial tissue trigger the inflammatory response by activating the plasma protein complement. This stimulation activates kinin and prostaglandin release that increases the permeability of blood vessels in the synovial membranes. This attracts several types of leukocytes and lym-phocytes to the synovial membrane.

The phagocytes of inflammation (neutrophils and macrophages) ingest the immune complexes that release powerful enzymes that degrade synovial tissue and articular cartilage. The immune system's B and T lymphocytes are also activated. The B lymphocytes are stimulated into producing more RFs, and the T lymphocytes produce enzymes that increase the inflammatory response. A microorganism, which may originally be responsible, can be killed off and removed from the body. However, in an autoimmune response, the newly targeted self-antigens (immunoglobulins) are in constant supply and unable to stop. They keep on perpetuating the formation of immune complexes indefinitely.

Inflammatory and immune processes have several damaging effects on the synovial membrane. Inflammation causes hemorrhage, coagulation, and fibrin deposits on the synovial membrane, in the intracellular matrix, and in the synovial fluid. Over denuded areas of the synovial membrane, fibrin develops into granulation tissue called *pannus*, which is the earliest tissue produced in the healing process. Pannus formation leads to formation of scar tissue that immobilizes the joint.

Along with the swelling caused by leukocyte infiltration, the synovial mem-brane undergoes hyperplastic thickening as its cells abnormally proliferate and enlarge. As synovial inflammation progresses to involve its blood vessels, small venules (a tiny vessel that collects blood from the capillaries and joins to form veins) become occluded by hypertrophied endothelial cells, fibrin, platelets, and inflammatory cells. These vascular derangements decrease blood flow to the synovial tissue and compromised circulation. This, coupled with increased metabolic needs due to hypertrophy and hyperplasia, causes hypoxia (oxygen depletion) and metabolic acidosis. Acidosis stimulates the release of hydrolytic enzymes from synovial cells into the surrounding tissue, initiating erosion of the articular cartilage and inflammation spreads into the supporting ligaments and tendons.

Joint change usually occurs in four general stages, but accompanying these changes is the atrophy of muscles, bones, and skin adjacent to the affected joint.

- *Stage 1*: Synovitis develops from congestion and edema of the synovial membrane and joint capsule.
- *Stage 2*: Formation of pannus occurs, covering the cartilage and eventually destroying the joint capsule and bone.
- *Stage 3*: Fibrous ankylosis, which is a fibrous invasion of pannus and scar tissue that fills the joint space, occurs. Bone atrophy and malalignment cause visible deformities and disrupt the articulation of opposing bones. This, in turn, causes muscle atrophy and imbalance that may also include partial dislocations (subluxations).
- *Stage 4*: Fibrous tissue begins to calcify, resulting in bony ankylosis (total immobility).

■ Risk factors

- Age: RA can occur at any age from childhood to old age, onset usually begins between the ages of 30-50.
- Gender: women are three times more likely than men to be afflicted.
- Smoking: heavy long-term smoking has shown to put patients at risk.

■ Clinical presentation

The disease usually presents gradually, but in some patients the onset is acute (Johnson & Quismorio, 2012). It is important to determine the course of the disorder, alleviating factors, and how the discomfort has affected the older patient's functioning (Johnson & Quismorio, 2012). Common patient complaints and physical findings include:

- Fatigue, occasional fevers, and a general sense of not feeling well
- Pain and stiffness lasting for more than 30 minutes in the morning or after a long rest
- Tender, warm, swollen joints
- Symmetrical pattern of affected joints
- Joint inflammation *often* affecting the wrist and finger joints closest to the hand

- Joint inflammation *sometimes* affecting other joints, including the neck, shoulders, elbows, hips, knees, ankles, and feet
- Symptoms that last for many years
- Variability of symptoms among people with the disease

Other symptoms that can occur in RA include:

- Low-grade fevers
- Loss of appetite
- Dry eyes and mouth from an associated condition known as Sjögren's syndrome: a systemic autoimmune disease in which immune cells attack and destroy the exocrine glands that produce tears and saliva
- Firm lumps, called rheumatoid nodules, which grow beneath the skin in areas such as the elbow and hands

▓ Nursing assessment

The physical examination findings may be as subtle as the clinical history. Assessment considerations include:

- *Neurologic*: assess for headaches or abnormal reflex patterns.
- *Cardiac*: inspect, auscultate and monitor for pleuritic pain, decreased chest expansion, poor perfusion to extremities, and peripheral pulses.
- *Abdomen*: assess for nausea, vomiting, and abdominal pain.
- *Musculoskeletal*: assess joints for range of motion and signs of inflammation.
- *Skin*: monitor for rashes, lesions, increased bruising, erythema, thinning or warmth.

▓ Diagnostics

RA can be difficult to diagnose because it may begin with only subtle symptoms, such as achy joints or a little stiffness in the morning. The American College of Rheumatology (1987) established criteria for the diagnosis of RA based on the symptoms described and physical examination findings such as warmth, swelling, and pain in the joints. Diagnosis is supported by laboratory testing and clinical criteria.

- RF: an antibody that is present eventually in the blood of most people with rheumatoid arthritis
- Anti-CCP antibodies: This blood test detects antibodies to cyclic citrullinated peptide (anti-CCP). This test is positive in most people with rheumatoid arthritis and can even be positive years before rheumatoid arthritis symptoms develop.
- Complete blood count (CBC) with differential
- Blood urea nitrogen (BUN), creatinine
- Liver function tests

- C-reactive protein
- Erythrocyte sedimentation rate may be elevated.
- Synovial fluid analysis

Imaging may include:

- Ultrasound and X-rays may not show any abnormalities in the first 3-6 months of arthritis.
- Magnetic resonance imaging (MRI)

■ Differential diagnosis

Patients may report that their symptoms are not present consistently often making diagnosis and treatment decisions difficult. Reports of intermittent joint inflammation can be confused with gout or pseudogout, proximal muscle pain and tenderness mimicking polymyalgia rheumatica, or diffuse musculo-skeletal pain seen in fibromyalgia.

■ Treatment

Although there is no cure for RA, the goal of treatment is the control of significant inflammatory synovitis, improvement of functional impairment, and reduction of joint damage. No single therapy is effective for all patients, and many will need to change treatment strategies during the course of their lifetime.

Successful management of RA requires early diagnosis and, at times, aggressive treatment. Patients with an established diagnosis of rheumatoid arthritis should begin treatment with disease-modifying antirheumatic drugs (DMARDs) (Grosser & Smyth, 2011).

DMARDs are often used in conjunction with NSAIDs and/or low dose corti-costeroids. DMARDs also include medications referred to as biologic response modifiers or "biologic agents", which specifically target parts of the immune system that lead to inflammation, joint, and tissue damage Grosser & Smyth, 2011).

The optimal treatment of RA often is combination therapy including medication, physical and occupational therapy.

■ Collaborative consultation

- Rheumatologists should be consulted.
- Physical therapy (PT) evaluation
- Occupational therapy (OT) evaluation

■ Complications

Medications used to treat RA all have the potential to cause serious complications. Rheumatoid arthritis can also affect other parts of the body as well as the joints. Some patients with severe disease may then be at higher risk for complications, such as the following:

- Anemia
- Heart disease
- Kidney
- Lung disease
- Lymphoma and other cancers
- Osteoporosis
- Periodontal disease
- Peripheral neuropathy
- Risk for infections
- Risk for skin problems
- Scleritis: a chronic, painful, and potentially blinding inflammatory disease that affects the white outer coating of the eye, known as the sclera
- Vasculitis (Amato & Barohn, 2012)

■ Prevention

- RA has no known prevention. However, research has shown that the risk of developing RA for smokers is nearly double compared to nonsmokers.
- Because RA may cause eye complications, patients should be have regular eye exams.

■ Patient/family education

- Teach patient and families techniques for relieving pain and morning stiffness, including:
  - Scheduling NSAIDs at equal intervals throughout the day
  - Performing range of motion (ROM) exercises in shower or bathtub
  - Applying local heat with paraffin dip or warm compress; using cold packs as needed
- Teach techniques to minimize joint stress while performing activities of daily living (ADLs).
- Review information about the disease process and its manifestations.
- Review prescribed medications and discuss side effects and the importance of notifying the physician if concerning side effects occur.
- Discuss importance of balancing rest and activity.

References

Amato A.A. & Barohn R.J. (2012) Chapter 384. Peripheral Neuropathy. In *Harrison's Principles of Internal Medicine*, 18e. (Longo, D.L., Fauci, A.S., Kasper, D.L., Hauser, S.L., Jameson, J.L., Loscalzo, J. eds), Online. Available from http://0-www.accessmedicine.com.library.simmons.edu/content.aspx?aID=9148461 (accessed 9 June 2012).

American College of Rheumatology (1987) The 1987 Classification Tree Criteria for Rheumatoid arthritis (RA). Online. Available from http://www.rheumatology.org/practice/clinical/classification/ra/ratree.asp; www.rheumatology.org/publications/classifications/ra/ratree.asp (accessed 9 June 2012).

Grosser T., & Smyth E. (2011) Chapter 34. Anti-inflammatory, Antipyretic, and Analgesic Agents; Pharmacotherapy of Gout. In L.L. Brunton, B.A. Chabner, B.C. Knollmann (Eds), *Goodman & Gilman's The Pharmacological Basis of Therapeutics*, 12e. Retrieved June 9, 2012 from http://0-www.accessmedicine.com.library.simmons.edu/content.aspx?aID=16670422.

Johnson, D.K. & Quismorio, Jr., F.P. (2012) Rheumatoid arthritis. In *Primary Care: A Collaborative Practice*, 4th edition. (Buttaro, T.M., Trybulski, J., Bailey, P.P., Sandberg-Cook, J. eds). Elsevier, St. Louis.

Further reading

Arnett, F.C., Edworthy, S.M., Bloch, D.A. *et al.* (1988) The American Rheumatism Association 1987 revised criteria for the classification of rheumatoid arthritis. *Arthritis and Rheumatism* **31**, 315–324.

Harris, E.D. Jr. (1990) Rheumatoid arthritis. Pathophysiology and implications for therapy. *New England Journal of Medicine* **322**, 1277.

Kelly, W.N., Harris, E.D. Jr, Ruddy, S. & Sledge, C.B. (eds) (1977) *Textbook of Rheumatology*, 5th edition. WB Saunders, Philadelphia.

Kiely, P.D., Brown, A.K., Edwards, C.J., *et al.* (2009) Contemporary treatment principles for early rheumatoid arthritis: a consensus statement. *Rheumatology* **48**, 765–772.

Lard, L.R., Visser, H., Speyer, I. *et al.* (2001) Early versus delayed treatment in patients with recent-onset rheumatoid arthritis: comparison of two cohorts who received different treatment strategies. *American Journal of Medicine* **111**, 446–451.

McCarty, D.J. & Koopman, W.J. (eds) (1993) *Arthritis and Allied Conditions*, 12th edition. Lea & Febiger, Philadelphia.

Nell, V.P., Machold, K.P., Eber, G. *et al.* (2004) Benefit of very early referral and very early therapy with disease-modifying anti-rheumatic drugs in patients with early rheumatoid arthritis. *Rheumatology* **43**, 906–914.

O'Dell, J.R. (2004) Therapeutic strategies for rheumatoid arthritis. *New England Journal of Medicine* **350**(25), 2591–2602.

Schumacher, H.R., Kippel, J.H. & Koopman, W.J. (1988) *Primer on the Rheumatic Diseases*, 10th edition. Arthritis Foundation, Atlanta.

Smolen, J.S., Aletaha, D., Koeller, M., Weisman, M.H. & Emery, P. (2007) New therapies for treatment of rheumatoid arthritis. *Lancet* **370**(9602), 1861–1874.

PART 4: SYSTEMIC LUPUS ERYTHEMATOSUS

Kate Roche

Systemic lupus erythematosus (SLE) is a chronic, autoimmune, multisystem disease that challenges patients and providers. It is a disease that can be difficult to identify because its presentation is highly individualized and symptoms can be vague occurring over years (Quismorio & Johnson, 2012). Patients are frequently burdened by a sense of uncertainty as they await diagnosis; then after diagnosis, patients often experience insecurity and anxiety around disease trajectory and prognosis.

SLE is one of many autoimmune disorders affecting women, particularly African-American women, more frequently than men. Though the cause of SLE is unclear, environmental triggers, genetics, and some medications have been associated with SLE (Quismorio & Johnson, 2012). The onset of SLE is generally between the ages of 15 to 45 with up to 20% of patients diagnosed after age 50 (Petri *et al.*, 2009). Clinical presentation in patients over 50 may be uncommon, making diagnosis even more challenging (Petri *et al.*, 2009).

SLE patients may experience symptoms that are physically uncomfortable, requiring patients and providers to work closely to find an optimal treatment regimen. The medications used to treat SLE can be complex. Patients with SLE may have a need for work modification or disability support due to disease progression. An awareness of the possibility of serious disease progression (e.g., organ failure) and death make this an especially difficult disease from a psychosocial standpoint. In light of these challenges, coping support and reassurance are critically important in the nursing care of SLE patients. Education is also crucial and should focus on signs and symptoms of an imminent flare is as well as flare, prevention, medication teaching and the management and minimization of complications.

Prior to, and following diagnosis, patients may suffer from symptoms that range in severity from mild to debilitating (Hahn, 2012). Treatment of SLE patients may involve medications as straightforward as nonsteroidal anti-inflammatory drugs (NSAIDs) and as complex as high-dose steroids or cytotoxic medications. While there are significant morbidity and mortality risks associated with SLE, survival rates have improved in recent years as now more than 90% of patients survive 10 years beyond diagnosis (Botwinik & Kessenich, 2006). Patients with SLE should be reassured by advances in treatments aimed at both symptom management and managing disease progression.

■ Risk factors

- African-American, Hispanic, Asian, or American Indian background
- Cigarette smoking
- Family history of SLE or other autoimmune disorders
- Female gender
- History of other autoimmune disorders

■ Clinical presentation

The American College of Rheumatology has identified eleven criteria (listed in Table 3.11.4.1) for diagnosing lupus. Of these eleven criteria, the patient must have at least four to be diagnosed with lupus. However, the symptoms do not need to occur simultaneously and are frequently experienced and assessed over a period of time (Petri *et al.*, 2009).

Table 3.11.4.1 Criteria for diagnosing lupus.

Criterion	Definition
1. Malar rash	Fixed erythema, flat or raised, over the malar eminences, tending to spare the nasolabial folds
2. Discoid rash	Erythematous raised patches with adherent keratotic scaling and follicular plugging; atrophic scarring may occur in older lesions
3. Photosensitivity	Skin rash as a result of unusual reaction to sunlight, by patient history or physician observation
4. Oral ulcers	Oral or nasopharyngeal ulceration, usually painless, observed by physician
5. Nonerosive arthritis	Involving two or more peripheral joints, characterized by tenderness, swelling, or effusion
6. Pleuritis or pericarditis	a. Pleuritis – convincing history of pleuritic pain or rubbing heard by a physician or evidence of pleural effusion *OR* b. Pericarditis – documented by electrocardiogram or rub or evidence of pericardial effusion
7. Renal disorder	a. Persistent proteinuria >0.5 grams per day or >than 3+ if quantitation not performed *OR* b. Cellular casts – may be red cell, hemoglobin, granular, tubular, or mixed.
8. Neurologic disorder	a. Seizures – in the absence of offending drugs or known metabolic derangements; e.g., uremia, ketoacidosis, or electrolyte imbalance *OR* b. Psychosis – in the absence of offending drugs or known metabolic derangements, e.g., uremia, ketoacidosis, or electrolyte imbalance
9. Hematologic disorder	a. Hemolytic anemia – with reticulocytosis *OR* b. Leukopenia – <4000/mm³ on ≥2 occasions *OR* c. Lymphopenia – <1500/mm³ on ≥2 occasions *OR* d. Thrombocytopenia – <100,000/mm³ in the absence of offending drugs

(Continued)

Table 3.11.4.1 (*Continued*)

Criterion	Definition
10. Immunologic disorder	a. Anti-DNA: antibody to native DNA in abnormal titer OR b. Anti-Sm: presence of antibody to Sm nuclear antigen OR c. Positive finding of antiphospholipid antibodies on: an abnormal serum level of IgG or IgM anticardiolipin antibodies, a positive test result for lupus anticoagulant using a standard method, or a false-positive test result for at least 6 months confirmed by *Treponema pallidum* immobilization or fluorescent treponemal antibody absorption test
11. Positive antinuclear antibody	An abnormal titer of antinuclear antibody by immunofluorescence or an equivalent assay at any point in time and in the absence of drugs

http://www.rheumatology.org/practice/clinical/classification/SLE/1997_update_of_the_1982_acr_revised_criteria_for_classification_of_sle.pdf
Reprinted from Hochberg, M.C. (1997) Updating the American College of Rheumatology revised criteria for the classification of systemic lupus erythematosus. *Arthritis & Rheumatism* **40**, 1725 with permission from John Wiley & Sons.

■ Nursing assessment

- The patient's health history and course of symptoms is important. Family history as well as medication and allergy history should be elicited. Further history includes a systems approach to the pain assessment as SLE can cause headaches, serositis (inflammation of the serous membranes that surround organs), and joint pain in addition to fatigue and myalgias. Determining the patient's energy level, mood, coping mechanisms, and social support are also important because of the vacillating, yet chronic, nature of this disorder (Quismorio & Johnson, 2012).

The physical assessment is ongoing because of the patient's autoimmune status and risk for infection, blood clots, and cardiovascular and cerebrovascular events. Important nursing considerations include:

- Vital signs:
  - A fever may indicate a disease flare or an underlying infection related to the immunocompromised state of SLE patients.
  - Dyspnea, increased heart rate, and/or change in blood pressure may be a sign of activity intolerance, infection, coronary ischemia, blood clot, or other disorder associated with lupus.
  - Increased blood pressure may be associated with increasing renal dysfunction.

- Skin
  - Inspect skin for bruises, rashes, purpura, petechiae, tender nodules, and ulcerations; evaluate location and evolution of affected areas (Quismorio & Johnson, 2012).
- Cardiac chest discomfort may be related to ischemia, thrombosis, costochondritis, pleurisy, pericarditis, myocarditis, or endocarditis.
- Pulmonary: assess shortness, of breath, dyspnea, cough, rales, wheezes, rhonchi, and rubs.
- Abdomen: monitor for pain.
- Kidneys: monitor blood urea nitrogen (BUN) and creatinine.
- Musculoskeletal: joint pain is common.
- Extremities: monitor for deep vein thrombosis (DVT).
- Neurological: observe for change in mental status, seizures, and signs of stroke.
- Assess response to therapies (medications and ointments).

■ Diagnostics

- There are many laboratory tests used to diagnose SLE. These tests are important initially to help exclude other disorders and to determine if the patient does have SLE. Many of these diagnostics will not be done again after the diagnosis is confirmed. Some diagnostics will be done with each hospitalization to help determine organ involvement (e.g., urinalysis, complete blood count (CBC) with differential, serum electrolytes, BUN, and creatinine). Initial diagnostics can include the following:
- Urinalysis
- CBC with differential to assess for the presence of:
  - Leukopenia, lymphopenia, thrombocytopenia, and hemolytic anemia with reticulocytosis
- Erythrocyte sedimentation rate (ESR)
- C-reactive protein (CRP)
- Rheumatoid factor
- Anti-DNA (antibody to native DNA)
- Anti-Sm (antibody to Smith nuclear antigen)
- Antinuclear antibody (ANA)
- Lupus anticoagulant
- Serum gamma globulins
- Anticardiolipin antibodies
- Antiphospholipid antibodies

■ Differential diagnosis

- Fibromyalgia
- Mixed connective tissue disease
- Multiple sclerosis
- Polymyositis
- Primary Sjögren's syndrome

- Psychiatric disorder
- Rheumatoid arthritis
- Systemic sclerosis

■ Treatment

Treatment for SLE often involves a multi-pronged approach. Treatment focuses on symptom management, the prevention of flares, and minimizing disease and treatment-related complications (Rooney, 2005; Quismorio & Johnson, 2012).

- Lifestyle changes include: regular, moderate exercise; avoiding sun exposure; and smoking cessation.
- NSAIDs:
  - NSAIDs are often used to manage the arthralgias associated with SLE.
  - Antimalarial drugs (hydroxychloroquine (Plaquenil) and chloroquine (Aralen) utilized to treat joint and skin-related symptoms
- Corticosteroids:
  - Steroids are utilized to treat skin-related symptoms, arthritis, peritonitis, pericarditis, and pleuritis.
  - High-dose steroids are often employed when there is serious organ involvement.
- Cytotoxic medications:
  - Cytotoxic medications may be necessary when serious complications arise. These include azathioprine (Imuran), cyclophosphamide (Cytoxan), methotrexate, and cyclosporine (Neoral and Sandimmune).

■ Collaborative consultation

- Patients with SLE should be followed by a rheumatologist.
- Patients being treated with antimalarial drugs should be evaluated every 6–12 months by an ophthalmologist to assess for potential retinal damage.
- Nurses caring for patients with SLE need to work closely with other members of the healthcare team to clarify patients' often complex medication regimens.

■ Complications

- Abnormal hepatic function
- Alopecia
- Ascites
- Cardiac complications include: pericarditis, myocarditis, and endocarditis
- Delirium
- Hematologic abnormalities including: anemia, leukopenia, thrombocytopenia, lymphopenia
- Intestinal vasculitis
- Pancreatitis
- Peripheral neuropathy

- Peritonitis
- Psychosis
- Rapid atherosclerotic changes; can cause myocardial infarction.
- Renal failure (may require dialysis or kidney transplantation).
- Seizures

■ Prevention

- Currently, there is no known means to prevent SLE.
- While it appears some environmental agents may trigger the onset of SLE (or a flare), it is impossible to predict which external stimuli would affect which patients and how.

■ Patient/family education

- Teach patient and families to monitor for symptoms that suggest a flare is imminent (fatigue, pain, rash, fever, or dizziness). Instruct patients and families to report the suspicion of an impending flare to their healthcare provider.
- Sun exposure may trigger a flare; the use of sunscreen and appropriate sun protective clothing is recommended.
- If a female patient with SLE wishes to become pregnant, she should consult with a high-risk obstetrician before conceiving.
- Regular, moderate exercise can help improve cardiovascular health, as well as mood.
- Smoking cessation is important; it is believed to improve both disease trajectory and response to therapy.
- SLE patients should avoid sulfa drugs; they are more likely to experience hypersensitivity reactions to sulfonamides.
- SLE patients may be on complex medication regimens that often change over time; provide patients and families with information about proper medication administration and side effects.
- Patients with SLE are at increased risk for infections:
  - Provide patients and families with education about hand hygiene as an important strategy to lessen this risk.
  - SLE patients should receive regular vaccinations, including influenza and pneumococcal vaccines.
- Encourage adequate omega 3 fatty acids, calcium, and Vitamin D in daily diet.
- Coping support is essential. Patients may benefit from joining a support group; more resources are available at www.lupus.org.

References

American College of Rheumatology webpage: http://www.rheumatology.org/practice/clinical/classification/SLE/1997_update_of_the_1982_acr_revised_criteria_for_classification_of_sle.pdf (accessed 27 March 2012).

Botwinik, J.J. & Kessenich, C.R. (2006) Systemic lupus erythematosus. *Advance for Nurse Practitioners* **14**(7), 51-53.

Hahn B.H. (2012) Chapter 319. Systemic Lupus Erythematosus. In D.L. Longo, A.S. Fauci, D.L. Kasper, S.L. Hauser, J.L. Jameson, J. Loscalzo (Eds), *Harrison's Principles of Internal Medicine*, 18e. Retrieved June 9, 2012 from http://0-www.accessmedicine.com.library.simmons.edu/content.aspx?aID=9136499

Petri, M., Abuav, R., Boumpas, D. *et al*. (2009) Systemic lupus erythematosus. In: J.H. Stone (ed.) *A Clinician's Pearls and Myths in Rheumatology*. Springer, New York, pp. 131-159.

Quismorio, F.P., Jr. & Johnson, D. (2012) Systemic lupus erytematosus. In Buttaro, T.B., Trybulski, J., Bailey, P.P. Sandberg-Cook, J. (Eds). *Primary Care: A Collaborative Practice* (4th edition). Elsevier: St. Louis.

Rooney, J. (2005) Systemic lupus: unmasking a great imitator. *Nursing* 2005 **35**(11), 54-60.

PART 5: TEMPORAL ARTERITIS

Kate Roche

Temporal arteritis (also referred to as giant cell arteritis) is a common type of vasculitis seen in older adults. The inflammatory changes that occur in blood vessels are often extensive; however symptomatic changes are usually confined to the cranial branches (Hoch, 2012; Salvarani *et al*., 2002). Hospitalization is generally not required for the diagnosis and treatment of temporal arteritis. However, the symptoms of temporal arteritis may manifest during a hospitalization for an unrelated co-morbidity. The nurse caring for hospitalized older adults needs to be familiar with the symptoms of temporal arteritis as the timely diagnosis and initiation of proper treatment is imperative to prevent permanent blindness. Liaison between a patient's primary provider and a rheumatologist is necessary to provide optimum treatment.

■ Risk factors

- Age greater than 50
- Caucasian women
- History of polymyalgia rheumatica

■ Clinical presentation

Temporal arteritis, for the most part, presents gradually, but the onset can be acute (Hoch, 2012). Most patients with temporal arteritis will ultimately seek treatment for a headache (often unilateral), scalp tenderness, ptosis, or visual changes (Levine, 2004). Pain with chewing (jaw claudication) is also associated with temporal arteritis (Hoch, 2012). Some patients will experience systemic symptoms including: fatigue, fever, hoarseness, cough, or sore throat (Kennedy-Malone & Enevold, 2001). If untreated, blindness can occur (Goadsby & Raskin, 2012; Hoch, 2012).

■ Nursing assessment

- Assess for the presence of a headache. Evaluate the onset, duration, location, severity, and quality of the headacheas well as associated, aggravating and alleviating factors. Question the patient about any recent visual changes.
- Baseline visual acuity should be established using a Rosenbaum or Snellen chart to allow quantification of further changes.
  - Partial to complete vision loss (may be one or both eyes) may be present.
- Note erythema or abnormal pulsation of temporal artery (diminished).
  - Pain with palpation of temporal artery may or may not be present.
- Vital signs:
  - A low-grade fever is often present; other vital signs are generally stable.
  - Approximately 15% of patients will experience a fever as high as 38.8-40°C (102-104°F) (Salvarani et al., 2002).

■ Diagnostics

- A markedly elevated erythrocyte sedimentation rate (ESR) is suggestive of temporal arteritis, though it is possible for patients to have temporal arteritis and have a normal ESR.
- C-reactive protein (CRP) is usually elevated.
- Mild anemia is common as is alkaline phosphatase increase.
- Temporal artery biopsy:
  - A negative biopsy result does not rule out temporal arteritis as not all sections of the artery are necessarily affected.
  - If temporal arteritis is strongly suspected, the timing of a biopsy should not delay the initiation of treatment with corticosteroids.

■ Differential diagnosis

- Consider primary systemic amyloidosis if there is not prompt improvement after initiation of treatment with corticosteroids.
- Symptoms may mimic Takayasu's arteritis and other systemic vasculitis disorders; however, these generally occur in younger patients, while temporal arteritis is most commonly seen in older adults >age 70 (Hoch, 2012).

■ Treatment

- Suspicion of temporal arteritis requires immediate physician consultation to avoid patient blindness.
- Oral corticosteroids are the gold standard for treatment of temporal arteritis.
  - Initial dose and length of therapy often vary according to provider preference. Most patients are started on high dose prednisone initially (40 to 60 milligrams by mouth daily), then require a slow taper of prednisone over a period of months or longer.

■ Collaborative consultation

- Consultation with a rheumatologist is recommended.
- Referral to an ophthalmologist may be indicated to evaluate changes in visual acuity.
- Discuss with physician addition of a proton pump inhibitor or H2 blocker to help decrease risk of a GI bleed, a risk for any patient on steroid therapy.
- All patients are at risk of developing steroid induced diabetes. Diabetic patients undergoing treatment with corticosteroids may experience increased serum glucose levels.
  - Monitor for and report elevated blood glucose levels to the provider managing the patient's insulin or oral hypoglycemic treatment regimen.
  - Adjustments to the patient's treatment regimen may be necessary to optimize blood glucose control.

■ Complications

- If untreated, temporal arteritis can lead to permanent blindness. Visual loss related to temporal arteritis is generally not reversible.
- Patients with a history of temporal arteritis are 17 times as likely to develop a thoracic aortic aneurysm; yearly screening in the form of a chest X-ray is recommended (Salvarani et al., 2002).
- Some patients with temporal arteritis may also develop polymyalgia rheumatica.

■ Prevention

- There is currently no known prevention for temporal arteritis.

■ Patient/family education

- Most patients experience significant improvement in symptoms quickly.
- Relapse may occur; review symptoms that may indicate a recurrence.
- Corticosteroids are often poorly tolerated; educate patients and families about side effects and timing of dosages.
- Encourage patients to take steroids with food.
- Explain to patients and families that steroids should not be stopped abruptly.

References

Goadsby, P.J., & Raskin, N.H. (2012) Chapter 14. Headache. In *Harrison's Principles of Internal Medicine*, 18th edition (Longo, D.L., Fauci, A.S., Kasper, D.L., Hauser, S.L., Jameson, J.L., Loscalzo, J. eds), Online. Available from http://0-www.accessmed icine.com.library.simmons.edu/content.aspx?aID=9094791 (accessed 10 June 2012).

Hoch, S. (2012) Polymyalgia rheumatica and giant cell arteritis. In *Primary Care: A Collaborative Practive*, 4th edition (Buttaro, T.M., Trybulski, J, Bailey, P.P.,& Sandberg-Cook, J. eds). Elsevier, St. Louis.

Kennedy-Malone, L. & Enevold, G. (2001) Assessment and management of polymyalgia rheumatica in older adults. *Geriatric Nursing* **22**(3), 152-155.

Levine, M. (2004) Giant cell arteritis (temporal arteritis) and polymyalgia rheumatica. In: Meldon, S., Ma, O.J., & Woolard, R. (eds), *Geriatric Emergency Medicine*. McGraw-Hill, New York, pp. 534-538.

Salvarani, C., Cantini, F., Boiardi, L., & Hunder, G. (2002) Polymyalgia rheumatica and giant-cell arteritis. *New England Journal of Medicine* **347**, 261-271.

PART 6: VASCULITIS

Kate Roche

Vasculitis (plural: vasculitides) is an umbrella term that includes a variety of inflammatory blood vessel disorders (Roane & Griger, 1999). The vasculitides are, by definition, uncommon. For example, estimates suggest only 23 cases of Wegener's granulomatosis per million adults and a mere 10 cases of Churg-Strauss syndrome per million adults (Semple *et al.*, 2005). The rarity of these disorders and the presence of symptoms potentially attributable to more common diseases can make timely diagnosis a challenge. A diagnosis of vasculitis requires a careful history, astute physical exam, judicious diagnostic testing, and a high index of suspicion when evaluating patients with constitutional symptoms and evidence of multisystem disease. Accurate diagnosis and prompt initiation of treatment are of paramount importance to optimize outcomes.

Currently, the causes of most vasculitides are unknown. It is clear, however, that vasculitis can affect any of the body's blood vessels: arteries, veins, and capillaries. Vasculitis involves inflammation of one or more of these blood vessels. The immune system, normally protective, becomes overactive in vasculitis and attacks blood vessels by mistake. This immune attack causes inflammation in blood vessel walls that lead to narrowing of the vessels. This narrowing results in diminished blood supply and subsequent damage to a tissue or organ. Complications and symptoms depend on the tissue or organ damaged and the extent of the damage (National Heart, Lung, and Blood Institute, 2011).

The vasculitides are often described in terms of the size of the affected blood vessels. Small-vessel diseases include Henoch-Schönlein purpura, cryoglobulinemic vasculitis, Wegener's granulomatosis, microscopic polyangiitis, Churg-Strauss syndrome, and cutaneous vasculitis (Stone, 2008). Medium-vessel diseases include polyarteritis nodosa, Kawasaki disease, and primary central nervous system angiitis (Stone, 2008). Large-vessel diseases include temporal arteritis, Takayasu's arteritis, and Behçet's disease (Stone, 2008).

Treatment varies, depending on the type and severity of vasculitis. However, virtually all treatment regimens present the risk of serious side effects and require close supervision and frequent monitoring. Regular laboratory tests are necessary to monitor response to therapy as well as side effects; periodic chest imaging may be indicated in patients with pulmonary involvement. The goal of vasculitis treatment is remission, prompt identification of and treatment for relapse, and minimizing medication side effects (Watts & Scott, 2010).

■ Risk factors

In most patients with vasculitis, the cause and risk factors are unknown.

- α_1-antitrypsin deficiency
- Connective tissue diseases
- Intestinal bypass surgery
- Medications: vasculitis sometimes occurs as a result of exposure to medication.
- Primary biliary cirrhosis
- Ulcerative colitis

Certain infections have been implicated in some types of vasculitis:

- Epstein-Barr virus infection
- Hepatitis B can trigger polyarteritis nodosa (Khasnis & Langford, 2009).
- Hepatitis C can trigger cryoglobulinemic vasculitis (Khasnis & Langford, 2009).
- HIV infection
- Rickettsias
- Subacute bacterial endocarditis (Langford & Fauci, 2012)

■ Clinical presentation

While all of the vasculitides involve blood vessel inflammation, the term vasculitis encompasses a wide variety of diseases. Consequently, the clinical presentation can vary significantly according to the type of vasculitis present. However, in almost every type of vasculitis, patients will experience constitutional symptoms such as musculoskeletal pain, fatigue, fever, and weight loss (Stone, 2008). All types of vasculitis are relatively rare; the vasculitides most likely to be seen in older adults are temporal arteritis, Wegener's granulomatosis, and microscopic polyangiitis (Roane & Griger, 1999; Khasnis & Langford, 2010).

- Small-vessel vasculitides will often display symptoms such as skin lesions (purpura, urticaria, etc.), alveolar hemorrhage, glomerulonephritis, and splinter hemorrhages.
  - Cutaneous vasculitis: skin lesions that are most often palpable purpura; may also be necrotic, urticarial, vesicular, or ulcerative.
  - Henoch-Schönlein purpura: Primarily affects children; presentation includes purpura, arthritis, and abdominal pain.

- Cryoglobulinemic vasculitis: palpable purpura and musculoskeletal symptoms
- Wegener's granulomatosis: Upper and/or lower airway symptoms (e.g., sinus pain, nosebleeds, and otitis media), hemoptysis, and hematuria
- Microscopic polyangiitis: ongoing cough and hemoptysis
- Churg–Strauss syndrome: elevated eosinophil count, pulmonary infiltrates, frequent allergic rhinitis, and asthma
- Medium-vessel vasculitides will often display symptoms such as digital gangrene, ulcers, cutaneous nodules, microaneurysms, or hypertension.
  - Polyarteritis nodosa: musculoskeletal symptoms, fever, hypertension, weight loss, fatigue, and postprandial abdominal pain
  - Kawasaki disease: The vast majority of cases are seen in children under the age of 5. Early symptoms (including fever, rash, bloodshot eyes, changes to oral mucosa, and brawny induration) progress to a peeling rash.
  - Primary central nervous system angiitis: headache and focal neurological deficits
- Large-vessel vasculitides will often display symptoms such as hypertension, asymmetric blood pressures, bruits, diminished/absent pulses, and aortic dilation.
  - Temporal arteritis: headache, scalp tenderness, and jaw pain with chewing
  - Takayasu's arteritis: headache, dizziness, and hypertension
  - Behçet's disease: recurrent aphthous ulcers

■ Nursing assessment

- Constitutional symptoms:
  - Presence, duration, and evolution of symptoms
- Cardiovascular:
  - Evaluate for hypertension, asymmetrical blood pressures, and bruits.
  - Assess for signs of impaired circulation: diminished/absent pulses, pallor, dusky extremities, and necrosis.
- Skin integrity:
  - Evaluate the presence, character, and evolution of ulcerations, purpura, or rashes; this may be a manifestation of disease or a medication side effect.
- Monitor for medication side effects:
  - Azathioprine: gastrointestinal upset and bone marrow suppression
  - Corticosteroids: alteration in skin integrity, risk for infection, and hyperglycemia
  - Cyclophosphamide: hemorrhagic cystitis, bone marrow suppression, leukopenia, and neutropenia
  - Methotrexate: bone marrow suppression, nausea, and oral ulcers
- Coping:
  - In the patient with an undiagnosed vasculitide, uncertainty and unresolved symptoms can be profoundly distressing. In the patient with a confirmed diagnosis of vasculitis, fear of disease progression and treatment side effects can be exhausting and frightening for patients and families.

An evaluation of psychosocial supports and life stressors is a vital nursing assessment; appropriate referral to support services can be beneficial.
- Knowledge deficit:
  - The vasculitides are, by definition, rare diseases. Patients and families most often experience a vasculitis diagnosis with little or no prior exposure to the disease or treatments. Patient and family teaching about disease trajectory, monitoring, medication administration, and side effects is critically important.

■ Diagnostics

- Urinalysis
- Complete blood count (CBC) with differential to assess for leukocytosis, leukopenia, or eosinophilia
- Liver function tests
- Creatinine
- Inflammatory markers: erythrocyte sedimentation rate (ESR), C-reactive protein (CRP)
- Rheumatoid factor
- Cryoglobulins
- Creatine phosphokinase
- Anti-neutrophil cytoplasmic antibody (ANCA)
- Biopsy
- Chest radiography
- Angiography

■ Differential diagnosis

- Antiphospholipid syndrome
- Atherosclerosis
- Atrial myxoma
- Cholesterol emboli
- Cocaine use
- Disseminated intravascular coagulopathy
- Major infection:
  - Sepsis
  - Tuberculosis
  - Endocarditis
  - *Legionella* infection
  - Atypical pneumonia
- Malignancy: lymphoma, leukemia, and paraneoplastic syndrome
- Rheumatoid arthritis
- Sarcoid
- Sjögren's syndrome
- Systemic lupus erythematosus
- Thrombotic thrombocytopenic purpura

■ Treatment

Treatment varies based on the type of vasculitis, disease severity, and co-morbidities. Common medications used to treat vasculitis include: cyclophos-phamide, glucocorticosteroids, azathioprine, and methotrexate.

- Cyclophosphamide:
  - This cytotoxic medication is often prescribed in addition to steroids in more severe cases.
  - Cyclophosphamide is usually given orally, but may also be given intravenously.
- Glucocorticosteroids:
  - Intravenous steroids may be necessary to treat a serious flare.
  - High-dose oral steroids are often utilized in an attempt to achieve remission.
- Azathioprine:
  - The safe, efficacious use of azathioprine (Imuran) is dependent on the patient possessing an adequate level of thiopurine-methyltransferase (TPMT), an enzyme necessary to safely metabolize the drug. TPMT levels are assessed through a lab test.
- Methotrexate:
  - Methotrexate is often given in conjunction with steroids.
  - Methotrexate is usually given orally, but may also be given intravenously.
  - Patients receiving methotrexate should also receive folic acid 1 milligram po daily.
- Infection prophylaxis:
  - Due to the immunosuppressed state of many patients being treated for vasculitis, single-strength sulfamethoxazole-trimethoprim (Bactrim) is prescribed to prevent *Pneumocystis jiroveci* pneumonia.

■ Collaborative consultation

- Patients with vasculitis should be followed closely by a rheumatologist or immunologist.
- In patients with both vasculitis and diabetes, treatment with corticosteroids may cause hyperglycemia and require treatment. Liaison with the patient's primary care provider or endocrinologist may be necessary to optimize regimens to provide tighter glycemic control.
- Pharmacists can be a valuable resource for the nurse caring for a vasculitis patient; they can advise on the proper administration and safe handling of the medications used to treat vasculitis.

■ Complications

Potential complications vary according to which type of vasculitis is implicated and the size of the affected vessels. Complications are generally inflammatory in nature.

- Cardiac complications may include endocarditis, myocarditis, or pericarditis with tamponade.
- Pulmonary complications may include pleural effusions or hemorrhage.
- Renal complications may include glomerulonephritis.
- Limb ischemia can occur in medium- and large-vessel vasculitides.
- Untreated vasculitis can lead to death.
- Many of the treatments for vasculitis have significant side effects and carry substantial risk. The most serious treatment complication is infection related to immunosuppression.
  - Careful monitoring of CBC is necessary.

Prevention

- For most types of vasculitis, there is no known prevention.
- In cases of vasculitis caused by a reaction to medication, avoiding that medication in the future may prevent a re-occurrence.

Patient/family education

- Medication teaching is critically important. Many of the therapies used to manage the vasculitides have significant side effects and the potential to cause complications. Patients and families need clear information about medication storage, administration, and side effects.
- Patients wishing to pursue conception will need fertility counseling: cyclophosphamide frequently induces infertility in both male and female patients. Female patients being treated with methotrexate should have a clear contraception plan in place as this agent causes miscarriage.
- Steroids are commonly used in the treatment of vasculitis. Patients often struggle with the sequelae of long-term steroid use: weight gain, skin problems, hyperglycemia, insomnia, and osteoporosis. Patient education around the management of these side effects can be crucial in terms of both physical and emotional wellbeing.
- Many of the medications used to treat the vasculitides have immunosuppressive effects; education about infection prevention is imperative. Influenza and pneumonia vaccines should be offered.
- Psychosocial support is vital. Patients may feel isolated and uncertain knowing that vasculitis is a rare disease with significant morbidity and mortality.

References

Langford, C.A., & Fauci A.S. (2012) Chapter 326. The vasculitis syndromes. In *Harrison's Principles of Internal Medicine*, 18th edition (Longo, D.L., Fauci, A.S., Kasper, D.L., Hauser, S.L., Jameson, J.L., Loscalzo, J. eds), Online. Available from http://0-www.accessmedicine.com.library.simmons.edu/content.aspx?aID=9138083 (accessed 9 June 2012).

Khasnis, A., & Langford, C.A. (2009) Update on vasculitis. *Journal of Allergy and Clinical Immunology* **123**(6), 1226-1236.

National Heart, Lung, and Blood Institute. (2011) What is vasculitis? Online. Available from http://www.nhlbi.nih.gov/health/health-topics/topics/vas/ (accessed 11 June 2012).

Roane, D.W. & Griger, D.R. (1999) An Approach to Diagnosis and Initial Management of Systemic Vasculitis. *American Family Physician* **60**(5), 1421-1430.

Semple, D., Keogh, J., Forni, L., & Venn, R. (2005) Clinical review: Vasculitis on the intensive care unit - part 1: diagnosis. *Critical Care* **9**(1), 92-97.

Stone, J.H. (2008) Vasculitis. In: Firestine, G., Budd, R., Harris, E., McInnes, I., Ruddy, S., & Sergent, J. (eds) *Kelley's Textbook of Rheumatology*. WB Saunders, Philadelphia, pp. 1401-1407.

Watts, R.A. & Scott, D.G.I. (2010) Vasculitis and related rashes. In: Adebajo, A. (ed.) *ABC of Rheumatology*. Blackwell, Hoboken, pp. 148-155.

Further reading

Langford, C.A. (2010) Vasculitis. *Journal of Allergy and Clinical Immunology* **125**(2), S216-S225.

Sejismundo, L. P. (2006) Vasculitis and biologic infusion therapies. *Journal of Infusion Nursing* **29**(5), 272-282.

Unit 12: The Surgical Patient

PART 1: THE SURGICAL PATIENT

Deanne C. Munroe

Older adults are susceptible to many postoperative complications. These range from mental status changes to chronic illness exacerbations, infections, and hospital related injuries. Physiologic aging changes also contribute to an elder's increased susceptibility postoperatively. These include cardiovascular changes, decreased lean body mass, increased adipose tissue, decreased total body water, plus diminished major organ function. Many changes attributed to physiologic deterioration may in fact be due to comorbid conditions such as type 2 diabetes mellitus, chronic obstructive lung disease, liver or renal disease, congestive heart failure, and medications. Nursing care of the older adult surgical patient is aimed at minimizing postoperative complications through careful monitoring for subtle changes along with anticipating and planning for more serious complications that may have an abrupt onset (e.g., myocardial infarction, congestive heart failure, pulmonary edema, stroke).

Preoperative functional status is predictive of postoperative functional status. Thus, the admission assessment is instrumental in assessing potential discharge needs postoperatively.

■ Risk factors

- Advanced age
- Comorbid medical conditions
- Depression
- Foley catheter
- Immunosuppression (cancer, diabetes, chronic illness, chronic immunosuppressive therapy including the use of glucocorticosteroids)
- Immobility
- Incontinence
- Intubation
- Low albumin

Special considerations:

- Bowel obstruction risk factors include intra-abdominal infection, decreased blood supply to the abdomen, multiple abdominal surgeries resulting in adhesions, chronic illness, malignancy, immobility (Kulaylat & Doerr, 2001).
- Incisional hernia risk factors include weight gain, activities causing an increase in intra-abdominal pressure (especially over the course of the healing period), as well as multiple abdominal surgeries.

- Pneumonia risk factors include surgery of the head, neck, chest, or abdomen, decreased level of consciousness, chronic illness, stroke or any neurologic disorder that affects the swallowing mechanism, compromised immune system, immobilization, poor dental hygiene, and malnutrition.
- Pulmonary embolism (PE)/deep vein thrombosis (DVT) risk factors include immobilization; genetic risk factors; obesity; surgery; hormone replacement therapy; trauma; disseminated intravascular coagulation (DIC); DVT (lower or upper extremity DVT); varicose veins; and history of cancer, chronic obstructive pulmonary disease, inflammatory bowel disease, ischemic heart disease, smoking, long dwelling central venous catheters, and previous history of DVT or PE.
- Wound infection risk factors include peripheral vascular disease, poorly controlled blood sugar, immunosuppression, and malnutrition, and any alteration in skin integrity.

■ Clinical presentation and nursing assessment

Physical assessment is essential to early identification and preemptive intervention in post-operative complications. For that reason it is necessary that the nurse continually assesses and reassesses each system. Every time you enter the patient's room, note how your patient looks. Does she/he have an unkempt or disheveled appearance? What is the general condition of the patient's immediate surroundings?

A cursory visual sweep of the room will reveal the intravenous fluids hanging as well as the rate of administration. Note any additional intravenous medications at the bedside and check the doctor's orders to ensure the correct fluids and/or medications are present. Intravenous tubing generally expires 96 hours from the time it is hung, though hospitals can have different protocols.

At least once each shift, perform a thorough head to toe physical assessment. More frequent assessments may be either warranted by the patient's condition or as ordered by the physician. Specific concerns include the changes noted below.

Mental status changes

- Changes in mental status occur for many reasons postoperatively and are fairly common in elders. "Sundowning" or late day confusion occurs as the afternoon and evening progresses and can be seen in various types of dementia and Alzheimer's disease. Late day confusion is exacerbated by the environmental change from familiar home surroundings to the hospital. The cause is not clear and may be multifactorial. Manifestations may include paranoia, delusions, agitation, anxiety, physical aggression, and wandering.
- Other issues that can affect mental status include:
  - *Depression* can manifest as a change in mental status. This type of depression tends to be more severe and may or may not have been recognized prior to hospitalization. Recognizing depression is important because it is an independent predictor of mortality in cardiac surgery

patients post-operatively in the setting of chronic illness (Connerney et al., 2001; Ho et al., 2005).

- *Alcohol withdrawal syndrome (AWS)* is another consideration if a change in mental status occurs in the postoperative patient. The admission interview may not reveal the true extent of habitual alcohol consumption because the patient may not view alcohol use as a problem or is embarrassed to disclose the information. Clinical manifestations include but are not limited to tachycardia, tremulousness, and delirium. Unrecognized AWS can be fatal.
- *Adverse drug reactions* present differently in older adults than in younger patients due to decreased organ function, comorbidity, and the concomitant use of multiple medications. Adverse drug reactions can present in ways other than the rash or breathing difficulties often associated with a drug allergy. In elders adverse drug reactions affect mental and/or functional status as well. Poly pharmacy (the use of multiple drugs) is frequently implicated in altered mental status or diminished cognitive functioning in elders. Common medication classes associated with cognitive changes include opioid narcotics, diuretics, digoxin, H_2 blockers, (especially cimetidine), neuroleptics, benzodiazepines, sedatives and anticholinergics.
  - Opioid analgesics and psychotropic drugs are associated with sedation. Antidepressants and antipsychotics may cause postural hypotension. Either of these adverse drug reactions may precipitate a fall resulting in a fractured hip, fractured pelvis, subdural or epidural bleed. Injuries related to a fall are preventable, adversely impact elder function, and increase health care costs. Hospital costs increase because hospital care for injuries related to a fall are not reimbursed by private insurers, Medicaid, and Medicare.

Vital signs

- Vital signs include temperature, heart rate and rhythm, respiratory rate, and oxygen saturation. Daily weights may also be indicated for patients receiving intravenous fluids and those receiving diuretic therapy.
- Postoperatively the patient may be tachycardic, hypotensive, and begin to show signs of shock.
  - Temperature increase may or may not be present. Noting subtle changes in a patient's baseline temperature from shift to shift or day to day is important as an increase from a usual temperature of 36.1°C (97°F) to 37.2°C (99°F) can indicate a significant change in status. Many patients, especially those over age 65, will not experience temperature elevation in the setting of a complicated infection or sepsis. In fact, patients may actually experience a decrease in temperature.
  - Tachycardia may be present if pain or infection is present.
  - Tachypnea may suggest pain, pneumonia, congestive heart failure, or a progressing infection process.

Skin

- Monitor for signs or symptoms of wound infection, secondary skin infection (cellulitis), signs of peripheral intravenous catheter infiltration, pain that is out of context with either an extremity injury or surgery (i.e., compartment syndrome). Monitor skin in overlying bony prominences for early signs of breakdown.
  - *Early signs of wound infection may include confusion, nausea, vomiting, purulent drainage, fever. Swelling of the wound may indicate either a hematoma or an abscess. Secondary infection manifests itself with lymphangitis and progressive signs of infection (i.e., erythema, warmth, tenderness of the surrounding skin).*
  - Note that not all redness (erythema) surrounding a wound is related to infection. Erythema may develop as a result of an allergic reaction to antibiotic ointment or adhesive tape. Pain is not usually associated with a localized allergic reaction.

Respiratory

- Auscultate for rales and wheezing that may indicate congestive heart failure. Rhonchi, wheezing, or decreased breath sounds may indicate atelectasis or pneumonia.
  - *Pneumonia*: hospital acquired pneumonia, by definition, occurs after the patient has been hospitalized for 48 hours. As with any infection in elders, the clinical presentation may be subtle and include acute confusion, delirium, a fall, a change in functional status, urinary incontinence, lethargy, anorexia or weakness. Fever may be present or patient may be hypothermic.
  - *PE*: the most common patient symptoms and clinical signs are dyspnea and tachycardia. Other manifestations of PE may include pleuritic chest pain, cough, shortness of breath, hemoptysis, tachypnea, low grade fever elevation, or a low oxygen saturation.

Cardiac

- Auscultate for S1, S2, presence of S3, S4, murmurs, rub, or gallops. Assess the cardiac rhythm for regularity or irregularity.
  - Myocardial infarction manifestations include chest pain/pressure, radiation of pain (jaw, back, neck, arms, abdomen), anxiety, palpitations, diaphoresis, shortness of breath, difficulty breathing, nausea, and epigastric discomfort. Women often experience atypical symptoms such as fatigue.

Gastrointestinal

- *Abdominal exam.* Observe the abdomen for masses, bruising. Auscultate for bowel sounds. Percuss for normal tympany. Palpate for pain, guarding, rebound/tenderness (concerning signs). Note each day when the patient last had a bowel movement.
- Abdominal hernias occur from abdominal wall weakness. The bulging may come and go. If the herniated bowel can be pushed back in, the hernia is reducible. A hernia that is not reducible is incarcerated and can progress to

strangulation. Strangulation is differentiated from an incarcerated hernia by the red or purple appearance of the overlying skin.

- Physical manifestations may include pain, nausea, vomiting, or constipation. Surgical repair of any hernia is indicated for increased pain, increased size, cosmetic reasons, or strangulation.
- *Bowel obstruction* symptoms include nausea, vomiting, abdominal distension/ fullness, pain, cramping, diarrhea or constipation. The four classic findings of bowel strangulation are tachycardia, fever, localized abdominal pain or tenderness, and leukocytosis.
  - If the patient is receiving feedings via a nasogastric tube, orogastric tube or percutaneous endoscopic gastrostomy tube check gastric residuals prior to increasing the rate of a tube feed or administering additional fluid or medications through the tube.

Genitourinary

- Monitor the total fluid intake and urinary output daily and document as this information helps determine intravenous fluid replacement.
- Additionally record how much the elder eats at each meal. Eating less than 50% of a meal can suggest impending infection in some elders.
- Be certain patients can reach fluids and drink safely.

Peripheral-vascular

The extremities are susceptible to pooling of fluids with inactivity and immobility. Fluid accumulation may be increased in patients with peripheral vascular disease and can result in thrombus formation in the deep veins. Thrombus formation in upper extremities is a risk because of intravenous catheterization/ infiltration. A low serum albumin may also result in peripheral edema.

- Assess the calves for erythema, warmth, tenderness of the skin, and swelling.
- Check pulses every shift and document. In some cases, a Doppler ultrasound will be necessary to determine peripheral pulses.
  - If the patient has had peripheral vascular surgery and a change in pulses occurs, report the change immediately to the surgeon.
- Check for Homan's sign by having the patient dorsiflex the foot. Homan's sign is a nonspecific test for the presence of DVT. Pain indicates a positive Homan's sign and may indicate a DVT, whereas the absence of pain is a negative Homan's sign.

Musculoskeletal

Fractures or any surgical procedure performed on an extremity requires a careful check of color, sensation, and movement (CSM) distal to the surgical site. Swelling may occur distal to the surgical site postoperatively, this can be minimized by elevation of the extremity above the level of the heart (as long as compartment syndrome is not suspected). If a cast or splint is applied, the distal extremity must also be monitored for numbness, tingling, decreased sensation, and weakness.

- *Compartment syndrome* is swelling of the fascia within a "compartment," or specific area resulting in the compression of nerves, blood vessels, and muscle. This complication most commonly occurs as a result of a traumatic injury or postoperatively. Physical manifestations of compartment syndrome are pain out of context with injury or what is expected postoperatively, swelling overlying the affected area, pallor of the skin over the affected area, and muscle weakness. The skin may appear taut, swollen and initially erythematous, but then progressing to pallor. Undiagnosed compartment syndrome leads to permanent nerve damage, decrease or absence of circulation to the area and distally, and necrosis of tissue.

  Early identification prevents permanent disability, a loss of function to amputation of the affected limb. Diagnosis is made by measuring the pressure in the compartment by the insertion of a needle directly into the compartment. A measurement of 45 mm of mercury or a measurement within 30 mm of the diastolic blood pressure indicates compartment syndrome. Treatment of Compartment syndrome involves a fasciotomy; long surgical incisions made through the affected fascia that is then left open to relieve pressure for up to 72 hours. At that point the wounds may be left open or surgically closed. Risk factors for developing Compartment syndrome include traumatic injury, crush injury, surgery, and anything that impedes causes increased pressure to the skin such as a tight cast or splint (National Library of Medicine, 2008).

■ Diagnostics

Serum electrolytes

It is especially important to monitor electrolytes postoperatively for those patients receiving intravenous fluids or for patients with a history of cardiac disease. The risk of cardiac arrhythmias will decrease in individuals with cardiac disease when potassium, magnesium and calcium are at the higher end of normal. Electrolytes must also be monitored closely in those affected by kidney disease and in patients receiving diuretics or any medication that affects electrolyte balance.

- *Anion gap* should be calculated when there is any suspicion for any acidotic state. Anion gap = (sodium) – (chloride + bicarbonate)
  - *Lactic acidosis* most commonly occurs in the setting of tissue hypoperfusion as seen in various states of shock. In the postoperative elder underlying disease increases the risk for development of lactic acidosis. These diseases include, but are not limited to, renal/hepatic disease, trauma, bowel ischemia, diabetes mellitus, carbohydrate malabsorption disorders, and dehydration either from fasting for contrast radiography or for surgery. There are several drug classes that may induce lactic acidosis including salicylates, biguanides, alcohols, and radiographic contrast.
    - ○ Type 2 diabetics should not receive Metformin within 48 hours preoperatively and should not restart Metformin until they are fully recovered

due to the risk for developing lactic acidosis. The underlying cause of acidosis must be determined in order to correct it (Nicks *et al.*, 2010).

Serum glucose should be monitored closely in all patients with diabetes for both hyperglycemia and hypoglycemia. Additionally patients who are not diabetic should have careful serum glucose monitoring if they are not eating well, are not receiving intravenous glucose, or if they are on antibiotic therapy as several antibiotics are associated with hypoglycemia (e.g., levofloxacin, sulfonamides). Any change in patient status requires a serum glucose blood check.

Blood urea nitrogen (BUN)/creatinine/glomerular filtration rate (GFR) to monitor fluid and renal status. Monitor BUN, creatinine ratio and glomerular filtration rate and report concerning changes to physician.

PT/INR – PTT

Prothrombin time (PT) is a measurement of extrinsic and common coagulation pathways (i.e., clotting factors I [fibrinogen], II [prothrombin], V, VII, and X [extrinsic system]). When there is a failure of any of these proteins, the PT is prolonged, which reflects a prolonged clotting time. A prolongation of PT is seen most commonly in liver disease, Vitamin K deficiency, malabsorption conditions, warfarin (Coumadin) therapy, obstructive biliary conditions, and DIC. Warfarin (Coumadin) directly affects the PT and International normalized ratio (INR) and is affected by foods, renal status, and medications (National Library of Medicine, 2010a).

Partial thromboplastin time (PTT) measures the intrinsic and common pathways of coagulation (i.e., clotting factors I [fibrinogen], II [prothrombin], V, VIII, IX, X, XI, and XII). PTT is prolonged due inadequate levels of these proteins. In addition to the conditions affecting the PT, a prolonged PTT may be seen in von Willebrand's disease, heparin therapy (heparin directly affects PTT and is the index to monitor for therapeutic anticoagulation, up to 2.5 times the normal) (National Library of Medicine, 2010b). Heparin is used for acute thromboembolic events such as PE and DVT.

INR is a standardized test. INR results are uniform and do not vary according to the testing procedure like the PT. The therapeutic goal INR ranges from 2.0 to 3.5 depending on the indication for anticoagulation. These indications include DVT or prophylaxis, pulmonary embolism, prosthetic cardiac valve prophylaxis, orthopedic surgery, and prophylaxis of emboli from atrial fibrillation (National Library of Medicine, 2010a, b). The concomitant use of intravenous heparin, subcutaneous heparin, or the low molecular weight heparins (e.g., Dalteparin or Fragmin) are frequently used in conjunction with warfarin (Coumadin) and serve as a "bridge" until the therapeutic INR is achieved.

D-dimers, the products of fibrin degradation, is a test used to diagnose DVT, PE, and DIC. In DIC, D-dimers will be elevated as are other fibrinogen degradation products. If a PE or DVT is suspected, D-dimer is not a specific test, but when negative, the test suggests that a DVT or PE is not present. If positive, a spiral CT or VQ scan is recommended. There is a qualitative portion of the test as well as a quantitative portion. If the qualitative is negative, the quantitative may be positive.

Serum albumin. Proteins are important components of hemoglobin, muscle, and transport proteins and play a role in many other physiologic functions. Proteins contribute to the maintenance of osmotic pressure within the vascular space thereby controlling fluid from leaking into the tissues and causing edema. Albumin is a protein that constitutes approximately 60% of the body's total protein.

There are several clinical implications for an elder with a low albumin. Albumin is a precursor to the development of surfactant in the lungs; low albumin contributes to atelectasis which in turn may precipitate pneumonia. Adequate albumin is required for wound healing. Many drugs are highly protein bound, thus, when albumin levels are low there is more free drug which may result in drug toxicity.

Complete blood count/differential
White blood cell count may be mildly elevated postoperatively due to physiologic stress. An elevated white blood cell count (i.e., leukocytosis) will usually occur within 48 hours of surgery if an infection is present. Other indices of infection include elevated neutrophils or an elevated absolute neutrophil count. The source of infection may be initially difficult to pinpoint and further diagnostics may be necessary.

Other sources of acute leukocytosis in the postoperative older patient include inflammation, tissue necrosis, trauma, or hemorrhage. A decrease in white blood cell count (i.e., leukopenia) may be noted in drug toxicity, sepsis, and nutritional deficiency such as vitamin B12.

Hemoglobin and hematocrit are obtained and compared to preoperative results keeping in mind the estimated blood loss during surgery. Hemoglobin is an indicator of oxygen binding capacity and is low in the setting of blood loss and hemodilution as seen in a patient that has received excessive intravenous fluids. Hematocrit is an indicator of circulating volume. A low hemoglobin and hematocrit (below 30) may precipitate a cardiovascular event due to the physiologic stress on the patient's system. A transfusion may be necessary to prevent a cardiovascular event. An elevation in hemoglobin and hematocrit is seen in dehydrated patients. Hemoglobin and hematocrit may be falsely low when white blood cells are high.

Platelets must be closely monitored in any patient receiving medications including postoperative anticoagulation. A decrease in platelets could suggest drug induced thrombocytopenia which may occur with the administration of many drugs ordered postoperatively (e.g., Heparin, Lovenox, Fragmin, or Zantac).

Cardiac biomarkers
- CK-MB
- Troponin levels (T and I).

Arterial blood gases. A blood gas may be useful to determine metabolic status and oxygen saturation.

Cultures
- Sputum cultures
- Wound cultures

A patient may need to be "pan-cultured" to determine an infection source. Pan-culturing includes obtaining a sputum culture, urine culture, wound culture, and at least two sets of blood cultures. The cultures are obtained prior to initiation of empiric antibiotic therapy and must be done expeditiously so the patient receives the antibiotics as soon as possible (usually within 2 hours of the physician's orders and sometimes sooner).

Cardiography
- Echocardiogram
- Electrocardiogram
  - Observe for rate changes, arrhythmias, ST elevation, Q wave changes.

Radiographic testing
Plain radiographs (X-rays) may be ordered postoperatively for a variety of reasons, but in some situations the information obtained from a plain radiograph is limited.

Chest X-ray may be ordered to rule out pneumonia, congestive heart failure, or pneumothorax. Chest X-rays are also ordered to confirm tube placement (e.g., endotracheal tubes, nasogastric tubes, orogastric tubes, chest tubes, peripheral inserted central catheters (PICC), and central lines). A chest X-ray may not reveal an early pneumonia in an older adult, therefore treatment is initiated based on the clinical presentation.

Kidneys, ureters, bladder (KUB) and upright or a X-ray of the abdomen may be ordered post percutaneous endoscopic gastrostomy tube (PEG) tube placement, to assess for kidney stones, evaluate for gross structural abnormalities of the abdominal or pelvic organs. A decubitus view evaluates the presence of free air in the abdomen.

Bone Radiographs. Postoperative X-rays of bones and joints evaluate hardware placement and alignment of fractures that have been reduced. These X-rays may also be used to evaluate for metastatic disease. Osteopenia is a common radiographic finding.

Ultrasound utilizes high frequency sound waves to reconstruct tissues and organs. Ultrasound is generally safe and does not expose the patient to unnecessary radiation. An ultrasound may be utilized as a screening tool for some of the following:

- Diagnose gallbladder disease or appendicitis.
- Diagnose nephrolithiasis.
- Evaluate infections such as an abscess.
- Evaluate blood flow of the heart to determine cardiac function or assess for cardiac valve disease.
- Evaluate blood flow of the extremities to rule out a deep vein thrombosis.

- Evaluate the thyroid gland.
- Evaluate both female and male reproductive organs.

Additional radiographic testing

Computerized tomography (CT) scans may be ordered with or without either oral or intravenous contrast depending on the differential diagnoses being considered. CT scans are more sensitive than plain radiographs at assessing for fluid collections, infection, fractures, chest, intraabdominal, and pelvic pathology. The issue for elders who receive oral or intravenous contrast dye is the impact of the dye on the kidneys. Acetylcysteine (Mucomyst) 600-1200 milligrams PO twice a day is given to help prevent contrast induced nephropathy.

Magnetic resonance imaging (MRI). MRIs are more sensitive than a CT scan, however MRIs are not always available. Additionally, a MRI requires the patient to be still for longer periods of time than a CT scan. A MRI cannot be performed on individuals with an implanted defibrillator, pacemaker, various surgically placed hardware such as surgical clips, plates, or screws, a cochlear implant, for obese individuals, and for those with a history of ocular injury related to metal.

Other diagnostics

- Test for compartment syndrome: diagnosis is made by measuring the pressure in the compartment by the insertion of a needle directly into the compartment. A measurement of 45 mmHg or a measurement within 30 mmHg of the diastolic blood pressure indicates compartment syndrome.
- VQ scan for suspected PE (CT scan is also used to diagnose PE).

■ Differential diagnosis

The differential diagnosis is dependent on the system affected. For example, chest pain can have multiple causes (e.g., myocardial infarction, a pulmonary embolus, or pericarditis) or an infection could be bacterial or fungal in nature.

■ Treatment

Preoperative considerations

- Cardiac and antihypertensive medications are generally given the day of surgery to prevent postoperative hypertension or cardiac decompensation.
- Intravenous antibiotics may be given either pre- or intraoperatively. Depending on the type of surgery and surgeon, a patient may receive a limited number of postoperative antibiotic doses for wound infection prophylaxis.
- Many patients are prescribed anticoagulation therapy to prevent deep vein thrombosis and pulmonary embolism.
- A histamine 2 blocker (e.g., ranitidine) or a proton pump inhibitor is commonly prescribed to prevent postoperative gastrointestinal stress ulcers. Cimetidine

(Tagamet) is usually avoided in elders because of potential confusion and drug-drug interactions.
- Assess the platelet count prior to administering ranitidine as thrombocytopenia is a potential side effect.

Postoperative considerations

- Assess mental status, reorient as needed to person, place, and time:
  - For confused patients with delirium, familiar items such as family pictures may help to minimize this phenomenon.
  - Providing a night light will help to illuminate the immediate surroundings for safety and will help to reorient the patient.
  - Repetitive activity such as folding laundry or rolling a skein of yarn may help keep some patients calm and occupied.
  - Often confused patients are placed near the nurse's station to be monitored closely.
  - Minimizing noise from the nurse's station, keeping television or radio sound low, and maintaining as quiet an environment as possible is helpful.
- Maintain a patient safe environment:
  - Hourly or more frequent visual checks
  - Maintain a safe environment.
  - Provide night time lighting and calendar with the correct date.
  - Side rails up; bed in the lowest position
  - Head of bed elevated to the appropriate degree
  - Keep potentially dangerous items that could be ingested off the bedside stand.
- Oral care:
  - Mechanically brush the teeth and tongue with toothpaste and toothbrush twice daily and prn.
  - Provide alcohol free, antiseptic oral rinse done after meals or twice daily at the minimum.
  - Moisturize the oral mucosa and lips with a water soluble moisturizer every 1-2 hours to maintain oral health.
- Skin care:
  - Wound check daily and as indicated. Document findings daily.
  - Assess skin surrounding intravenous angiocatheters and any surgical tubes.
  - Turn and reposition patient every 2 hours if the patient is unable to do so.
  - Inspect skin overlying bony prominences including the scalp, monitor the ears for breakdown due to respiratory equipment such as tubing of the nasal cannula.
- Cardiac:
  - Auscultate heart sounds and assess cardiac rhythm.
  - Monitor serum electrolytes. The heart is electrolyte sensitive and high normal levels of potassium, magnesium, and calcium help to maintain cardiac homeostasis.

- ECG immediately to identify arrhythmias or ST elevation changes.
- If chest pain is present, relieve chest discomfort with oxygen and indicated pain medications, immediately contact emergency medical team.
  - Usual treatment includes aspirin, 325 milligrams, chewed as well as nitroglycerin and morphine as indicated.
  - Nitroglycerin is contraindicated in patients who have critical aortic stenosis or hypotension.
- Respiratory:
  - Monitor lung sounds every 8 hours or as the patient's condition warrants.
  - Encourage deep breaths and coughing and/or incentive spirometry every hour while awake to prevent atelectasis and pneumonia.
- Gastrointestinal/genitourinary:
  - Monitor bowel sounds and bowel movements to prevent constipation.
  - Develop a bladder and bowel protocol for patients (e.g., toileting every 2 hours while awake to prevent incontinence, falls).
- Musculoskeletal:
  - Discuss with physician early mobilization of patient to chair and ambulation to prevent muscle loss, weakness, and DVT. For patients able to do so, encourage leg exercises in bed.

Specific treatment considerations

- Surgical repair of a hernia is indicated for increased pain, increased size, cosmetic reasons, or strangulation.
  - *Strangulation is a surgical emergency and must be corrected in order to prevent bowel necrosis.*
    - Nonsurgical treatment of an incisional hernia includes weight loss, the use of a truss or binder to maintain counter pressure over the hernia.
- *Compartment syndrome* treatment involves a fasciotomy, long surgical incisions made through the affected fascia left open to relieve pressure for up to 72 hours. At that point the wounds may be left open or surgically closed.
- *Pneumonia* is treated with the appropriate antibiotic therapy, inhaled bronchodilators, and/or cough expectorants or suppressants (if indicated).
- *PE* treatment consists of immediate anticoagulation therapy. A vena cava filter may be placed in patients at high risk for reoccurrence of thromboembolism.

■ Collaborative consultation

Nutrition

The dietician generally assesses a patient's *nutritional status*; however, you can quickly ascertain nutritional status by determining the BMI and the albumin level. Regardless of the BMI if the albumin level is low you may conclude that the individual is in a malnourished state and may be at risk for drug toxicities.

Postoperatively, diet is resumed per doctor's orders. Once bowel sounds have returned the patient usually first starts with clear liquids and advances as tolerated to the prescribed diet. Monitor intake and output. Monitor the abdomen for increased pain, distension, bowel sounds, and for bowel movements.

New tube feeds are advanced as tolerated to the goal rate. The physician will order the type of tube feed, generally after a dietician has evaluated the patient's current nutritional status and determines nutritional needs. Tube feeds delivered via nasogastric tube (NGT), oral gastric tube (OGT), or PEG tube all must be checked for residual tube feed prior to increasing the rate and should be checked prior to administering medications. The head of bed should be maintained at 30° when a tube feed is being administered. If the head of bed is to be lowered for patient care the tube feed must be shut off to decrease the risk of aspiration. A "J" tube or tube placed into the jejunum does not have to be checked for residuals or placement as there is no risk of aspiration.

Physical therapy to assess ability to ambulate safely, climb stairs and fall risk.

■ Complications

Abdominal surgery complications include bleeding, which may be the result of a missed bleeding source at time of incisional closure or an inadvertent wound to a blood vessel or organ that was sustained unknowingly intraoperatively. Postoperatively the patient may be tachycardic, hypotensive, and begin to show signs of shock. Other complications include:

- Bowel obstruction is a complication of abdominal surgery that occurs either for a mechanical reason or is the result of a functional obstruction in which the bowel malfunctions and is unable to move along contents. A bowel obstruction may be partial or complete. A small bowel obstruction (SBO) may occur at anywhere along the small bowel with varying symptoms depending on location. A SBO may progress to become either strangulated or gangrenous and is a surgical emergency. Another type of bowel obstruction is intussusception, the result of a segment of bowel telescoping into itself (Kulaylat & Doerr, 2001).
- Dehiscence
- Evisceration
- Herniation:
  - Incisional hernia or ventral hernia
- Peritonitis results in spilling of bowel contents into the peritoneum.
- Stress ulceration of the gastrointestinal tract, esophageal varices, may be other sources of blood loss.

Cardiovascular complications include arrhythmias, myocardial infarction and stroke. Decompensation of chronic cardiac disease can result in congestive heart failure or pulmonary edema which in some cases may be related to the patient receiving excessive fluid volume.

Musculoskeletal complications:

- Anemia/bleeding
- Compartment syndrome

Other complications

- Deep vein thrombosis, pulmonary embolus
- Hospital-acquired infections, MRSA, MSSA, VRE
- Infections precipitated by antibiotic use (e.g., candidiasis, *Clostridium difficile*)
- Pneumonia complications include adult respiratory distress syndrome (ARDS), respiratory failure requiring mechanical ventilation, sepsis, lung abscess or empyema (National Library of Medicine, 2010c).
- Sepsis
- Stress ulceration of the gastrointestinal tract, esophageal varices, may be other sources of blood loss.
- Urinary tract infection
- Wound dehiscence occurs when the wound edges begin to separate, the degree of which varies. Sutures or staples may fail. Contributing factors to wound complications include low albumin, poorly controlled blood sugar, malnutrition, and chronic illness.
- Wound infection – Postoperative wound complications include infection, bleeding, draining, or wound dehiscence. Surgical wounds are monitored for the progress of healing, approximation of wound edges and for complications. Early signs of infection are confusion, nausea, vomiting, purulent drainage, fever. Swelling of the wound may indicate either a hematoma or an abscess. Secondary infection manifests itself with progressive signs infection, erythema, warmth, tenderness of the surrounding skin, and lymphangitis. Diagnosis is made clinically based on presentation. A wound culture is obtained to determine the specific microorganism and informs antibiotic choice. Any break in skin integrity increases the risk of secondary infection. Risk factors for developing a wound infection include peripheral vascular disease, poorly controlled blood sugar, immunosuppression, and malnutrition.

The Centers for Medicaid and Medicare Services (CMS), as well as many private insurance companies, will not pay for expensive hospital care related to the following hospital-acquired infections and injuries. These conditions are deemed to be preventable when evidence based nursing and medical practice is employed:

- Hospital-acquired infections
  - Many hospital acquired infections are multidrug resistant affecting wounds, the lungs, urinary tract, gastrointestinal tract, and wounds.
  - Infection in an elder increases overall mortality.
- Injuries related to falls and trauma:
  - Fractures
  - Dislocations

- Intracranial injuries
- Burns
- Electric shock
- Crush injuries
- Manifestations of poor glycemic control:
  - Diabetic ketoacidosis
  - Nonketotic hyperosmolar coma
  - Hypoglycemic coma
  - Secondary diabetes with ketoacidosis or hyperosmolarity
- Surgical site infection following:
  - Coronary artery bypass graft (CABG)
  - Bariatric surgery to include laparoscopic gastric bypass, gastroenterostomy, laparoscopic gastric restrictive surgery
  - Orthopedic procedures involving the spine, neck, shoulder, or elbow
- DVT/PE following knee or hip replacement surgery
- Vascular catheter-associated infection
- Catheter-associated urinary tract infection
- Air embolism
- Blood incompatibility
- Stage III and IV pressure ulcers
- Retained foreign body postoperatively (CMS, 2012)

■ Prevention

Simple hand washing, maintaining universal precautions, and maintaining prescribed precautions help prevent the transmission of pathogens.

■ Patient/family education

Patient and family education depends on the patient's illness and needs. The following are potential teaching considerations.

- If the patient is unable to effectively deep breathe/cough or use the incentive spirometer then chest physiotherapy should be performed every two hours while awake. Suction oral secretions as needed. Deeper suctioning may be needed to assist patient in clearing secretions.
- Monitor the abdomen for bowel sounds, new or worsening pain or tenderness on palpation.
- Antiembolism stockings and/or pneumo boots for DVT prophylaxis
- A back rub will help you to connect with your patient, decrease stress the patient is experiencing and reduce the need for pain medication.
- Encourage the patient to use the call light for any needs.
- Encourage the patient to report pain utilizing a 1-10 numeric scale.
- Encourage aggressive pulmonary toilet; deep breaths, coughing/incentive spirometer every hour while awake.

- Encourage patient to report urinary symptoms.
- Explain potential medication side effects and stress the importance of reporting side effects.
- Explain all procedures prior to and during the procedure.
- Encourage family to provide family pictures or a familiar object for patient's room.
- Explain that an abdominal incision can take up to 6 months to heal.

References

Centers for Medicaid and Medicare Services (CMS) (2012) Hospital-acquired conditions (HAC) in acute inpatient prospective payment system (IPPS) hospitals. Online. Available from http://www.cms.gov/HospitalAcqCond/06_Hospital-Acquired_Conditions (accessed 16 June 2012).

Connerney, I., Shapiro, P.A., Mclaughlin, J.S., Bagiella, E. & Sloan, R.P. (2001) Relation between depression after coronary artery bypass surgery and 12-month outcome: a prospective study. *Lancet* **358**(9295), 1766-1771.

Ho, P.M., Masoudi, F.A., Spertus, J.A. *et al.* (2005) Depression predicts mortality following cardiac valve surgery. *Annals of Thoracic Surgery* **79**, 1255-1259.

Kulaylat, M.N., & Doerr, R.J. (2001). Small bowel obstruction. National Center for Biotechnology Information. Online. Available from http://www.ncbi.nlm.nih.gov/bookshelf/br.fcgi?book=surg&part=A918 (accessed 28 March 2012).

National Library of Medicine. National Institutes of Health. Medline plus (2008) Compartment syndrome. Online. Available from http://www.nlm.nih.gov/medlineplus/ency/article/001224.htm (accessed 28 March 2012).

National Library of Medicine. National Institutes of Health. Medline plus (2010a) Prothrombin time. Online. Available from http://www.nlm.nih.gov/medlineplus/ency/article/003652.htm (accessed 28 March 2012).

National Library of Medicine. National Institutes of Health. Medline plus (2010b) Partial thromboplastin time. Online. Available from http://www.nlm.nih.gov/medlineplus/ency/article/003653.htm (accessed 28 March 2012).

National Library of Medicine. National Institutes of Health (2010c) Pneumonia. Medline plus. Online. Available from http://www.nlm.nih.gov/medlineplus/ency/article/000145.htm (accessed 28 March 2012).

Nicks, B.A., McGinnis, H.D., Borron, S.W. & Mégarbane, B. (2010) Lactic acidosis. eMedicine. Online. Available from http://emedicine.medscape.com/article/768159-overview (accessed 28 March 2012).

Further reading

Bratzler, D.W. & Hunt, D.R. (2006) The Surgical Infection Prevention and Surgical Care Improvement Projects: National Initiatives to Improve Outcomes for Patients Having Surgery. Online. Available from http://www.journals.uchicago.edu/doi/pdf/10.1086/505220 (accessed 28 March 2012).

Centers for Disease Control and Prevention (2010) Facts about deep vein thrombosis. Online. Available from http://www.cdc.gov/ncbddd/dvt/facts.html (accessed 28 March 2012).

Peters, M.L. (2010) The older adult in the emergency department: aging and atypical illness presentation. *Journal of Emergency Nursing* **36**(1), 29-34.

Sopena, N., & Sabria, M. (2005) Multicenter study of hospital acquired pneumonia in non-ICU Patients. *Chest* **127**(1), 213-219.

Weitzel, T., Robinson, S., & Holmes, J. (2006) Preventing nosocomial pneumonia: Routine oral care reduced the risk of infection at one facility. *American Journal of Nursing* **106**(9), 72a-72e.

Unit 13: Fluid and Electrolytes

PART 1: DEHYDRATION AND OTHER HYPOVOLEMIC FLUID DISORDERS

Terry Mahan Buttaro

Fluid and electrolyte disorders in older adults are common. Dehydration, also known as hypertonic hypovolemia, is the most common fluid disorder. This disorder is usually related to a fever, but older patients can easily become dehydrated in hot weather or if exercising and not drinking enough fluids. Associated with hypernatremia, the serum sodium is greater than 145 mEq/l and serum osmolality is greater than 295 mOsm/l in patients with dehydration.

There are other causes of fluid losses besides fever, excess heat, and exercise however. Isotonic hypovolemia is associated with vomiting and diarrhea and is characterized by a normal serum osmolality (275-295 mOsm/l) and normal serum sodium (135-145 mEq/l). Hypotonic hypovolemia is associated with diuretic therapy. In hypotonic hypovolemia, the serum sodium is less than 135 mEq/l and the serum osmolality is less than 275 mOsm/l.

Nurses can easily calculate the serum osmolality based on the patient's current serum electrolytes, glucose, and blood urea nitrogen (BUN). Calculated serum osmolality:

$$2 (NA) + serum\ glucose/18 + BUN/2.8.$$

■ Risk factors

- Aging changes:
  - Age >85 years
  - Decreased body water
  - Decreased lean body mass
  - Dietary restrictions
  - Dysphagia
  - Organ changes: heart, lungs, kidneys (i.e., reduced renal sodium and water conservation capacity, decreased glomerular filtration rate [GFR])
- Antidiuretic hormone deficiency
- Comorbid disorders:
  - Central diabetes insipidus
  - Dementia
  - Heart failure
  - Nephrogenic diabetes insipidus
  - Primary aldosteronism
- Cultural and patient preferences
- Deceased oral intake
- Decreased thirst

- Dietary restrictions: low salt or fluid restrictions
- Diuretic and laxative medications
- Excessive IV normal saline
- Fluid restrictions
- High solute tube feedings
- Immobility-inability to reach or drink fluids without assistance
- Impaired cognition
- Increased insensible losses
- Nothing by mouth (NPO) status for diagnostic evaluation

Clinical presentation

Some patients may be asymptomatic despite significant fluid and electrolyte changes. Most often patients become symptomatic once the serum sodium rises above 150 mEq/l. The symptoms are often nonspecific and include:

- Agitation
- Cognitive or functional changes
- Delirium
- Lethargy
- Lightheadedness
- Muscle twitching
- Personality changes
- Polyuria
- Seizures

Nursing assessment

Determining the history of the present illness is essential, though if the elder is confused, the history might be obtained from a family member or caregiver. Questions might include:

Has the elder had pain or been ill with nausea, vomiting, or diarrhea?

Is the patient taking diuretics? Antibiotics?

Was the patient drinking fluids? Last oral intake? Last void and bowel movement?

The patient's past medical history, allergies, and current medications are also necessary to determine the cause of the patient's symptoms.

Assessment of the patient's weight (noting any weight loss), vital signs, and appearance is of utmost importance. A focused exam may reveal some of the following changes.

- Vital signs:
  - Fever
  - Hypotension, postural changes:
    - Blood pressure should be checked lying, sitting, and standing within 3 to 5 minutes and with 3 to 5 minute intervals between positions.

A 20 mmHg drop in systolic blood pressure is positive for orthostatic hypotension, though older patients may be symptomatic (i.e., light-headed, dizzy) with a smaller drop in blood pressure.

- Tachycardia
- Recent weight loss
- Cognitive changes:
  - Agitated, confused, delirious, or lethargic
- Skin:
  - Poor skin turgor
  - Temporal wasting
- Mucous membranes (dried, cracked)
- Cardiac:
  - Flattened neck veins
  - Tachycardia
- Respiratory rate may be normal or increased.
- Abdomen: may be normal depending on cause of patient illness. Examine for presence and quality of bowel sounds as well as tenderness, rebound, or guarding.
- Genitourinary:
  - Diminished urinary output or polyuria, if diabetes insipidus or osmotic diuresis
- Hyperreflexia, muscle twitching, seizures, or spasticity

■ Diagnostics

The history and physical examination determine which diagnostics will be helpful. Serum electrolytes, glucose, BUN, and creatinine are absolutely necessary to determine fluid and electrolyte status and calculate the serum osmolality (see above).

Other diagnostics may include:

- Complete blood count (CBC) with differential
- Urine:
  - Urine volume: hourly and daily urine output
  - Urinalysis and urine culture and sensitivity (C&S) if suspected urinary tract infection (UTI) (frequent cause of dehydration in older adults)
  - Urine sodium:
    - <25 mEq/l = volume depletion associated with water loss
    - >100 mEq/l = excessive oral or intravenous sodium intake
  - Urine osmolality:
    - Urine osmolality < serum osmolality indicates possible diabetes insipidus.
    - Urine osmolality >200 mOsm/kg suggests hypovolemic dehydration.
  - Urine specific gravity (SG)
    - Normal urine SG:
      - 1.020 to 1.028
      - Elevated urine SG >1.035 = severe dehydration

- Decreased urine SG <1.005 suggests diabetes mellitus, diabetes insipidus, excessive water intake or renal disease (e.g., acute tubular necrosis, glomerulonephritis, and pyelonephritis).

Imaging may be necessary in some instances, but will depend on patient history.

◼ Differential diagnosis

The differential diagnosis is concerned with determining the cause of the patient's dehydration.

◼ Treatment

Treatment is based on identifying the cause of the dehydration (e.g., does the patient have an infection or is there another cause of the hypovolemia). Additionally, the patient's fluid and electrolyte balance need to be restored to normal, though caution is necessary to prevent too quickly a return to the patient's normal fluid and electrolyte status. To do this the physician will calculate the patient's fluid deficit and replace the fluid deficit and patient's ongoing fluid and insensible losses over 48 to 72 hours; only half the fluid deficit is corrected in the first 24 hours.

Oral rehydration is the safest way of restoring an older patient's fluid losses, though this is not always possible as the patient may be hypovolemic (hypotensive) and/or unable to drink fluids. Sometimes, fluid replacement with free water via a nasogastric tube is used for rehydration. Intravenous fluid resuscitation with 0.9% N/S may be indicated until the patient's blood pressure is restored to normal levels. Then, a hypotonic solution (D5W or 0.45% N/S) is usually indicated for 24 hours. Frequent evaluation of the serum sodium is necessary as serum sodium cannot be corrected more than 0.5 mEq/hour with hypotonic intravenous fluids or cerebral edema can occur. Other treatment modalities may include:

- Treat underlying cause (e.g., bowel obstruction, infection, diabetes insipidus, etc.).
- Medications such as diuretic and laxatives should be reviewed with the physician to determine if they should be held or discontinued until homeostasis is achieved.
- Sodium restricted diet, if indicated
- Calculating fluid deficit in older adults:

$$0.45 \times (\text{current weight in kg}) \times \left(\left[\frac{\text{serum Na}}{140} \right] - 1 \right)$$

◼ Collaborative consultation

The physician should always be contacted when the nurse notices a change in a patient's cognitive or functional status or other concerning change in patient status. Awareness of weight changes, vital signs, hourly urine output and, when possible, the patient's intake and output over the last three days will guide treatment of the underlying disorder.

The registered dietician should be consulted for a diet and fluid review.

■ Complications

- Arrhythmias
- Cerebral edema if fluid balance is corrected too quickly
- Coma
- Death
- Falls
- Hypovolemic shock
- Kidney failure
- Permanent neurologic deficits
- Seizures

■ Prevention

- Monitor patient cognitive and functional changes as these may be first signs of dehydration.
- Monitor daily fluid and electrolytes.
  - Most patients need approximately 2000 milliliters PO daily though elders rarely drink this much and some patients do require fluid restrictions.
  - Review patient intake and output over three days to assess fluid status and discuss potential fluid deficit with physician.
- Monitor fluid resuscitation carefully to be certain that hypernatremia is not corrected too quickly.
- Include adequate daily fluid intake in the nursing care plan.
- Avoid prolonged periods of NPO.
- Consider individual and patient preferences when offering food and fluids.
- Offer small amounts of oral fluids frequently.
- Consider patient inability to ask for fluids or drink without assistance.
- Provide mouth care for all patients at least twice a day, but more frequently for patients with dehydration.

■ Patient/family education

- Explain the cause and treatment of the disorder to the patient, family, and caregivers.
- Prior to discharge, discuss preventive measures to avoid future episodes of dehydration (e.g., adequate fluid intake).
- Explain that older adults often lose their thirst sensation and therefore may not think to drink fluids as frequently as they should. Some patients may need to consume fluids on a regularly scheduled basis.

Further reading

Buttaro, T.M. (2012) Hypernatremia and hyponatremia. In: Buttaro, T.M., Trybulski, J., Polgar-Bailey, P.P. & Sandberg-Cook, J. (eds) *Primary Care: A Collaborative Practice*, 4th edition. Mosby, St. Louis.

Buttaro, T.M., Aznavorian, S. & Dick, K. (2006) Fluid and electrolyte disorders. In: Buttaro, T.M., Aznavorian, S. & Dick, K. (eds) *Clinical Management of Patients in Sub-Acute and Long-Term Care Settings*. Mosby, St. Louis.

Leeuwen, A.M. & Poelhuis-Leth, D.J. (2009) *Davis's Comprehensive Handbook of Laboratory and Diagnostic Tests with Nursing Implications*. F.A. Davis Company, Philadelphia.

Philips, L.D. (2010) *Manual of IV Therapeutics: Evidenced-Based Practice for Infusion Therapy*, 5th edition. F.A. Davis Company, Philadelphia.

Tareen, N., Martins, D., Nagami, G. *et al.* (2005) Sodium disorders in the elderly. *Journal of the National Medical Association* **97**(2), 217–224.

PART 2: HYPERCALCEMIA AND HYPOCALCEMIA

Nancy A. Kelly

Extracellular fluid calcium levels play an important role in cellular function, neuromuscular signaling, cardiac contractility, hormone secretion, blood coagulation with the conversion of prothrombin to thrombin, and proper functioning of ion channels of the neurological presynaptic membrane and neurotransmitter release (Kee, 2004). Hypercalcemia can be life threatening due to decreased neuromuscular excitability and risk for cardiac arrhythmias. Hypocalcemia increases the excitability of nerve and muscle membranes leading to skeletal muscle spasms. Normal calcium levels are maintained by mechanisms involving parathyroid hormone (PTH) and vitamin D metabolite (1,25-dihydroxyvitamin D) through signaling mechanisms involving the parathyroid gland, kidney, small intestine, and bone. The mechanisms for calcium regulation require multiple signaling steps (Table 3.13.2.1), which collectively lead to normal calcium levels (Sundeep, 2008).

Hypercalcemia and hypocalcemia are diagnosed by measurement of serum calcium levels. Approximately 40%–45% of calcium is bound to albumin. Ionized calcium is the physiologically active form of calcium, and is not influenced by protein concentrations, renal failure, nephrotic syndrome, multiple myeloma or malabsorption. If calcium levels are abnormal, albumin levels should be obtained to determine if the calcium defect is related to an abnormal albumin level. Calcium levels can be corrected for albumin (Box 3.13.2.1). Alternatively, the ionized calcium level may be checked, and may be more accurate.

The cause of hypercalcemia or hypocalcemia is determined through evaluation of factors involved in the regulatory process for maintaining normal

Table 3.13.2.1 Examples of the multiple signaling steps for calcium regulation.

Low ECF calcium →
Increase PTH secretion →
Increase tubular renal reabsorption of calcium with decreased renal calcium excretion →
Increase bone resorption of calcium →
Increase renal production of vitamin D 1,25(OH$_2$) →
Increase intestinal absorption of calcium →
Normal ECF calcium

High ECF calcium →
Decrease PTH secretion →
Decrease tubular renal reabsorption of calcium with increased renal calcium excretions →
Decrease bone resorption of calcium →
Decrease renal production of vitamin D 1,25(OH$_2$) →
Decrease intestinal absorption of calcium →
Normal ECF calcium

Box 3.13.2.1   Calcium correction for albumin formula

Observed calcium (mg/dl) + 0.8×[(normal albumin − observed albumin (g/dl))] = corrected calcium
Normal albumin = 4 g/dl

calcium levels. Laboratory testing for diagnosis of the primary cause of hyper- or hypocalcemia is imperative for appropriate treatment.

■ Risk factors

Older adults and people with abnormal renal function are at higher risk for hypercalcemia due to changes in glomerular filtration rate (GFR). When GFR falls below 60 milliliters per minute, PTH may not be fully excreted leading to hypercalcemia. All persons with impaired renal function should have calcium levels monitored (Patel & Wiggins, 2007). Hypercalcemia is also associated with hyperparathyroidism, hyperthyroidism, malignancy, milk alkali syndrome (a condition in which there are high levels of calcium and a shift towards metabolic alkalosis caused by drinking too much milk (which is high in calcium) and taking certain antacids, especially calcium carbonate or sodium bicarbonate (baking soda), over a long period of time), medications (e.g., thiazide diuretics, calcium, and vitamin D), and prolonged periods of immobility.

Elders who have limited exposure to sunlight are at higher risk for vitamin D deficiency and associated hypocalcemia. Also, poor dietary intake of calcium, history of small bowel surgery or malabsorption, and renal failure increase the risk for hypocalcemia.

▪ Clinical presentation

Hypercalcemia

Patients with mild hypercalcemia (calcium levels 11–11.5 mg/dl) may be asymptomatic, and the diagnosis based on routine laboratory evaluation. Other symptoms and medical problems associated with hypercalcemia may include:

- Poor concentration
- Change in personality
- Depression
- Gastroesophageal reflux
- Decreased peristalsis: hypoactive or absent bowel sounds
- Nephrolithiasis

Severe hypercalcemia (calcium levels over 12 mg/dl) symptoms may include:

- Lethargy
- Coma
- Nausea, vomiting
- Anorexia
- Constipation
- Abdominal pain
- Nocturia, polyuria, polydipsia
- Bone pain or fracture
- Electrocardiogram changes including bradycardia, atrioventricular block (AV block), shortened QT interval, cardiac arrest (Malabanan, 2012)
- Pancreatitis

Hypocalcemia

- Fatigue
- Change in mental status
- Muscle weakness and cramps (Malabanan, 2012)
- Spasms of skeletal muscles causing cramps or tetany
- Bronchospasm, laryngospasm with stridor
- Seizures
- Parathesia of the lips and extremities
- Increased peristalsis: hyperactive bowel sounds, diarrhea, abdominal cramping
- Associated hyperphosphatemia and/or hypomagnesia
- Electrocardiogram changes including bradycardia, prolongation of QT interval
- Cataracts

▪ Nursing assessment

Though the patient with hypocalcemia or hypercalcemia may be asymptomatic, the patient history is always important and often can help explain the cause of the disorder. A thorough medication and dietary review including over the counter medications (e.g., TUMS) is always helpful. The physical assessment for these disorders includes the following:

Hypercalcemia
- Determine patient's baseline mental status.
- Cardiac assessment: assess blood pressure and pulse.
- Cardiac monitoring: monitor for bradycardia, AV block, and shortened QT interval.
- During the abdominal exam note if the abdomen is soft, firm, or distended. Determine if bowel sounds are present in all four quadrants. Note the quality of bowel sounds (tinkling or diminished). Note any tympany or dullness with percussion. Determine if there is abdominal tenderness and its location.
- Monitor intake and output. Strain urine if nephrolithiasis suspected.

Hypocalcemia
- Determine dietary history: intake of calcium-containing foods and supplements.
- Assess for parathesia, muscle twitching, cramps, and spasms.
- Cardiac monitoring: monitor for bradycardia and prolonged QT interval.
- During the abdominal exam note if the abdomen is soft, firm, or distended. Determine if bowel sounds are present in all 4 quadrants. Note the quality of bowel sounds (tinkling or diminished). Note any tympany or dullness with percussion. Determine if there is abdominal tenderness and its location.
- Chvostek's sign. Tested by tapping the facial nerve, anterior to the ear, that causes contraction of the facial muscle
- Trousseau's sign. Tested by occluding the brachial artery for 3 minutes with a blood pressure cuff that causes carpal spasm

▧ Diagnostics
Calcium levels should be routinely monitored for patients with renal insufficiency or renal failure, and in patients who have cancer. If the serum calcium is abnormal, further evaluation for the cause should focus on the underlying etiology of the abnormality. Laboratory testing may include:

- Ionized calcium
- Serum albumin
- Vitamin D25OH
- Renal function (Blood urea nitrogen (BUN), creatinine, GFR)
- Intact PTH:
  - Suppressed PTH suggests a non-parathyroid mediated cause of hypercalcemia. Most commonly seen with non-parathyroid malignancy.
  - Increased PTH with hypophosphatemia is suggestive of renal impairment with lack of renal clearance of PTH; or, familial hypocalciuric hypercalcemia (FHH).
- Phosphorus, which is inversely related to calcium level

- Magnesium
- Thyroid function
- Cortisol level
- Parathyroid related peptide (PTHrp) which is elevated in skeletal malignancy but normal in hyperparathyroidism
- Electrocardiogram to assess impact of hyper/hypocalcemia on cardiac status
- Radiological exams to evaluate for lytic skeletal lesions

■ Differential diagnosis

The underlying cause of hypercalcemia/hypocalcemia must be determined for proper treatment as the primary cause of calcium deregulation guides treatment.

Hypercalcemia

- Primary hyperparathyroidism due to parathyroid malignancy, adenoma, or hyperplasia, causing elevated parathyroid hormone. This is the most common cause of hypercalcemia (Sundeep, 2008; Malabanan, 2012).
- Malignancy, particularly skeletal lytic lesions (Malabanan, 2012)
- FHH leading to impaired calcium level sensing by parathyroid and kidney
- Tertiary hyperparathyroidism caused by long-term stimulation of PTH due to renal insufficiency
- Excessive 1,25 vitamin D production, which may occur with lymphoma, sarcoidosis, tuberculosis, silicosis, vitamin D intoxication
- Primary bone resorption related to hyperthyroidism, or immobility
- Excessive calcium intake in diet, total parental nutrition, or milk alkali syndrome (Malabanan, 2012)
- Endocrine disorders such as adrenal insufficiency and pheochromocytoma
- Medications such as thiazides, vitamin A, antiestrogens, and lithium (Sundeep, 2008)

Hypocalcemia

- Renal failure due to *decreased production* of vitamin D3 and hyperphosphatemia (Fukawa *et al.*, 2006)
- Decreased calcium intake or absorption related to small bowel bypass or vitamin D deficiency
- Increased calcium losses due to alcoholism, renal failure, or loop diuretics
- Alkalosis increases calcium binding to protein leading to lower ionized calcium (Metheny, 1996).
- Endocrine disease:
  - Hypoparathyroidism
  - Pseudohypoparathyroidism due to renal resistance to PTH and PTH receptor mutations
  - Thyroid malignancy which releases calcitonin leading to calcium return to bone
  - Familial hypocalcemia
- Acute pancreatitis associated hypocalcemia occurs in 40-75% of patients with acute pancreatitis (Fernandez & Kerman, 2012; Metheny, 1996). Acute

pancreatitis causes release of proteolytic and lipolytic enzymes leading to release of fatty acids through lyposis which bind to calcium ions decreasing the serum calcium concentration. Also, there may be inadequate PTH response to the hypocalcemia caused by acute pancreatitis.

■ Treatment

Hypercalcemia

- Mild asymptomatic hypercalcemia (calcium level less than 11.5 mg/dl) may only require evaluation and treatment of the underlying cause of hypercalcemia.
- Mild persistent asymptomatic hypercalcemia (calcium levels greater than 10.5 mg/dl) may require endocrine and oncology evaluation (Fukagawa *et al.*, 2006; Malabanan, 2012).
- Symptomatic hypercalcemia requires urgent assessment and treatment of the underlying disorder. Additional interventions include:
  - Hydration with intravenous normal saline to increase renal excretion of calcium. Sodium and calcium are excreted in the loop of Henle. Loop diuretics may be given simultaneously to enhance calcium excretion. Large volumes of intravenous fluids should be used cautiously for patients with congestive heart failure or who are at risk for volume overload; these patients may require loop diuretics.
  - Zoledronic acid may be given for patients with skeletal malignancy associated hypercalcemia to inhibit bone resorption of calcium.
  - Glucocorticoids may be given for patients with excessive vitamin 1,25D mediated hypercalcemia to decrease production of vitamin 1,25D.
- Nursing interventions include:
  - Monitor calcium level. Patients who are taking thiazide diuretics, lithium, high doses of vitamin A or D, and/or calcium carbonate are at higher risk for hypercalcemia.
  - Obtain EKG to monitor for shortened QT interval.
  - Encourage oral fluids to prevent dehydration related to hypercalcemia. If signs and symptoms of dehydration are present, discuss with medical providers.
  - Encourage mobility to decrease bone loss of calcium. If a patient is bed-bound, obtain physical therapy evaluation for range of motion activities.
  - Prevent falls due to risk for fracture if there has been long-term hypercalcemia that may cause changes in bone structure.
  - Low calcium diet
  - Digoxin levels should be monitored as there is an increase risk for Digoxin toxicity with hypercalcemia.

Hypocalcemia

- Intravenous calcium gluconate diluted in dextrose is given intravenously. Calcium gluconate should not be diluted in normal saline because saline increases renal excretion of calcium (Kee, 2004).

- Intravenous calcium is given slowly to prevent hypotension, bradycardia or other cardiac arrhythmia.
- Calcium chloride is not given intravenous due to high risk of tissue sloughing if there is infiltration of calcium chloride into the subcutaneous tissue.
- Oral calcium with vitamin D
- Treatment of other abnormal electrolytes may influence calcium levels.
- Nursing interventions include:
  - Monitor calcium level. In particular, patients with malabsorption, poor nutrition, and/or receiving loop diuretics, are at higher risk for hypocalcemia.
  - Obtain EKG to monitor for prolonged QT interval.
  - When administering intravenous calcium gluconate, use dextrose as diluant and administer calcium gluconate slowly (Kee, 2004).
  - Give oral calcium one hour before meals to enhance calcium absorption.

■ Collaborative consultation

- Discuss changes in mental status and inability to maintain oral hydration or oral medications with collaborating medical providers to determine treatment plan.
- Discuss Physical Therapy consultation if patients are immobile or at risk for falls.
- Develop a treatment plan for associated symptoms of hyper/hypocalcemia such as treatment of constipation or bone pain.

■ Complications

Hypercalcemia
- Bone pain and/or fractures
- Cardiac arrhythmia including bradycardia, AV block, and shortened QT interval
- Dehydration and azotemia
- Mental status changes
- Nausea, anorexia
- Nephrolithiasis
- Pancreatitis
- Peptic ulcer disease

Hypocalcemia
- Abdominal pain
- Cataracts
- Laryngospasm with stridor
- Muscle spasms and/or tetany
- Seizures

■ Prevention

Hypercalcemia

Patients with renal failure, immobility, or malignancy should be followed for hypercalcemia. Patients with prolonged hypercalcemia and patients with skeletal bone malignancy are at higher risk for bone fracture due to changes in the bone structure. Fall prevention for these patients is important due to the higher risk for fractures. Older adults are particularly at risk for falls due to age related changes in balance, and comorbities that increase fall risk.

Patients with prolonged immobility should have exercises such as range of motion activities to decrease calcium loss from bones and risk for hypercalcemia.

Hypocalcemia

Patients who have a history of small bowel bypass surgery, malabsorption, or risk for vitamin D deficiency should be followed for hypocalcemia.

■ Patient/family education

Hypercalcemia

- Diet should be low in calcium with liberal fluid intake to 2 liters per day.
- Regular activity is important to maintain bone health, decrease risk for calcium loss from bone, and decrease risk for falls and fracture.
- Changes in mental status should be immediately reported to health care providers.
- Thiazide diuretics, vitamin A supplements, and antiestrogen medication increase calcium levels.

Hypocalcemia

- Diet should contain calcium rich foods, and alcohol should be avoided.
- Muscle cramping or spasm should be immediately reported to health care providers.
- Loop diuretics should be avoided as they increase the risk for calcium loss.
- Calcium carbonate supplements should include vitamin D and be taken 1 hour before meals to improve absorption; gastric acid secretion is required for optimal absorption.
  - Calcium citrate preparations do not require gastric acid for absorption.
  - Large doses of oral calcium carbonate have unpredictable absorption related to neutralizing effects on gastric acid, and divided smaller doses are recommended.

References

Fernandez, H.J. & Kerman, D. (2012) Pancreatitis. In: Buttaro, T.M., Trybulski, J., Bailey, P.P. & Sandberg-Cook, J. (eds). *Primary Care: A Collaborative Practice.* Mosby, St. Louis.

Fukagawa, M., Kurokawa, K. & Papadakis, M.A. (2006) Hypocalcemia. In: Papadakis M. & McPhee S. (eds) *Current Concepts of Medicine*. McGraw Hill, New York.

Kee, J. (2004) Calcium balance. In: Kee, J., Paulanka, R.B. & Purnell, L. (eds) *Fluids and Electrolytes with Clinical Applications*, *A Programmed Approach*, 7th edition. Delmar Cengage Learning, Florence, KY.

Malabanan, A. (2012) Hypercalcemia and hypocalcemia. In: Buttaro, T.M., Trybulski, J., Bailey, P.P. Sandberg-Cook, J. (eds) *Primary Care: A Collaborative Practice*. Mosby, St. Louis.

Malone, M.L. (eds) *Practice of Geriatrics*, 4th edition. Saunders Elsevier, Philadelphia.

Metheny, N.M. (1996) Calcium imbalances. In: Metheny, N.M., Stead, L., Vaugh, C. *et al.* (eds) *Fluid and Electrolyte Balance: Nursing Considerations*, 7th edition. Lippincott, Williams & Wilkins, Philadelphia.

Patel, S.J. & Wiggins, J. (2007) Renal and electrolyte disorders. In: Duthie, E.H., Katz, P.R. & Malone, M.L. (eds) *Practice of Geriatrics*, 4th edition. Saunders Elsevier, Philadelphia.

Sundeep, K. (2008) Hypercalcemia and hypocalcemia. In: Fauci, A.S., Braunwald, E., Kasper, D.L. *et al.* (eds) *Harrison's Principles of Internal Medicine*. McGraw Hill, New York.

PART 3: HYPERKALEMIA AND HYPOKALEMIA

Grace A. Good

Potassium is critical for the normal functioning of the muscles, heart, and nerves. It plays an important role in controlling activity of smooth muscle (such as muscles found in the digestive tract) and skeletal muscle (muscles of the extremities and torso), as well as the muscles of the heart. It is also important for normal transmission of electrical signals throughout the nervous system within the body. Normal blood levels of potassium are critical for maintaining normal heart electrical rhythm. Both low blood potassium levels (hypokalemia) and high blood potassium levels (hyperkalemia) can lead to abnormal heart rhythms (Elliot *et al.*, 2010; Whelan, 2012).

Depending on the laboratory the normal value assigned to potassium is 3.5 to 5.0 mEq/l.

Hypokalemia is a condition that is present when the blood level of potassium is abnormally low.

- Mild to moderate hypokalemia is present when blood serum levels of potassium are 3 to 3.5 mEq/l.
- Severe hypokalemia is present when serum levels fall below 3 mEq/l.

Hyperkalemia is defined as a potassium level greater than 5.5 mEq/l. Potassium levels greater than 5.5 mEq/l require attention; levels greater than 6 mEq/l require urgent medical intervention (Elliot *et al.*, 2010).

Hypokalemia and hyperkalemia are common findings in hospitalized patients (Elliot *et al.*, 2010; Lippi *et al.*, 2010). Older adults are especially prone to developing hypokalemia and hyperkalemia due to age related reduction in kidney function and the number of medications effecting potassium levels that the elder may be taking. Salt substitutes, consisting primarily of potassium chloride, represent an unintended source of exogenous potassium and are often recommended in older persons with hypertension or heart disease to decrease sodium. These salt substitutes may be an unintentional cause of hyperkalemia (Zarowitz & Lefkovitz, 2008). There are hereditary skeletal muscle diseases that can also affect potassium levels (i.e., primary hyperkalemic periodic paralysis and primary hypokalemic periodic paralysis) (Amato & Brown, 2012).

The serum potassium concentration is determined by the relationship between potassium intake, the distribution of potassium between the cells and the extracellular fluid, and the urinary potassium excretion. Normally, dietary potassium is largely excreted in the urine.

Kidneys adapt to acute and chronic alterations in potassium intake. When potassium intake is chronically high, potassium excretion also is increased. In the absence of potassium intake, obligatory renal losses are 10–15 mEq/day. Thus, chronic losses occur in the absence of any ingested potassium. The kidney maintains a central role in the maintenance of potassium homeostasis, even in the setting of chronic renal failure. Renal adaptive mechanisms allow the kidneys to maintain potassium homeostasis until the glomerular filtration rate drops to less than 15–20 ml/min.

■ Risk factors

Hyperkalemia
- Adrenal insufficiency
- Cancer
- Decreased renal excretion of potassium: renal insufficiency
- Diabetes
- Extremes of life: Premature infants and older adults
- Excessive intake of potassium: uncommon cause
- Gender: male
- Genitourinary disease
- Impaired responsiveness of the distal tubule to aldosterone
- Intracellular to extracellular space shift, an uncommon cause
- Medications:
  - Angiotensin-converting enzyme (ACE) inhibitors
  - Potassium-sparing diuretics
  - Nonsteroidal anti-inflammatory drugs (NSAIDs)
- Polypharmacy
- Pseudohyperkalemia:
  - Traumatic venipuncture
  - Venipuncture from a vein where intravenous potassium is currently being infused
  - Leukocytosis
  - Thrombosis

Hypokalemia

- Acute increase in hematopoietic cell production
- Barium intoxication resulting from ingestion of contaminated foods.
- Cushing's syndrome
- Decreased potassium intake
- Diarrhea
- Diuretic use
- Excessive licorice ingestion
- Hypothermia
- Increased availability of insulin
- Increased sweating
- Liddle's syndrome
- Medications:
  - Chloroquine intoxication
  - Diuretics that act proximal to the potassium secretory site
  - Risperidone
  - Quetiapine
  - Cesium
  - Amphotericin B
- Metabolic acidosis
- Polyuria
- Respiratory acidosis
- Stress-induced release of epinephrine (adrenaline)
- Vomiting

■ Clinical presentation

Hyperkalemia can be asymptomatic, meaning that some patients will not experience symptoms. Sometimes, patients with hyperkalemia report vague symptoms including nausea, fatigue, muscle weakness, or tingling sensations. More serious symptoms of hyperkalemia include bradycardia and a weak pulse. Severe hyperkalemia can result in fatal cardiac standstill (Hollander-Rodriquez & Calvert, 2005). Generally, a slow rising potassium level (e.g., with chronic kidney failure) is better tolerated than an abrupt rise in potassium levels. Unless the rise in potassium has been very rapid, symptoms of the hyperkalemia are usually not apparent until potassium levels are typically 7.0 mEq/l or higher. Symptoms may also be related to the disorder causing the hyperkalemia.

Signs and symptoms of hypokalemia tend to be related to the degree and duration of the condition and include severe muscle weakness or paralysis, cardiac arrhythmias and electrocardiogram (ECG) abnormalities, rhabdomyolysis, and renal abnormalities.

Patients may not be symptomatic and signs of hypokalemia may not be apparent until the serum potassium is below 3.0 mEq/l unless the serum potassium falls rapidly or the patient has a potentiating factor such as a predisposition to arrhythmia due to the use of digitalis. Symptoms usually resolve with the correction of the hypokalemia.

▪ Nursing assessment

Careful attention should be given to the patient's history, as causes of hypokalemia and hyperkalemia may be discovered. Pertinent information should include:

- Medication review
  - Hyperkalemia is associated with NSAIDs, ACE inhibitors, amiloride, azole antifungals, beta-blockers, heparin, penicillin, trimethoprim-sulfamethoxazole, spironolactone, potassium supplements, and some herbal products.
  - Hypokalemia may be related to some antibiotics and non-potassium-sparing diuretics.
- Nutrition history
  - Hypokalemia: alcohol ingestion
  - Excessive licorice ingestion
- Past medical history of hypokalemia and hyperkalemia, as well as existing conditions that could contribute to potassium disturbances (e.g., Bartter syndrome, bulimia, Cushing syndrome, diarrhea, Fanconi syndrome, Liddle syndrome, hyperaldosteronism, vomiting, and certain antibiotics [amphotericin B, carbenicillin, and gentamicin]).

The physical examination should be done with careful attention to even vague complaints, as findings may be subtle, depending on the severity of the potassium level.

- Vital signs: assess hemodynamic instability
- Cardiac examination:
  - Hyperkalemia: evaluate ECG for peaked T waves, PR interval and QRS widening, atrioventricular block (AVB), and bundle branch block.
  - Hypokalemia: evaluate ECG for sinus bradycardia, premature atrial contractions, premature ventricular contractions, paroxysmal atrial tachycardia, AVB, U waves, prolonged QT interval, ventricular tachycardia, and ventricular fibrillation.
- Neurological examination:
  - Hyperkalemia: may reveal muscle weakness, tingling, and in severe cases, paralysis.
  - Hypokalemia: may reveal muscle weakness.
- It is essential that nurses monitor kidney function, but particularly so in older adults because kidney function begins to diminish after age 40. Daily awareness of a patient's BUN, creatinine, and glomerular filtration rate (GFR) is essential not only to prevent potassium disorders but also to assure proper renal dosing for all medications.
  - Hyperkalemia: check BUN/Cr, GFR, assess for signs of edema.
  - Hypokalemia: check BUN/Cr, GFR.

■ Diagnostics

Hyperkalemia

The history and physical exam directs diagnostic testing. Initially, the serum potassium is immediately rechecked to be certain the serum potassium is not related to a laboratory error, traumatic venipuncture, or other cause of falsely elevated potassium. Additionally, the patient's medications are reviewed to determine if there is a history of medications associated with hyperkalemia such as angiotensin-converting enzyme inhibitors, Bactrim, heparin and beta-blockers, and conditions associated with hyperkalemia.

- Rechecking potassium level is recommended because of potentially falsely elevated potassium levels.
- Laboratory:
  - serum potassium level
  - BUN/Cr

Other potential diagnostics include:

- Serum glucose
- If indicated: digoxin level
- Arterial blood gases (ABG)
- Aldosterone level
- ACTH cosyntropin stimulation test
- 24 hour urine for creatinine clearance
- 12 lead ECG for changes or arrhythmias; continuous cardiac monitoring may be required.

Hypokalemia

Review history and physical examination to determine if the patient is taking medications such as non-potassium sparring diuretics and beta-adrenergic agonists, or has a past medical history conditions associated with hypokalemia.

Laboratory tests for:

- Serum electrolytes, focusing on the potassium
- BUN/creatinine
- Serum glucose
- Serum magnesium
- Urinary potassium
- If indicated: 24 hour urine collection for potassium
- Urine osmolality
- Plasma rennin
- Plasma aldosterone
- Arterial blood gases
- 12 lead EKG for changes or arrhythmias. Continuous cardiac monitoring may be necessary.

■ Differential diagnosis

Abnormal potassium levels should always be rechecked to rule out incorrectly reported results. Further differential diagnosis is concerned with the cause of the altered potassium.

Hyperkalemia

- Medications: ACE inhibitors, NSAIDs, ARBs, potassium sparing diuretics, potassium supplements
- Pseudohyperkalemia
- Acute or chronic renal disease
- Addison's disease
- Rhabdomyolysis
- Severe burns or trauma

Hypokalemia

- Medications: antibiotics (penicillin and some other cillins, gentamicin); antifungals (amphotericin B); antivirals (foscarnet); diuretics; laxatives
- Vomiting, diarrhea
- Eating disorder
- Chronic renal disease
- Primary aldosteronism
- Bartter syndrome
- Fanconi syndrome
- Liddle syndrome
- Cushing syndrome
- Magnesium deficiency
- Licorice (large amount)

■ Treatment

It is important to determine the underlying cause of the potassium disturbance (i.e., hyperkalemia or hypokalemia) and treat the cause of potassium disturbance accordingly. Whether treating hypokalemia or hyperkalemia, repeat potassium levels should be checked frequently (i.e., every 1-2 hours) until a normal serum potassium level is obtained and maintained (Elliot *et al.*, 2010).

- The severity of the potassium excess or deficit will help determine the treatment.

Hyperkalemia

Determine and validate the serum potassium to determine the appropriate intervention as improper handling of blood samples and traumatic venipuncture can result in elevated serum potassium.

- Obtain ECG to assess cardiac changes.
- Acute, severe hyperkalemia should be treated quickly. If the hyperkalemia is life-threatening and hyperkalemic ECG changes are present, calcium gluconate 1 gram intravenously is the initial treatment of choice (Elliot et al., 2010). Intravenous glucose combined with intravenous regular (short-acting) insulin and nebulized beta agonist therapy (i.e., salbutamol 10 milligrams) is another option (Elliot et al., 2010). Hemodialysis and rarely sodium bicarbonate, are recommended treatments in specific situations (Elliot et al., 2010).
- Less severe levels of hyperkalemia could be treated with albuterol nebulizer treatments, diuretic therapy, or Kayexalate.
- Hold or discontinue medications that may have caused or contributed to hyperkalemia (e.g., NSAIDs, potassium supplements, ACEIs/ARBs, aldosterone antagonists, potassium-sparing diuretics, beta-blockers, heparin, digoxin toxicity, and Bactrim) (Zarowitz & Lefovitz, 2008).

Hypokalemia

Severe hypokalemia should be treated with an intravenous potassium chloride infusion. The potassium fluid concentration will be determined by hospital policy and the type of intravenous access available. The rate is usually 10 mEq per hour. *IV potassium is NEVER given by IV push.*

Less severe hypokalemia could be treated with oral potassium supplementation. The dose will depend on the serum potassium level.

■ Collaborative consultation

Discussion with a physician is essential. The physician may elect to consult a nephrologist or pharmacist.

■ Complications

Potassium abnormalities are potentially life threatening. Cardiac conduction defects, arrhythmias, metabolic alkalosis, constipation, ileus, paralysis, muscle weakness, increased blood pressure, and renal injury are consequences of hypokalemia. Hyperkalemia also causes cardiac arrhythmias, as well as heart block, ventricular fibrillation, muscle weakness, and paralysis (Whelan, 2012).

■ Prevention

Obtaining a careful health history, serial serum monitoring of potassium levels, especially when the patient is taking medications that potentially alter serum potassium levels, and awareness of a condition that can alter serum potassium levels are essential components of patient safety and nursing care.

■ Patient/family education

- Patient education for hypokalemia or hyperkalemia should center on diet education and awareness of the importance of continued chronic supplementation therapy and laboratory monitoring.

- Education regarding potential drug effects causing hypokalemia or hyperkalemia is also important.
- Patients need to understand that chronic laxative use should be avoided, since this has been associated with potassium loss. Patients with chronic hypokalemia should avoid large amounts of licorice, since licorice has also been associated with hypokalemia.
- Patients taking potassium supplements should be advised not to crush the potassium tablets and also to swallow the tablet with a large glass of fluid.
- If untoward effects of potassium occur, the patient/family should be advised to call or see a primary care provider (Whelan, 2012).

References

Amato A.A. & Brown, R.H. (2012) Chapter 387. Muscular dystrophies and other muscle diseases. In *Harrison's Principles of Internal Medicine*, 18th edition (Longo, D.L., Fauci, A.S., Kasper, D.L., Hauser, S.L., Jameson, J.L., Loscalzo, J. eds), Online. Available from http://0-www.accessmedicine.com.library.simmons.edu/content.aspx?aID=9148971 (accessed 10 June 2012).

Elliott, M.J., Ronksley, P.E., Clase, C.M., Ahmed, S.B. & Hemmelgarn, B.R. (2010) Management of patients with acute hyperkalemia. *CMAJ* **182**(15), 1631-1635.

Hollander-Rodriquez, J.C., & Calvert, J.F. (2005) Hyperkalemia. *American Family Physician* **73**(2), 283-290.

Lippi, G., Favaloro, E.J., Montagnana, M. & Guidi, G.C. (2010) Prevalence of hypokalaemia: the experience of a large academic hospital. *Internal Medicine Journal* **40**(4), 315-316.

Whelan, C. (2012) Hypokalemia and hyperkalemia. In: Buttaro, T.M., Trybulski, J., Bailey, P. & Sandberg-Cook, J. (eds) *Primary Care: A Collaborative Practice*, 4th edition. Mosby, St. Louis.

Zarowitz, B.J. & Lefkovitz, A. (2008) Recognition and treatment of hyperkalemia. *Geriatric Nursing* **9**(5), 333-339.

Further reading

Harvey, S. & Jordan, S. (2010) Diuretic therapy: Implications for nursing practice. *Nursing Standard* **24**(43), 40-50.

PART 4: HYPONATREMIA AND HYPERNATREMIA

Grace A. Good

Hyponatremia

Hyponatremia is an acute or chronic electrolyte disorder identified by a serum sodium concentration below <135 mEq/l. There may be no signs or symptoms of hyponatremia present until the sodium level falls below 125 mEq/l. As the sodium level decreases, there is increased risk of adverse outcomes, including longer hospital stays and increased morbidity and mortality (Waikar *et al.*, 2009).

There are many causes of hyponatremia including: adverse drug effects, acquired immune deficiency syndrome (AIDS), endocrine disorders, infections, traumatic brain injuries, malignancy, endurance exercise, psychogenic polydipsia, the syndrome of inappropriate antidiuretic hormone (SIADH), and other disorders. Renal insensitivity to antidiuretic hormone (ADH) or a disturbance in ADH release is associated with the lowered serum sodium in these disorders. Other causes of hyponatremia are associated with adrenal insufficiency, hypothalamic dysfunction, and hyperglycemia. As a result of normal aging changes, older patients may be at increased risk for hyponatremia.

Acute hyponatremia is associated with volume overload and can occur in patients after a surgical procedure. The onset of acute hyponatremia occurs within 48 hours, is considered a medical emergency, and has been associated with permanent brain damage and death (Haskal, 2007).

Chronic symptomatic hyponatremia occurs over a longer period of time (i.e., more than 48 hours), but can also result in serious adverse outcomes. There are numerous causes of chronic hyponatremia, but medications remain a frequent cause.

The pathophysiology of hyponatremia is varied and depends on the cause of the lowered sodium. There are four classifications of hyponatremia. Three causes of hyponatremia are usually associated with a decreased serum plasma osmolality, and are determined by extracellular fluid volume (ECFV) status. The plasma osmolarity in the fourth category of hyponatremia, pseudohyponatremia, can be varied with either normal or increased serum osmolality.

- Hypervolemic hyponatremia is characterized by excess water retention or increased ECFV. Cirrhosis, congestive heart failure, nephrotic syndrome, or advanced renal failure are the fluid overload volume disorders associated with hypervolemic hyponatremia.
- Hypovolemic hyponatremia is associated with excessive loss of sodium or decreased ECFV. This condition can be caused by renal or nonrenal precipitants. Renal-associated disorders include chronic renal disease, osmotic diabetic diuresis, mineralocorticoid deficiency, angiotensin-converting enzyme (ACE) inhibitors, and diuretics. Nonrenal causes include dehydration related to diarrhea and vomiting, burns, diaphoresis, and third-space fluid losses (Buttaro, 2012).
- Euvolemic hyponatremia is associated with normal ECFV.
  - SIADH is a potential cause of euvolemic hyponatremia. SIADH precipitates an increase in water reabsorption, an increase in glomerular filtration rate, and a decrease in sodium reabsorption (Buttaro, 2012).
  - Other causes of euvolemic hyponatremia include beer potomania, psychogenic polydipsia, reset thermostat, and postoperative fluid replacement with hypotonic intravenous fluids.

Pseudohyponatremia, the fourth category of hyponatremia, is associated with either an increased or normal plasma osmolality. In pseudohyponatremia, ECFV may vary. Potential causes include hyperglycemia, glycerol therapy, hyperlipidemia, hyperproteinuria, or sorbitol.

■ Risk factors

- Advanced renal failure
- Adrenal insufficiency
- Beer drinker's potomania
- Brain injury
- Cirrhosis
- Extreme exercise with excessive water intake
- Heart failure
- Hyperglycemia
- Hypothyroidism
- Low sodium intake
- Malignancy
- Medications: thiazide diuretics, mannitol administration, sorbitol, nonsteroidal anti-inflammatory drugs (NSAIDs), corticosteroids, and selective serotonin reuptake inhibitors (SSRIs)
- Nephrotic syndrome
- SIADH
- Poor oral intake
- Primary polydipsia
- Pulmonary disorders
- Reset osmotic
- Severe gastrointestinal disturbances such as severe diarrhea or vomiting
- Extreme exercise with excessive water intake

■ Clinical presentation

The signs and symptoms of hyponatremia are related to the cellular edema of brain cells and depend on the severity of the decrease in serum sodium. A change in mental status, headache, nausea, irritability, lethargy, malaise, and falls are common. If the serum sodium decreases abruptly or falls below 120 mEq/l, seizures, coma, and death are possible (Singer & Brenner, 2008). In chronic hyponatremia, patients can be asymptomatic or develop subtle neurologic changes. Most patients will exhibit mental status changes, nausea, dizziness, lethargy, and muscle cramps if the serum sodium falls below 120 mEq/l. The history is essential to determine the patient's medications, past medical history, and recent and co-morbid illnesses.

■ Nursing assessment

The history is focused to determine potential causes of the sodium alteration. The physical exam requires attentiveness, because the neurologic changes can be subtle and misinterpreted particularly in older adults.

Important aspects of the physical exam include:

- *Mental status*:- may reveal mild forgetfulness to extreme confusion and agitation.
- *Vital signs*: hypo- or hypertension. Check for orthostatic changes.
- *Weight*: there may be a decrease in weight if there is dehydration or low volume status present, or weight gain if there is volume excess.
- *Skin*: poor skin turgor if there is dehydration or poor volume status present. Anasarca (generalized edema) possibly present in fluid overload
- *Cardiac*: assess for S3, which may indicate fluid overload. Determine if neck veins are distended or flat.
- *Lungs*: auscultate for wheezes, rales or rhonchi, which may be present in fluid volume overload.
- *Abdomen*: percuss for tympany and dullness which could indicate ascites. Percuss, feel and measure for hepatomegaly.
- *Extremities*: assess for edema, indicating fluid retention or overload.
- Monitor intake and output.

■ Diagnostics

- Initial diagnostics help determine both the serum sodium and the serum osmolality. These include:
  - Serum electrolytes
  - Serum glucose
  - Blood urea nitrogen (BUN), creatinine
- Serum osmolality determines the extracellular fluid status and directs treatment of the underlying cause of the hyponatremia. To calculate serum osmolality:

  2(Na [mEq/l]) + K (mEq/l) + (BUN [in mg/dl]/2.8) + (glucose [in mg/dl]/18).

  - Normal serum osmolality is 275-295 mOsm/kg indicating an isotonic state
  - Serum osmolality >295 mOsm/kg indicates a hypertonic state
  - Serum osmolality <275 mOsm/kg indicates a hypotonic state

Additional diagnostics may include

- Complete blood count (CBC) with differential
- Calcium, magnesium, phosphorus
- Liver function tests (LFTs)
- Thyroid-stimulating hormone (TSH)
- Fasting lipid profile
- Uric acid
- Urine for sodium, specific gravity, and osmolality:
  - Urine sodium concentration – a low urine sodium can help confirm intravascular volume depletion.
  - Low urine osmolality may indicate primary polydipsia, beer drinker's potomania and reset osmostat.

Osmolality >300 mOsm/kg helps rule out primary polydipsia or low solute diet.

■ Differential diagnosis

Hyponatremia is determined by sodium laboratory values. The differential diagnoses are focused on the various classifications and causes of hyponatremia.

■ Treatment

Most patients will have mild serum sodium changes requiring careful monitoring. Treatment of hyponatremia is dependent on the underlying cause. Medications associated with the low serum sodium should be discontinued when possible. For some patients a water restriction will be necessary. If volume depletion is present, the administration of isotonic saline may be indicated. Vasopressin receptor antagonists also may be helpful.

Patients with critically lowered serum sodium require vigilant care. For these patients, cautious use of intravenous hypertonic saline is indicated. The serum sodium must be increased gradually to prevent neurologic damage and death. Vasopressin receptor antagonists can be used in these situations also.

Patients with low sodium levels should be monitored carefully. Seizure precautions are recommended.

■ Collaborative consultation

Discussion with the physician about fluid status recommendations (e.g., whether restricting water or giving intravenous or oral fluid), is essential. Be certain to discuss existing medications and underlying disorders contributing to the hyponatremia as well as the treatment for these illnesses.

■ Complications

- Death
- Permanent neurologic damage
- Seizures

■ Prevention

- Obtaining a careful health history will help identify medications and existing disease processes that increase the risk of hyponatremia.
- Careful attention to fluid volume status, and discussion with the physician when either fluid volume excess or depletion is suspected

■ Patient/family education

- Discuss the symptoms of hyponatremia and the need for careful assessment. If the patient is on a water restriction, discuss the need to adhere to the restriction, and the importance of measuring all water ingested.
- Inform the patient and family of the need for any procedure that will be done (e.g., laboratory diagnostics and urine samples). If intravenous fluids are to be administered, explain the rationale.

● Explain the need for safety precautions, as the patient may be confused, and therefore at increased risk for injury.

Hypernatremia

Patients with hypernatremia have a serum sodium level greater than 145 mEq/l. Hypernatremia is most often due to water losses. These losses can occur from the gastrointestinal or respiratory tracts or in the urine. Hypernatremia can also be acute or chronic, and serious long term effects are possible, particularly in frail elders. In older adults, thirst is often decreased and in 66% of elders with hypernatremia, thirst is absent (Chassagne et al., 2006). Why thirst is decreased in older adults is not clear, but for nurses it is an important concept to understand. Older adults may also have decreased mobility, function, and cognition-all factors that increase the risk of hypernatremia in this population.

Hypernatremia is usually related to a water deficit (e.g., dehydration), but this electrolyte disorder can also be related to excess sodium intake or chronic kidney disease. Like hyponatremia, hypernatremia indicates an abnormality in water homeostasis evidenced by an increase in serum osmolality greater than 295 mOsm/kg. Most often, hypernatremia is mild, but illness, medications, heat, cognitive status, and other factors can increase the severity of this disorder. Elders are especially at risk because of the diminished renal concentrating ability that occurs with aging (Buttaro, 2012).

■ Risk factors

● Antidiuretic hormone deficiency
● Central diabetes insipidus
● Decreased level of consciousness
● Decreased thirst
● Diarrhea/vomiting
● Fluid restrictions
● High solute tube feedings
● Illness
● Immobility
● Impaired kidney excretion
● Infection
● Intravenous isotonic or hypertonic saline
● Nephrogenic diabetes
● Poor oral intake
● Primary aldosteronism

■ Clinical presentation

Lethargy, lightheadedness, weakness, irritability, and change in mental status are common presenting symptoms of hypernatremia. In severe hypernatremia (i.e., serum sodium >158 mEq/l), muscle twitching, seizures, and coma are possible. Severely elevated levels of serum sodium are associated with death.

■ Nursing assessment

The nursing history is focused on determining the cause of the hypernatremia and should include discussion of excess fluid loss (e.g., diarrhea, excessive sweating, or polyuria), the use of current or recent medications, and the presence or absence of thirst.

The physical exam is focused, but requires careful attention. Findings may be subtle, depending of the severity of the sodium excess.

- *Neurologic exam*: altered mental status is often the first sign of a sodium disorder, but, weakness, lethargy, neuromuscular irritability, and seizures are possible. In extreme cases coma may be present.
- *Vital signs*: the patient may be febrile, hyper/hypotensive, tachycardic, or even tachypneic depending on the cause of the elevated serum sodium. Postural vital signs should be obtained to assess for hypovolemia.
- *Weight*: patients should be weighed on admission and daily, as in older adults, daily fluid repletion orders are based on initial weight loss and daily water losses (i.e., urine, emesis, drainage tubes, and insensible water losses). There may be weight fluctuation depending on fluid status.
- Monitor daily fluid intake and output carefully and discuss with health care provider.
- Monitor sodium intake.

■ Diagnostics

- Initial diagnostics include:
  - Serum electrolytes
  - Serum glucose
  - BUN, creatinine
  - Calculated serum osmolality
- Depending on patient presentation further diagnostics may include:
  - CBC and differential
  - Serum protein
  - Urine osmolality
  - Urine specific gravity
  - Computed tomography scan (CT scan), magnetic resonsnce imaging (MRI) if indicated

■ Differential diagnosis

Causes may include volume depletion due to:

- Diuretic therapy
- Fever

- Fluid restrictions
- Heat
- Illness/infection
- Impaired thirst
- Polyuria
- Sweat losses
- Tube feedings without adequate free water supplementation
- Vomiting/diarrhea

Other potential causes of hypernatremia include:

- Chronic renal failure
- High-solute tube feedings
- Water loss from peritoneal dialysis
- Abnormal thirst mechanism
- Diabetes insipidus
- Hypodipsia – a primary hypothalamic lesion affecting thirst or osmoreceptors
- Osmotic diuresis due to hyperglycemia or mannitol
- Severe exercise
- Severe heat
- Sodium overload (e.g., intravenous isotonic or hypertonic saline)

■ Treatment

Treatment for hypernatremia is dependent on the fluid status accompanying the increased sodium and the cause of the hypernatremia. Most often, it is necessary to hold diuretics and laxatives until the patient's water balance is restored.

The goals of therapy are to increase total body water and extracellular fluid volume, thereby returning the serum sodium to normal. In patients able to take oral fluids, the safest route of administration of water is by mouth or in some cases via a nasogastric tube or other feeding tube.

For hypotensive patients, with hypernatremia, intravascular fluid volume resuscitation with intravenous fluids is necessary. Once the blood pressure is normal, 5% dextrose in water or 0.45% saline can be given intravenously (Singer & Brenner, 2008). The rate of the sodium correction depends on whether the hypernatremia is chronic or acute, but high serum sodium levels should not be corrected too quickly especially in older patients. Acute, mild hypernatremia (less than 24 hours duration) can be corrected over 24 hours, but water deficit corrected slowly over 24 to 48 hours helps to prevent cerebral edema (Buttaro, 2012). Reductions of serum sodium by no more than 1-2 mEq/l/hr is recommended to avoid cerebral consequences (Buttaro, 2012).

If the cause of the hypernatremia is central diabetes insipidus then desmopressin acetate (DDAVP) or vasopressin is given in order to decrease renal water losses. If nephrogenic diabetes insipidus is the cause, then a thiazide diuretic and a 2 gram sodium-restricted diet is the treatment of choice (Buttaro, 2012).

Collaborative consultation

Discussion with the physician/nurse practitioner/physician assistant about fluid status, and recommendations for giving or restricting free water is essential. There should also be discussion about the underlying cause of the hypernatremia.

Consultation with the nutritionist would be helpful, if a sodium restricted diet is to be implemented.

Complications

- Cerebral vascular damage
- Coma
- Death
- Seizures
- Shock from volume depletion

Prevention

Since older adults have a decreased sensation of thirst, there should be attention paid to their fluid volume status, in particular, free water intake. There is also a need to be attentive to medications that elders may be taking, as many of them are on diuretics, and other agents which could lead to hypernatremia, including the use of NSAIDs.

Dietary intake of sodium may need to be monitored, and so diet teaching may be beneficial.

Patient/family education

Attention to fluid intake, in particular free water, should be stressed with the elderly patient. Since the sensation of thirst decreases with age, it may be necessary to teach the patient to keep a daily chart with the number of glasses of fluid consumption outlined on it.

The family should also be taught the importance of fluid intake. If the older patient has a cognitive deficit, this becomes even more important, as the family may be the ones monitoring fluid intake.

Both patient and family should be made aware of the initial signs of hypernatremia, stressing any change in mental status, lethargy, weakness, and confusion. They should be taught to report these signs to the patient's health care provider.

References

Buttaro, T.M. (2012) Hypernatremia and hyponatremia. In: Buttaro, T.M., Trybulski, J., Bailey, P.P. & Sandberg-Cook, J. (eds) *Primary Care: A Collaborative Practice*, 4th edition. Mosby, St. Louis.

Chassagne, P., Druesne, L., Capet, C., Menard, J.F., & Bercoff, E. (2006) Clinical presentation of hypernatremia in elderly patients: a case control study. *Journal of the American Geriatrics Society* **54**, 1225-1230.

Haskal, R. (2007) Current issues for nurse practitioner: hyponatremia. *Journal of the American Academy of Nurse Practitioners* **19**, 563-579.

Singer, G.G. & Brenner, B.M. (2008) Chapter 46. Fluid and electrolyte disturbances. In: *Harrison's Principles of Internal Medicine*, 17th edition (Fauci AS, Braunwald E, Kasper DL, *et al*. eds). Online. Available from http://accessmedicine.com/resource TOC.aspx?resourceID=4 (accessed 29 March 2012).

Waikar, S.S., Mount, D.B. & Curhan, G.C. (2009) Mortality after hospitalization with mild, moderate, and severe hyponatremia. *American Journal of Medicine* **122**(9), 857-865.

PART 5: HYPOMAGNESEMIA AND HYPERMAGNESEMIA

Nancy A. Kelly

Intracellular magnesium is involved in over 300 enzymatic reactions and metabolic processes, especially those involving the production and utilization of adenosine triphosphate (ATP), and is considered vital to normal cellular function (Methaney, 2000; Torii *et al*., 2009). A possible factor in age-related disease, magnesium may reduce reactive oxygen species in addition to being a cofactor for the enzymes, transporters, and nucleic acids necessary for cellular function, replication, and energy metabolism (Torii *et al*., 2009). Magnesium is required for cardiac contractility, transport of sodium and potassium across cell membranes, activation of enzymes for carbohydrate and protein metabolism and influences utilization of potassium, calcium and protein. Magnesium is similar to potassium in function, concentration, and manifestation of imbalance (Kee, 2004).

Approximately 49% of the body's magnesium is intracellular; 50% stored in bone, and only 1% of total body magnesium is in extracellular fluid. Serum magnesium levels may not reflect total body magnesium levels. Approximately 30% of magnesium is protein bound, and the remainder is ionized or free for utilization in cellular function (Kee, 2004). Normal magnesium levels range from 1.7 to 2.4 mg/dl (Bringhurst, 2012).

Magnesium levels are regulated by renal reabsorption and intestinal absorption. Renal reabsorption of magnesium is affected by sodium chloride through creation of a negative potential that influences reabsorption, and by parathyroid hormone (PTH) and calcium levels. PTH increases magnesium reabsorption, and hypercalcemia inhibits magnesium reabsorption. Dietary sources of magnesium are absorbed in the jejunum and ileum. Magnesium absorption is stimulated by vitamin D (1,25[OH$_2$]), and vitamin D can improve intestinal magnesium absorption from the typical range of 30–40% of dietary sources, to up to 70% of dietary sources during magnesium deprivation (Bringhurst, 2012). Dietary sources of magnesium are found in green vegetables, grains, nuts, and seafood (Methaney, 2004).

■ Risk factors

Hypomagnesemia

Risk factors for hypomagnesemia are diseases or conditions that impair intestinal absorption or renal reabsorption of magnesium. Patients with impaired intestinal absorption may have malabsorption syndromes, inflammatory bowel disease, surgery affecting absorption from the ileum or jejunum, protracted vomiting or diarrhea, intestinal drainage, or poor nutrition. Loss of fluid from the lower gastrointestinal tract poses a higher risk for hypomagnesia than losses from the upper gastrointestinal tract (Methaney, 2000). Impaired renal tubular reabsorption of magnesium can be related to genetic magnesium wasting syndromes, acquired renal disease, drugs or toxins. Older adults have normal age related changes in the kidney that can affect reabsorption of electrolytes; thus, they may be at higher risk for changes in renal reabsorption of magnesium (Wiggins, 2000). Drugs associated with hypomagnesemia include loop diuretics, aminoglycosides, amphotericin B, cyclosporine, chemotherapy agents such as cisplatin, foscarnet, and pentamidine, and alcohol. Diuresis during the recovery phase of acute renal failure increases the risk for hypomagnesemia. Poorly controlled diabetes may affect renal reabsorption of magnesium by glucose induced osmotic diuresis. Expansion of extracellular fluid volume will lower magnesium levels and may occur with metabolic acidosis, hypercalcemia, and hyperthyroidism. Shifts of extracellular magnesium to intracellular fluid may be seen in refeeding syndrome, recovery from diabetic ketoacidosis, correction of respiratory acidosis, pancreatitis, burns, excessive sweating, and during the third trimester of pregnancy and lactation. Accelerated bone formation will also cause shifts of extracellular magnesium to intracellular fluid, and this may occur during treatment of vitamin D deficiency, bone metastasis, or following parathyroidectomy (Bringhurst, 2012). Alcoholism may increase the risk for hypomagnesemia, and may aggravate alcohol withdrawal symptoms (Methaney, 2000).

Patients with hypomagnesemia are at higher risk for digoxin toxicity. Additionally hypomagnesemia may increase insulin resistance (Mehaney, 2000).

Hypermagnesemia

Risk factors for hypermagnesemia are related to impairment of renal excretion or excessive dietary intake of magnesium. Magnesium is excreted by the kidneys (40%), or through the stool (60%) (Kee, 2004). Renal causes of hypermagnesemia are related to renal failure, and familial hypocalciuric hypercalcemia. Excessive magnesium intake may occur with high doses of magnesium based laxatives or parenteral administration of magnesium. Elders are at risk for hypermagnesemia due to age related changes in glomerular function, and are at higher risk for hypermagnesemia due to decreased renal excretion (Wiggins, 2000). Diseases associated with hypermagnesemia include adrenal insufficiency, hypothyroidism, and hypothermia. Conditions which cause a shift of magnesium from tissues such as burns, trauma and sepsis may also be causes of hypermagnesemia (Bringhurst, 2012).

■ Clinical presentation

Hypomagnesemia

Symptoms of hypomagnesia are due to changes in neuromuscular function. Patients are usually asymptomatic at magnesium levels above 1.2 mg/dl. Signs and symptoms related to decreased serum magnesium include:

- Apathy
- Ataxia
- Cardiac arrhythmia:
  - Tachycardia, sinus or supraventricular tachycardia
  - Ventricular arrhythmia
  - Prolonged pr or qt interval, torsades de pointes
  - Wide qrs
  - St segment depression
  - T wave flattening or inversion
- Dysphagia
- Delirium
- Depression
- Irritability
- Muscle weakness
- Nystagmus
- Psychosis
- Seizures
- Stridor
- Tetany
- Tremor
- Vertigo

Hypermagnesemia

Symptoms of hypermagnesemia are due to vasodilation and neuromuscular blockade. Signs and symptoms of hypermagnesemia may not be noticed until magnesium levels are greater than 4.8 mg/dl.

- Facial flushing
- Dilated pupils
- Hypotension that is unresponsive to volume expansion

- Cardiac arrhythmia:
  - Bradycardia
  - Shortened QT interval
  - Prolonged PR, QRS
  - Heart block
  - If magnesium levels extremely elevated, asystole may occur.
- Coma
- Decreased deep tendon reflexes
- Ileus or gastrointestinal hypomotility
- Lethargy
- Nausea
- Paralysis
- Respiratory failure

■ Nursing assessment

Hypomagnesemia

Nursing assessment for patients includes identifying patients at risk for hypomagnesemia and patients with hypomagnesemia. Hypomagnesemia is often under diagnosed due to lack of symptoms until magnesium levels are very low, less than 1.2 mg/dl (Kee, 2004; Bringhurst, 2012). Patients with malabsorption syndrome, vomiting, diarrhea, poor nutrition, alcohol abuse, or are receiving chemotherapy or diuretics should have magnesium levels monitored routinely. Older patients who are receiving loop diuretics, have a poor diet, use laxatives to induce bowel movements, and have concomitant calcium and vitamin D deficiency are at higher risk for hypomagnesemia and require regular magnesium level monitoring.

Patients who have hypomagnesemia must be closely monitored for laryngeal stridor or respiratory distress, dysphagia, or weakness. Seizure precautions and cardiac monitoring are indicated if magnesium level is 1.2 mg/dl.

Hypermagnesemia

Nursing assessment for patients with hypermagnesemia includes monitoring respiratory status and blood pressure. Elevated magnesium levels can lead to apnea and hypotension. Mental status can also be affected with resultant lethargy and coma. Deep tendon reflexes will be depressed, and may be followed by nurses if the nurse is confident in physical assessment of deep tendon reflexes.

■ Diagnostics

Laboratory evaluation of serum magnesium levels determines if hypo- or hypermagnesemia is present. Normal magnesium levels range from 1.7 to 2.4 mg/dl (Bringhurst *et al.*, 2012). Diagnosis cannot be made by physical exam or symptoms alone.

■ Differential diagnosis

Concurrent electrolyte disturbances may be seen with disturbance of magnesium levels, and monitoring of calcium and potassium should occur if magnesium levels are abnormal. Hypomagnesemia is diagnosed when serum magnesium levels are less than 1.2 mg/dl, and hypermagnesemia is diagnosed with magnesium levels are greater than 4.8 mg/dl (Bringhurst, 2012).

■ Treatment

Hypomagnesia

Mild or asymptomatic hypomagnesia can be treated with oral magnesium supplements. Oral supplements are recommended to be given in low and divided doses to prevent diarrhea.

For severe hypomagnesia or for patients unable to tolerate oral magnesium, intravenous supplementation is necessary. Administration of intravenous magnesium requires dose adjustment for patients with impaired renal function, and the dose should be reviewed with a pharmacist if renal impairment is present. Typically, the dose will be reduced by 25% to 50% if a patient has chronic kidney disease or renal dysfunction. Administration of parenteral magnesium sulfate may exacerbate hypocalcemia by binding of sulfate to calcium ions, but magnesium chloride may not. Approximately 50-75% of the administered parenteral dose is retained, and 25-50% renally excreted. Levels should be monitored over days to insure adequate repletion that may be slow due to renal excretion and slow repletion of intracellular magnesium (Bringhurst, 2012). Normal serum magnesium levels may not reflect intracellular repletion (Methaney, 2004).

Nurses must not accept an order for magnesium written for number of vials or ampules as magnesium concentrations vary, and if total dose is not indicated, there is a high risk for administering the wrong dose with subsequent patient injury. Also, the written orders should specify the dilution of magnesium and rate of administration. Questions about correct dose or orders can be reviewed with a pharmacist prior to contacting the ordering clinician if there are questions on the dose, dilution and infusion rate (Mehaney, 2000). Intramuscular administration is not recommended due to limited dose available in the injection and pain related to the injection (Bringhurst, 2012).

Simultaneous correction of other electrolytes and vitamin D is recommended to assure correction of all electrolytes. In magnesium deficient patients, potassium may not respond to repletion if magnesium is not also repleted. If magnesium is repleted without correcting calcium and phosphorus deficiencies, PTH stimulation and other neuromuscular symptoms may occur (Bringhurst, 2012).

Administration of intravenous magnesium should be given slowly with monitoring at frequent intervals for hypotension, flushing and sweating as parenteral magnesium produces vasodilation (Methaney, 2000). The patient should be informed prior to initiating intravenous magnesium that these symptoms may occur. If hypotension or respiratory distress occurs during infusion, immediately stop the infusion and notify the physician or nurse practitioner. Cardiac monitoring may be indicated during parenteral administration of magnesium.

Hypermagnesemia

The focus of treatment of hypermagnesemia should focus on the cause of the elevation and concurrently increase renal clearance of magnesium. If there was a large oral ingestion of magnesium, magnesium free laxatives may be given to clear the magnesium from the gastrointestinal tract. Intravenous fluids and calcium gluconate administration will aid renal clearance (Methaney, 2000). If a patient has poor renal function, hemodialysis may be needed for treatment of hypermagnesemia.

■ Collaborative consultation

Physician or nurse practitioner consultation should occur for patients who have risk factors for hypo- or hypermagnesemia to determine if monitoring magnesium levels is indicated. Collaborative consultation should occur especially for older patients who are taking magnesium based laxatives, loop diuretics, or have concomitant vitamin D deficiency as magnesium levels may need to be monitored. If a patient has potassium or calcium imbalances, they may be at higher risk for magnesium imbalance and if magnesium is not being monitored, this should be discussed with the physician or nurse practitioner. Patients with impaired renal function should not receive magnesium-based laxatives, and discussion for alternate laxatives should occur if these types of laxatives are ordered.

Consultation with a registered dietician may assist in improving dietary sources of magnesium and limit the need for oral or parenteral supplementation. If a patient is unable to take enteral nutrition, collaborative consultation with the physician should include discussion about parenteral electrolytes; intravenous fluids or parenteral nutrition may require frequent adjustment of electrolytes to insure proper electrolyte balance (Methaney, 2000).

■ Complications

Hypomagnesemia

Complications related to undertreatment of hypomagnesemia include symptoms of hypomagnesemia:

- Acute confusion
- Aspiration due to weakness, dysphagia
- Cardiac arrhythmia, including torsades de pointes
- Death
- Falls due to muscle weakness, ataxia, tremor, vertigo
- Respiratory decompensation due to stridor, seizures

Hypermagnesemia

Complications associated with hypermagnesemia, or administration of excessive magnesium supplements include:

- Cardiac arrest
- Coma
- Death
- Hypotension not responsive to volume expansion
- Respiratory failure
- Vomiting with associated electrolyte disturbance, pain, and risk for aspiration

■ Prevention

Prevention of magnesium disturbance is related to understanding the risk factors for a magnesium disturbance, monitoring patients at risk, and implementing treatment when needed.

■ Patient/family education

Hypomagnesemia

Patients with risk factors for hypomagnesemia should be instructed on their risk factors, dietary sources of magnesium (green vegetables, meat, seafood, dairy products), symptoms of hypomagnesemia, and the need for regular serum magnesium monitoring. Patients at risk for hypomagnesemia may include patients with:

- Loop diuretic therapy
- Excessive laxative use with frequent bowel movements
- Chemotherapy
- Inflammatory bowel disease
- Malabsorption or surgery impairing ileal and jejunum absorption
- Alcohol abuse

Hypermagnesemia

Patients most at risk for hypermagnesemia are patients with renal failure. All patients with renal failure should be instructed on their risk factors and be instructed not to take magnesium containing laxatives. Patients with renal dysfunction should always discuss use of over the counter medications or remedies with their health care provider(s).

References

Bringhurst, F.R., Demay, M.B., Krane, S.M., & Kronenberg, H.M. (2012) Chapter 352. Bone and Mineral Metabolism in Health and Disease. In, *Harrison's Principles of Internal Medicine*, 18th edition (Longo, D.L., Fauci, A.S., Kasper, D.L., Hauser, S.L.,

Jameson, J.L., Loscalzo, J. eds). Online. Available from http://0-www.accessmed-icine.com.library.simmons.edu/content.aspx?aID=9142739 (accessed 11 June 2012).

Kee, J. (2004) Magnesium balance. In: Kee, J., Paulanka, R.B. & Purnell, L. (eds) *Fluids and Electrolytes with Clinical Applications*, 7th edition: a programmed approach. Delmar Cengage Learning, Florence, KY.

Metheny, N.M. (2000) Magnesium imbalance. In: *Fluid and Electrolyte Balance: Nursing Considerations*, 7th edition (Metheny, N.M., Stead, L., Vaugh, C. *et al.* eds). Lippincott, Williams & Wilkins, Philadelphia.

Torii, S., Kobayashi, K., Takahashi, M. *et al.* (2009) Magnesium deficiency causes loss of response to intermittent hypoxia in paraganglion cells. *Journal of Biological Chemistry* **284**(28), 19077-19028.

Wiggins, J. (2000) Approach to the elderly patient with disorders of fluid and osmolarity balance. In: *Kelley's Textbook of Internal Medicine* (Dupont, L. ed.). Lippincott, Williams & Wilkins, Philadelphia.

Unit 14: Psychological Issues

PART 1: ANXIETY DISORDERS

Constance Cruz, Sara A. Fisher, Mary Lussier-Cushing
and Jennifer Repper-DeLisi

The prevalence of anxiety disorders in older adults is estimated to range from 1% to 19% (Pinquart & Duberstein, 2007). Anxiety symptoms in this population are associated with a diminished sense of well-being, increased disability, and increased health care utilization. The most common anxiety disorder experienced by older people is generalized anxiety disorder (GAD) (Flint, 2007). Phobic disorders, post-traumatic stress disorder, obsessive–compulsive disorder, and panic are identified to a lesser degree (Flint, 2007; Pinquart & Duberstein, 2007). Researchers have placed the rate of GAD to be as high as 70% among patients with Alzheimer's disease (Starkstein *et al.*, 2007).

The *Diagnostic and Statistical Manual of Mental Disorders-Text Revised* (DSM-IV_TR), defines GAD as "excessive anxiety and worry" (APA, 2000, p. 476) about a variety of events and situations. Lenze & Wetherell (2009) stress that

> it is the amount of worry, the difficulty the individual has in stopping it, and the degree of distress or functional impairment related to the worry that is critical, not the degree to which the worry is realistic (p. 336).

An anxiety disorder may manifest itself cognitively, as excessive worry or fear, behaviorally as hyperkinesis or phobic avoidance, or physiologically through numerous somatic symptoms. Often, a patient will interpret the physiological symptoms of tension, muscle aches, fatigue, gastrointestinal distress, and excess autonomic nervous system activity as an indication of acute medical illness.

The pathophysiology of anxiety is multifactorial. It is thought to be caused by a combination of genetics, biochemistry, and environmental stressors. Some have suggested that individuals inherit a genetic characteristic, "like a hyperactive autonomic nervous system, anxiety sensitivity, behavioral inhibition, or shyness" (Laraia, 2001, p. 111). When a person with this type of genetic loading is confronted with trauma or even mild life stressors, they may become symptomatic. The biochemistry of anxiety disorders includes the activity of **gamma-aminobutyric acid** (GABA), norepinephrine and serotonin, which are several neurotransmitters active in the emotion centers of the brain (the amygdala and the hippocampus) as well as in the cerebral cortex.

It is believed that there is reduced transmission of neuronal messages in the aging brain. Overall, the aging brain has fewer neurons and it is assumed that there is a decrease in the activity of norepinephrine, dopamine, and serotonin. It is thought that it is this reduced neuroactivity associated with the multiple stressors of aging such as cognitive changes, loss of independence, loss of loved ones, or illness that is responsible for some of the more prevalent emotional, behavioral, and cognitive disorders.

■ Risk factors

- Alzheimer's disease
- Care giving responsibilities
- Chronic illness
- Depression
- Diminished economic resources
- Disability
- External locus of control
- Female gender
- Frailty
- Neurotic personality
- Pharmacology/medication side effects (anticholinergics, psychostimulants, steroids, etc.)
- Social isolation
- Traumatic life events
- Unanticipated life changes

■ Clinical presentation

Identification of late life anxiety can be a challenge. Older adults may be unable to identify their feelings as 'anxiety' and may present with a multitude of somatic complaints making it difficult for the clinician to diagnose anxiety as being at the root of the problem. Anxiety disorders can present in a variety of ways. Smith *et al.* (2009) suggest that

> any person age 60 or older who expresses worry or fear and who is identified as being at risk (e.g., physical illness, recent psychosocial stress, depression, cognitive impairment, and somatic complaints for which no cause can be identified) should be evaluated for anxiety (p. 12).

GAD is described by the DSM IV-TR as

A. Six months of excessive anxiety and worry
B. Difficulty in controlling the anxiety and worry
C. The presence of three or more of the following symptoms:
   (1) Feeling wound-up, tense, or restless
   (2) Becoming easily fatigued or worn-out
   (3) Concentration problems
   (4) Irritability
   (5) Significant tension in muscles
   (6) Difficulty with sleep
D. The symptoms are not part of another mental disorder.
E. The symptoms cause "clinically significant distress" or problems functioning in daily life.
F. The condition is not due to a substance or medical issue.

Source: APA (2000).

■ Nursing assessment

The nursing assessment of a patient with an anxiety generally consists of both clinical interview and behavioral observation. The interview should be conducted in a quiet area to minimize extra stimulation and allow the client to focus. The mental status exam is part of the assessment. Ask both direct questions about the nature of patient's pains or fears as well as open ended questions. Assessment involves gathering data about anxiety symptoms, triggers, and personal as well as family history of anxiety. Determine how the anxiety has interfered with the client's daily functioning and how the patient understands the illness. Take a history of prescribed and over-the-counter medications, drug and alcohol use as well as caffeine intake.

Behavioral observations will include noting restlessness that may take the form of psychomotor agitation, easy startle, frequent sighing, or irregular respirations. Ask for permission to speak with family members about their thoughts and observations. The physical exam is important and should include evaluating the patient for thyroid abnormalities, tremor, arrhythmias, heart murmurs, tachycardia, and tachypnea.

■ Diagnostics

The contribution of comorbid illness is an essential consideration during the evaluation of anxiety. A diagnostic workup should include careful consideration of the contribution of other medical conditions or medication that the patient is currently receiving. Laboratory screening may include complete blood count, chemistries, and thyroid function panel.

■ Differential diagnosis

There are numerous medical conditions that may first present as anxiety symptoms. The following list is not all inclusive.

- Cardiovascular
  - Angina, arrhythmia, pulmonary embolism, congestive heart failure, mitral valve prolapse
- Endocrine
  - Cushing's syndrome, hypo- and hyperthyroidism, hypo and hyperparathyroidism, vitamin B12 deficiency
- Metabolic
  - Acidosis, hypercalcemia, dehydration
- Neurological
  - Cerebral anoxia, delirium. dementia, Parkinson's disease
- Respiratory
  - Chronic obstructive pulmonary disease, hypoxia, asthma
- Medications
  - Over the counter as well as prescription

- Withdrawal syndromes
  - Intoxication
  - Toxic exposure

■ Treatment

The treatment of anxiety disorders can include both nonpharmacologic and pharmacologic interventions. Nonpharmacologic interventions include cognitive-behavioral, supportive therapy, psychodynamic therapy, relaxation techniques, guided imagery, and meditation.

Pharmacologic interventions include antidepressants such as selective serotonin reuptake inhibitors, tricyclic antidepressants, and monoamine oxidase inhibitors. Because of an increased sensitivity to benzodiazepines in older patients, the decision to use benzodiazepines should be cautiously made. If used, smaller doses of short-acting benzodiazepines may be effective as well as safer. Long-acting benzodiazepines should be avoided as these drugs have a long half-life in elders potentially causing prolonged sedation and increasing the risk of falls and fractures (Fick & Semla, 2012).

Nursing care starts with the establishment of a trusting relationship. Always approach the patient with calm demeanor and accept a patient's psychological defenses. Avoid making personal judgments or becoming confrontational. Allow time for client to express their thoughts and feelings, use empathy. Help the client to determine if there are clear precipitants to the anxiety and remove sources of anxiety when possible. Establish daily schedules with clients so they will know what to expect in a given day, explain all procedures using language the patient will understand.

■ Collaborative consultation

Patients with anxiety disorders benefit from a multidisciplinary approach that includes consultation with mental health professionals (e.g., psychiatric nurses, social workers, psychologists, and psychiatrists), primary care providers, and the hospital care team to aid in evaluation and treatment.

■ Complications

- Memory impairment
- Poorer cognitive reasoning
- Poorer verbal reasoning
- Reduced attention
- Reduced learning
- Reduced quality of life
- Risks associated with side effects of antidepressants and benzodiazepines
- Risks associated with withdrawal symptoms of antidepressants and benzodiazepines (GI distress, joint and muscle aches, aggression, agitation, irritability, increased anxiety, perceptual disturbances, seizure)

■ Prevention

Early identification and treatment of an anxiety disorder may spare the patient from excess suffering and limit functional disability. Early identification can be achieved by attending to risk factors, nursing assessment of patient symptoms and including collateral information from family and caretakers.

■ Patient/family education

The nurse can be instrumental in educating the patient and family about the symptoms of anxiety disorders, risk factors, and the importance of early intervention to prevent escalation of symptoms (Flood, 2009). Family can be educated regarding the importance of supportive communication such as maintaining a calm and rational response to symptoms. Nonpharmacological interventions require teaching coping skills such as relaxation, meditation and cognitive-behavioral strategies. If medications are prescribed, the patient will need medication teaching.

References

American Psychiatric Association (2000) *Diagnostic and Statistical Manual of Mental Disorders* (4th Ed., Text Revision). American Psychiatric Association, Washington, DC.

Fick, D.M., & Semla, T.P. (2012) AGS Updated Beers Criteria for Potentially Inappropriate Medication Use in Older Adults. Online. Available from http://www.americangeriatrics.org/health_care_professionals/clinical_practice/clinical_guidelines_recommendations/2012 (accessed 11 June 2012).

Flint, A.J. (2007) Anxiety disorders in later life: from epidemiology to treatment. *American Journal of Geriatric Psychiatry* **15**(8), 635–638.

Flood, M. & Buckwalter, C. (2009) Recommendations for mental health care of older adults Part 1 – an overview of depression and anxiety. *Journal of Gerontological Nursing* **35**(2), 26–33.

Laraia, M.T. (2001) Biological context of psychiatric nursing care. In: Stuart, G.W. & Laraia, M.T. (eds) *Principles and Practice of Psychiatric Nursing*, 7th edition. Mosby, St. Louis, MO, pp. 88–119., Inc.

Lenze, E.J. & Loebach Wetherell, J. (2009) Anxiety disorders. In: Blazer, D.G. & Steffens, D.C. (eds) *The American Psychiatric Publishing Textbook of Geriatric Psychiatry*. American Psychiatric Publishing, Inc., Arlington, VA, pp. 333–345.

Pinquart, M. & Duberstein, P.R. (2007) Treatment of anxiety disorders in older adults: a meta-analytic comparison of behavioral and pharmacological interventions. *American Journal of Geriatric Psychiatry* **15**(8), 639–651.

Smith, M., Ibgram, T., Brighton, V. & Adams, S. (2009) Evidence-based guideline: detection and assessment of late-life anxiety. *Journal of Gerontological Nursing* **35**(7), 9–15.

Starkstein, S.E., Jorge, R., Petracca, G. & Robinson, R.G. (2007) The construct of generalized anxiety disorder in Alzheimer disease. *American Journal of Geriatric Psychiatry* **15**(1), 42–49.

Further reading

Andreescu, C., Herbeck Belnap, B., Rollman, B.L. *et al.* (2008) Generalized anxiety disorder severity scale validation in older adults. *American Journal of Geriatric Psychiatry* **16**(10), 813-818.

Beekman, A.T.F., de Beurs, E., van Balkom, A.J.L.M., Deeg, D.J.H., Dyck, R. & van Tilburg, W. (2000) Anxiety and depression in later life: co-occurrence and communality of risk factors. *The American Journal of Psychiatry* **157**(1), 89-95.

Boddice, G., Pachana, N.A. & Byrne, G.J. (2008) The clinical utility of the geriatric anxiety inventory in older adults with cognitive impairment. *Nursing Older People* **20**(8), 36-40.

Dada, F., Sethi, S., & Grossberg, G.T. (2001) Generalized anxiety disorder in the elderly. *Psychiatric Clinics of North America* **24**(1), 155-163.

Mantella, R.C., Butters, M.A., Dew, M.A. *et al.* (2007) Cognitive impairment in late-life generalized disorder. *American Journal of Psychiatry* **15**(8), 673-679.

Smith, M. (2005) Nursing assessment and treatment of anxiety in late life. In: Devereaux Melillo, K. & Crocker Houde, S. (eds.) *Geropsychiatric and Mental Health Nursing*. Jones and Bartlett, Sudbury, MA, pp. 151-172.

Zarit, S.H. & Zarit, J.M. (2007) *Mental Disorders in Older Adults: Fundamentals of assessment and treatment*. 2nd edition. Guilford Press; New York, NY.

PART 2: DEPRESSION

Jennifer Repper-DeLisi, Constance Cruz, Sara A. Fisher and Mary Lussier-Cushing

Depression in late life is a disabling condition that may affect up to 15% percent of those 65 years or older (Blazer & Williams, 1980; National Institute of Mental Health, 2012). Medically ill older adults are a particularly vulnerable group with rates as high as 25% percent (Geriatric Mental Health Foundations, ND). Episodes in the elder population tend to last longer (Twedell, 2007) and significantly impact health and well-being. Depression increases the likelihood of death from medical causes (Schulz *et al.*, 2002), is associated with functional decline (Djernes, 2006), and contributes to noncompliance with medical care (DiMatteo *et al.*, 2000). The risk of suicide is a serious concern among those with late life depression. Elder rates of suicide are higher than for any other age group and highest for those over the age of 85 (National Institute of Mental Health, 2007).

While treatment outcomes are optimistic, only a small fraction of older patients are identified and treated (Steffens, 2009). Patients or their families may mistakenly view depressive symptoms as a natural part of aging and fail to report the condition. Depression in patients with complex medical and functional problems may remain undetected by care providers. Nurses at the bedside are in a pivotal position to identify the syndrome, facilitate further evaluation by a mental health professional, monitor response to pharmacologic treatment, and initiate nursing care measures to support recovery.

■ Risk factors

Risk factors for late life depression are numerous and include genetic factors, medical co-morbidities, psychological characteristics, and social stressors (Heok & Ho, 2008; Cole *et al.*, 2008; Djernes, 2006; Blazer, 2006).

- Genetic risk factors:
  - Previous depressive episodes or other psychiatric illness
  - Female sex
  - Functional decline
- Medical comorbidities:
  - Chronic illness
  - Cognitive impairment
  - Medications
  - Pain
  - Substance use
- Psychological risk factors include:
  - Pessimistic view of the world
  - Poor coping abilities
  - Poor life satisfaction
  - Unresolved bereavement
- Social risk factors:
  - Absence of religious affiliation
  - Living alone or in an institution
  - Stressful life events (loss of loved one, loss of home and familiar surroundings, loss of independence, loss of social supports)
  - Pessimistic view of the world

■ Clinical presentation

Late life depression is a chronic illness characterized by relapses and remissions (Callahan, 2001). There are many signs and symptoms associated with the disorder. While the clinical picture may vary among patients, a pattern of symptoms emerges during the course of the illness (Beck, 2009; APA, 2000). These include:

- An enduring low mood: There may be crying spells, withdrawal from relationships, persistent hopelessness/helplessness, worthlessness, and guilt or negative feelings about oneself.
- Decrease in motivation: Loss of interest in pleasurable activities, decreased energy, and alterations in self care
- Cognitive impairment: Poor concentration, memory problems, and difficulty making decisions
- Physical manifestations: Sleep/wake cycle disruption, change in appetite (with weight loss or gain), decreased libido, psychomotor changes (either slowing or agitation) and increase in somatic complaints

Table 3.14.2.1 Symptoms of depression: SIG: E CAPS.

> S   Sleep disturbance (insomnia or hypersomnia)
> I   Interest (loss of interest in pleasurable activities)
> G   Guilt (recurrent guilty or morbid thoughts)
> E   Energy (loss of energy, persistent fatigue)
> C   Concentration (difficulty sustaining attention)
> A   Appetite changes (with resulting weight loss or gain)
> P   Psychomotor changes (agitation or retardation)
> S   Suicidal thoughts or actions

- Psychotic symptoms: Delusions of worthlessness, excessive or inappropriate guilt, and paranoid thoughts
- Suicidal thoughts: Thoughts of death, suicidal plans, and suicidal acts

■ Nursing assessment

The diagnosis may be made as part of a health assessment on admission to the hospital and/or when patient reports or demonstrates symptoms associated with depression. Brief screening tools may be easily integrated into the nursing assessment process. The short form of the Geriatric Depression Scale (GDS) includes 15 yes/no questions, is easily administered and scored in a few minutes, and has been validated in the medically ill geriatric population (Kurlowicz & Greenberg, 2007; Marc et al., 2008, Yesavage et al., 1983). The mnemonic SIG: E CAPS is widely used as a helpful reminder when screening for depression (see Table 3.14.2.1) (Caplan & Stern, 2008). Both of these tools may be used to evaluate progress over time. A positive screen should trigger a complete diagnostic evaluation by a mental health professional.

■ Diagnostics

The contribution of comorbid illness is an essential consideration during the evaluation of depression. A diagnostic workup should include careful consideration of the contribution of other medical conditions or medication that the patient is currently receiving (Cassem et al., 2004). Laboratory screening may include complete blood count, chemistries, and thyroid function panel (Blazer et al., 2009).

■ Differential diagnosis

- Bereavement
- Delirium
- Dementia
- Physical manifestations may be related to underlying medical cause.

◼ Treatment

Treatment may include medication, psychotherapy, and electroconvulsive therapy (ECT) (see Box 3.14.2.1). Studies have demonstrated that a flexible individualized approach provided by knowledgeable clinicians may be most effective (Callahan *et al*., 2005).

Selective serotonin reuptake inhibitors (SSRIs) are effective and generally well tolerated by older patients. These drugs have largely replaced the tricyclic antidepressants (TCAs) as first-line agents due to their comparative cardiac safety, tolerability, and low lethality in overdose. However, not all patients tolerate SSRI medications and may experience symptoms including gastrointestinal side effects, headache, sleep disturbance, anxiety, and sexual dysfunction (Varcarolis, 2006). Other agents including tricyclics, psychostimulants, and mood stabilizers may be employed based on the patient's individual needs. Of note, older adults may resist use of medications. Nursing interventions should include exploration of patient barriers to taking medication and include education and support (Buckwater, 2009).

Brief psychotherapies have also demonstrated benefit for treatment of depression in the older adult. Cognitive behavioral therapy may provide substantial benefit (either alone or in conjunction with psychopharmacologic agents) to depressed patients. Family therapy may also be useful to help loved ones understand the experience of the depressed individual as well as learn therapeutic interventions. For those patients who have a religious affiliation, counseling from a clergy member may provide the needed support (Blazer *et al*., 2009).

Box 3.14.2.1 Electroconvulsive treatment

Electroconvulsive therapy (ECT) is a well-established treatment in which brief seizures are electrically induced to relieve depressive symptoms. Patients who receive ECT usually include those who fail to respond to medication management, who have had a previous good response to ECT, who are at immediate medical risk, or who are catatonic.

The number of treatments necessary to effectively treat a depressive episode is estimated between 6 and 12 separate treatments although some patients require more. The schedule of treatments is typically 3×/week. Side effects may include confusion, disorientation, agitation, headache, muscle aches, and nausea. Difficulty remembering new information during treatment is common, but usually resolves over time following completion of treatment. Some memory problems may remain, particularly those just prior to and following treatment. Patients usually receive antidepressant therapy to maintain treatment response/reduce risk of relapse although some patients receive maintenance ECT therapy (Welch, 2004).

The primary goal of nursing care is to support the recovery process through: (1) therapeutic interpersonal communications, (2) treatment of the physiological symptoms of depression, and (3) manipulation of the hospital environment to promote safety and well-being.

Communication

- Keep the patients interpersonally engaged: Interact at frequent intervals, encouraging verbal expression of thoughts and feelings. Instill a sense of hope for the future with each interaction.
- Provide realistic feedback to negative thinking. "I know it's hard for you to get out of bed this morning, but it's going to get easier."
- Assist the patient to identify healthy coping mechanisms. Ask the patient how he has dealt with stress in the past and help him to translate those positive efforts to the here and now.
- Encourage religious practice and refer to hospital chaplain for patients with religious affiliations/spiritual beliefs/spiritual distress.
- Encourage reminiscences of positive experiences.
- Provide education regarding the nature of depression as a treatable medical disease. Remind patients of the gradual process of recovery, discouraging any expectations that they "snap out of it".
- Discourage major life decisions in the social realm, and encourage informed medical decisions.
- Employ relaxation therapies such as therapeutic touch, relaxation breathing, and guided imagery.
- For the patient with comorbid suicide risk, assess the patient's suicide risk daily and with any observable decrease in level of engagement or increased anxiety. Patients with increased risk are those with a workable suicide plan and expressed intent to act on that plan.

Physiological

- Maintain activities of daily living: Determine patient's current capacity, schedule activities in collaboration with the patient, and reinforce efforts. Set a pace in nursing care that matches the patient's current abilities.
- Encourage physical activity: Assist patient to plan daily schedule of activities. Encourage patient to spend time out of bed and out of room as appropriate.
- Facilitate sleep: Determine the patient's baseline sleep patterns, implement strategies which have been in useful in past, and utilize medication as appropriate. Decrease the amount of time patient spends in bed during the day. Provide a warm drink or back rub at bedtime.
- Facilitate adequate nutrition and hydration: Encourage and monitor intake at each meal. Provide snacks if patient unable to consume adequate quantities. Monitor weight weekly.
- Address elimination problems: Maintain normal bowel pattern by increasing activity level, altering diet, and/or inclusion of a bowel regimen, if indicated.
- Monitor for effects and side effects of medications.

Environment

- Provide stimulation during the day (lights on, door open, curtains open).
- Decrease environmental stimuli in the late evening and night (close door, lights low).
- Minimize hazards in room. Remove clutter, and provide for a clear path to the bathroom.
- Encourage family to bring objects from home that may promote positive emotion and familiarity.
- For management of suicide risk: Move the patient to a room with easy access to staff and with increased visibility. Create a safe environment by removing objects from the room that may be used for self destructive purposes. Provide frequent ongoing assessment and constant observation when indicated to minimize risk (Psychiatric Nursing Consultation Service Nursing Care Guidelines, Massachusetts General Hospital, 2010).

Nursing interventions

- Prior to treatment:
  - Provide education to the patient regarding NPO status.
  - Note and implement medication order changes. Certain medications are contraindicated during ECT, some will be discontinued for the duration of treatment, others will be held just prior to each treatment.
- Following each ECT treatment:
  - Turn patient on their side to help prevent aspiration.
  - Monitor vital signs regularly.
  - Assess patient mental status and implement safety measures for the patient with agitation, disorientation, or confusion. Reorient the patient as needed.
  - Provide medication as ordered for postoperative symptoms of nausea and headache.
- During treatment course:
  - Monitor treatment response, noting specific changes in symptom presentation and patient's subjective response.
  - Monitor patient mental status for evidence of cognitive impairment, particularly memory loss.

■ Collaborative consultation

- Patients with depression benefit from a multidisciplinary approach (Harpole et al., 2004) during a hospitalization that may include consultation with mental health professions (psychiatrists, social workers, and psychiatric nurses), primary care providers, and the hospital care team to aid in evaluation and treatment.
- Discharge planning should include:
  - Referrals to receiving institutions with information about patient's depression, treatment, and clinical course
  - Communication with primary care provider (PCP) regarding diagnosis and treatment, evaluation of need for additional outpatient supports

■ Complications

There appears to be a complex relationship between the incidence and persistence of depression, functional status, medical illness, and morbidity and mortality of elder patients (Reynolds *et al.*, 2008).

- Elder patients with depression are at a much higher risk of death (from suicide, and as a result of co-morbid medical illness) (Reynolds *et al.*, 2008).
- Physical symptoms associated with depression (e.g., poor nutrition, poor sleep, and impaired bowel function) may contribute to functional decline.
- Treatment of depression improves physical functioning in older adults. (Callahan, 2005).
- Depression is an independent risk factor for poorer cognitive function (Sachs-Ericsson *et al.*, 2005; Han *et al.*, 2008). Presence of comorbid cognitive impairment further diminishes functional status and may represent impending onset of Alzheimer's disease (Alexopoulos *et al.*, 1993).
- Depression contributes to noncompliance with medical treatment (DiMatteo *et al.*, 2000).

■ Prevention

- Early identification of symptoms and prompt treatment to help prevent the complications associated with depression.
- Interventions to address modifiable risk factors (Djernes, 2006; Cole *et al.*, 2008) include:
  - Increased emotional and family support
  - Substance abuse treatment
  - Maximize functional status.
  - Maximize social engagement/relieve loneliness.

■ Patient/family education

- Depression is not a sign of personal weakness, but a complex and serious medical diagnosis that requires treatment.
- Depression should not be ignored. The disease negatively impacts other health conditions as well as the functional status of elder patients.
- Depression may intensify the experience of physical symptoms. Suspect the diagnosis of depression with persistent somatic complaints, particularly when other clinical indicators are limited or absent.
- Failure to diagnose is the biggest problem associated with the treatment of depression. Once the diagnosis is made, treatment outcomes are optimistic.
- Patients and families need to understand the multifaceted treatment needs for getting better and staying better.

References

Alexopoulos, G.S., Meyers, B.S. & Young, R.C. (1993) The course of geriatric depression with "reversible dementia": a controlled study. *American Journal of Psychiatry* **150**, 1693–1699.

American Psychiatric Association (2000) *The Diagnostic and Statistical Manual of Mental Disorders-IV TR*. APA, Washington, DC.

Beck, A. (2000) *Depression: Causes and Treatment*, 2nd edition. University of Pennsylvania Press, Philadelphia, PA, and APA, Washington, DC.

Blazer, D.G. (2006) Spirituality, depression, and the elderly. *Southern Medical Journal* **99**, 1178–1179.

Blazer, D. & Williams, C.D. (1980) Epidemiology of dysphoria and depression in an elderly population. *American Journal of Psychiatry* **137**, 439–444.

Blazer, D.G., Steffens, D.C. & Koenig, H.G. (2009) Mood disorders. In: *Textbook of Geriatric Psychiatry* (Blazer, D.G., Steffens, D.C. eds). American Psychiatric Publishing,, Arlington, VA, pp. 275–299.

Buckwater, K.C. (2009) Recommendations for mental health care of older adults: Part1 – An overview of depression and anxiety. *Journal of Gerontological Nursing* **35**, 26–34.

Callahan, C.M. (2001) Quality improvement research on late life depression in primary care. *Medical Care* **39**, 772–784.

Callahan, C.M., Kroenke, K., Counsell, S.R. et al. (2005) Treatment of depression improves physical functioning in older adults. *Journal of the American Geriatrics Society* **53**, 367–373.

Caplan, J.P. & Stern, T.A. (2008) Mnemonics in a nutshell: 32 aids to psychiatric diagnosis. *Current Psychiatry* **7**, 27–33.

Cassem, N.H., Papakostas, G.I., Fava, M. & Stern, T.A. (2004) Mood-disordered patients. In: *Handbook of General Hospital Psychiatry*, 5th edition (Stern, T.A. ed.). Mosby, St. Louis, pp. 69–92.

Cole, M.G., McCusker, J., Ciampi, A. & Belzile, E. (2008) Risk factors for major depression in older medical inpatients: a prospective study. *American Journal of Geriatr Psychiatry* **16**, 175–178.

DiMatteo, M.R., Lepper, H.S. & Croghan, T.W. (2000) Depression is a risk factor for noncompliance with medical treatment. *Archives of Internal Medicine* **160**, 2101–2107.

Djernes, J.K. (2006) Prevalence and predictors of depression in populations of elderly: a review. *Acta Psychiatrica Scandinavica* **113**, 372–387.

Geriatric Mental Health Foundations. Late life depression: a fact sheet. Online. Available from http://www.gmhfonline.org/gmhf/(accessed 29 March 2012).

Han, L., McCusker, J., Cole, M., Abrahamowicz, M. & Capek, R. (2008) 12-month cognitive outcomes of major and minor depression in older medical patients. *American Journal of Geriatric Psychiatry* **16**, 742–751.

Harpole, L.H., Williams, J.W., Olsen, M.K. et al. (2005) Improving depression outcomes in older adults with comorbid medical illness. *General Hospital Psychiatry* **27**, 4–12.

Heok, K.E. & Ho, R. (2008) The many faces of geriatric depression. *Current Opinion in Psychiatry* **21**, 540–545.

Kurlowicz, L. & Greenberg, S.A. (2007) The Geriatric Depression Scale (GDS). The Hartford Institute for Geriatric Nursing 4, 2007. Online. Available from http://www.hartfordign.org/Practice/Try_This/ (accessed 29 March 2012).

Marc, L.G., Raue, P.J. & Bruce, M.L. (2008) Screening performance of the 15-item Geriatric Depression Scale in a diverse elderly home care population. *American Journal of Geriatric Psychiatry* **16**, 914–921.

National Institute of Mental Health: Older adults: depression and suicide (fact sheet). Online. Available from www.nimh.nih.gov/health/publications/older-adults-depression-and-suicide-facts-fact-sheet/index.shtml (accessed 29 March 2012).

Psychiatric Nursing Consultation Service Nursing Care Guidelines, Massachusetts General Hospital (2010).

Reynolds, S.L., Haley, W.E. & Kozlenko, N. (2008) The impact of depressive symptoms and chronic diseases on active life expectancy in older Americans. *American Journal of Geriatric Psychiatry* **16**, 425–432.

Sachs-Ericsson, N., Joiner, R., Plant, E.A. & Blazer, D.G. (2005) The influence of depression on cognitive decline in community-dwelling elderly persons. *American Journal of Geriatric Psychiatry* **13**, 402–408.

Schulz, R., Drayer, R.A. & Rollman, B.L. (2002) Depression as a risk factor for non-suicide mortality in the elderly. *Biological Psychiatry* **52**, 205–225.

Steffens, D.C. (2009) A multiplicity of approaches to characterize geriatric depression and its outcomes. *Current Opinion in Psychiatry* **22**, 522–526.

Twedell, D. (2007) Depression in the elderly. *Journal of Continuing Education in Nursing* **38**, 14–15.

Varcarolis, E.M. (2006) Mood disorders: depression. In: Varcarolis, E.M., Carson, V.B. & Shoemaker, N.C. (eds) *Foundations of Psychiatric Mental Health Nursing: A Clinical Approach*, WB Saunders, Philadelphia, pp. 228–251.

Welch, C.A. (2004) Electroconvulsive therapy in the general hospital. In: *Handbook of General Hospital Psychiatry*, 5th edition (Stern, T.A., Fricchione, G., Cassem, N.H., Jellinek, M.S. & Rosenbaum, J.F. eds). Mosby, St. Louis, pp. 105–112.

Yesavage, J.A., Brink, T.L. & Rose, T.L. *et al.* (1983) Development and validation of a geriatric depression screening scale: A preliminary report. *Journal of Psychiatric Research* **17**, 37–49.

Chapter 4
Special Considerations

Hallie S. Greenberg

Age-related changes in the immune system put older adults at increased risk for nosocomial (hospital-acquired) infections (NI). These changes include thinning skin, decreased T-lymphocyte production and proliferation and therefore lower cell-mediated immunity, reduced antibody production, and diminished cough reflex (Strausbaugh, 2001). Other physiologic changes involved in the aging process include decreased filtration through the portal and renal systems. The reduced ability to detoxify and cleanse the system puts the older adult at increased risk for an accumulation of toxins from medications, ingested substances, and infectious processes. Combined with decreasing mobility and polypharmacy, older adults are at far greater risk for nosocomial infections than other patient populations.

To further confound the issue of NI in older adults, the strict definition and criteria for NI applied by the Centers for Disease Control (CDC) may not always be applicable to elders. Older patients often have atypical clinical presentations and prompt empirical treatment may be necessary for this cohort (Lim *et al.*, 2008) even in an age when the CDC is recommending less is more with antibiotic therapy.

■ Risk factors

"Infections account for approximately 75% of nosocomial febrile illnesses in hospitalized patients" (Trivalle *et al.*, 1998, p. 1560). Worldwide, the literature has noted an increasing incidence of methicillin-resistant *Staphylococcus aureus* (MRSA), vancomycin-resistant *Enterococcus* (VRE), and *Clostridium-difficile* diarrhea (C-diff) (also called *Clostridium difficile*-associated disease/CDAD) across all populations (Anderson & Rasch, 2000; Duffy, 2002; Durai *et al.*, 2006; Hamilton Spectator, 2008a, b; Trowbridge, 2009). These three agents, now collectively referred to as "super bugs", increase length of hospital stay, increase

Nursing Care of the Hospitalized Older Patient, First Edition. Edited by
Terry Mahan Buttaro and Kate A. Barba.
© 2013 John Wiley & Sons, Inc. Published 2013 by John Wiley & Sons, Inc.

treatment costs, and can be life ending in elders and other vulnerable populations. Treatment choices for these three infectious agents can also potentially harm patients with already compromised hepatic and renal systems.

Golliot *et al*. (2001) in a French study noted that the patient characteristics for an elder at risk for NI include the following:

- At least one of the following medical devices:
  - Urinary catheter
  - Nasogastric tube
  - Intravenous line
  - Percutaneous gastrostomy
- Open bedsore
- Swallowing disorder
- Surgery within the previous 30 days (or year in the case of a prosthesis)
- Transfer from another hospital or department within the previous three months
- Fecal or urinary incontinence
- Inability to move without assistance
- Immunodeficiency

The age-old adage "an ounce of prevention is worth a pound of cure" is certainly an essential consideration in preventing NI (see Appendix). Hand hygiene noncompliance continues to be a major cause of NI. A study done at Duke University was designed to show what the annual savings could be with improved hand hygiene. The Duke study showed that the mean cost per noncompliant event in hand hygiene was $52.53 and a 200-bed hospital would incur a total of $1,779,283 in annual MRSA infection-related expenses attributed to hand hygiene noncompliance. A 1% increase in compliance in this same hospital would lead to a savings of $39,650 (Cummings *et al*., 2010). The cost of human suffering cannot be estimated into these costs.

Because Medicare no longer reimburses the costs associated with NI, the potential cost saving for large academic medical centers is staggering. Healthcare facilities are now responsible for the entire cost of hand hygiene noncompliance, so improving hand hygiene compliance across all healthcare disciplines is of paramount importance.

Methicillin-resistant *Staphylococcus aureus* (MRSA)

MRSA, the most frequent cause of health care-associated infection, can be life threatening in immunocompromised and vulnerable populations (Wang & Barrett, 2007). It is a Gram-positive coccus with a protein (i.e., penicillin-binding protein 2a {PBP2a}) found in the wall of the bacterium that causes its resistance to methicillin (Palavecino, 2007). Diagnosis is made by wound or nasal swab culture and direct implantation onto a nutrient medium plate. MRSA is resistant to commonly used antibiotics and if the patient has had previous exposure to antibiotics, the risk of acquiring MRSA is doubled (Taconelli, 2008). MRSA is spread by either direct or indirect contact and the highest prevalence within a healthcare facility is usually found in burn and orthopedic units as well as transplant units. High burdens of MRSA can be spread by skin-to-skin contact from healthcare workers who have been infected with the organism.

Clinical signs of MRSA in a patient who has acquired this type of infection are areas that are erythematous (red), edematous, painful, and warm to the touch. Wounds are often purulent and the patient frequently has a fever. If untreated, the infection may enter the bloodstream and cause septicemia. This is especially true of those patients with weakened immune systems.

Hospitalized orthopedic patients who have urinary catheters are at increased risk for a surgical wound infection as well as a catheter-associated urinary tract infection (CAUTI). While MRSA is not the major causative agent of infections, it is estimated that approximately 40% of healthcare-associated infections are CAUTI and some of these are MRSA related (CDC, 2009). Thus, it should be noted that patients with MRSA and urinary catheters are at greater risk for CAUTI. The CDC (2009) now recommends that appropriate indwelling catheterization includes treatment for urinary retention, bladder outlet obstruction, essential monitoring of urinary output, specific surgical procedures, treatment of sacral/perineal wounds in incontinent patients, necessary immobilization (e.g., multiple trauma), and comfort care. Indwelling urinary catheters should be removed as soon as possible and unnecessary catheterization avoided to help prevent CAUTI.

MRSA treatment should be multimodal and include systemic antibiotics, topical treatments and nonmedication therapy. First line antibiotic therapy is usually vancomycin. Other antibiotics considered include doxycycline, rifampin, linezolid, cotrimoxazole, and ciprofloxacin (Durai et al., 2010). The interaction of these medications with medications already prescribed for the elder patient will be of major importance when choosing the appropriate pharmacologic therapy. Close observation of the older adult in the first few days of vancomycin therapy for major side effects is an important nursing function (e.g., monitor for hearing loss and decreased renal function).

Vancomycin-resistant *Enterococcus* (VRE)

Enterococcus is a Gram-positive round-shaped bacterium normally present in the human intestinal tract and the female genital tract.

Enterococci, in general, are much less capable of causing disease than staphylococcus or *Escherichia coli* (*E. coli*) but still can complicate and prolong hospital stays (NIH, 2009).

It is because of its lack of virulence that physicians are much less concerned about VRE causing a pandemic outbreak than CDAD or MRSA (NIH, 2009).

VRE is an opportunistic disease that preys almost exclusively on hospitalized individuals (CDC, 2010). Enterococcal infections are also more common in elders; especially those in skilled care facilities because they are more likely to be exposed to infection risk factors such as medical instruments (NIH, 2009). VRE is one of the four most common infections present in CAUTI (CDC, 2009). As of 2007, scientists in the United States had reported seven cases of vancomycin-resistant *Staphylococcus aureus*; in one of these cases there was confirmation of the transfer of a key antibiotic resistance gene from *Enterococcus* to *Staphylococcus* (NIH, 2009). The ramifications of this for future antibiotic treatment of infectious diseases are still unfolding.

Clostridium difficile-associated disease (CDAD)

CDAD continues to be the most common infectious cause of nosocomial diarrhea worldwide (Cherifi *et al.*, 2006; Zar *et al.*, 2007). C-diff, a Gram-positive spore-forming rod type bacterium, is related to antibiotic therapy. Diagnosis is made by stool culture with enzyme immunoassay (EIA). However, this test is less specific and sensitive than the cell cytotoxin assay. Older adults are particularly vulnerable to CDAD as the associated diarrhea causes dehydration, loss of electrolytes, anemia (if there is associated bleeding) and malnutrition. In addition to these problems, dehydration and electrolyte losses also greatly increase the risk of delirium for the elder who frequently is taking medications (e.g., diuretics) that already affect homeostasis. Loss of fluid, potassium, and sodium may affect cognition, balance, and increase the risk for falls, skin breakdown, and serious injury that can be as life threatening as the actual CDAD infection.

Morbidity and mortality

Zoutman *et al.* (2003) stated, "NI is second only to medication errors in frequency among adverse events befalling hospitalized patients" (p. 266). Despite great advances in medical care over the last 20 years and advances in infection control, patients admitted to inpatient healthcare facilities are at great risk to acquire healthcare-associated infections. As our ability to diagnose and treat medical conditions increases, the longevity of many of our citizens increases. However, many of them do spend time within the confines of a healthcare facility increasing their risk of a hospital-acquired infection. Identifed risk factors for acquired healthcare-associated infections include, poor nutrition, complex co-morbidities, and an impaired immune system.

The ability to identify NI accurately and in a timely fashion is of paramount importance in older adults as this population is especially vulnerable to poorer outcomes when diagnosis is delayed (Bourdel-Marchasson *et al.*, 2001; Beaujean *et al.*, 1997). Additionally, elders often present atypically with NI.

The morbidity and mortality of MRSA, VRE, and CDAD extends far beyond the actual infection and possible treatment side effects. Currently, each of these infections requires that the patient be placed on some type of isolation precaution while hospitalized. The isolation may also take a toll on the already vulnerable elder. Isolation can result in functional decline, as the patient is not able to ambulate as much as he/she needs. Isolation can also result in cognitive changes and loss of sensory input from environmental isolation. This may also cause emotional isolation and may lead to confusion and delirium in an older adult. As a result, many elders with physiologic decline who are still able to perform self-care and be independent in the community may not be able to do so when ready for discharge from the hospital environment. Additionally, the physical decline associated with isolation combined with the healthcare-acquired infection frequently results in a long periods of rehabilitation for reconditioning.

The three specific organisms discussed in this chapter are multidrug-resistant organisms (MDROs). In many cases, drug resistance is related to over use of antibiotics. In the European community the eradication of CDAD can be attributed to the strict reduction in the use of antibiotics and the use of intensive infection control measures. The CDC cautions physicians and prescribers about antibiotic use to decrease drug resistance in this country (CDC, 2010). Indiscriminate use of broad-spectrum antibiotics more than doubles an individual's chance of acquiring future infection with a resistant organism. When combined with the spiraling costs of healthcare, the cost savings of a propitious use of antibiotics for all people will be of benefit.

References

Anderson, B.M. & Rasch, M. (2000) Hospital-acquired infections in Norwegian long-term-care institutions, a three-year survey of hospital-acquired infections and antibiotic treatment in nursing/residential homes, including 4500 residents in Oslo [Electronic Version]. *Journal of Hospital Infection* **46**, 288–296.

Beaujean, D., Blok, H., Vandenbroucke-Grauls, C., Weersink, A., Raymakers, J.A. & Verhoef, J. (1997) Surveillance of nosocomial infections in geriatric patients. *Journal of Hospital Infection* **36**(4), 275–284.

Centers for Disease Control and Prevention (2009) Guideline for prevention of catheter-associated urinary tract infections 2009. Online. Available from http://www.cdc.gov/hicpac/pdf/CAUTI/CAUTIguideline2009final.pdf (accessed 29 March 2012).

Centers for Disease Control and Prevention (2010) Controlling the spread of resistance. Online. Available from http://www.cdc.gov/ncidod/aip/research/ar.html (accessed 29 March 2012).

Cassel, B.G., Parkers, V., Poon, R. & Rae, H. (2008) Quality improvement: Best practices and long-term indwelling urinary catheters. *Perspectives: The Journal of the Gerontological Nursing Association* **32**(1), 13–17.

Cherifi, S., Delmee, M., Van Broeck, J., Beyer, I., Byl, B. & Mascart, G. (2006) Management of an outbreak of clostridium difficile-associated disease among geriatric patients. *Infection Control and Hospital Epidemiology* **27**(11), 1200–1205.

Creditor, M.C. (1993) Hazards of hospitalization of the elderly. *Annals of Internal Medicine* **118**(3), 219–223.

Cummings, K.L., Anderson, D.J. & Kaye, K.S. (2010) Hand hygiene noncompliance and the cost of hospital-acquired methicillin-resistant *Staphylococcus aureus* infection. *Infection Control & Hospital Epidemiology* **31**(4), 357–364.

Dowell, S.F. & Schwartz, B. (1997) Resistant pneumococci: Protecting patients through judicious use of antibiotics. *American Family Physician* **55**, 1647–1654, 1657–1658.

Durai, R., Ng, P.C. & Hoque, H. (2010) Methicillin-resistant *Staphylococcus aureus*: An update. *AORN Journal* **91**(5), 599-606.

Golliot, F., Astagneau, P., Cassou, B., Okra, N., Rothan-Tondeur, M. & Brücker, G. (2001) Nosocomial infections in geriatric long-term-care and rehabilitation facilities: Exploration in the development of a risk index for epidemiological surveillance. *Infection Control & Hospital Epidemiology* **22**(12), 746-753.

Hamilton Spectator (2008, May 23). C. diff blamed for deaths in Oakville: Hospital reports 18 patients with bug died in 5 months. Online. Available from http://www.thespec.com/Breaking News/article/373797 (accessed 13 June 2012).

Hamilton Spectator (2008a, May 14). An explosion of C. diff deaths, 125 known dead in five outbreaks over 20 months. Online. Available from http://wwthespec.com.burlingtonlife/artide/068862 (accessed 13 June 2012).

Hamilton Spectator (2008b, July 4). 463 C.diff deaths, 22 hospitals, 2 year figures from a fraction of Ontario hospitals hint how enormous the scope of lethal superbug outbreaks may turn out to be. Online. Available from http://www.thespec.com/BreakingNews/article/400388 (accessed 13 June 2012).

Lim, P.L., Barkham, T.M.S., Ling, L.M., Dimatatac, F., Alfre, T. & Ang, B. (2008) Increasing incidence of *Clostridium difficile*-associated disease, Singapore. *CDC EID Journal*; (14):9. Online. Available from http://www.cdc.gov/eid/content/14/9/1487.htm (accessed 29 March 2012).

National Institutes of Health (2009) Understanding *E. coli*. Online. Available from http://www.niaid.nih.gov/topics/ecoli/Understanding/Pages/overview.aspx (accessed 29 March 2012).

Palevecino, E. (2007) Clinical, epidemiological, and laboratory aspects of methicillin-resistant *Staphylococcus aureus* (MRSA) infections. *Methods in Molecular Biology* **391**, 1-19.

Strausbaugh, L.J. (2001) Emerging health care-associated infections in the geriatric population. *Emerging Infectious Diseases* **7**(2), 268-271.

Taconelli, E. (2008) Methicillin-resistant *Staphylococcus aureus*: risk assessment and infection control policies. *Clinical Microbiology and Infection* **14**(5), 407-410.

Trivalle, C., Chassagne, P., Bouaniche, M. *et al.* (1998) Nosocomial febrile illness in the elderly; frequency, causes and risk factors. *Archives of Internal Medicine* **158**, 1560-1565.

Trowbridge, S. (2009) Hospital-acquired infections and infection control practices: What are the consequences to the elderly patient? *Perspectives: The Journal of the Gerontological Nursing Association* **33**(1), 16-22.

Walsh, K.A. & Bruza, J.M. (2007) Hospitalization of the elderly. *Annals of Long Term Care* **15**(11), 18-23.

Wang, L. & Barrett, J.F. (2007) Control and prevention of MRSA infections. *Methods of Molecular Biology* **391**, 209-225.

Zoutman, D.E., Ford, B.D., Bryce, E. *et al.* (2003) The state of infection survallance and control in Canadian acute care hospitals. *American Journal of Infection Control* **31**(5), 266-273.

Further reading and resources

At a glance. Hospital rates of C diff surpassing MRSA. (2010) *OR Manager* **26**(5), 32-32.

Bader, M. (2006) *Staphylococcus aureus* bacteremia in older adults: Predictors of 7-Day mortality and infection with a Methicillin-resistant strain. *Infection Control and Hospital Epidemiology* **27**(11), 1219-1225.

Centers for Disease Control and Prevention (www.cdc.gov) has frequent updates about nosocomial infections and suggestions about the control of hospital acquired infections.

Gould, C.V., Umscheid, C.A., Agarwal, R.K., Kuntz, G. & Pegues, D.A. (2010) Guideline for prevention of catheter-associated urinary tract infections 2009. *Infection Control & Hospital Epidemiology* **31**(4), 319–326.

Hamel, M., Zoutman, D. & O'Callaghan, C. (2010) Exposure to hospital roommates as a risk factor for health care-associated infection. *American Journal of Infection Control* **38**(3), 173–181.

LeDell, K., Muto, C.A., Jarvis, W.R., & Farr, B.M. (2003) SHEA guideline for preventing nosocomial transmission of multidrug-resistant strains of staphylococcus aureus and enterococcus. *Infection Control & Hospital Epidemiology* **24**(9), 639–641.

Lescure, F., Locher, G., Eveillard, M. *et al.* (2006) Community-acquired infection with healthcare-associated methicillin-resistant *Staphylococcus aureus*: The role of home nursing care. *Infection Control and Hospital Epidemiology* **27**(11), 1213–1218.

Madaras-Kelly, K., Remington, R.E., Lewis, P.G. & Stevens, D.L. (2006) Evaluation of an intervention designed to decrease the rate of nosocomial methicillin-resistant *Staphylococcus aureus* infection by encouraging decreased fluoroquinolone use. *Infection Control & Hospital Epidemiology* **27**(2), 155–169.

National nosocomial infections surveillance (NNIS) system report, data summary from January 1992 through June 2004, issued October 2004 (2004) *American Journal of Infection Control* **32**(8), 470–485.

National Institutes of Health (www.nih.gov) has full text articles on the ongoing concerns and statistics on NI.

Paillaud, E., Herbaud, S., Caillet, P., Lejonc, J., Campillo, B. & Bories, P. (2005) Relations between undernutrition and nosocomial infections in elderly patients. *Age & Ageing* **34**(6), 619–625.

Patel, M. (2009) Community-associated methicillin-resistant *Staphylococcus aureus* infections: Epidemiology, recognition and management. *Drugs* **69**(6), 693–716.

Pop-Vicas, A., Mitchell, S.L., Kandel, R., Schreiber, R. & D'Agata, E. (2008) Multidrug-resistant gram-negative bacteria in a long-term care facility: Prevalence and risk factors. *Journal of the American Geriatrics Society* **56**(7), 1276–1280.

Rothan-Tondeur, M., Meaume, S., Girard, L., *et al.* (2003) Risk factors for nosocomial pneumonia in a geriatric hospital: A control-case one-center study. *Journal of the American Geriatrics Society* **51**(7), 997.

Ruben, F.L., Dearwater, S.R., Norden, C.W. *et al.* (1995) Clinical infections in the noninstitutionalized geriatric age group: Methods utilized and incidence of infections: The Pittsburgh good health study. *American Journal of Epidemiology* **141**(2), 145–157.

Spore wars: C. diff rise tied to drug resistance: Will U.S. hospitals ban fluoroquinolones? (2010) *Hospital Infection Control & Prevention* **37**(5), 51–51.

Zarl, F.A., Bakkanagari, S.R., Moorthi, K.M.L.S.T. & Davis, M.B. (2007) A Comparison of vancomycin and metronidazole for the treatment of *Clostridium difficile*-associated diarrhea, Stratified by disease severity. *Clinical Infectious Diseases* **45**(3), 302–307.

Appendix: Preventing hospital-acquired infections

- Universal precautions
- Careful hand washing before and after each patient and patient environment encounter (e.g., touching bedrails, linens, patient care items or room surfaces).
- Identify patients with history of nosocomial infections and institute contact precautions and need for surveillance cultures.

- Contact and /or droplet precautions for patients with MRSA, VRE and other infectious processes
- Discuss need for surveillance cultures for pre-operative patients, patients admitted to the intensive care unit, and patients with a history of MRSA, VRE, or other infectious process with nursing supervisor, physician, and infection control coordinator.
- Discourage urinary catheterization unless absolutely necessary. When necessary, discuss with physician advisability of intermittent urinary catheterization.
- Encourage discontinuation of urinary catheterization as soon as possible.
- Scrupulous aseptic technique for central venous catheters, intravenous insertion, and urinary catheterization
- Monitor IV sites and all dressings.
- Replace all wet or soiled dressings immediately and all dressings on a regular schedule.
- Wash stethoscope and other equipment aggressively with 70% isopropyl alcohol or facility approved cleaner between all patient encounters.
- Aggressive room and environment cleaning daily

Adapted from Centers from Disease Control. Infection Control Guidelines. Online. Available from http://www.cdc.gov/ncidod/dhqp/guidelines.htm (accessed 29 March 2012).

PART 2: ELDER ABUSE AND NEGLECT

Margaretta Byrne

Elder abuse and neglect are defined as the maltreatment of an individual who is 60 years of age or older (Centers for Disease Control, 2009). The abuse can be physical, sexual, emotional, or financial (CDC, 2009). Abandonment, another type of abuse, occurs when the caregiver leaves an elder at home alone or no longer provides care for the individual (CDC, 2009).

It is estimated that between 1 and 2 million Americans age 65 or older have been injured, exploited, or otherwise mistreated by someone they depend on for care or protection (DHHS, 2010). Despite these alarming numbers, there is no nationwide reporting for elder mistreatment, a major health concern. In the community, the expected prevalence of elder abuse ranges from 2 to 10% (Lachs & Pilleme, 2004; Teaster *et al.*, 2006; Halphen & Dyer, 2009). The most common types of elder abuse include self-neglect (27%) and caregiver neglect (24%) (Teaster *et al.*, 2006). Other types include financial exploitation (21%) and emotional (14%), physical (13%), and sexual abuse (0.7%) (Teaster *et al.*, 2006).

Elder abuse victim profile:

- 66% are female.
- 43% are 80 years of age or older.

- 75% are Caucasian.
- 89% of elder abuse occurs in a domestic setting.

Perpetrator profile:

- 75% are under age 60.
- 53% are female.
- 33% are an adult child of the victim.
- 22% of perpetrators are other family members (Teaster *et al.*, 2006).

Neglect is the failure to meet an elder's basic needs including food, housing, clothing, and medical care (CDC, 2009). Neglect can be further classified as caregiver-inflicted or self-inflicted (Teaster *et al.*, 2006). Self-inflicted neglect is described as (1) the person's inability to perform essential self-care tasks (to obtain food, shelter, health care) and/or (2) their inability to obtain goods or services necessary to maintain physical health, mental health, or general safety and/or (3) as in the inability to manage financial affairs due to physical or mental impairment or diminished capacity (Teaster *et al.*, 2006). Choice of lifestyle or living arrangement by itself is not evidence of self-neglect (Teaster *et al.*, 2006).

Physical abuse is any intentional hitting, slapping, kicking, burning, pushing, or other show of force against an elderly person which results in injury (CDC, 2009). Sexual abuse includes forcing an elder to engage in sexual activity when the individual does not or cannot consent (CDC, 2009). Emotional or psychosocial abuse is any behavior that causes harm to an elder's emotional state or self-worth (CDC, 2009). Financial abuse or exploitation involves withholding or misusing an elder's money, property, or assets (CDC, 2009). Elder mistreatment may also include administration of inappropriate types of medications, inappropriate doses of medications (insufficient or excessive), or neglecting to monitor drug therapy (Halphen & Dyer, 2009). Diverting medications or administering medications negligently or in excess to render the elder docile is also considered abuse (Halphen & Dyer, 2009).

All elders should be assessed for signs of abuse, but it is particularly important to assess elders who have been victims in the past to determine risk factors for future abuse. According to the National Center on Elder Abuse (NCEA) (2009) possible indicators of abuse include bruises, pressure marks, broken bones, abrasions, and burns which could be an indication of physical abuse, neglect, or mistreatment. When caregiver abuse is suspected, individuals should be interviewed without family members present.

■ Risk factors of abuse

- Age >85 years
- Belittling, threats, or uses of power and control by caregivers
- Decreased mental capacity
- Depression
- Frequent bladder incontinence

- Lack of a trusted family member or friend
- Living alone
- Low socioeconomic status (lower education and income levels)
- Social isolation
- Strained or tense relationships such as frequent arguments between the caregiver and elderly person
- Sudden changes in financial stability or transfer of property by an elder who lacks the capacity to consent to a transfer may indicate exploitation.
- Unexplained withdrawal from normal activities, social isolation, and sudden change in alertness
- Unfavorable caretaker characteristics (related to substance abuse, history of violence or antisocial behavior, depression, or financial dependency on the victim)

■ Risk factors of neglect
- Being single
- History of hip fracture or stroke
- Institutional staffing shortages
- Living with a family member who is not a partner
- Malnutrition
- Mental impairment: dementia/disability
- Social isolation/living arrangements
- Unfavorable caretaker characteristics (related to substance abuse, history of violence or antisocial behavior, depression or financial dependency on the victim)

■ Clinical presentation
As a clinician, it especially important to be alert during an assessment as it is common for a patient to suffer in silence. Changes in behavior or personality require further investigation (NCEA, 2009). Unfortunately, the elderly will sometimes neglect their own care which can lead to injury or illness (NCEA). Since self-neglect represents the majority of cases reported to protective services, it is important to include this in the assessment for elder abuse (NCEA, 2009). Frequently, self-neglect correlates with declining health, isolation, Alzheimer's disease or dementia, or drug and alcohol dependence (NCEA, 2009).

Signs of self-neglect

- Confusion
- Dehydration
- Failure to take essential medications
- Hoarding
- Inability to attend to housekeeping

- Leaving a burning stove unattended
- Poor hygiene
- Refusal to seek medical treatment for serious illness
- Wearing inappropriate clothing for the weather

Screening and assessment

Controversy remains on the protocol for recommended screening (Halphen & Dyer, 2009). The US Preventive Services Task Force noted a lack of proven effectiveness for screening instruments and lack of evidence that screening improves clinical outcomes (Nelson *et al.*, 2004). Recommended screening tools include The Conflict Tactics Scale, The Brief Abuse Screen, and The Elder Assessment Instrument (Halphen & Dyer). Although these tests do not address self-neglect, a tool, the Self-Neglect Severity Scale, is currently being evaluated (Halphen & Dyer, 2009). Other experts recommend that clinical judgment and raising awareness of clinicians may improve screening success (Lachs & Pilleme, 2004).

The major aim of screening and assessment is to determine the following:

- Is someone who is expected to help and/or protect the elder abusing, neglecting or exploiting him or her?
- Does the elderly person have an impaired capacity for self-care and protection making him or her vulnerable and in need of additional support?
- Is the elder identified as vulnerable? Is there a condition or behavior that may cause harm to that elder?
- Is the elder socially isolated?

Social isolation and mental impairment can put an individual at increased risk for abuse. Neglect abuse is positively associated with social isolation and living arrangements (Garre-Olmo *et al.*, 2009). Individuals who are single, older than 85 years of age, or who have decreased mental capacity are at increased risk for financial abuse (Garre-Olmo *et al.*, 2009). Living alone may be a risk factor for other types of abuse (Garre-Olmo *et al.*, 2009; NCEA, 2009). Frequent bladder incontinence, depression, social isolation or not having access to a trusted person may increase the likelihood of other types of abuse, including emotional abuse and physical abuse (Garre-Olmo *et al.*, 2009; NCEA, 2009). Neglect-abuse has been associated with social isolation, being single, or living with a family member who is not a partner (Garre-Olmo *et al.*, 2009). If a patient is malnourished, this may also be indicative of neglect-abuse (Garre-Olmo *et al.*, 2009).

Patients should be interviewed by themselves if possible to avoid intimidation by possible abusers (Halphen & Dyer, 2009). Patients should be questioned about family composition and living arrangements (Halphen & Dyer, 2009). Also they should be asked directly about abuse including questions such as:

- Do you feel safe where you live?
- Who prepares your meals?
- Who handles your checkbook?

If abuse is suspected, a more specific follow-up inquiry should be made. Suggested questions include:

- Has anyone at home ever hurt you?
- Has anyone ever touched you without your consent?
- Has anyone taken anything of yours without asking?
- Has anyone ever threatened you?
- Have you been forced to sign any documents that you didn't understand?
- Are you afraid of anyone at home?
- Are you alone a lot of the time?

Additional interview questions that address supports in the community will help reveal the capacity of the patient to live on their own if neglect or abuse is suspected (NCEA, 2009). For possible victims who are fearful or cognitively impaired, physical exam findings may need to be corroborated or information may need to be obtained from persons whose motives are not in question (Halphen & Dyer, 2009).

In addition to topics addressing the risk factors, other specific questions to ask when collecting the history include:

- Are there any known medical problems including confusion and memory loss?
- What kind of family and social supports are there?
- Have you heard or seen any incidents of yelling, hitting, or other abusive behavior?

The US Medicare program requires nursing facilities to monitor residents for neglect and abuse by means of the minimum data set (MDS) instruments (CMMS, 2008). In 1992, the AMA proposed for clinicians in all practice settings to screen geriatric patients for elder abuse (Aravanis et al., 1993).

■ Nursing assessment

An assessment of cognitive and functional ability is a significant part of the exam to determine capacity for self-care and self-protection (Halphen & Dyer, 2009).

Physical examination findings will most likely indicate physical violation if abuse is present. Assessment considerations include:

- General:
  - Dehydration may also indicate neglect if the elder needs assistance to take in fluids.
  - Malnutrition may indicate neglect if the elder prepares his or her own meals or requires feeding or financial exploitation if the elder does not have the funds to obtain food.
  - Poor hygiene, lack of medical compliance, and unusual weight loss may indicate neglect.

- Skin:
  - Intentional failure to follow the standard of care to prevent pressure ulcers is abuse.
  - Pressure ulcers are common for older patients who are hospitalized acutely or in long-term care. Pressure ulcers do not indicate neglect by themselves but may occur more often when the standard of care for prevention is not followed for a patient at risk.
  - Skin tears, abrasions, burns, and bruises that are inadequately explained or in unusual locations (usually found on arms and hands)
- Breasts/abdomen/genital/anal area:
  - Bruises, lacerations, or pain in this location may indicate sexual abuse.
  - Evidence of venereal disease in the oral or anal-genital areas may indicate sexual abuse.
  - Vaginal or rectal bleeding are possible signs of sexual abuse.
- Musculoskeletal:
  - Hip fractures and other fractures may indicate self-neglect.
  - Spiral fractures on long bones and fractures other than common areas (such as wrist, hip, and vertebrae) may indicate physical abuse in an elderly person with good mental health (i.e., nonalcoholic).
  - Vertebral fractures can be spontaneous and are common.

Management

Clinicians are best qualified to distinguish normal aging from the manifestations of abuse (Lachs & Pilleme, 2004). When an elder is determined to be a victim of elder abuse or mistreatment, medical, social, and legal interventions should be offered (Halphen & Dyer, 2009). Family members should be interviewed to determine more details about the suspected abuse and solicited for help when appropriate. Elders who are evaluated as having the mental capacity to understand and to consent to protective services have the right to reject offered interventions (Halphen & Dyer, 2009). Legal requirements vary according to the state of residence (Halphen & Dyer, 2009). Generally, if a patient maintains mental capacity, they are entitled to remain in their home regardless of a neglectful situation and health care workers and legal officials may not intervene (Halphen & Dyer, 2009).

Whenever elder abuse is suspected, the primary responsibility of a health care worker is to assure the safety of the elder in conjunction with community agencies and social workers (Halphen & Dyer, 2009). A home visit may be required to determine elder abuse (Halphen & Dyer, 2009). If financial exploitation, neglect, or self-neglect is suspected, a health care worker should promptly report the situation (Halphen & Dyer, 2009).

Statutes to protect elders from mistreatment exist in all states (Halphen & Dyer, 2009). Adult protective services and long term care ombudsman are present in all US jurisdictions and will provide or assist with the necessary protocol for reporting (Halphen & Dyer, 2009). In 38 states, penalties exist for failure to report suspected abuse (Halphen & Dyer, 2009).

As a clinician it may be important to contact Adult Protective Services if elder abuse or neglect is suspected where the patient is incapacitated or the power of attorney is the suspected abuser (Halphen & Dyer, 2009). Inadequate housing, inadequate food, shut off utilities, financial or physical inability to obtain medications, or the lack of capacity to negotiate the health care system to arrange for medical visits or follow a treatment plan all threaten the elder's capacity to safe and comfortable living (Halphen & Dyer, 2009). Adult Protective Services should be able to provide resources or activate outside resources to help an elder when a living situation is suspected as unsafe (Halphen & Dyer, 2009). If a state enforces mandatory reporting, a clinician is required to report suspected abuse even if a competent elder patient specifically asks that the abuse not be reported (Wei & Herbers, 2004).

In practically every state, medical directors and other nursing home medical practitioners are mandatory reporters for elder abuse in nursing homes (Lindbloom *et al.*, 2007). Physicians make up a small number of those who refer for suspicion of mistreatment (Lindbloom *et al.*, 2007). Suspicions of abuse should be made to the local ombudsmen associated with the nursing home. It is important for clinicians to remember that a report of suspicion is just that. It is a suspicion or concern rather than a conviction (Lindbloom *et al.*, 2007). Those individuals who receive the report will then investigate further and search for evidence (Lindbloom *et al.*, 2007). Documentation that may aid investigations include quotes from the resident and possible perpetrator, photographs or drawings, description of general appearance, full body surface exam, and neurological assessment including cognitive status and affect (Lindbloom *et al.*, 2007). Contact information for reporting by state including a separate institutional/nursing home contact, when applicable, is available at this website: http://www.ncea.aoa.gov/NCEAroot/Main_Site/Find_Help/State_Resources.aspx (Lindbloom *et al.*, 2007). Lawyers and police officers are now specifically trained on elder abuse and specifically the best way to prosecute a perpetrator if necessary (NCEA, 2009). State law and protective service contact information is available on the National Center on Elder Abuse website at http://www.ncea.aoa.gov/NCEAroot/Main_Site/Index.aspx (NCEA, 2009).

If reporting is generated by reasonable suspicion without evidence, government resources will assist with investigation (Halphen & Dyer, 2009). A clinician who reports elder abuse will help mobilize these resources and interventions from the adult protective services (Halphen & Dyer, 2009). Services provided from this agency include housing assistance, nursing home placement, reactivation of utilities, medications, home safety repairs, transportation and personal care services (Halphen & Dyer, 2009; NCEA, 2009).

Guardianship

Medical intervention may successfully treat some conditions related to elder abuse such as depression, diabetes, hypertension, infection, and malnutrition (Halphen & Dyer, 2009; NCEA, 2009). In some cases if the problem of abuse is severe enough, a guardian may be appointed (NCEA, 2009). Medical evaluation and treatment can be required if the elder is unable to consent (Halphen & Dyer, 2009).

If an individual is showing signs of diminished capacity for self-care or protection, a clinician may be asked to determine a need for guardianship (APA, 2006). Areas to be considered when assessing a need for guardianship include:

- Cognitive impairment (i.e., short-term memory, communication, attention, planning, decision-making, adaptation and implementation)
- Consideration of the individual's preferences and values
- Determination of whether less restrictive means of guardianship are possible
- Difficulty performing activities of everyday living
- Medical condition that might produce functional disability
- Risk of harm and level of necessary supervision

Decision making, planning, implementation and adaptive skills can be evaluated during the history and physical examination (Halphen & Dyer, 2009). Referral for neuropsychological testing may be useful in cases where self-care or self-protection capacity is still in question (Halphen & Dyer, 2009). Specific capacities that a clinician may need to assess in an elder include the capacity to consent to sexual activity, make a will, vote, drive, transfer property, consent to participate in research, and consent to treatment (Halphen & Dyer, 2009).

Follow-up of medical treatment can be challenging in a situation of elder abuse (Halphen & Dyer, 2009). An abuser may resist or try to sabotage medical interventions if hostility towards the agency or medical office responsible for identifying the abuse exists (Halphen & Dyer, 2009). Transfer of care to new medical providers, in agreement with the family and the patient, may be necessary (Halphen & Dyer, 2009). Adult protective services should also follow-up with court required interventions to ensure the patient is being taken to the medical provider and the treatment plan is being followed up (Halphen & Dyer, 2009).

If an agency determines that a victim lacks the capacity to understand and consent to protective services, the agency may petition a court for emergency order for protective services that a situation is unsafe (Halphen & Dyer, 2009). A majority of the states (all but 13) have statutes providing for emergency or involuntary protective services for those without the capacity to consent (Stiegle & Klem, 2007). Courts may require a statement from a clinician to support a finding for lack of capacity in order to consent to protective services before an emergency order is issued (Halphen & Dyer, 2009).

References

American Psychological Association: American Bar Association Commission on Law and Aging (2006) Judicial Determination of Capacity of Older Adults in Guardianship Proceedings. Online. Available from http://www.apa.org/pi/aging/resources/guides/judges-diminished.pdf (accessed 29 March 2012).

Aravanis, S.C., Adelman, R.D., Breckman, R. *et al.* (1993) Diagnostic and treatment guidelines on elder abuse and neglect. *Archives of Family Medicine* **2**(4), 371–388.

Centers for Disease Control and Prevention (2009) Understanding elder maltreatment. Online. Available from www.cdc.gov/violenceprevention/pdf/em-factsheet-a.pdf (accessed 29 March 2012).

Centers for Medicare and Medicaid Services (2008) MDS 2.0 for Nursing Home Nursing Home Quality Initiative. Online. Available from https://www.cms.gov/NursingHomeQualityInits/downloads/MDS20MDSAllForms.pdf (accessed 29 March 2012).

Department of Health and Human Services: Administration on Aging (2010) Justification of Estimates for Appropriations Committee. Online. Available from @http://www.aoa.gov/AoARoot/Program_Results/docs/2010/FY2010 AoACongressionalJustificationFinal.PDF (accessed 29 March 2012).

Garre-Olmo, J., Planas-Pujol, X., López-Pousa, S., Juvinya, D., Vilà, A. & Vilalta-Franch, J. (2009) Prevalence and risk factors of suspected elder abuse subtypes in people aged 75 and older. *Journal of the American Geriatrics Society* **57**(5), 815–822.

Halphen, J.M. & Dyer, C.B. (2009) Elder mistreatment: abuse, neglect, and financial exploitation. In: *UpToDate* (Schmader, K.E. ed.). UpToDate, Waltham, MA.

Lachs, M.S. & Pilleme, K. (2004) Elder abuse. *Lancet* **364**(9441), 1263–1272.

Lindbloom, E.J., Brandt, J., Landon, D.H. & Meadows, S.E. (2007) Elder mistreatment in the nursing home: a systematic review. *Journal of the American Medical Director's Association* **8**, 610–616.

National Center on Elder Abuse (2009) National Center on Elder Abuse: Administration on Aging Website. Online. Available from http://www.ncea.aoa.gov/NCEAroot/Main_Site/Index.aspx (accessed 29 March 2012).

Nelson, H.D., Nygren, P., McInerney, Y. & Klein, J. (2004) Screening women and elderly adults for family and intimate partner violence. US Preventive Services Task Force. Online. Available from www.ahrq.gov/clinic/3rduspstf/famviolence/famviolrev.htm (accessed 29 March 2012).

Stiegle, L. & Klem, E. (2007) Explanation of the "Emergency or involuntary services to victims: Comparison Chart of Provisions in Adult Protective Services Laws with Citations by State" Chart. American Bar Association Commission on Law and Aging. Online. Available from www.abanet.org/aging/about/pdfs/emergency_or_involuntary_services_explanation.pdf (accessed 29 March 2012).

Teaster, P., Dugar, T., Mendiondo, M., Abner, E. & Cecil, K. (2006) 2004 Survey of State Adult Protective Services: Abuse of adults 60 years of age and older. Report to the National Center on Elder Abuse. Administration on Aging, Washington, DC.

Wei, G.S. & Herbers, J.E. (2004) Reporting elder abuse: a medical, legal, and ethical overview. *Journal of the American Medical Womens Association* **59**(4), 248–254.

PART 3: ADVANCE DIRECTIVES

Anita M. Coppola-Ash

Advance directives are an individual's health care wishes in the event an individual is unable to communicate his or her medical decisions regarding care and treatment. Advance directives come in many forms including a living will, health care proxy, and power of attorney. This particular aspect of medical care is often overlooked by individuals and health care providers until an emergency situation arises. "A review of current literature indicates that approximately 85% to 95% of the population does not have adequate advance directives or palliative care measures written in their medical record" (Alfonso, 2009, p. 42). There, any many ethical dilemmas surrounding advance directives which can lead to costly, unwanted medical treatment, stress to family members and caregivers faced with making end-of-life decisions, and stress to health care professionals providing care during acute care hospitalizations.

Definitions of advance directives

Advance directives are recognized by the United States government to guide medical care for individuals. Each state, however, has its own laws and documents, which are recognized according to state regulations. Therefore, advance directives formulated in one state may not be legal in another. This is important to note as the demographic structure of family has changed over the past century and fewer families live in close proximity to their siblings and parents. While some advance directives require an attorney and fee to be drawn up, others can be free of charge and require only a witness. In order to invoke an advance directive, a physician must deem the patient incompetent to make his or her own health care decisions.

Living will

Living wills are a map of an individual's health care wishes when planning for future medical treatment and end-of-life care. Living wills can be drawn up by attorneys or can be as easy as writing down one's wishes and having the document notarized. Living wills may include, but are not limited to decisions regarding life sustaining treatment. Life sustaining treatments include mechanical ventilation, supplemental nutrition such as peg tubes, dialysis, and cardiopulmonary resuscitation. Living wills can help both health care providers and family members when faced with difficult decisions as the decision has already been made by the individual prior to becoming ill. Having your wishes in writing can relieve the burden of decision making for the caregiver. Living wills, like other advance directives, can be changed at any time by the individual implementing them.

Health care proxy

Health care proxies are much different than living wills. A health care proxy is the appointment of another individual to make health care decisions in the event you are unable to make decisions for yourself. A health care proxy is invoked only when a physician has determined that an individual is incapable of making their own decisions. The appointment of a health care proxy may also include an alternate proxy in the event the primary individual is not available and/or capable or able to act as proxy. A health care proxy usually only requires the signature of two witnesses to be recognized as a legal document. Again, each state and its laws are individual. Although the health care proxy does not outline an individual's wishes, it is the responsibility of the proxy to know the individual's wishes regarding medical care.

Power of attorney

A durable power of attorney (DPA) is another example of an advance directive. This particular document is a legal document recognized in every state in the United States. DPAs are usually established to appoint an individual to make financial decisions. However, a power of attorney (POA) can also include a health care clause which is designed to designate the POA to make both financial and medical decisions. The durable power of attorney is only executed when the individual is incapacitated and is unable to make financial and health care decisions (Crane & Wittink, 2005, p. 1265). A power of attorney is also often responsible for an individual's estate planning following death. In addition to the appointment of the power of attorney and health care clause, DPAs can also include specific health care instructions for the POA. Instructions regarding health care decisions may include an individual's wishes regarding Do-not-Resuscitate orders, Do-not-intubate orders, feeding tubes, and hemodialysis. Advance planning for end-of-life care significantly decreases the stress and guilt associated with making decisions for loved ones in the absence of advance directives.

Case study

Mrs. Riley has come into the emergency room from home after the family called 911. According to the family's report, Mrs. Riley was sitting at the kitchen table with her husband when he noticed his wife's speech was garbled. When her husband tried to engage her in conversation, Mrs. Riley spoke with a thick tongue and her words did not make sense. Mrs. Riley then dropped her fork and seemed to drift off, staring in a gaze. When her husband went to her side and tried to stand her, Mrs. Riley was noted to have weakness on her left side and was unable to stand. Mr. Riley immediately called 911 and Mrs. Riley was rushed to the emergency room.

At the time of arrival to the emergency room, Mrs. Riley was unresponsive. Paramedics performed cardiopulmonary resuscitation (CPR) en route to the hospital, and were able to get a pulse. Electrocardiography (ECG) monitoring revealed atrial fibrillation, and a heart rate of 65 beats per minute. Her family remained at her bedside as the emergency room staff worked vigilantly to keep her alive. Intravenous lines were established, blood pressure, oxygen saturations, pulse and ECG monitoring was ongoing, and the history was obtained from the family. The time of onset of symptoms was established and Mrs. Riley was rushed to computed tomography scan (CAT scan) to confirm whether or not she had suffered a hemorrhagic or ischemic stroke. If the stroke was not hemorrhagic, than Mrs. Riley was a candidate for tissue plasminogen activator (TPA). TPA is only used in acute ischemic strokes as a clot busting agent.

The entire family had assembled and waited anxiously for the results of the CAT scan. The family included her spouse and six children, with one who lived out of state and could only be reached by phone. The emergency room physician met with the family to discuss medical management, diagnosis, and prognosis. The family was faced with so many questions, none of which they had considered before this day. Like most families, end-of-life treatment and life sustaining measures are not discussed until a crisis occurs. And in time of crisis, emotions and fear can take over rational thinking. In larger families, it is inevitable that not everyone will agree on the course of treatment for end-of-life care. The physician notified the family of the CT scan results. Mrs. Riley had suffered a hemorrhagic stroke; chance of survival was only 50% (Zomorodi, 2011).

Case study review

This is a common scenario often seen by health care providers. In an acute care setting, decisions often have to be made with urgency as an individual's life is dependent on it. The family has suffered a tremendous loss and is now faced with having to make a decision regarding treatment, knowing the prognosis of survival is only 50%. In this particular case, there has been no advance directive established. The spouse and children must come to an agreement on end-of-life care based on the information that has been provided to them. It is the role of the physician to determine who the primary decision maker is, which often defaults to the spouse. It is inevitable in larger families that not everyone will come to an agreement regarding end-of-life care. However, all family members closest to the patient must be involved in order to support the primary decision maker (Meehan, 2009). It is the role of the health care professional to step in and provide guidance, education, and support to the family.

The role of the nurse

Nurses play an important role with families during end-of-life care and decision making. Education is a pivotal piece of the advance directive process. Education for nurses regarding advance directives begins in school but is not often implemented until nurses enter the workforce. The importance of advance planning is seen in all areas of health care including primary care offices, outpatient clinics, hospitals, and long term care facilities. Regardless of the scope of practice, advance directives should be initiated and discussed at time of admission. Nurses must have a thorough understanding of advance directives appropriate to their state regulations in order to initiate the first conversation. The use of brochures, pamphlets, and examples of various advance directives will be helpful when initiating this discussion (Alfonso, 2009). Having basic knowledge in this area will empower nurses to feel more comfortable when discussing end-of-life care with patients.

The role of the nurse is much greater than education when discussing advance directives. Initiating a plan of care after careful, individualized evaluation and assessment of each situation is the next step in advance directive planning. Care plans are established to provide an outline for treatments and goals agreed upon by the medical professionals, patients and family members. There are a multitude of factors to consider when working with families during end-of-life, including cultural and religious beliefs. These must be carefully considered when adopting a plan of care. Assessment of the families understanding of the patient's medical status is also important to the planning process (Lang & Quill, 2004). It is the role of the physician and the nurse to provide the family with accurate information regarding the patient's medical condition while at the same time assessing the families understanding of the information provided. If the health care professionals and family members cannot reach an agreement, it is unlikely that end-of-life care planning can be established.

Communication and support are an integral part of the nursing process when initiating and implementing advance directives. Advance planning in the absence of illness is highly recommended but is not often the case. Often when advance directives are discussed, the health or the competency of the patient is compromised, leaving the decision making to family members. Illness and death lead to feelings of fear, anxiety, guilt, anger, and depression. The role of the nurse to provide emotional support under these circumstances is very important. Providing support by establishing rapport, open communication and empathy will provide a safe environment for families during these difficult times.

References

Alfonso, H. (2009) The Importance of living wills and advance directives. *Journal of Gerontological Nursing* **35**, 42–45.

Crane, M.K. & Wittink, M. (2005) Respecting end-of-life treatment preferences. *American Family Physician* **72**(7), 1263–1268.

Zomorodi, M. (2011) Stroke. In Lewis, S.M., Dirksen, S.R. Heitkemper, M.M Bucher, L. & Camera, I.M. (2011) *Medical Surgical Nursing Assessment and Management of Clinical Problems*. Mosby, St. Louis, MO.

Lang, F. & Quill, T. (2004) Making decisions with families at the end of life. *American Family Physician* **70**(4), 719–723.

Meehan, K.A. (2009) Advance directives: the clinical nurse specialist as a change agent. *Clinical Nurse Specialist* **23**(5), 258–264.

Messinger-Rapport, B., Baum, E.E. & Smith, M.L. (2009) Advance care planning: beyond the living will. *Cleveland Clinic Journal of Medicine* **76**(5), 276–285.

Further reading

Dash, T. & Mailloux, L.U. (2007) Ethical Issues in the care of the patient with end-stage renal disease. Online. Available from http://www.uptodate.com/contents/ethical-issues-in-the-care-of-the-patient-with-end-stage-renal-disease (accessed 30 March 2012).

PART 4: NUTRITION AND OLDER ADULTS

Deborah A. D'Avolio

Body composition and energy changes related to normal aging can impact several systems; gastrointestinal (GI), central nervous system, metabolic, renal, musculoskeletal, and sensory. In general, body fat increases and total water decreases as we age. In the GI system there can be decreased hepatic function, gastric and colonic motility, and anorectal function. The consequences of these age related changes include delayed absorption of some drugs, decreased calcium absorption, and constipation.

Alterations in nutrition are common among older adults, particularly malnutrition. The energy needs of an adult with an acute illness increase as protein and fat stores are utilized. The increased caloric and protein requirements are dependent upon the injury, illness, or stress. The increased requirements can increase slightly in mild illness with a much higher requirement in severe illness or stress.

Data show that 55% of hospitalized older adults are found to be undernourished on admission (Milne *et al.*, 2006). Malnutrition is defined as inadequate nutritional status and undernourishment, particularly protein energy undernutrition. The common characteristics include insufficient dietary intake, poor appetite, muscle wasting, and weight loss (Chen *et al.*, 2001). Malnutrition among older adults is a serious problem which contributes to complications, longer hospitalizations, and increased morbidity and mortality. Survival rates among older hospitalized patients who are malnourished and at risk for malnourishment are significantly lower than in well nourished patients (Kagansky *et al.*, 2005). Older people with dementia experience difficulty with feeding which leads to further physical and functional decline.

Nutritional syndromes among older adults also include obesity which is increasing among older adults. Excess body weight and weight gain are associated with medical co morbidities including hypertension, cardiovascular disease, diabetes, osteoarthritis, and increased mortality. In obese older adults, a careful evaluation of a safe weight loss program's risks and benefits should be considered.

Dehydration is the most common fluid or electrolyte imbalance among older adults. In normal aging there may be decreased thirst, impaired serum osmolarity, and reduced ability to concentrate urine flow when fluid intake decreases. Decreased fluid intake can also be the result of diseases that reduce the mental or physical ability to recognize thirst. The typical fluid needs of older adults are 30 milliliters per kg of body weight per day. Fluid needs may be altered during fever, infection, and the use of diuretics and laxatives.

■ Risk factors for alterations in nutrition

- Availability of protein, high quality food
- Changes in dietary intake
- Changes in taste
- Chronic illness

- Decreased muscle mass
- Dementia
- Depression
- Eating less than two meals per day
- Frail and ill older adults
- Functional disabilities which impact ability to shop and prepare food
- Inadequate intake of nutrients
- Injury
- Involuntary weight loss
- Lack of appetite
- Lack of transportation to purchase food
- Limited income to purchase food
- Loneliness, social isolation
- Nothing by mouth (NPO) ordered while hospitalized
- Pain
- Poor oral health; cavities, gum disease, dry mouth
- Problems with chewing or swallowing
- Recent surgery
- Sepsis
- Side effects of medications; dry mouth, decreased appetite

Nutritional screening and assessment

Assessment of nutritional problems in older adults has been recommended in routine screening and as part of a comprehensive geriatric assessment (CGA). During routine nursing assessment the nutritional status of older adults should be evaluated as part of a comprehensive geriatric assessment to identify risk factors.

In clinical practice, assessment for nutrition would include present illness, symptoms, and past medical history. Assessment includes the patient's ability to eat, GI function, weight history, change in clothing size, a 3 day food intake history, and functional status. Obtain a history of alcohol use and medications, including self-prescribed dietary and vitamin supplements.

A complete physical exam would include assessment of the patient's oral cavity, subcutaneous fat, muscle wasting, and body mass index (BMI). During the physical assessment, it is important to assess for common signs of dehydration. These symptoms may include decreased urine output, fever, orthostatic changes, skin turgor changes, constipation, mucosal dryness, and confusion or change in mental status. Altered fluid status including over hydration can affect lab values resulting in an inaccurate interpretation of results.

Mini Nutritional Assessment

The Mini Nutritional Assessment (MNA) is one of the most widely used geriatric nutritional tools (Beck et al., 2001; Vellas et al., 2006). An MNA score of less than 17 usually indicates that the patient has a protein caloric malnutrition and nutritional intervention is necessary. Scores between 17 and 23.5 indicate that the patient is at risk for malnutrition. The MNA is used in conjunction with other assessment information such as the patient's food preferences, cultural background, and symptoms.

Anthropometrics

An unintended weight loss of 4.5 kg (10 pounds) in the preceding several months is an indicator of morbidity. Weight loss is usually defined as 5% or more in the past 6 months. BMI is also assessed. Other anthropometrics include skin fold and circumference measurements, but these are done by trained personnel.

Laboratory tests

Serum albumin has been recognized as a risk indicator for morbidity and mortality. In community dwelling older adults, hypoalbuminemia has been associated with functional decline, sarcopenia (the degenerative loss of skeletal muscle mass and strength associated with aging) and increased health care utilization. In the hospitalized older adult it has been associated with prolonged hospitalization, complications, readmissions, and mortality. Prealbumin can indicate short term changes in protein status. Serum cholesterol is checked because low cholesterol can indicate poor health and an inflammatory condition. Other laboratory data would include thyroid-stimulating hormone (TSH), transferrin, total lymphocyte count, hemoglobin, hematocrit, serum electrolytes, blood urea nitrogen (BUN) and creatinine.

■ Complications of malnutrition
- Critically obese patients are at increased risk.
- Delayed wound healing
- Immune dysfunction
- Increased morbidity
- Organ dysfunction
- Vitamin and mineral deficiencies
- Weight loss in older adults is associated with increased risk of mortality.

Nutritional interventions

Strategies focus on interventions to increase intake, if the gastrointestinal system is functioning properly. In an acute care hospitalization, the NPO status of older adults should be carefully monitored to avoid iatrogenic malnutrition or dehydration. Nutritional interventions have been shown to be effective in improving weight, MNA score, and muscle mass. Protein and energy nutritional supplements have been shown to have beneficial effects on mortality and length of stay among hospitalized patients. Nutritional interventions should be started as soon as possible.

Many oral supplementation formulas are available, most are milk based and have approximately 1–1.5 calories per milliliter. Supplements should be given between meals rather than with meals. Dietary recommendations for older adults include multivitamins, supplements of protein, calcium, vitamin D, vitamin E, zinc, and other micronutrients

Note: drugs should not be used as a first-line intervention in older adults.

Interventions

- Dentures should be assessed for fit and oral cavity checked for lesions.
- Incorporate food preferences as much as possible.
- Prepare patients for meals with appropriate mouth and hand care.
- Ensure oral health.
- If possible have the patient take all meals out of bed in a chair.
- Provide smaller meals more frequently.
- Those needing assistance should be helped.
- The use of herbs and spices may be used to help compensate for changes in taste/smell.
- Allow adequate time for meals.
- Encourage exercise.

Enteral or tube feedings

Enteral nutrition (EN) or tube feedings may be indicated to ensure adequate intake of macronutrients, micronutrients, and water. Special consideration is given to the patient's condition, the theoretical benefits, and patient's desires and concerns. Formulas contain between 0.5 and 2.0 calories per milliliter. Most contain no milk products. For those patients who have fluid restrictions, there are higher concentrated formulas available but they may cause diarrhea. In older adults, special consideration is the protein content and possible reduced kidney function associated with aging. There are important drug-enteral interactions to consider, check with your pharmacist to review the patient's medications and the best way to administer sustain released, enteric coated, and micro-encapsulated medications (e.g., lansoprazole, diltiazem, omeprazole, verapamil).

Gastrostomy/jejunostomy tube feedings may be initiated in some instances. However, chronic artificial nutrition and hydration is not a basic intervention. It has been shown to be associated with uncertain benefit, risks and discomfort.

Prior to initiating the use of artificial support the patient's advanced directives should be reviewed. Total parenteral nutrition (TPN) may be indicated in those who have digestive dysfunction precluding enteral feeding. It provides protein, amino acids, fat as lipids, and dextrose. It is important to follow hospital policies and procedures related to safe administration of artificial feeding.

Indications for EN or TP

- Chronic debilitation
- Delays in feeding
- Alcohol abuse
- Inability to use GI tract (e.g., esophageal cancer, radiation therapy to head or neck)
- Inadequate ability to feed or take food or fluids
- NPO status, especially three 3 days or more
- Recent major surgery, trauma, stress, pain, and steroids
- Sepsis, acute respiratory failure, acute respiratory distress syndrome, and severe pancreatitis.

Collaborative strategies

- Enhancing older adults' nutritional status or targeted nutritional goals are developed in collaboration with interdisciplinary colleagues.
- Refer to dietician and nutritional support team those patients who are at risk for or have under-nutrition.
- Consult with the pharmacist to review medications which may cause possible drug/nutrition interactions.
- Speech and swallow pathologists can evaluate swallowing difficulties. Strategies focus on ways to increase nutritional intake and prevent complications from nutritional problems.

■ Patient/family education

If a patient has been identified as having a nutritional problem or at risk the patient's family should receive education on the targeted nutritional interventions to support a safe transition to home. It is important for families to know simple strategies which may improve intake. For example; small frequent meals, increasing the nutritional density of food, and providing supplements between meals. They can assist with enhancing the environment during meal time. Family members can arrange to eat meals with their older adults to help increase their enjoyment of food and intake.

References

Beck, A.M., Ovesen, L. & Schroll, M. (2001) A six months' prospective follow-up of 65+-y-old patients from general practice classified according to nutritional risk by the mini nutritional assessment. *European Journal of Clinical Nutrition* **55**(11), 1028–1033.

Chen, C.C., Schilling, L.S. & Lyder, C.H. (2001) A concept analysis of malnutrition in the elderly. *Journal of Advanced Nursing* **36**(1), 131–142.

Kagansky, N., Berner, Y., Koren-Morag, N., Perelman, L., Knobler, H. & Levy, S. (2005) Poor nutritional habits are predictors of poor outcome in very old hospitalized patients. *The American Journal of Clinical Nutrition* **82**(4), 784–91; quiz 913–4.

Milne, A.C., Avenell, A. & Potter, J. (2006) Meta-analysis: Protein and energy supplementation in older people. *Annals of Internal Medicine* **144**(1), 37–48.

Vellas, B., Villars, H., Abellan, G., *et al.* (2006) Overview of the MNA® – Its History and Challenges. *Journal of Nutrition and Health in Aging* **10**, 456–465.

Further reading

Beck, A.M., Balknas, U.N., Furst, P. *et al.* (2001) Food and nutritional care in hospitals: How to prevent undernutrition – report and guidelines from the Council of Europe. *Clinical Nutrition (Edinburgh, Scotland)* **20**(5), 455–460.

Berrut, G., Favreau, A.M., Dizo, E. *et al.* (2002) Estimation of calorie and protein intake in aged patients: Validation of a method based on meal portions consumed. *The Journals of Gerontology. Series A, Biological Sciences and Medical Sciences* **57**(1), M52–6.

Bleda, M.J., Bolibar, I., Pares, R. & Salva, A. (2002) Reliability of the mini nutritional assessment (MNA) in institutionalized elderly people. *The Journal of Nutrition, Health & Aging* **6**(2), 134–137.

DiMaria-Ghalili, R.A. (2008) Nutrition. In: *Evidence-Based Geriatric Nursing Protocols for Best Practice*, 3rd edition (Capezuti, E., Zwicker, D., Mezey M. & Fulmer, T. eds). Springer Publishing Company, New York, pp. 353–357.

Green, S.M. & Watson, R. (2006) Nutritional screening and assessment tools for older adults: Literature review. *Journal of Advanced Nursing* **54**(4), 477–490.

Guigoz, Y., Jensen, G., Thomas, D. & Vellas, B. (2006) The mini nutritional assessment (mna®) review of the literature – what does it tell us?/discussion. *The Journal of Nutrition, Health & Aging* **10**(6), 466.

Janssen, I., Heymsfield, S.B. & Ross, R. (2002) Low relative skeletal muscle mass (sarcopenia) in older persons is associated with functional impairment and physical disability. *Journal of the American Geriatrics Society* **50**(5), 889–896.

Kyle, U.G., Pirlich, M., Schuetz, T., Lochs, H. & Pichard, C. (2004) Is nutritional depletion by nutritional risk index associated with increased length of hospital stay? A population-based study. *JPEN. Journal of Parenteral and Enteral Nutrition* **28**(2), 99–104.

National Collaborating Centre for Acute Care (2006) *Nutrition support in adults: Oral nutritionsupport, enteral tube feeding and parenteral nutrition*. Clinical guideline number 32. Online. Available from http://guidance.nice.org.uk/CG32/Guidance/pdf/English (accessed 30 March 2012).

Pichard, C., Kyle, U.G., Morabia, A., Perrier, A., Vermeulen, B. & Unger, P. (2004) Nutritional assessment: Lean body mass depletion at hospital admission is associated with an increased length of stay. *The American Journal of Clinical Nutrition* **79**(4), 613–618.

Rubenstein, L.Z., Harker, J.O., Salva, A., Guigoz, Y. & Vellas, B. (2001) Screening for undernutrition in geriatric practice: Developing the short-form mini-nutritional assessment (MNA-SF). *The Journals of Gerontology* **56A**(6), M366.

Salvà, A., Corman, B., Andrieu, S., Salas, J. & Vellas, B. (2004) Minimum data set for nutritional intervention studies in elderly people. *The Journals of Gerontology* **59A**(7), 724.

Sullivan, D.H., Roberson, P.K. & Bopp, M.M. (2005) Hypoalbuminemia 3 months after hospital discharge: Significance for long-term survival. *Journal of the American Geriatrics Society* **53**(7), 1222–1226.

PART 5: FALL PREVENTION

Deborah A. D'Avolio

Among older adults, falls are the leading cause of injury-related deaths. The incidence of fall-related deaths among older adults rose significantly over the past decade (Centers for Disease Control and Prevention (CDC), National Center for Injury Prevention and Control (NCIPC)). Falls are also the most common cause of nonfatal injuries and trauma related hospital admissions (CDC, 2012). In 2008, 19,700 people 65 and older died from injuries related to unintentional falls; in 2009 about 2.2 million people 65 and older were treated in emergency departments for nonfatal injuries from falls, and more than 581,000 of these patients were hospitalized (CDC, 2012).

There are several definitions of a fall and nurses should refer to their hospital policy and procedures for an organizational definition. The National Database for Nursing Quality Indicators (NDNQI) defines a fall as "an unplanned descent to the floor (or extension of the floor, e.g., trash can or other equipment) with or without injury. All types of falls are included, whether they result from physiological reasons or environmental reasons" (American Nurses Association, 2009).

The negative outcomes of falls are significant. Those who suffer moderate to severe injuries may experience an impact to their ability to ambulate and maintain activities of daily living. Even those not injured may develop a fear of falling. This fear can limit activities, which may lead to decreased mobility and function, and as a result an increased risk of falling. Decreased mobility also leads to imbalance, loss of postural reflexes, skin breakdown, and multiple problems for older adults.

Falls are a leading cause of death for older adults and can contribute to early death. Hip fractures are one of the serious consequences of falls. They are a contributing factor in nursing home admissions. Recurrent falls are a common reason for admission of previously independent older persons to long-term care facilities. Falls are the most common cause of traumatic brain injuries (TBI) and accounted for 46% of fatal falls among older adults (CDC, 2012;

Jager et al., 2000). In addition to the physical and psychological outcomes of falls, the medical costs are significant, $0.2 billion ($179 million) for fatal falls and $19 billion for nonfatal fall injuries (CDC, 2012; Stevens et al., 2006).

Falls were once considered an accident or a part of normal aging process. However, we now know that falls should not be viewed as accidental or normal. Balance and walking require complex interactions of cognition, senses, neurological and muscular systems. As persons age, these systems undergo changes which predispose older adults to increased risks for falls and fall injuries. Thus, falls are rarely the result of one risk factor and prevention involves intrinsic and environmental risk factors. Hospitalization places most patients at higher risk for falls because of the complex interaction of vulnerability, impairment, and environment. Acute illness, surgery, immobility, treatments, medications, and an unfamiliar environment are some of the common risk factors which can contribute to falls.

One of the Joint Commission on Accreditation Healthcare Organization (JCAHO) goals focuses on reducing the risk of patient harm resulting from falls. JCAHO organizations are directed to have their healthcare providers assess and reassess each patient's risk and potential risks for falls and take action to address any identified risks (Joint Commission on Accreditation of Health Care Organizations).

In 2008, the Centers for Medicare and Medicaid determined that hospital falls are one of eight conditions that should not occur after admission to the hospital and Medicare can withhold payment for costs incurred from a fall. Patient falls are at the top of the list of nursing quality challenges and are recognized as nursing sensitive by the National Quality Forum, the Agency for Healthcare Research and Quality, JCAHO, and the National Database of Nursing Quality Indicators (NDNQI).

An effective organizational response to fall prevention is a program which includes at least three major elements: fall risk assessment, post-fall assessment, and use of fall reduction tools. All of these fundamental elements are implemented or coordinated by nurses and included in policy and practice. Nurses provide individualized assessment and reassessment, manage the environment, and develop and implement individualized plans of care. Nurses play an important role in identifying the risk factors that contribute to older adults' risk for falls and serious injury and utilize this knowledge to develop nursing care plans to prevent falls (Morse, 2009).

■ Risk factors

Research has shown that falls among hospitalized older adults are multifactorial and a combination of several risk factors. Those occurring within the person are referred to as intrinsic factors while risks occurring in the environment are extrinsic risk factors. Some medications can cause significant side effects in older adults (e.g., sedatives, benzodiazepines, hypnotics, alcohol, antidepressants, neuroleptics, digoxin, anti-arrhythmics, diuretics, and/or taking four or more medications).

The side effects of medications can increase fall risks. These side effects may include low blood pressure, postural hypotension, dizziness, drowsiness, confusion, and problems with balance. It is important to remember that some risk tools do not assess for injury risk. Patients at particular risk for fall related injuries include those who have a low BMI, osteoporosis, vitamin D deficiency, are on antiplatelet therapy, or are frail.

Person-intrinsic risk factors:

- Age 75 or older
- Arthritis
- Balance impairment
- Comorbidities
- Decreased cognition
- Delirium
- Depression
- Fear of falling
- Gait impairment
- History of falls
- Impaired activities of daily living
- Lower extremity weakness
- Sensory impairment; neuropathies, hearing loss, impaired vision, impaired sensation
- Urinary incontinence
- Use of an assistive device
- Weakness

Environment-extrinsic risk factors:

- Call bell not within easy reach
- Clutter
- Improper footwear
- Lack of handrails in patient rooms, bathrooms, and hall ways
- Lack of safe, comfortable, proper seating
- Physical restraint use
- Poor lighting or lighting which causes high glare
- Poorly maintained equipment; wheelchairs, walkers
- Side rails
- Uneven, cracked, wet, slippery, or shiny floor surfaces
- Use of IV pole as assistive ambulatory device

■ Nursing assessment

In addition to reviewing the patient's history of present illness, past medical history, past history of falls, and external and internal risk factors, there are several other components of a fall risk assessment. Assessment tools are used to identify risk for falling and support fall prevention interventions. When selecting a fall risk tool, it is essential to use the instrument as intended by the researcher who developed it. Any changes to the tool can change the reliability and validity of the instrument. A useful tool should be reliable, valid, and brief in length. The Morse tool is one of commonly used assessment tools (Morse, 2009). Assessment tools are always used in conjunction with other components of patient assessment and evaluation. Patient reassessment should occur at regular intervals. If the patient has been identified to be at risk for falling, it is essential to communicate the fall risk among team members and include the fall assessment and plan in verbal and written reports. It is also essential to provide fall risk identification (e.g., signage, electronic medical record, and patient identification bands). The patient and, if appropriate, the family should be informed of the fall risk and the fall prevention plan of care.

Interventions

One of the most important interventions for hospitalized older adults is fall prevention, but it is important to avoid bed rest whenever possible. Interventions are multimodal and targeted to the individual patient's underlying disorders and risk factors as outlined in the section above. Most intrinsic and extrinsic/environmental risk factors can be modified. It is important to review and monitor all medications for side effects.

- Older adults may have reduced visual acuity and dark adaptation, as well as reduced hearing.
  - Cerumen removal and audiology or ophthalmology evaluation may be indicated.
- Older adults need twice the illumination as younger people. It is important to reduce glare and remove shadows.
- Review and monitor all medications for side effects.
- Monitor for signs and symptoms of delirium and provide appropriate prevention and intervention measures.
- Provide accessible switches, grab bars, a clear path, and a night light in the bathroom.
- The bathroom should have a non-skid shower area and raised toilet seat.
- Spills on the floor must be cleaned promptly and assistive ambulatory devices should be available.
- A bladder and bowel protocol will establish a toileting regime to eliminate urgency and incontinence.
- Utilize chair and bed alarms for patients who need assistance to ambulate and may forget to request assistance.
- Use proper footwear to aid ambulation. Shoes with firm, nonskid soles and low heels should be worn and walking in stocking feet or loose slippers should be avoided.
- Musculoskeletal disorders need appropriate evaluation. Interventions may include strength and gait training; muscle strengthening exercises, and assistive walking devices.

- If foot disorders are a contributing factor; calluses, bunions, and toe nail deformities can be corrected.
- Postural vital signs should be routinely assessed in older adults because postural hypotension is common.
- Medication assessment and fluid status should be continually reassessed.
- Physical therapy consultation
- Educate patient and family on how to gradually change position when changing position from resting to standing.

Post fall management

All patients who fall should receive a post fall assessment and have their plan of care revised. By conducting a root cause analysis of the interacting factors it is possible to learn those factors that may have caused the fall. This information can help us prevent future falls. Basics of post fall management include:

- Remain with the patient and summon help.
- Provide reassurance.
- When the patient's status allows, obtain information from the patient about the incident and any pain experienced.
- Depending on the condition and stability of the patient, take measures to control bleeding, then assess level of consciousness, airway, vital signs, and oxygen status.
- Examine the patient carefully for signs of external injury:
  - Hip fracture: leg shortening, external rotation
  - Pelvic fracture: pain in the groin, hip, or lower back
  - Subdural hematoma: changes in neurological status
- Notify MD and appropriate personnel as soon as possible and provide an update on the patient's condition.
- Observe for evidence of head or neck injury, abnormal neurological responses, change in mental status, uncontrolled bleeding, fever, unstable vital signs, pain, extremity swelling, discolored skin, laceration or contusion, incontinence, or decreased range of motion.
- Note location, activity, position of patient, and time of fall.
- Assist for further evaluation, diagnosis, and treatment.
- Evaluate environment and equipment.
- Review possible causes.
- Review medications.
- Reassess intrinsic and extrinsic risk factors.
- Revise the plan of care.
- Implement fall prevention strategies.
- Implement general safety measures.

Continue to assess the patient's sensory and functional status and review and report pertinent findings. Following a fall the presence of injury may not be apparent for days. Remember to continue observations of patient status with attention to subtle or significant changes that can signal an underlying injury. The development of acute delirium or post fall confusion can signal the possibility of injury. Provide a continuous loop of communication.

■ Patient/family education

If a patient is identified to be a fall risk in the hospital, risk reduction should continue to support the older adult's safe transition to home. The older adult and their family should receive education about fall prevention at home and in the community. There are excellent fall prevention resources available on line through the Centers for Disease Control and Prevention web site. Additionally, Visiting Nurses can do a Home Safety Evaluation to help the patient and family make home environment changes to help decrease the risk of falls.

References

American Nurses Association (2009) American Nurses Association national database for nursing quality indicators: Guidelines for data collection and submission on American Medical Directors Association (AMDA). (1998) *Falls and fall risk*. AMDA, Columbia, MD.

Centers for Disease Control and Prevention (2012) Fall among older adults: an overview. Online. Available from http://www.cdc.gov/HomeandRecreationalSafety/Falls/adultfalls.html (accessed 13 June 2012).

Injury Surveillance Program, Bureau of Health Information, Statistics, Research, and Evaluation (2007) *Fall-related injuries: Deaths, hospital discharges, observation stays, and emergency department visits*. Massachusetts Department of Public Health.

Jager, T.E., Weiss, H.B., Cohen, J.H. & Pepe, P.E. (2000). Traumatic brain injuries evaluated in U.S. emergency departments, 1992-1994. *Academic Emergency Medicine* **359**(7), 134-140.

Joint Commission on Accreditation of Health Care Organizations *Sentinal event alert: Fatal falls: Lessons for the future*. Online. Available from http://www.jointcommission.org/SentinelEvents/SentinelEventAlert/sea_14.htm (last accessed 17 February 2009).

Morse, J.M. (ed.) (2009) *Preventing Patient Falls: Establishing a Fall Prevention Program*, 2nd edition. Springer Publishing Company, New York.

Stevens, J.A., Corso, P.S., Finkelstein, E.A. & Miller, T.R. (2006) The costs of fatal and non-fatal falls among older adults. *Injury Prevention* **12**(5), 290-295.

Further reading

Boushon, B., Nielsen, G., Quigley, P., Rutherford, P., Taylor, J. & Shannon, D. (2008) *Transforming care at the bedside how-to guide: Reducing patient injuries from falls*. Institute for Healthcare Improvement, Cambridge, MA.

Capezuti, E., Evans, L., Strumpf, N. & Maislin, G. (1996) Physical restraint use and falls in nursing home residents. *Journal of the American Geriatrics Society* **44**(6), 627-633.

Capezuti, E., Maislin, G., Strumpf, N. & Evans, L.K. (2002) Side rail use and bed-related fall outcomes among nursing home residents. *Journal of the American Geriatrics Society* **50**(1), 90-96.

Capezuti, E., Zwicker, D., Mezey, M. & Fulmer, T. (2008) In: Gray-Miceli, D. & Kluger, M. (eds) *Evidence Based Geriatric Nursing Protocols for Best Practice*, 3rd edition. Springer Publishing Company, New York.

Centers for Disease Control and Prevention (CDC) National Center for Injury Prevention and Control (NCIPC) *Preventing falls among older adults*. Online. Available from http://cdc.gov/ncipc/duip/preventadultfalls.htm (accessed 30 March 2012).

Chang, J.T., Morton, S.C., Rubenstein, L.Z. *et al.* (2004) Interventions for the prevention of falls in older adults: Systematic review and meta-analysis of randomised clinical trials. *BMJ* **328**(7441), 680.

Colon-Emeric, C., Schenck, A., Gorospe, J. *et al.* (2006) Translating evidence-based falls prevention into clinical practice in nursing facilities: Results and lessons from a quality improvement collaborative. *Journal of the American Geriatrics Society* **54**(9), 1414-1418.

Coussement, J., De Paepe, L., Schwendimann, R., Denhaerynck, K., Dejaeger, E. & Milisen, K. (2008) Interventions for preventing falls in acute- and chronic-care hospitals: A systematic review and meta-analysis. *Journal of the American Geriatrics Society* **56**(1), 29-36.

Dellinger, A.M. & Stevens, J.A. (2006) The injury problem among older adults: Mortality, morbidity and costs. *Journal of Safety Research* **37**(5), 519-522.

ECRI Institute (2006) *Falls Prevention in the Healthcare Settings Guide*. ECRI Publishers, Plymouth Meeting, PA.

Fernandez, H.M., Callahan, K.E., Likourezos, A. & Leipzig, R.M. (2008) House staff member awareness of older inpatients' risks for hazards of hospitalization. *Archives of Internal Medicine* **168**(4), 390-396.

Fischer, I.D., Krauss, M.J., Dunagan, W.C. *et al.* (2005) Patterns and predictors of inpatient falls and fall-related injuries in a large academic hospital. *Infection Control & Hospital Epidemiology* **26**(10), 822-827.

Gray-Miceli, D.L., Strumpf, N.E., Johnson, J., Draganescu, M. & Ratcliffe, S.J. (2006) Psychometric properties of the post-fall index. *Clinical Nursing Research* **15**(3), 157-176.

Haines, T.P., Bennell, K.L., Osborne, R.H. & Hill, K.D. (2006) A new instrument for targeting falls prevention interventions was accurate and clinically applicable in a hospital setting. *Journal of Clinical Epidemiology* **59**(2), 168-175.

Haines, T.P., Massey, B., Varghese, P., Fleming, J. & Gray, L. (2009) Inconsistency in classification and reporting of in-hospital falls. *Journal of the American Geriatrics Society* **57**(3), 517-523.

Healey, F., Monro, A., Cockram, A., Adams, V. & Heseltine, D. (2004) Using targeted risk factor reduction to prevent falls in older in-patients: A randomised controlled trial. *Age & Ageing* **33**(4), 390-395.

Hendrich, A., Nyhuis, A., Kippenbrock, T. & Soja, M.E. (1995) Hospital falls: Development of a predictive model for clinical practice. *Applied Nursing Research* **8**(3), 129-139.

Kim, E.A., Mordiffi, S.Z., Bee, W.H., Devi, K. & Evans, D. (2007) Evaluation of three fall-risk assessment tools in an acute care setting. *Journal of Advanced Nursing* **60**(4), 427-435.

Koh, S.S., Manias, E., Hutchinson, A.M., Donath, S. & Johnston, L. (2008) Nurses' perceived barriers to the implementation of a fall prevention clinical practice guideline in singapore hospitals. *BMC Health Services Research* **8**, 105.

Krauss, M.J., Evanoff, B., Hitcho, E. *et al.* (2005). A case-control study of patient, medication, and care-related risk factors for inpatient falls. *Journal of General Internal Medicine* **20**(2), 116–122.

Krauss, M.J., Tutlam, N., Costantinou, E., Johnson, S., Jackson, D. & Fraser, V.J. (2008) Intervention to prevent falls on the medical service in a teaching hospital. *Infection Control & Hospital Epidemiology* **29**(6), 539–545.

Leipzig, R.M., Cumming, R.G. & Tinetti, M.E. (1999) Drugs and falls in older people: A systematic review and meta-analysis: I. psychotropic drugs. *Journal of the American Geriatrics Society* **47**(1), 30–39.

Lyons, S.S. (2005) Evidence-based protocol: Fall prevention for older adults. *Journal of Gerontological Nursing* **31**(11), 9–14.

MacCulloch, P. A., Gardner, T. & Bonner, A. (2007) Comprehensive fall prevention programs across settings: A review of the literature. *Geriatric Nursing* **28**(5), 306–311.

McCarter-Bayer, A., Bayer, F. & Hall, K. (2005) Preventing falls in acute care: An innovative approach. *Journal of Gerontological Nursing* **31**(3), 25–33.

Milisen, K., Staelens, N., Schwendimann, R. *et al.* (2007) Fall prediction in inpatients by bedside nurses using the st. thomas's risk assessment tool in falling elderly inpatients (STRATIFY) instrument: A multicenter study. *Journal of the American Geriatrics Society* **55**(5), 725–733.

Morgan, R.O., Devito, C.A., Stevens, J.A. *et al.* (2005) A self-assessment tool was reliable in identifying hazards in the homes of elders. *Journal of Clinical Epidemiology* **58**(12), 1252–1259.

Moylan, K.C. & Binder, E.F. (2007) Falls in older adults: Risk assessment, management and prevention. *American Journal of Medicine* **120**(6), 493.e1–493.e6.

Murphy, T.H., Labonte, P., Klock, M. & Houser, L. (2008) Falls prevention for elders in acute care: An evidence-based nursing practice initiative. *Critical Care Nursing Quarterly* **31**(1), 33–39.

Oliver, D., Connelly, J.B., Victor, C.R. *et al.* (2007) Strategies to prevent falls and fractures in hospitals and care homes and effect of cognitive impairment: Systematic review and meta-analyses. *BMJ* **334**(7584), 82.

Rapp, K., Lamb, S.E., Buchele, G., Lall, R., Lindemann, U. & Becker, C. (2008) Prevention of falls in nursing homes: Subgroup analyses of a randomized fall prevention trial. *Journal of the American Geriatrics Society* **56**(6), 1092–1097.

Resnick, B. (2003) Preventing falls in acute care. In: Mezey, M., Fulmer, T., Abraham I. & Zwicker, D. (eds) *Geriatric Nursing Protocols for Best Practice*, 2nd edition. Springer Publishing Company, New York.

Rubenstein, L.Z. & Josephson, K.R. (2006) Falls and their prevention in elderly people: What does the evidence show? *Medical Clinics of North America* **90**(5), 807–824.

Rush, K.L., Robey-Williams, C., Patton, L.M., Chamberlain, D., Bendyk, H. & Sparks, T. (2009) Patient falls: Acute care nurses' experiences. *Journal of Clinical Nursing* **18**(3), 357–365.

Schwendimann, R., Milisen, K., Buhler, H. & De Geest, S. (2006) Fall prevention in a swiss acute care hospital setting reducing multiple falls. *Journal of Gerontological Nursing* **32**(3), 13–22.

Stevens, J.A. (2005) Falls among older adults-risk factors and prevention strategies. *Journal of Safety Research* **36**(4), 409–411.

Tanner, E.K. (2003) Assessing home safety in homebound older adults. *Geriatric Nursing* **24**(4), 250–254.

Tzeng, H.M. & Yin, C.Y. (2008) The extrinsic risk factors for inpatient falls in hospital patient rooms. *Journal of Nursing Care Quality* **23**(3), 233–241.

US Department of Veteran Affairs: National Center for Patient Safety (2004) *Fall prevention toolkit: Falls policy*. Online. Available from http://www.patientsafety.gov/SafetyTopics/fallstoolkit/notebook/05_fallspolicy.pdf (accessed 30 March 2012).

van der Helm, J., Goossens, A. & Bossuyt, P. (2006) When implementation fails: The case of a nursing guideline for fall prevention. *Joint Commission Journal on Quality & Patient Safety* **32**(3), 152-160.

von Renteln-Kruse, W. & Krause, T. (2007) Incidence of in-hospital falls in geriatric patients before and after the introduction of an interdisciplinary team-based fall-prevention intervention. *Journal of the American Geriatrics Society* **55**(12), 2068-2074.

Wagner, L.M., Capezuti, E., Clark, P.C., Parmelee, P.A. & Ouslander, J.G. (2008) Use of a falls incident reporting system to improve care process documentation in nursing homes. *Quality & Safety in Health Care* **17**(2), 104-108.

PART 6: PAIN AND OLDER ADULTS

Deborah A. D'Avolio

Pain is a significant problem for older adults. It has been shown that persistent pain is common in elders. The discomfort is often related to musculoskeletal disorders, such as degenerative joint or spine disease and arthritis (American Geriatrics Society, 2009). In addition, up to 80% of older adults diagnosed with cancer reported pain during their illness (Rao & Cohen, 2004). Pain impacts health, daily functioning, and quality of life. Undetected pain or inadequate treatment is associated with a number of adverse outcomes. These adverse outcomes include functional impairment, delirium, falls, depression, withdrawal, anxiety, sleep, appetite disturbances, and increased health care utilization. It is distressing for older adults, caregivers, and their loved ones. Despite the prevalence and adverse consequences, pain is often undetected and poorly managed (Horgas & Dunn, 2001; Horgas, 2003).

There are several contributing factors to undetected or untreated pain. These include individual, caregiver, and health care provider based factors. Older adults may be concerned about being labeled a hypochondriac or complainer, and may fear that pain indicates disease progression. Patients may worry about health care costs and believe their pain is not important to health care providers. Health care providers may not effectively assess pain among their older adult patients or be concerned about the adverse effects associated with pain medications (Coker *et al.*, 2010). Both patients and health care providers may believe that pain is a part of normal aging and may fear addiction or adverse reactions to medication.

Older adults may have a combination of acute and persistent pain and they are more vulnerable to persistent pain after an acute illness or injury. Persistent musculoskeletal pain may be associated with musculoskeletal disorders that are common in aging, such as degenerative spinal conditions and arthritis. The American Geriatric Society (AGS) has published clinical practice guidelines for older adults about managing persistent pain and osteoarthritis pain (American Geriatrics Society, 2009).

An additional concern is that older adults may have an elevated threshold and rate mild pain as less intense and unpleasant than younger adults. Older adults can also present with absent, vague, or atypical patterns and symptoms when ill. Instead, their presenting symptoms may include confusion, restlessness, aggression, anorexia, or fatigue. For example, an older adult with an acute myocardial infarction (MI) may be asymptomatic.

With evidence to support that pain limits function in older adults it is imperative to help older adults remain active, socially engaged, and functioning. Their pain needs to be assessed and managed more effectively.

Assessment of pain in older adults

The approach to assessment and pain management in older adults is different than that for younger people. Pain assessment among older adults can be challenging due to multiple co-morbidities, persistent pain, polypharmacy, cognitive and sensory impairments. An older person may experience acute pain, persistent pain, or a combination of pain. Acute pain is defined by recent onset, short duration, usually following an injury or trauma. There are often vital sign changes and the cause is frequently known. However, in older adults, persistent pain is more common. Persistent pain lasts longer than three months or is continuous, or recurring from a chronic condition, such as arthritis. Usually there are no detectable changes in the patient's vital signs and it can cause complications and functional decline.

There are several effective assessment strategies that can be employed. The patient's report of pain is the most effective measurement of pain. It must include the intensity and effect of the pain on daily function. The use of standardized pain assessment tools is essential in evaluating pain. Older adults with normal cognition can have difficulty with quantitative pain scales and may prefer a word scale. When assessing those with mild to moderate cognitive impairment, simple questions and screening tools have been proven effective. The Faces, Numeric Rating, and Verbal Descriptor Scales may be used with older adults who have normal and impaired cognition. The Faces Pain Scale asks patients to view facial expressions and chose one which closely relates to their pain. The Numeric Rating Scale asks patients to rate their pain by a number with zero indicating no pain and 10 as the worst pain. The Verbal Descriptor Scale asks the patient to describe their pain as "no pain" to pain as bad as it could be." Examples of these tools can be seen at www.ConsultGeriRN.org.

In the presence of cognitive impairment be sure to discuss the patient's history and behavioral clues with the health care providers, family, or care givers who are familiar with the patient. There are specific tools designed for those who are non-verbal or cognitively impaired. For older adults who can't report pain, behavioral observation pain indicators are used (Horgas, 2007; Horgas & Miller, 2008). Examples of observed pain indicators are guarded movement, changes in normal activity or mental status, grimacing, painful noises, sleeplessness, decreased appetite, withdrawal, respiratory changes, and restlessness. Examples of pain assessment tools used in cognitive impairment are available on www.ConsultGeriRN.org.

When asking older adults about pain, it is helpful to also use other words such as "hurt, ache, or discomfort." Simple assessment questions are best. "Do you have pain or do you hurt? What does it feel like? How severe is the pain? Does the pain come and go? What makes it better, what makes it worse?" Pain assessment tools should be simple, easy to understand, have larger print, and clear contrast. It is important to be sure the patient has their hearing and visual devices in place. Evaluate the intensity, character, quality, frequency, pattern, location, duration, and precipitating/alleviating factors. The mnemonics OLD CARTS and WILDA may be used (OLDCARTS = onset, location, duration, characteristics, course, associated, aggravating, relieving, treatments, and severity; WILDA = words to describe the pain, intensity 0-10, location, duration, aggravating and alleviating factors).

Pain management strategies

A major barrier to treatment is inadequate assessment. A comprehensive assessment is necessary to the development of a treatment plan. In managing pain among older adults the main goal is to maximize function and quality of life by minimizing or eliminating pain. A multidimensional tailored approach is best. A combination of pharmacological and non-pharmacological strategies helps reduce pain and increase comfort. This in turn leads to improved function, interpersonal/social interactions, and improved mood.

Pharmacological interventions

General principles to pain treatment

When treating pain in older adults there are several important principles to consider. Pain treatment requires a careful assessment of the risks vs. benefits of medication and a careful review of current medications. The nurse and interdisciplinary team should have clear goals of drug therapy. Consider frequency of medication use, duration, and cost of medication. Older adults are at a higher risk of side effects due to normal physiologic changes and decreased homeostatic resilience. Normal aging impacts organ function. This in turn causes pharmacodynamic and pharmacokinetic changes which may affect safety. Because of these age related changes, older adults are more prone to adverse drug events, side effects, toxicity, falls, and death.

Mild to moderate pain can be treated with acetaminophen or cautious use of anti-inflammatory drugs (NSAIDs). Acetaminophen has been shown to provide adequate pain relief in many pain syndromes, especially musculoskeletal pain. No more than 4 grams of acetaminophen should be administered in 24 hours to patients with normal hepatic and renal function, due to the risk of hepatoxicity- and this dose should not usually be continued for a long period of time. For those patients with hepatic disease, the dose should be lowered by 50%. Since acetaminophen is common in many over the counter and prescription products, knowledge of all the medications the patient is taking is critical. NSAIDs are effective and may be used in an acute exacerbation of pain that is not controlled with acetaminophen. However, there are significant potential adverse effects. These adverse effects include renal dysfunction, gastrointestinal bleeding, fluid retention, and platelet dysfunction.

Moderate to severe pain that is chronic often requires opioid medication. Continuous pain should be treated with a 24-hour pain medication in sustain released formulation after a trial of a short-acting agent. Opioids are metabolized in the liver and excreted by the kidneys. In the presence of renal dysfunction, active metabolites can accumulate, which places the patient at risk for sedation. A common adverse effect of opioid treatment is constipation. Education on the probable need for a laxative is important. Older patients may experience sedation, fatigue, and mild cognitive impairment with opioids. They need to be educated about the risks of adverse effects and warned of the increased risk of falls and asked not to drive or operate heavy equipment when the medications are initiated. Older adults are at risk of respiratory depression when the doses are increased too rapidly. This adverse outcome can be avoided when the medication is titrated upward slowly and response to dosage is carefully evaluated.

Older adults may have concerns about addiction and tolerance to opioids. It has been shown that this rarely occurs when opioids are used as medications for pain control The fear of addiction and tolerance can be addressed by a honest discussion of the patient's concerns.

In deciding upon a pharmacological pain treatment plan it is best to start at the lowest effective dose. Slowly titrate dosage upward with short acting drugs to obtain the desired effect. Chose drugs with the shortest half life and the fewest side effects. The geriatric theme of "start low and go slow" is an effective reminder when planning a pain treatment plan. If pain is treated before it occurs, less medication is required. Strategies include around the clock dosing, medication prior to a painful treatment, and administering the next dose before the last dose wears off.

There are several drugs which should be avoided in the older adult because they are not effective or may cause side effects. These drugs include propoxyphene (Darvon) (no longer available in the US) and combination products, trimethobenzamide (Tigan), meperidine (Demerol), pentazocine (Talwin), muscle relaxants, and antispasmodics. They may cause hallucinations and confusion. Sedatives, antihistamines, and antiemetics should also be avoided. For the complete list of potentially inappropriate medications, see *Beers Criteria for Potentially Inappropriate Medication Use in Older Adults*; Part 1 and Part II at www.ConsultGeriRN.org.

Nonpharmacological interventions

The following approaches should be considered as adjuvants to pharmacological management when appropriate.

- Acupuncture
- Application of cold or heat (cautiously to prevent skin burns)
- Cognitive-behavioral interventions
- Hypnosis
- Imagery
- Massage
- Music therapy
- Over the counter muscle creams
- Physical or occupational therapies
- Relaxation training
- Splints or braces
- T'ai Chi
- Therapeutic touch
- Transcutaneous electrical nerve stimulation (TENS)
- Weight reduction if indicated

Collaborative strategies

Pain management should be tailored to the individual patient in collaboration with interdisciplinary colleagues. Refer to physical and occupation therapists those patients who are at risk for persistent pain. Consult with the pharmacist and the prescriber to review medications which may cause possible drug/drug interactions. Patients with persistent pain that do not respond to treatment plans should be referred to a pain clinic that has an interdisciplinary approach. Regular physical activity has been shown to improve mood, function, and stabilize gait. Referral to the Arthritis Foundation or community resources such as the Senior Center or YMCA can be considered. Focus pain management strategies on ways to increase daily activities and prevent complications. To help older adults remain independent and function fully, pain needs to be managed effectively.

■ Patient/family education

Engage the older adult and their family as active participants in the development of the treatment plan and ongoing monitoring of potential side effects of medications.

Older adults and their families should receive education on the proper use of medications to reduce medication related adverse events. They should understand the targeted interventions that help eliminate or decrease pain. It is important for families to know simple strategies that may improve pain; relaxation techniques, pacing of tasks, and proper use of medications. Ensure that the patient and family know the name of each medication, its purpose, the correct dose, when and how to take it, and when to call their health care provider. Older adults are at high risk of medication related adverse events immediately after hospital discharge. Medication education and discharge planning are essential to reduce adverse events.

References

American Geriatrics Society Panel on the Pharmacological Management of Persistent Pain in Older,Persons (2009) Pharmacological management of persistent pain in older persons. *Journal of the American Geriatrics Society* **57**(8), 1331-1346.

Coker, E., Papaioannou, A., Kaasalainen, S., Dolovich, L., Turpie, I. & Taniguchi, A. (2010) Nurses' perceived barriers to optimal pain management in older adults on acute medical units. *Applied Nursing Research* **23**(3), 139-146.

Horgas, A.L. (2003) Pain management in elderly adults. *Journal of Infusion Nursing* **26**(3), 161-165.

Horgas, A.L. (2007) Assessing pain in persons with dementia. *MEDSURG Nursing* **16**(3), 207-208.

Horgas, A.L. & Dunn, K. (2001) Pain in nursing home residents. comparison of residents' self-report and nursing assistants' perceptions. incongruencies exist in resident and caregiver reports of pain; therefore, pain management education is needed to prevent suffering. *Journal of Gerontological Nursing* **27**(3), 44-53.

Horgas, A. & Miller, L. (2008) Pain assessment in people with dementia. *American Journal of Nursing* **108**(7), 62-70.

Rao, A. & Cohen, H.J. (2004) Symptom management in the elderly cancer patient: Fatigue, pain, and depression. *Journal of the Naionatl Cancer Institute Monographs* **2004**(32), 150-157.

Further reading

Elliott, A.F. & Horgas, A.L. (2009) Effects of an analgesic trial in reducing pain behaviors in community-dwelling older adults with dementia. *Nursing Research* **58**(2), 140-145.

Feldt, K.S., Warne, M.A. & Ryden, M.B. (1998) Examining pain in aggressive cognitively impaired older adults. *Journal of Gerontological Nursing* **24**(11), 14-22.

Feldt, K.S. (2000) The checklist of nonverbal pain indicators. *Pain Management Nursing* **1**(1), 13-21.

Gagliese, L. (2009) Aging and the management of cancer pain. *Annals of Oncology* **20**(10), 1752.

Gagliese, L., Gauthier, L.R. & Rodin, G. (2007) Cancer pain and depression: A systematic review of age-related patterns. *Pain Research & Management* **12**(3), 205-211.

Gagliese, L. & Melzack, R. (1997) Chronic pain in elderly people. *Pain* **70**(1), 3-14.

Gagliese, L. & Melzack, R. (2003) Age-related differences in the qualities but not the intensity of chronic pain. *Pain* **104**(3), 597-608.

Gordon, D.B., Dahl, J., Phillips, P. *et al.* (2005) The use of 'as-needed' range orders for opioid analgesics in the management of acute pain: A consensus statement of the american society for pain management nursing and the American Pain Society. *Home Healthcare Nurse* **23**(6), 388-396.

Hadjistavropoulos, T., Marchildon, G.P., Fine, P.G. *et al.* (2009) Transforming long-term care pain management in North America: The policy-clinical interface. *Pain Medicine* **10**(3), 506-520.

Hadjistavropoulos, T., Herr, K., Turk, D.C. *et al.* (2007) An interdisciplinary expert consensus statement on assessment of pain in older persons. *Clinical Journal of Pain* **23**(1 Suppl), S1-43.

Herr, K., Coyne, P.J., Key, T. *et al.* (2006). Pain assessment in the nonverbal patient: Position statement with clinical practice recommendations. *Pain Management Nursing* **7**(2), 44-52.

Horgas, A.L., Nichols, A.L., Schapson, C.A. & Vietes, K. (2007).Assessing pain in persons with dementia: Relationships among the non-communicative patient's pain assessment instrument, self-report, and behavioral observations. *Pain Management Nursing* **8**(2), 77-85.

Horgas, A.L., Yoon, S.L., Nichols, A.L. & Marsiske, M. (2008) The relationship between pain and functional disability in black and white older adults. *Research in Nursing & Health* **31**(4), 341-354.

Kaasalainen, S. (2007) Pain assessment in older adults with dementia: Using behavioral observation methods in clinical practice. *Journal of Gerontological Nursing* **33**(6), 6-10.

Rodin, G., Lo, C., Mikulincer, M., Donner, A., Gagliese, L. & Zimmermann, C. (2009) Pathways to distress: The multiple determinants of depression, hopelessness, and the desire for hastened death in metastatic cancer patients. *Social Science & Medicine* **68**(3), 562-569.

PART 7: PALLIATIVE CARE

Jennifer R. Howard

Palliative care is a philosophy of care, one which encompasses the physical, emotional, spiritual, cultural and social aspects of the whole person. The focus of palliative care is to achieve the best quality of life, and relieve pain and suffering in both the non-hospice and hospice realm of health care. Palliative care is appropriate at any stage of disease (Sepulveda *et al.*, 2010). Individuals who may be entering their final days, weeks, months of life, as well as those who seek curative measures or life-prolonging therapies, benefit from early intervention of palliative care (National Consensus Project, 2010). Quality of life is the main goal of palliative care; that is, what quality of life means for that particular individual. The World Health Organization, the first to endorse palliative care, defines palliative care as:

> an approach that improves the quality of life of patients and their families facing the problems associated with life-threatening illness, through the prevention and relief of suffering by means of early identification and impeccable assessment and treatment of pain and other problems; physical, psychosocial, and spiritual (Sepulveda *et al.*, 2010).

In the palliative care model, the patient and family are considered the unit of care. A comprehensive interdisciplinary team works together to coordinate all care for the best possible outcome for the patient and family. Ideally, palliative care should be introduced early to work collaboratively with all disciplines, whether the goal is curative, life prolonging or hospice and end of life focused (Kelley & Meier, 2010). Unfortunately, often the palliative care team is recommended when the patient is no longer responsive to curative treatments or has advanced and end-stage illness.

When considering palliative care for patients, the team addresses numerous aspects of care. These include, disease-modifying and supportive compassionate therapies; such as pain and symptom management, as well as assisting patients and families to discuss and make difficult decisions regarding their plan of care.

Palliative care is best provided by an interdisciplinary team, which includes, but is not limited to:

- Physicians; primary care and specialists
- Nursing
- Social work
- Chaplaincy/spiritual caregivers
- Nutrition/dieticians
- Rehabilitation; physical/occupational/speech therapy

Over the past century there has been a significant shift in where palliative and hospice care is delivered. For those age 65 and over this care is primarily provided in hospital or nursing home settings (Bruce & Boston, 2008). Palliative care in older adults is focused not only on pain and symptom management, but also on maintaining the highest degree of functional status, reducing treatment burden, and addressing family member concerns. Older adults often experience an adverse event causing an unexpected hospitalization, plus many elders have a higher symptom of burden related to chronic illness (Long *et al.*, 2010). These issues create challenges and force elders to make difficult decisions. For this reason, it is important to start the conversation as to what the goal of care is for the elder client. Throughout our lifespan, adapting to health status changes are not always easy, often requiring in depth discussions about the best choice considering the available options. Approaching "old age" comes with significant losses, and this most often is the time in our lives where we have to make some of the most difficult decisions (Hanks *et al.*, 2010).

When a geriatric patient enters the acute hospital setting, having an immediate discussion with the client and or family member is the first step in understanding what the individual's wishes are. When an elder person, who may have multiple comorbidities, is hospitalized for an acute illness, a palliative care consult should be recommended earlier rather than later in their hospitalization. This is not only in the patient's best interest, but also provides the hospital staff with a clear understanding of how to best treat and care for this individual. Knowing the goals of care will also help decrease burdens on family caregivers, and reduce costly ineffective therapies if there is advanced disease and or progressive chronic illness when the patient's goal is no longer curative, but care and comfort (Fadul *et al.*, 2009). To assist in addressing difficult topics, a palliative care referral by the physician is recommended. Once an order is given, the palliative care team can initiate dialogue with the patient or family as to what his/her goals of care are and what quality of life means to them. For those hospitals and nursing facilities that do not have a palliative care team, a referral to a home care agency is another option. Many home care hospices and visiting nurse associations (VNAs) have nurses or physicians who provide palliative care consultations.

Goals of care

The approach to difficult discussions with geriatric patients differs from younger patients because of functional, psychological, and physiological changes that occur with aging. The history and the physical exam must address not only the acute illness, but also the multiple chronic diseases that an elder patient may have (Hanks et al., 2010). An example is an 88-year-old woman with a new diagnosis of small cell lung cancer, yet other health problems include a history of chronic obstructive pulmonary disease (COPD), Type II diabetes, and congestive heart failure (CHF). Goal setting should take priority over the problem list. This is important because all treatment options will be based on whether or not the patient wishes to pursue aggressive care; to fight towards cure or whether comfort with the best quality of life at this stage is the goal. The patient and family should be informed of all options. This list may include:

- Diagnostic testing
- Financial costs that may incur outside of insurance (assuming the patient has insurance)
- Treatment available
- Undesired side effects of treatments
- Statistics regarding favorable and unfavorable outcomes
- Time and travel commitments

These issues address the risks versus the benefits of care. The discussions during this time can be lengthy and time consuming. Based on the acuity of the patient's illness and cognitive status, the options and the risks and benefits need to be repeated over a number of visits. Further discussions may include:

- Artificial nutrition and hydration
- Blood transfusions
- Financial concerns other than medical costs
- Laboratory and diagnostic testing
- Living arrangements, home environment and/or possible increased need for assistance with personal care
- Physical exams (which may cause pain or distress)

Discussions about Do Not Resuscitate (DNR), Do Not Intubate (DNI) and Do Not Hospitalize (DNH) choices, and what they mean, can be troublesome conversations, both emotional and stressful.

Finally, it is important to learn who the patient wishes to be involved with these decisions and what support services are important to the patient. Additional information necessary includes:

- Are there specific family members involved or excluded?
- Are there any wills and/or legal documents available?
- Does the patient have spiritual and/or religious beliefs and desires?
- Is there an assigned Health Care Proxy (HCP) if the patient can no longer speak for him/herself?

This process can be overwhelming and stressful, yet these conversations are necessary to provide appropriate care based on the patient's wishes. Goals of care are about what is valued by the patient.

Initiating the dialog

Present illness is often clear, for this is the acute episode that brought the patient to the hospital. Factors to consider when initiating the discussion about goals of care include:

- Present illness
- Past medical history
- Past functional status
- Social assessment

Past medical history not only is important in assessing if the patient will be able to tolerate treatment of present illness, but will allow you to review how well the patient has managed his/her chronic disease at home and for what duration. This will provide helpful information in considering if the patient is a candidate for treatment of the current acute illness, and as to how successful it may be.

Past functional status is essential in determining baseline information about the elder's ability to care for him/herself at home. We cannot assume that the patient's functional level in the acute care setting is equivalent to their functional capability before the hospitalization. If the patient had limited mobility at home and had significant homecare services prior to the new adverse event, this information will impact the new treatment plan, and possibly limit options. However, healthcare professionals should not underestimate a patient's potential for recovery. Goal setting is based on presenting the most realistic options for the patient, so that he/she is able to make an informed decision as to the direction of his/her care.

Social assessment is an equally important aspect of the patient's history. Understanding how the individual has been managing at home with a chronic illness, is beneficial when having a realistic discussion to prepare an appropriate plan of care. The social assessment is more than patient's functional status, it includes all aspects of daily living; social, financial, spiritual, and legal. Important questions to be answered include:

- Has the patient been living home alone?
- Is there a healthy and involved spouse/partner or other individual who is the caregiver?
- Does the patient have other support systems available (e.g., friends)?
- Is the caregiver ill with his/her own chronic or debilitating disease?
- Is the home environment safe? Are there safety measures in place?
- Are there any financial concerns?
- Is the patient religious or spiritual? Are there concerns regarding treatments?

Quality of life is not the same for everyone. Taking the time to ask the question about what that means to a geriatric individual is of utmost importance. This question changes throughout our lifespan. One person may opt to live in pain, no matter how much education has been presented to alleviate it, in order to have full control over all decisions. Another may request a feeding tube for nutrition if this will extend his/her life a little longer to see a grandchild born. Quality of life can be a different discussion for an elder person compared to a younger one.

Pain and symptom management

Pain and symptom management is a key component to palliative care. Often the palliative care team is called in to alleviate a certain symptom. A thorough pain and/or symptom assessment is required for all patients. In elders this may be particularly challenging due to multiple health and/or cognitive issues. In hospitals and long term settings, older patients experience pain that is often unrecognized and or under treated (Long *et al.*, 2010). There have been numerous pain assessment tools developed to assist with identifying patient's discomfort, however, older patients may not be able to express or describe their pain as well as younger patients. Unfortunately, there are areas of concern with medication management in older adults. These include allergies, adverse side effects, the ability to metabolize and excrete the drug efficiently, and safety issues (McLean & Le Couteur, 2004). Although these are reasonable concerns, it is not acceptable to leave any patient in pain if they wish to be as pain free as possible.

Some of the physiological changes to be addressed prior to preparing an appropriate plan of care include:

- Bowel and bladder: constipation, renal function
- Cardiorespiratory compromise: congestive heart failure, chronic obstructive pulmonary disease
- Dysphasia/swallowing: cerebrovascular accident

- Gastrointestinal: gastroesophageal reflux disease, bleeding, alcoholism, liver disease
- Infections: urinary tract, pneumonia
- Mental status changes; dementia
- Musculoskeletal disorders: arthritis, osteoporosis, disseminated joint disease
- Skin breakdown: wounds, ulcers
- Tremors: seizure disorder, Parkinson's disease

Whether it is an existing condition, onset related to new diagnosis, or progressing disease, pain and symptom management is a priority in providing appropriate and best practice palliative care interventions. It is essential to assess the past and present function of major body systems so that the plan is realistic and the patient will not only benefit from the medication or therapy, but also not be harmed. Medications that should be discussed and used cautiously due to high side effect profiles include:

- Adrenergic bronchodilators
- Anticholinergics
- Antihistamines
- Antidepressants
- Barbiturates
- Cardiovascular drugs; e.g., beta-blockers, angiotensin II converting enzyme inhibitors
- Corticosteroids
- Gastrointestinal antispasmodics
- Long-acting benzodiazepines
- Muscle relaxants
- Nonsteroidal anti-inflammatory agents
- Opioids

Older patients tend to have more trouble with metabolizing and excreting drugs, therefore drugs may linger in their system longer, increasing the risk for side effects (McLean & Le Couteur, 2004). Once the goals of care are established, the benefit of the pharmacological treatment may outweigh the possible concerns of long term adverse side effects.

Barriers to care

Palliative care for elders in a hospitalized setting should begin early in order to provide the best care in response to the patient's wishes. There are numerous barriers to effective palliative care for elders, many of these are out of the patient's or family's control (Hanks *et al.*, 2010). These include:

- Difficulties in assessing pain and symptoms in cognitively impaired patients
- Disagreement on specific advanced disease/end of life issues among family members

- Failure to implement a timely plan
- Failure to recognize end of life; prognostication difficult
- Failure to recognize treatment futility; physician hesitancy to discuss end of life care, and/or lack of knowledge, experience and comfort level of health care team to discuss end of life issues
- Fear and anxiety of patient and family to discuss advanced disease/patient decline
- Lack of clinician skills in providing symptom management
- Lack of health care assessment to recognize need for palliative care referral
- Poor communication between patient/caregiver, physician and health care team

Respecting an elder patient's wishes once they enter a hospitalized setting is the primary goal of all health care individuals caring for the patient. Beginning the conversation about palliative care, understanding the patient's goals, and implementing a care plan is challenging, and time consuming. Communication and collaboration with all health care providers and family involvement are integral to success. Obtaining the referral for the palliative care team is helpful to both the patient and hospital staff. Education is essential in achieving the appropriate interventions for each patient. These include:

- Ability to provide support and compassion to the elder patient
- Identifying the need for various assessment tools
- Knowledge and understanding of effective assessment of the patient's pain and symptoms
- Managing medication side effects
- On going communication with family and team members
- Titrating analgesics
- Understanding non verbal behavioral manifestations of pain
- Utilizing interdisciplinary team members

Palliative care is not only appropriate, but highly beneficial for the geriatric hospitalized patient, and should be initiated as early as possible upon admission.

References

Bruce, A. & Boston, P. (2008) The changing landscape of palliative care. *Journal of Hospice and Palliative Nursing* **10**(1), 49–55.
Center for Disease Control National Vital Statistics Reports. Nov. 7 2007 52 (9).
Fadul, N., Elsayem, A., Palmer, J.L. *et al.* (2009) Supportive versus palliative care: what's in a name? A survey of medical oncologists and midlevel providers at a comprehensive cancer center. *Cancer* **115**, 2013–2021.
Hanks, G., Cherney, N.I., Christakis, N.A., Fallon, M., Kassa, S. & Portenoy, R.K. (2010) *Oxford Textbook of Palliative Medicine*, 4th edition. Oxford University Press, New York: Oxford University Press; 2010.

Kelley, A.S., & Meier, D.E. (2010). Palliative care-a shifting paradigm. *The New England Journal of Medicine* **363**(8), 781-782.

Long, C.O., Morgan, B.M., Alonzo, T.R., Mitchell, K.M., Bonnell D.K., & Beardsley, M.E. (2010) Improving pain management in long-term care. *Journal of Hospice and Palliative Nursing.* **12** (3), 148-155.

McLean, A.J. & Le Couteur, D.G. (2004) Aging biology and geriatric clinical pharmacology. *Pharmacology Review* **56**, 163-184. Online. Available at www.pharmrev.aspetjournals.org/cgi/content/full/56/2/163 (accessed 3 August 2010).

National Consensus Project (2010) Online. Available from http://www.nationalconsensusproject.org (accessed 3 April 2012).

Sepulveda, C., Marlin, A., Yoshida, T. *et al.* (2002) Palliative care: The World Health Organization's global perspective. *Journal of Pain and Symptom Management*, **24**(2), 91-96.

Additional resources

Centers for Disease Control National Vital Statistics Reports. Nov. 7 2007, 52(9).
Academy of Hospice and Palliative Medicine. 2010. http://www.aahpm.org/
HPNA; Hospice and Palliative Nursing Association. http://www.hpna.org
NHPCO; National Hospice and Palliative Care Organization. http://nhpco.org
American Pain Society. http://ampainsoc.org

PART 8: MEDICATIONS AND OLDER ADULTS

Deborah A. D'Avolio

Older adults are particularly vulnerable to medication-related problems because of the prevalence of chronic illness and the numbers of medications taken. These factors along with metabolic changes predispose older adults to adverse drug events (ADEs) and adverse drug reactions (ADRs). During care transitions, including hospital admission and discharge, drug related problems may appear. Older adults have more emergency department visits and hospitalizations from medication related problems than those below the age of 65 (Hartford Institute for Geriatric Nursing, 2011). This is due to a variety of age related physiologic changes. These changes result in sensitivity to medications, and an altered ability to metabolize and excrete medications. Changes in the gastrointestinal tract include decreased hepatic function, gastric acidity, colonic motility, and as a result, delayed absorption of drugs. Changes in the cardiovascular system can result in hypotensive responses, volume depletion, and impaired blood pressure response can be further exacerbated by some cardiac medications. Decreased kidney filtration rate can result in impaired excretion of some medications. The volume distribution of drugs can be affected due to a decrease in body water and increase in body fat. Therefore, water soluble drugs can become more concentrated and fat soluble drugs can have longer half-lives. In addition to impaired drug clearance, older patients can have altered responses to drugs. They are more sensitive to some drugs such as opiates and anticoagulants and less sensitive to others. Older patients with multiple conditions can be taking several drugs, thus increasing their risk for ADEs and ADRs.

It is estimated that more than 75% of older adults take medications with nearly half taking five or more drugs. In addition to prescribed medications, older adults are also taking over the counter (OTC) medications (Hanlon *et al.*, 2001). The combination of prescription and OTC medications can lead to adverse drug and drug-drug reactions.

Although there is no universal definition for ADEs and ADRs, it is generally understood that an ADE is harm which results from the use of medication and includes appropriate use, inappropriate use, poor adherence, or self medication. ADEs can include medication errors. An ADR is unexpected harm that results from the normal use of medication at a normal dose.

Some medications are known to be inappropriate for older adults as they increase an older adult's risk of developing an ADE or ADR. These medications include: warfarin, antihypertensives, cardiotonics, and psychoactive drugs including sedatives, hypnotics, antidepressants and OTCs. The Beers Criteria (AGS, 2012; Fick *et al.*, 2003) lists the criteria for inappropriate medication use in older adults. It includes comprehensive information related to medications, medication classes, diagnoses to consider, and severity ratings of high or low. It is important that nurses reference this list when reviewing an older adult's medication list or when any new medication is ordered. Unfortunately, it has been shown that up to 23% of older adults are taking at least one drug listed on the Beers Criteria (Fick *et al.*, 2003).

Examples of potentially inappropriate medications

- Amitriptyline
- Amphetamines
- Anticholinergics and antihistamines
- Barbiturates
- Benzodiazepines
- Chlorpropamide
- Doxepin
- Fluoxetine
- Flurazepam
- Indomethacin
- Ketorolac
- Methyldopa
- Muscle relaxants and antispasmodics

Once a medication is decided upon, the prescribing clinician should check to be sure that the symptoms being treated are not due to another drug. Precautions should be taken to avoid toxicity and medication should begin at less than the usual adult dose and the dose should be increased slowly. The geriatric saying "start low and go slow" is important to remember in the management of medications.

■ Risk factors for medication problems

- Drug-disease interaction
- Drug-drug interaction
- Iatrogenic causes
- Incorrect dosage; over and/ or under dosages
- Multiple medications
- Multiple prescribers
- Nonadherence
- Self medication
- Unreported herbal or OTC medications

■ Nursing assessment and interventions

The nurse should conduct a complete medical and medication history including medication allergies and type of reaction, prescription medications, OTCs, vitamins, and nutritional supplements. Ask how long the patient has been taking each medication. Also inquire about medications which they may have stopped and why. In addition, assess alcohol, illicit or recreational drugs, smoking, and immunization status. It is important to perform a medication reconciliation to verify actual medications before hospitalization and during hospitalization. The Joint Commission on Accreditation of Health Care Organizations (JACHO) requires medication reconciliation across all practice settings. This ensures that regardless of where the patient receives care, a complete and current list of medications will be communicated. Since medications can be very expensive, it is also important to ask about cost concerns. If cost is identified as a barrier to medication adherence, resources should be explored to support cost of medications. It is essential to assess cognitive and functional abilities to ensure that the older adults can safely manage their medications.

It is well known that polypharmacy is a risk factor for delirium. In addition, many individual medications found on the Beers list can cause delirium. With any changes in behavior or cognition a thorough medication review should be completed to rule out medication as a cause of the change. Discharge planning should include medication reconciliation, review of the treatment plan, and home follow up strategies. If new symptoms develop, one should suspect an adverse drug reaction and monitor for possible drug toxicity. Many medications can contribute to fall risk. If a fall should occur it is important to review medications to determine if they are contributing to fall risk.

Below you will find some commonly used tools to evaluate medication use among older adults.

Commonly used tools to evaluate older adults' medication use

AGS (2012);

- Drug-drug interactions
- Functional capacity tools used to assess physical and cognitive ability to administer medications
- Cockroft-Gault Formula used to assess creatinine clearance

Collaborative strategies

Nurses are in a key position to closely monitor the effects of medications. Collaboration with interdisciplinary colleagues including pharmacist, physicians, social workers, and others is essential to preventing or decreasing adverse drug events and drug reactions.

■ Patient/family education

The patient and family should understand the reason for each medication, the correct dose, and possible adverse reactions. They should be instructed to call their primary care provider if they should have any questions about their medications. A medication chart has been shown to be an effective tool to help older adults and their families manage the medication regime. Ongoing monitoring at home is essential to ensure safe administration and therapeutic response to medications. Patients and families should be instructed to always carry a list of current medications. If admitted to the emergency department or other care settings, be sure their primary care provider has been contacted. Their pharmacist is another resource to help them learn more about their medications and medication safety.

References

American Geriatrics Society (AGS). (2012) AGS Beers Criteria for Potentially Inappropriate Medication Use in Older Adults. Online. Available from http://www.americangeriatrics.org/files/documents/beers/2012AGSBeersCriteriaCitations.pdf (accessed 13 June 2012).

Fick, D.M., Cooper, F.W., Wade, W.E., Waller, J.L., Maclean, J.R., & Beers, M.H. (2003) Updating the Beers criteria for potentially inappropriate medication use in older adults. *Archives of Internal Medicine* **163**(22), 2716-2724.

Joint Commission on Accreditation of Health Care Organizations Patient Safety Goals Related to Medications (2007) Online. Available from http://www.jointcommission.org/standards_information/npsgs.aspx (accessed 3 April 2012).

Hanlon, J.T., Fillenbaum, G.G., Ruby, C.M., Gray, S., & Bohannon, A. (2001) Epidemiology of over-the-counter drug use in community-dwelling elderly.

United States perspective. *Drugs & Aging* **18**(2), 123-131. Evidence Level V: Literature Review.

Hartford Institute for Geriatric Nursing (2011). A practice brief from the Hartford Institute of geriatric nursing: Medication safety for older adults. *Hartford Institute for Geriatric Nursing Report* 1(1). New York University College of Nursing, New York.

Further reading

AHRQ Patient Safety Network. Online. Available from http://www.psnet.ahrq.gov/glossary.aspx (accessed 3 April 2012).

Capezuti, E., Zwicker, D., Mezey, M., & Fulmer, T. (2008) In: Gray-Miceli, D. & Kluger, M (eds) *Evidence Based Geriatric Nursing Protocols for Best Practice*, 3rd edition. Springer Publishing Company, New York.

Corbett, C.F., Setter, S.M., Daratha, K.B., Neumiller, J.J. & Wood, L.D. (2010) Nurse identified hospital to home medication discrepancies: Implications for improving transitional care. *Geriatric Nursing* **31**(3), 188-196.

Fick, D.M., Mion, L.C., Beers, M.H., & L Waller, J. (2008) Health outcomes associated with potentially inappropriate medication use in older adults. *Research in Nursing & Health* **31**(1), 42-51.

Flood, K.L. (2010) Improving medication safety in older adults. An interview with Dr. Kellie L. Flood, by Scott Bugg. *Geriatric Nursing* **31**(6), 472-473.

Howland, R.H. (2009) Effects of aging on pharmacokinetic and pharmacodynamic drug processes. *Journal of Psychosocial Nursing & Mental Health Services* **47**(10), 15-16.

Howland, R.H. (2009). Prescribing psychotropic medications for elderly patients. *Journal of Psychosocial Nursing & Mental Health Services* **47**(11), 17-20.

Joanna Briggs Institute (2009) Strategies to reduce medication errors in older adults. *Australian Nursing Journal* **17**(3), 30-33.

Lindsey, P.L. (2009) Psychotropic medication use among older adults: What all nurses need to know. *Journal of Gerontological Nursing* **35**(9), 28-38.

Mager, D.D., & Madigan, E.A. (2010) Medication use among older adults in a home care setting. *Home Healthcare Nurse* **28**(1), 14-21.

Meurer, W.J., Potti, T.A., Kerber, K.A. *et al.* (2010) Potentially inappropriate medication utilization in the emergency department visits by older adults: Analysis from a nationally representative sample. *Academic Emergency Medicine* **17**(3), 231-237.

Molony, S.L. (2009) Monitoring medication use in older adults. *American Journal of Nursing* **109**(1), 68-78.

Murray, L.M., & Laditka, S.B. (2010) Care transitions by older adults from nursing homes to hospitals: Implications for long-term care practice, geriatrics education, and research. *Journal of the American Medical Directors Association* **11**(4), 231-238.

Perhats, C., Valdez, A.M., & St Mars, T. (2008) Promoting safer medication use among older adults. *Journal of Emergency Nursing* **34**(2), 156-158.

Phillips, R.M. (2011) The challenge of medication management in older adults. *Nursing made Incredibly Easy!* **9**(1), 24-31.

Planton, J., & Edlund, B.J. (2010) Strategies for reducing polypharmacy in older adults. *Journal of Gerontological Nursing* **36**(1), 8-12.

Rolita, L., & Freedman, M. (2008) Over-the-counter medication use in older adults. *Journal of Gerontological Nursing* **34**(4), 8-17.

Ruppar, T.M., Conn, V.S., & Russell, C.L. (2008). Medication adherence interventions for older adults: Literature review. *Research & Theory for Nursing Practice* **22**(2), 114-147.

Snowden, A. (2008) Medication management in older adults: A critique of concordance. *British Journal of Nursing* **17**(2), 114-119.

Swanlund, S.L., Scherck, K.A., Metcalfe, S.A., & Jesek-Hale, S.R. (2008) Keys to successful self-management of medications. *Nursing Science Quarterly* **21**(3), 238-246.

Van Leuven, K. (2010) Psychotropic medications and falls in older adults. *Journal of Psychosocial Nursing & Mental Health Services*, **48**(9), 35-43.

Zivin, K., Ratliff, S., Heisler, M.M., Langa, K.M., & Piette, J.D. (2010) Factors influencing cost-related nonadherence to medication in older adults: A conceptually based approach. *Value in Health* **13**(4), 338-345.

PART 9: SLEEP DISORDERS

Donna M. Glynn

Sleeping disorders are a common complaint reported by older patients. Sleep needs change with the aging process and may be associated with medical, pharmaceutical, and environmental factors. The National Institute of Aging states that more that 50% of men and women over the age of 65 report sleep disturbances (Subramanian & Surani, 2007). The International Classification of Sleep Disorders has identified more than 90 different sleep disorders which include insomnia, depression, sleep apnea, and restless leg syndrome (AASM, 2001). Therefore, thorough screening and initiation of appropriate interventions may improve the quality of sleep and well-being of older patients.

Insomnia is a subjective perception of the quality and duration of sleep. Insomnia may be classified as primary or secondary. Primary insomnia is not related to other diagnoses or health care concerns. Secondary insomnia is attributed to a medical condition, which may include arthritis, heart disease, cancer, pulmonary etiologies, medications, depression, dementia, or anxiety (Subramanian & Surani, 2007). Types of insomnia include difficulty falling asleep, difficulty maintaining sleep, nonrestorative sleep, and early morning awakening which may lead to increased napping during the day for older patients (Fisher & Valente, 2009). Sleep disturbances may lead to increased fatigue and increased risk of falls in elderly patients. Insomnia may be short term or long term. Short-term insomnia is typically related to changes in environment including hospitalization and changes in medications, including the withdrawal of benzodiazepines.

Several studies have correlated insomnia with depression in older patients. Depression has also been linked to an increase in daytime napping which further impacts the ability to obtain a restful night sleep (Roberts *et al.*, 2000). Other psychiatric conditions have been linked to insomnia and include dementia and anxiety disorders. Patients with dementia will exhibit nocturnal behaviors which include confusion, hallucinations, and repeatedly getting out of bed. These behaviors increase the risk of falls and injury.

Typically adults require 7 to 8 hours of sleep per night. A determinant of sleep is an individual's biological clock which regulates circadian rhythm. Disruption in a patient's circadian rhythm may lead to disturbed sleep patterns. Sleep is divided into two components: non-rapid eye movement (non-REM) and rapid eye movement (REM). During the non-REM stage of sleep, a patient will experience a slowing of respirations and heart rate. During REM sleep, brain wave activity is described as short, rapid wave patterns similar to wave patterns during waking hours. REM sleep is essential for elder patients. During REM sleep neurotransmitters are replenished and this phase of sleep is critical for elders and impacts the daily tasks of remembering and problem solving. REM sleep is critical for the transfer of short-term memories to become long-term memories and plays a major role in maintaining cognitive function in elderly patients (Townsend-Roccichelli, Sanford & VandeWaa, 2010).

It is reported that 25% of older patients may experience sleep apnea. Sleep apnea is defined as a respiratory disturbance of greater than 10 episodes of apnea per hour of sleep in patients over age 60 (Barthlen, 2002). Effective treatment of sleep apnea includes continuous positive airways pressure (CPAP) to improve upper airway flow and augmented restorative sleep patterns.

Restless leg syndrome has also been identified as a cause of sleep disturbances in approximately 20% of older adults (Townsend-Roccichelli, Sanford & VandeWaa, 2010). Polypharmacy may contribute to the symptoms of restless leg syndrome and warrant an accurate and thorough review of the patient's current medications including prescription and over-the-counter medications.

Several common medications also contribute to sleep disturbances in elder patients. Beta-blockers have been associated with nightmares, increased waking, and insomnia (Ahmed et al., 2010). Decongestants, CNS stimulants, anticholinergics, corticosteroids, and beta-agonists may also contribute to sleep disturbances.

Hospitalized older adults may develop sleep disturbances due to environmental changes and altered health function. The necessary interruptions in the sleep process associated with vital sign assessment, physical examinations, medication administration, roommates, lighting, telephones, and call lights may lead to sleep disturbances, sleep deprivation, and changes in mental status. The hospitalized elder is at risk for increased fall and injury.

■ Risk factors for sleep disturbances
Physical
- Anxiety
- Dementia
- Depression
- Nocturia
- Osteoarthritis (pain)
- Restless leg syndrome
- Sleep apnea

Environmental
- Hospital setting
- Light, noise

Medications
- Alcohol
- Anticholinergics
- Central nervous system (CNS) stimulants
- Beta-agonists
- Beta-blockers
- Corticosteroids

■ Clinical presentation

Older patients may present to the hospital setting and report difficulty sleeping. If a sleep disorder is not accurately evaluated, the patient may develop sleep deprivation, change in mental status, risk of injury, and failure to thrive. A thorough nursing assessment is critical to determine the causative factors related to the sleep disturbance and to establish an effective treatment approach.

■ Nursing assessment

A thorough assessment of the patient who is experiencing a sleep disorder is critical to an effective plan of care. Patient assessment should include a sleep history including length of time to fall asleep, difficulties staying asleep, nocturia, early wakening, daytime napping, and daytime fatigue. The patient assessment should include the patient's perceptions of the quality of sleep. A medication history needs to include prescription medication, over-the-counter medications, sleep aids, caffeine, and alcohol intake. The Epworth Sleepiness Scale is a reliable sleep scale to assess sleepiness in older adults (Hartford Institute for Geriatric Nursing, 2007). Physical examination should include mental status assessment, cardiac, and pulmonary evaluation. The nurse should also assess the patient's ambulatory status and evaluate for risk of falls.

■ Diagnostic studies

Diagnostic studies related to sleep disturbances are based on the patient's medical conditions and medication profile. Laboratory testing may include complete blood count, chemistries, thyroid function, and urinalysis. A sleep study may be considered to evaluate for sleep apnea and determine the need for CPAP (Fisher & Valente, 2009).

■ Differential diagnosis

Differential diagnoses related to sleep disturbances include many medical conditions that may interrupt the elderly patient's ability to sleep. The following list is not all inclusive:

- Angina, congestive heart failure
- Chronic obstructive pulmonary disease, asthma, pulmonary embolism
- Delirium, dementia, Parkinson's disease, anxiety disorder
- Hyperparathyroidism
- Osteoarthritis, degenerative joint disease, chronic back pain
- Urinary tract infection, benign prostatic hyperplasia

■ Treatment

The treatment of sleep disorders includes both nonpharmacologic and pharmacologic interventions.

It has been reported that nonpharmacologic therapy has been underutilized by healthcare providers related to sleep disorders in hospitalized elders. Behavioral therapy should include environmental controls, avoidance of caffeine, limiting fluids prior to bedtime, and restricting TV watching. The nurse should evaluate the room and provide the patient with a calm, quiet environment to encourage sleep and coordinate the necessary tasks to encourage prolonged rest periods. Environmental controls are challenging in the acute care setting. The nurse should be aware of daytime napping and if possible napping should be avoided.

Pharmacologic interventions must be managed cautiously in older patients. Prescription medications for sleep disorders include benzodiazepines, nonbenzodiazepines, and antidepressant medications. Benzodiazepines (e.g., triazolam, flurazepam, and temazepam) should be utilized short-term only as discontinuation after prolonged treatment may result in rebound insomnia and withdrawal effects. Benzodiazepine therapy also increases the risk of falls and prolonged sedation in older patients (Townsend-Roccichelli, Sanford & VandeWas, 2010). Nonbenzodiazepine medications include eszopiclone, zolpidem, and zaleplon. These medications appear safer for long-term use in the elderly, but require patient assessment related to risk of falls and increased daytime sleepiness. If the patient has a coexisting diagnosis of depression, antidepressant therapy may be effective to promote improved sleeping patterns.

Over the counter melatonin has been proven helpful to promote sleep in patients. Melatonin assists patient to fall asleep when taken 1-2 hours prior to bedtime. However, melatonin has not been shown to increase the time spent in REM sleep. Melatonin is considered safe for long-term use (Buscemi *et al.*, 2004).

■ Complications

- Anxiety
- Daytime drowsiness
- Delirium
- Depression
- Increased risk of falls
- Memory impairment

- Reduced quality of life
- Risks associated with benzodiazepine, nonbenzodiazepine, and antidepressant therapy

■ Collaborative consultation

Patients with sleep disorders benefit from a multidisciplinary approach and thorough assessment. As polypharmacy is a concern, medication management of the disorder must be initiated with caution to avoid changes in mental status and injury. Consultation with the patient, patient's family, primary care provider, and the hospital team will establish a comprehensive plan to improve sleep patterns.

■ Patient/family education

Sleep disorders are a common concern for older patients. However, nonpharmaceutical approaches are underutilized and the patients and their families need to be educated on proper sleep hygiene. Nutrition, exercise, avoidance of caffeine and alcohol, and decreasing stimulating activities prior to bedtime will improve the patient's ability to sleep and feel rested. After initiation of non-pharmacologic interventions, education should include pharmacologic approaches and potential adverse reactions. Most sleep disorders are treatable and accurate diagnosis and an effective plan of care may potentially improve sleep, decrease daytime napping, and improve cognition for elderly patients.

References

Ahmed, A., Van Mierlo, P., Jansen, P. et al. (2010). Sleep disorders, nightmares, depression and anxiety in an elderly patient treated with low-dose metoprolol. *General Hospital Psychiatry* **32**(6).

American Academy of Sleep Medicine (2001) The international classification of sleep disorders 2001. Online. Available from http://www.esst.org/adds/ICSD.pdf (accessed 3 April 2012).

Barthlem, G. (2002) Sleep disorders: Obstructive sleep apnea syndrome, restless legs syndrome and insomnia in geriatric patients. *Geriatrics* **57**(11), 34–39.

Buscemi, N., Vandermeer, B., Pandya, R. et al. (2004) Melatonin for treatment of sleep disorders. Summary, evidence report/technology assessment. Prepared by the University of Alberta, AHRZ Publication No. 05-E002-1. Agency for Healthcare Research and Quality, Rockville, MD.

Fisher, D. & Valente, S. (2009) Evaluating and managing insomnia. *The Nurse Practitioner* **34**(8), 20–26.

Hartford Institute for Geriatric Nursing (2007) Best practices in nurse care to older adults. The Epworth Sleepiness Scale. Online. Available from http://hartfordign.org/Practice/Try_This/ (accessed 3 April 2012).

Roberts, E., Shema, S., Kaplan, G. & Strawbridge, W. (2000) Sleep complaints and depression in an aging cohort: a prospective perspective. *American Journal of Psychiatry* **157**(1), 81–88.

Subramanian, S. & Surani, S. (2007) Patient handout: Sleep disorders in the elderly. *Geriatrics* **62**(12).

Townsend-Roccichelli, J., Sanford, J. & VandeWaa, E. (2010) Managing sleep disorders in the elderly. *The Nurse Practitioner* **35**(5), 30-37.

PART 10: URINARY INCONTINENCE

Mary L. McDonough

Urinary incontinence (UI) is the involuntary or the accidental release of urine that many patients describe as leaking. It can be transient or "established in nature". It can also range from a minor inconvenience with minimal leaking to having a major impact on lifestyle when there is a complete lack of control (Weiss & Barry, 1998). UI can happen to anyone at any age, although it is more common for women than men and is most commonly found within the older adult population. There is also a higher chance of urinary incontinence among older adults who are institutionalized.

The Department of Health and Human Service estimates that urinary incontinence affects 26 million adults in the US (NY Times Health, 2009). Experts believe that urinary incontinence has been and continues to be underreported, under diagnosed, and under treated. Urinary incontinence in many cases is a symptom of an underlying problem which can take time to identify. There can be several contributing factors. But in the end when an individual's ability to urinate normally is compromised, their life style is significantly disrupted.

Since many older adults believe that urinary incontinence is a normal part of the aging process they make adjustments in their daily routines to accommodate for this change. Their focus becomes managing the leaking by wearing a continence pad, by staying close to a bathroom, by limiting what they drink, by decreasing the time spent away from home, or by not taking the medications that cause them to urinate more frequently. They often struggle with the fact that their bodies are letting them down. Gradually, these adjustments begin to impact quality of life, causing depression, social isolation, a potential for skin breakdown, and adding cost to what may be a limited budget.

Thinking that it is normal or due to what is perceived as an embarrassing problem, many of those suffering from UI do not talk to their health care providers about this problem. As nurses, it is important to understand their reluctance and begin the conversation. It is essential for the health care provider and nurse to ask the right questions and obtain the most accurate information to identify, treat, and manage urinary incontinence.

The genitourinary system (GU) consists of two kidneys, two ureters, a bladder, two sphincters muscles (around the urethra), and the urethra. The function of this system is to collect, store, and transport waste in the form of urine. Although it sounds simple these are big responsibilities. The kidneys collect waste and produce urine. The urine is transported from the kidneys via the ureters to the bladder, where it is stored.

As the bladder begins to fill, signals travel along the nerves initiating the contraction of the destructor muscles in the bladder wall. This contraction creates pressure, which in turn causes the sphincter muscles to relax allowing for the passage of urine through the urethra and out of the body.

Successful elimination of urine requires that the structures of the GU system work effectively. There must also be an effective communication pathway between the muscles of the bladder, urethra, and the central nervous system if the GU system is to function properly. Any deviation from normal functioning of the bladder, sphincters, urethra, or the communication pathway, can increase the individual's risk of developing urinary incontinence.

■ Risk factors

- Advanced age
- Certain medications (e.g., diuretics) Lasix, hydrochlorothiazide)
- Comorbidities (e.g., diabetes, obesity, smoking, or chronic obstructive pulmonary disease)
- Constipation
- Dietary factors (e.g., caffeine or fluid intake)
- Environment
- Female gender
- Genitourinary disorder (e.g., benign prostatic hyperplasia, bladder, or prostate cancer)
- Institutionalization
- Multiple pregnancies or vaginal atrophy (hormonal imbalance)
- Neurologic disorder (e.g., multiple sclerosis, Parkinson's disease, or stroke)
- Reduced or limited mobility
- Urinary tract infections

■ Clinical presentation

The clinical presentation of urinary incontinence is subtle and not easily disclosed, especially with older adults. Since the older adult is not apt to share their experiences with urinary incontinence, it is the nurse's responsibility to begin the discussion .

The assessment and evaluation of any patient, especially older adults, begins when first meeting the patient. What is first observed can provide the first clue to a potential problem with continence. Obesity, immobility, gender, and age that are possible risk factors. The outline of a continence product through an individual's clothing or the scent of urine suggest the possibility of urinary incontinence. Nurses can also ask specific questions focused on voiding patterns such as; do you ever leak urine when you sneeze, cough or laugh? How many times do you get up during the night to go to the bathroom?

Types of incontinence

It is essential to accurately identify the type of incontinence being experienced in order to design and implement a plan of care that is specific to the type of UI.

- *Transient incontinence* has a sudden onset and is considered a reversible change in an individual's voiding pattern. This can occur with a urinary tract infection, a cold with a cough, or the addition of a medication which increases the need to urinate.
- *Established incontinence* has been a gradual voiding pattern change which over time has become the new normal. The following types of incontinence are categorized as established:
  - *Urge incontinence* is the strong sudden urge to urinate. The bladder is over sensitive and contracts more often than normal. The result is an overactive bladder.
  - *Stress incontinence* is the leaking of urine with an increase in abdominal pressure which then puts pressure on an impaired urethral sphincter. This can occur with sneezing, coughing, laughing, doing a sit up, running, squatting, or lifting.
  - *Mixed incontinence* is the combination of both urge and stress incontinence.
  - *Overflow incontinence* occurs when an individual urinates frequently but only passes a small amount of urine with each void. It is usually caused by a urethral blockage limiting the bladder's ability to empty properly. One example of overflow incontinence is an enlarged prostate.
  - *Functional incontinence* is associated with mental or physical impairment and occurs when an individual recognizes the urge to urinate, but is physically unable to go to the bathroom independently.

▓ Nursing assessment

As discussed, the clinical presentation of urinary incontinence is subtle and not easily disclosed. It is the nurse's responsibility to encourage an honest discussion around voiding patterns and urinary incontinence. Important patient history includes the patient's medical history including comorbidities, medications, bowel pattern, and dietary and fluid intake. Additional information to determine includes the following:

- Voiding pattern: Asking the right questions is an important part of assessing voiding patterns and establishing the type of incontinence the patient has. In the outpatient setting the voiding diary is the gold standard in assessment tools. A patient uses the tool so they can record the details of how they void at home for 5 to 7 days. During a hospitalization, the nurse needs a more practical way to obtain this information quickly. The following tools can be helpful in this assessment. The International Prostate Symptom Score (Barry *et al.*, 1992) is a set of questions design to help assess a man's voiding pattern. The more frequent the symptoms the more likely the patient is experiencing overflow incontinence. The questions may need to be reworded for the patient to understand.

- Do you feel like you want to empty your bladder when you take a bath? How often?
- Do you urinate more often than every 2 hours?
- When you urinate how often do you stop and have to start again?
- How often do you find it difficult to postpone urination?
- Do you have a weak or strong urinary stream?
- Do you feel as though you have to push or strain to urinate?
- How many times do you get up at night to urinate?

There are also tools that have been developed that can assist the nurse in assessing established urinary incontinence. The questionnaires can either guide a discussion by a nurse or be completed by the patient. If the nurse was to discuss continence with a patient it would be important to ask about strength of stream, frequency, urgency, leakage, the number of times up at night and emptying of bladder. Another essential question to ask the older adult is how has the leaking changed your life or impacted your daily activities (Uebersax *et al.*, 1995).

The physical exam requires assessing the patient's skin for evidence of skin breakdown and checking for abdominal and bladder distention.

▪ Diagnostics

- Urinalysis
- Urine culture
- Bladder ultrasound used to measure the amount of urine left in the bladder after a patient voids (post void residual).
- Uroflowmetry
- Bladder stress test
- Urodynamic study
- Cystoscopy

▪ Differential diagnosis

- DIAPPERS and TOILETED are mnemonics that have been identified to help a nurse remember the possible reason for incontinence.
  - When using DIAPPERS think of delirium, infection, atrophic urethritis or vaginitis, pharmacology, psychological disorders, endocrine disorders, restricted mobility, and stool impaction.
  - When using TOILETED think of thin, dry vaginal or urethral epithelium, obstruction (constipation), infection, limited mobility, emotional (depression), therapeutic medications, endocrine disorders, and delirium (Resnick & Yalla, 1985).

■ Treatment

Urinary incontinence can be treated and managed effectively. Once the type of urinary incontinence has been identified, it is important to begin to develop a plan for the patient. Interventions fall into three categories: behavioral, pharmacological or surgical. When implementing interventions, start with the least invasive approach then progress slowly based on the individual's response.

Behavioral interventions

- Bladder training gradually increases the time between voiding.
- Timed or prompted voiding
- Kegel exercises are recommended to help strengthen the pelvic floor muscles. Identify the muscle used to stop the stream.
- Dietary modification: limit caffeine and alcohol intake while increasing water intake.
- Maintenance of a healthy weight
- Encourage life style changes.

Pharmacological interventions

- Medications (e.g., Enablex, Sanctura, Ditropan, and Vesicare)
  - Some medications used for incontinence can cause dry mouth, constipation, confusion, falls, and other side effects in older adults.
- Botox, when injected into the bladder wall, helps to relax it.

Surgical interventions (see Table 4.10.1)

- Pessaries placed into the vagina to support a bladder's natural position
- Bulking agents are injected into the sphincter.
- InterStim: uses electrical stimulation to relax or increase resistance in pelvic floor.
- Slings: reposition urethra and bladder.
- Artificial sphincters
- Decreasing the size of the prostate: photo-selective vaporization of the prostate (with the green light laser) or transurethral resection of the prostate (TURP)
- Intermittent self catheterization

■ Collaborative consultation

- Consult urologist
- Physical therapist

Table 4.10.1 Suggested interventions for specific types of incontinence.

Urge incontinence	Stress incontinence	Overflow incontinence	Functional incontinence
Timed voiding Kegel exercises Weight & diet modification Medications Pessaries (if prolapse) Interstim (stimulation to relax)	Timed voiding Kegel exercises Weight & diet modification Bulking agent Botox (into bladder wall) Pessaries (if prolapse) Sling procedure	Flomax, Avodart, Proscar TVT green light laser Intermittent self catheterization.	Consult physical therapy. Organize environment to support independent toileting.

- Dietitian (as appropriate)
- Smoking cessation (as appropriate)

■ Complications

- Depression
- Potential dehydration
- Potential injury (fall)
- Skin breakdown
- Social isolation
- Urinary tract infection

■ Prevention

- Proactive managing of risk factors
- Discussion about voiding patterns at annual appointment with PCP
- Increase awareness of urinary incontinence with individuals and families
- Proactively manage urinary incontinence (Kegel, timed voiding).
- Encourage healthy diet and a normal weight.
- Maintain a bowel regime.
- Manage fluid intake by limiting coffee and alcohol, drink six glasses of water daily.
- Maintain an active lifestyle.

■ Patient/family education

- Provide written information on urinary incontinence.
- Provide informative websites.
- Identify potential support group.
- Encourage independence and self management.

References

Barry, M.J., Fowler, F.J. Jr, O'Leary, M.P. *et al.* (1992) The American Urological Association symptom index for benign prostatic hyperplasia. The Measurement Committee of the American Urological Association. *Journal of Urology* **148**(5), 1549-15457; discussion 1564 Medical Practices Evaluation Center, Massachusetts General Hospital, Boston.

NY Times Health (2009) Incontinence In-Depth Report. Online. Available from http://health.nytimes.com/health/guides/symptoms/urinary-incontinence/print.html (accessed 3 April 2012).

Resnick, N.M. & Yalla, S.V. (1985) Management of urinary incontinence in the elderly. *New England Journal of Medicine* **313**(800-804).

Uebersax, J.S., Wyman, J.F., Shumaker, S.A., McClish, D.K., Fantl, J.A. & The Continence Program for Women Research Group (1995) Short forms to assess life quality and symptom distress for urinary incontinence in women: the Incontinence Impact Questionnaire and the Urogenital Distress Inventory. *Neurology and Urodynamics* **14**(2), 131-139.

Weiss, M.D. & Barry, D. (1998) Diagnostic evaluation of urinary incontinence in geriatric patients. *American Family Physician*. Online. Available from http://aafp.org/afp/980600ap/weiss.html (accessed 3 April 2012).

Further reading

Dowling-Castronovo, A. & Bradway, C. (2008) Urinary incontinence: Nursing Standard of Practice Protocol: Urinary incontinence (UI) in the older adults admitted to acute care. Online. Available from http://consultgerirn.org/topics/Urinary_Incontinence/want_to_know_more (accessed 3 April 2012).

Dowling-Castronovo, A. & Spiro, E.L. (2008) Urinary incontinence assessment in older adults: Part II – Established urinary incontinence. Online. Available from http://consultgerirn.org/uploads/File/trythis/try_this_11_2.pdf (accessed 3 April 2012).

Dowling-Castronovo, A. (2008) Urinary incontinence assessment in older adults: Part I – Transient urinary incontinence. Online. Available from http://consultgerirn.org/uploads/File/trythis/try_this_11_1.pdf (accessed 3 April 2012).

Kuchel, G.A. & DuBeau, C.E. (2009) urinary incontinence in the elderly. Chapter 30: Geriatric Nephrology Curriculum. Online. Available from http://www.asn-online.org/education_and_meetings/distancelearning/curricula/geriatrics/Chapter30.pdf (accessed 3 April 2012).

National Guideline Clearinghouse Guideline Synthesis. (updated 2007) Evaluation and management of urinary incontinence in women. Online. Available from http://www.guidelines.gov/content.aspx?id=10931 (accessed 3 April 2012).

US National Institutes of Health. National Institute on Aging (2008) Urinary Incontinence. Online. Available from http://www.nia.nih.gov/health/publication/urinary-incontinence (accessed 3 April 2012).

PART 11: DISCHARGE PLANNING AND TEACHING

Arlene J. Lowenstein

Discharge planning needs to start early in a hospital stay. When a patient is admitted it is important to carry out a teaching assessment in addition to the nursing assessment. Much information needs to be gathered to be sure your patient will be able to be successful in understanding how to care for him/herself outside of the hospital, and to reduce the need to return to the hospital shortly after discharge for a worsening condition. The objective for effective discharge and disease management should be to assist patients to understand, manage, and live well with their illness, and it can also be an opportunity to work with family members to support the patient and encourage them to establish healthy living to prevent their own potential illnesses.

Rose and Haugen (2010) identified four main components in effective discharge planning, effective being the key word:

(1) Assessment of the patient's post-hospital needs.
(2) Collaboration with the health care team to determine an appropriate discharge date and disposition.
(3) Identification and coordination of necessary resources for ongoing care.
(4) Assurance that the necessary paperwork, prescriptions, and patient education were completed.

The researchers conducted patient and nursing staff surveys and observed discharge teaching procedures and sessions. They found that the primary issues delaying the discharge process were a lack of complete and accurate hospital dismissal summaries, incomplete prescriptions, inconsistent dismissal education, and lack of communication regarding the patient's dismissal date, time, and disposition (Rose & Haugen, 2010).

Teaching assessment

The first step in a teaching assessment is an understanding of who the person is that has the need for your teaching. What is his/her family structure, and is there an opportunity to do individual or family teaching? What are the major cultural, ethnic, educational, and social backgrounds of the patients you work with, and are you aware of cultural and ethnic issues that may impact their understanding and care? What is his/her living facility (urban, rural, apartment, home, institution, etc.)? Understanding the patient's prehospitalization social life is also important. Does your patient have families, friends or neighbors that can be contacted in case of need for assistance, and how will that contact take place, or how isolated is the patient's living style, especially when single and a contact person is not available?

If your patients are very ill or handicapped, what will they need to be able to go home, or will they need to go to another institution, such as a rehab center or nursing home. If another site, either temporary or permanent, is the case, what will that mean for them and their families? If they can go home, will they be caring for themselves or who will be assisting in their care? Working with caregivers is a very important piece of discharge planning and knowing if a caregiver is involved or a patient will be caring for him/her self is crucial.

What are the physical facilities where your patients live? Are there stairs in the home; what are their toilet and bathing facilities, and are they handicap accessible if needed, or even just have grab bars to make bathing and toileting safer? How do they plan to get their food and other shopping and transportation needs?

What is the overall financial status of your patients? Can they afford what they need? What type of insurance programs are they enrolled in, and will insurance companies provide funds for services? How much do their medications cost? Have you gone to the pharmacy lately to check out the price of gauze bandages, specific medications and other common medical supplies? You may be shocked when you see the prices patients may need to pay.

What type of medical care do they get and with whom? How many health professionals are involved in their care? Most importantly, what is the chain of communication between those health professionals and between patients and their health professionals? What type of communication issues could there be for your patients for emergencies or just for general communication and information seeking? What is their ability to have their questions asked, or learn more about their condition? How can your patients reach you or other health care personnel if they need you? What access do they have to phones, internet, transportation for appointments, TV and DVD, etc.? Can they use e-mail and/or the internet (we live in a world of incredibly fast-growing technology), what is their exposure to it and will it help them or not to have access and learn how to use it? Knowing your patient populations, are there any other issues that you can think of?

Teaching and learning issues

These are some of the major issues to consider about patient learning (Lowenstein et al., 2009):

(1) Literacy – how do your patients read, understand and make meaning of the words and graphics? It is important that handout literature be developed with an assessment of reading levels. Some patients are at low levels of reading (but also be aware that some cannot read, but often don't like to admit it and try to hide it). Others have higher reading levels but may (or may not) want simplified handouts. Graphics and color can often make the material more memorable. Try not to crowd the pages. Knowing their computer literacy is also important (Pugliese & Janowski, 2009a, b).

There are health literature, health knowledge games and other health teaching tools to be found on the internet that can help patients and families.

(2) Cultural diversity and English as a second language includes understanding the different meanings of words, rituals, and patterns of behaviors. Besides learning about our patients, this also offers us the opportunity to learn about other cultures. When speaking with patients who have English as a second language, *talk slowly*, but not loudly (they are not deaf). It can be difficult to ask them to repeat something because you did not understand completely. Be careful of smiles – all of us, patients and health professionals, tend to smile if we don't understand something but are ashamed to ask again. A smile does not necessarily mean they understand the point you are trying to make (Scrimshaw, 2009).

(3) Poverty – what choices are available for patients with limited resources? Consider the cost of medication, supplies, services, healthy food, heat, transportation, housing, recreation (Collard & Sowell, 2009). Choice is an important word. How much can we deprive ourselves when we have limited resources? With all the stress on advertisements that encourage people to buy, it can be very difficult to not have "things" when others have them. Do they need to buy medicine instead of a piece of clothing or a dinner at a restaurant, and how will they make that choice?

(4) Stress and illness – anxiety, pain and discomfort reduce focus, and caregiving issues, family and work issues may interfere with the ability for patients to manage their illness (Romano, 2009). It is difficult to listen when you don't feel well. Attention is diverted to the area of discomfort. Stress can cause fatigue due to lack of sleep, which can also cause lack of focus. It is important to explore with your patients what causes them stress and look for stress reducing techniques to help them.

Foundations of teaching and learning

- Know your learner, which includes the teaching assessment and the background medical issues. Most importantly, know what your learners want to learn, before you begin teaching them what you want them to learn. When you can answer their questions and satisfy what they see as important, then they can listen, focus on what you are saying and potentially learn what you want them to learn.
- Learning needs to be active and interesting. Keep them involved in the learning conversation. Return demonstrations and asking them to answer questions about what you have taught can be important. Know your PVC's, tell them your *Perception* of what you think they said, *Validate* those perceptions and *Clarify* any misconceptions.
- Activity directed around learning helps retention. People forget quickly and may need reinforcement and/or teaching aids or information to take with them. Be sure to review those aids and information with them.

- People are responsible for their own learning; they make their own decisions to learn, either consciously or unconsciously. To encourage learning, they need to understand the importance of the material you want them to learn and why it is important.
- We cannot force learning. We can encourage learning with a goal of making it easier for patients to learn, and we can reinforce learning to enhance retention.

Know what you need to teach and how you plan to do it

Once you know who your patient is, use your teaching assessment to help define your objectives for the teaching experience. Are you looking for understanding of medications, side effects and what to do if those occur? Will you be teaching about treatments that need to be continued at home? Are you looking for behavior change and lifestyle changes for health promotion and disease prevention? What content do you need to teach? What methods would you like to use to do that teaching? What teaching resources do you have, and what can you make available to your patients. Finally, how will you determine if objectives will be met? Will you be able to follow up outside of the hospital to help get feedback about your teaching? Did you refer your patient for follow up and communicate to the referral contact person what you were able to teach, but what, if anything still needs follow up, reinforcement and additional teaching? Answering these questions will help you to develop a basic lesson plan for how you plan to work with your patients in this endeavor.

Health behavior models

There are four health behavior models that can be very helpful to understand and use in patient teaching. These models deal with illness to wellness behaviors and particularly with behaviors important to health promotion. These models are often the cornerstones of health education and health promotion. Information is readily available in the literature and on the internet:

(1) *Health Belief Model* (Strecher & Rosenstock, 1997) – what do patients believe and how can some of those beliefs be changed for the better? The major terms include susceptibility, perceived severity, perceived benefits, perceived barriers, cues to action and self-efficacy (the confidence to successfully perform an action).

(2) *Mersey Harm Reduction Model* – you may not get patients to change all behavior, but may be able to reduce some harmful behaviors (Ritter & Cameron, 2005). This model poses that you may not be able to get people to abandon their habits, but if you can help them make small changes instead of overwhelming ones, it may reduce the level of harm.

(3) *Prochaska stages of behavioral change* – precontemplation; contemplation; preparation; action; maintenance and termination (Prochaska *et al.*,

1992). This model is one of the best known to define how behavior change develops and strategies for encouraging behavior change.

(4) *Pender Health Promotion Model* – this is a nursing model (Srof & Velsor-Friedrich, 2006). Health promotion is approach motivated, whereas health protection is avoidance motivated. Discusses factors involved in thinking prospectively about healthy lifestyles.

Important teaching points

As previously mentioned, discharge assessment and teaching needs to start early in a hospital stay. Teaching opportunities can arise when least expected, and it is important to be aware of this potential and to try to capitalize on them. Every interaction is an opportunity to teach. Listen to patients and families – there may be a teaching opportunity with families as well as patients. It is important to keep communication lines open to reinforce and clarify. Be sure to communicate with others on the interdisciplinary team who can enhance and reinforce the patient's learning.

The day of discharge is the worst possible day to provide discharge teaching that has not been provided before. The patients and families are restless and thinking about home. It is hard to concentrate on what is being said. If you must do this, be sure to provide clear written instructions for patients to take home. If at all possible, provide a contact phone number or internet access to get other questions answered. Think of teaching assessments as you do nursing assessments and find ways to communicate those findings to appropriate practitioners.

Teaching strategies and techniques: making learning
stick (Lowenstein & Reeder, 2009)

Understand the difference between the patient's objectives versus your teaching objective. This is extremely important. Assess what your patients know about their conditions and what they want to know before you begin giving information. That will allow you to correct misconceptions, and once you know what the patient knows or doesn't know, you can adjust your teaching. Once you are able to provide answers that the patient wants to hear, you can expand in the direction that you would like them to learn, and they will be more attuned to the health information they need and understand. From your teaching assessment you will be knowledgeable about the patient's situation in life and home background, and can devise ways to make the teaching doable for the patient.

Assessing literacy, sensory, and memory issues is very important. Does your patient have problems with hearing or eyesight that interferes with understanding or reading? Ask your patient to read back an instruction or short paragraph to help determine their level of literacy and understanding. Your teaching may need to be adapted, depending on age related memory changes. Teaching strategies to enhance recall may include reflection, recall and personalization. Reflection can be very helpful to get patients to recall important experiences and feelings that may be discussed and worked with. You may want to explore what happened in previous hospitalizations, if appropriate. People often respond well to personalization. They see themselves being important in this equation, especially in relationship to how to work with medications and treatments. Allow them to work up their own plan with guidance and support from you (Lowenstein & Reeder, 2009).

Scaring patients into behavior change may have the opposite effect. The patient might think that the possibilities are so bad that there is nothing that can be done anyway, so why try? It is also difficult for patients to think about the future, when they are dealing the with current issue. But humor can help reduce anxiety and stress, increase interest and make learning a pleasant experience. Humor can provide a more comforting environment, but be careful not to overdo it.

Use your PVCs - *perception, validation* and *clarification*. Ask your patients if what you think you are hearing is correct (your *perception*) and *validate* what is correct, *clarifying* questions and final statements. Return demonstrations can be helpful, but it often takes more than one return to make a memorable impact in what to do, and it can be easily forgotten if there is a long wait before that action is needed at home, leading to forgetting and confusion. Be sure you follow up with written instructions in easy to understand language. Graphics and pictures can help memory and retention.

A vast array of teaching tools and technologies are available, but tools are not a replacement for the teacher. Teaching tools and technologies provide visual, auditory and tactile components that can encourage learning retention (Pittman, 2009). Good teaching tools and technologies can assist in memory retention, and they can be used to enhance and reinforce the teaching. Effective tools and technologies often tap into emotional involvement and may address the patient's learning style to assist in behavior change. The emotional piece is important, because patients can often remember those emotions and relate them to the teaching.

Evaluating and reporting

Evaluation is critical for identification of teaching objectives. Evaluate teaching and learning -what was said and what was left out, what was accepted by the learner, what learner needs were not met, and what learner needs can be met as well as how to meet those needs. Take a few minutes after the teaching session to write down your impressions, and record them for others to read who are authorized to read this (don't forget privacy issues). Report your experience to the patient's contact or referral contact as appropriate for addition to, reinforcement, and follow up of learning.

If possible, follow up with your patient to provide feedback about your teaching. Patients often will not understand, but are reluctant to tell that to the person teaching. It is very helpful to know if your patient is having or had difficulty following a posthospital teaching plan and why that happened. Follow up can give you insights into how you can improve your teaching methods and make you teaching more effective.

References

Collard, C.S. & Sowell, R.L. (2009) Impact of poverty on learning. In: *Teaching Strategies for Health Education and Health Promotion: Working with Patients, Families and Communities* (Lowenstein, A.J., Foord, L. & Romano, J.C. eds). Jones and Bartlett, Boston, pp. 43–56.

Lowenstein, A.J., Foord, L. & Romano, J.C. (eds) (2009) *Teaching Strategies for Health Education and Health Promotion: Working with Patients, Families and Communities*. Jones and Bartlett, Boston.

Lowenstein, A.J. & Reeder, J.A. (2009) Making learning stick. In: *Teaching Strategies for Health Education and Health Promotion: Working with Patients, Families and Communities* (Lowenstein, A.J., Foord, L. & Romano, J.C. eds). Jones and Bartlett, Boston, pp. 151–178.

Pittman, T.J. (2009). Teaching tools. In: *Teaching Strategies for Health Education and Health Promotion: Working with Patients, Families and Communities* (Lowenstein, A.J., Foord, L. & Romano, J.C. eds). Jones and Bartlett, Boston, pp. 197–228.

Prochaska, J.O., DiClemente, C.C. & Norcross, J.C. (1992) In search of how people change: applications to addictive behaviors. *American Psychologist* **47**, 1102–1114.

Pugliese, M.E. & Janowski, K. (2009a) Supporting patient literacy using technology. In: *Teaching Strategies for Health Education and Health Promotion: Working with Patients, Families and Communities* (Lowenstein, A.J., Foord, L. & Romano, J.C. eds). Jones and Bartlett, Boston, pp. 69–88.

Pugliese, M.E. & Janowski, K. (2009b) Technology in teaching. In: *Teaching Strategies for Health Education and Health Promotion: Working with Patients, Families and Communities* (Lowenstein, A.J., Foord, L. & Romano, J.C. eds). Jones and Bartlett, Boston, pp. 229–254.

Ritter, A. & Cameron, J. (2005) Monograph No. 06: A systematic review of harm reduction. *DPMP Monograph Series*. Turning Point Alcohol and Drug Centre, Fitzroy.

Romano, J.C. (2009) Stress and illness. In: *Teaching Strategies for Health Education and Health Promotion: Working with Patients, Families and Communities* (Lowenstein, A.J., Foord, L. & Romano, J.C. eds). Jones and Bartlett, Boston, pp. 89–104.

Rose, K.E. & Haugen, M.B. (2010) Discharge planning: Your last chance to make a good impression. *MEDSURG Nursing* **19**(1), 47–53.

Scrimshaw, S.C. (2009) Methodologies for working with cultural diversity. In: *Teaching Strategies for Health Education and Health Promotion: Working with Patients, Families and Communities* (Lowenstein, A.J., Foord, L. & Romano, J.C. eds). Jones and Bartlett, Boston, pp. 57–68.

Srof, B.J. & Velsor-Friedrich, B. (2006) Health promotion in adolescents: A review of Pender's Health Promotion model. *Nursing Science Quarterly* **19**(4), 366–373.

Strecher, V.J. & Rosenstock, I.M. (1997) The Health Belief Model. In: *Health Behavior and Health Education: Theory, Research, and Practice* (Glanz, K., Lewis, F.M. & Rimer, B.K. eds). Jossey-Bass, San Francisco, pp. 41–59.

Resources

The Rapid Estimate of Health Literacy in Medicine Tool. Online. Available from http://www.ahrq.gov/populations/sahlsatool.htm (accessed 3 April 2012).
National Patient Safety Foundation. The AskMe3™ website http://www.npsf.org/ for-healthcare-professionals/programs/ask-me-3/ (accessed 3 April 2012).

PART 12: SBAR COMMUNICATION

Eva Beliveau

Good communication between healthcare providers is necessary to insure quality patient care and positive outcomes. This is especially true with older patients as they often have complex medical histories and/or mental status and memory deficits that can impact their current treatment. Most healthcare providers, including nonprofessional caregivers, do receive communication training as part of their core curriculum or orientation. Unfortunately though, communication breakdown is often cited as the cause of medical errors. This may be true because the communication training may be inconsistent and nonsystematic.

According to the Joint Commission (2007), the organization that provides healthcare organizations certification, communication breakdown has often been cited as the root cause for almost every sentinel event that occurred over the past decade. This alarming information caused the Joint Commission in 2007 to designate improved communication as one of their National Patient Safety Goals. This standard required all healthcare facilities to improve the effectiveness of communication between caregivers. Strategies such as eliminating disruptive and intimidating behaviors between healthcare providers (e.g., nurses and physicians) and creating a culture that stresses open communication are now required to receive Joint Commission accreditation. Another component of this goal is to develop a standardized process for the transfer of information between healthcare providers, often called hands off communication (Nadzam, 2009).

The Joint Commission does not recommend a specific technique for hands-off communication to meet the standard but rather, is looking for healthcare facilities to implement systemwide strategies aimed at preventing communication failures. The SBAR (situation, background, assessment, recommendation) method provides a format that can easily be adapted to caregivers across the healthcare system and is often used effectively to meet this safety standard (Nadzam, 2009). SBAR is actually a method modeled after aviation and military hands off communication and adapted to the healthcare environment (Eden & Willingham, 2007). SBAR provides a standardized framework for reporting patient's progress or changes between healthcare workers. The technique is easy to remember and helps systematically frame conversation, that can be used at end of shift, when transferring patients or reporting changes to physicians and practitioners. It provides a focused way to set expectations for what will be communicated between healthcare workers thus fostering a culture of patient safety (Amato-Vealey et al., 2008).

■ Risk factors

There are many factors that may contribute to ineffective communication and compromise patient safety such as:

- Cultural differences
- Differences in ways physicians (disease focused) and nurses (holism focused) approach patient care
- Intimidation by healthcare workers
- Lack of experience
- Lack of organizational skills
- Language barriers
- Sudden critical changes in patient conditions
- Workload stress

Theoretical framework

Theoretically, SBAR is composed of four components: situation, background information, assessment and recommendation and is broken down as follows:

- Situation (what is presently going on with the patient):
  - Identify yourself and your relationship to the patient
  - Patient condition at present
  - Signs and symptoms the patient is experiencing
- Background (pertinent patient information related to the situation):
  - Significant medical surgical history
  - Current medications and/or treatments that maybe be related to the situation
  - Baseline data pertinent to the situation (e.g., mental status, vital signs, urinary output)
- Assessment (subjective and objective data relevant to the situation):
  - Vital signs (temperature, pulse, respirations, pulse oximetery)
  - Level of consciousness
  - Mental status
  - Brief focused assessment related to the situation (e.g., lungs sounds, apical pulse)
- Recommendation (what you think needs to be done about the situation):
  - Request the physician or practitioner to come evaluate the patient.
  - Recommend specific medications.
  - Recommend specific tests.
  - Recommend the patient be transferred.
  - Recommend the patient just be observed.

Operationalizing SBAR

The following case scenario provides a specific clinical example to demon-strate how to use SBAR in practice.

Mrs. Smith is a 78-year-old patient admitted to the medical-surgical floor 7 hours ago from the long-term facility where she has been a resident for 2 years. She was sent to the emergency room with new and unexplained left lower leg edema, pain, erythema, and warmth. Admitting diagnosis is to rule out deep vein thrombosis (DVT). Left leg ultrasound and D-dimer blood tests are pending. Subcutaneous Lovenox, a low molecular weight heparin, was started and compression stockings were applied to her legs. She has a significant past medical history of hypertension, controlled with a beta-blocker and ACE-inhibitor, and a left hemisphere stoke with deficits of right sided hemiplegia and expressive aphasia. Her mental status, difficult to assess due to the expressive aphasia, is reported to be calm, cooperative on admission and she is reportedly able to follow commands well. Mrs. Smith's admitting vital signs were as follows: Temperature 36.3°C (97.3°F); pulse 68 and regular; blood pressure 118/78 and pulse oximetery 98% on room air. She is a full code.

While making rounds, the primary nurse finds Mrs. Smith to be extremely anxious, tachypnic and holding her chest with her left arm. Her blood pressure is 182/98, apical pulse is 72 and regular, respiratory rate 32 and shallow, and pulse oximetery is 89% on room air. The nurse immediately calls for assistance and places a 100% nonrebreather oxygen mask on Mrs. Smith. After two other nurses arrive to Mrs. Smith's room, the primary nurse prepares to call the physician and nursing supervisor using SBAR communication technique. She proceeds as follows:

- **Situation**
  - Identify herself as the primary nurse.
  - Describes finding Mrs. Smith anxious, tachypnic and clutching her chest.
  - Explain that she put 100% oxygen on Mrs. Smith and have 2 nurses pres-ently with her.
- **Background**
  - Admitted 7 hours ago with nonconfirmed but probable symptoms of DVT from a long-term care facility
  - Baseline vital signs of temperature 36.3°C (97.3°F); pulse 68 and regular; blood pressure 118/78 and pulse oximetry 98% on room air
  - Past medical history of a left-sided stroke with hemiparesis and hypertension
  - Full code status
- **Assessment**
  - Blood pressure is 182/98, apical pulse is 72 and regular, respiratory rate 32 and shallow, and pulse oximetry is 89% on room air, lungs appear clear bilaterally.
  - Mrs. Smith developed sudden onset acute respiratory distress with oxygen desaturation and hypertension.

- Based on the situation, tachypnea and oxygen desaturation, and background history, past stroke and decreased activity level, the primary nurse believes Mrs. Smith has ineffective cardiopulmonary tissue perfusion possibly caused by PE.
- **Recommendation**
  - Transfer to the Intensive Care Unit for hemodynamic monitoring.
  - The physician comes in to see the patient.
  - Family notification
  - Ventilation perfusion lung scan or CAT scan
  - Screening laboratory tests (complete blood count, chemistries, coagulation panel)

The primary nurse should use the SBAR format to call report to the physician, the nursing supervisor and to the accepting ICU nurse. When used consistently across the entire system, caregivers understand how to quickly and concisely gather, organize and report pertinent information and the recipients can anticipate how the information will be delivered.

SBAR can be used in all situations that require a hands off report such as at the end of shift or when transporting to the X-ray department. When the patient is stable that is in fact the situation. The background is a brief history of present illness, the assessment is the latest vital signs and/ or focused assessment and the recommendation may be to continue to monitor the patient's symptoms and response to treatment.

Correlation to the nursing process

The nursing process is the critical thinking model that forms the foundation for decision-making and actions that nurses take while caring for their patients. It consists of five interrelated steps; assessment, diagnosis, planning, implementation, and evaluation designed to organize and prioritize care. Assessment encompasses the collection of subjective and objective data. A nursing diagnosis is then formed based on the data collected. Desired patient outcomes are identified and a plan of care is developed to meet the outcomes. The plan is implemented and evaluated to determine if the outcomes have been met (Alfaro-Lefebvre, 2006). The nursing process is based on scientific reasoning and determines how the patient responds to illness, treatments and wellness.

SBAR communication format can easily be adapted to the nursing process.

- **Situation**
  - subjective and objective data collection
  - patient report and/or what the nurse observes
- **Background**
  - subjective and objective data collection
  - obtained through patient history, patient reports and the patients chart

- **Assessment**
  - subjective and objective data specific to the situation
  - utilization of critical thinking skills to anticipate focused assessment
- **Recommendation**
  - derived from outcome of the collected subjective and objective assessments
  - based on the nursing diagnosis

Referring back to the case scenario with Mrs. Smith, the primary nurse, using the nursing process and critical thinking skills, deducted that this patient's DVT may have dislodged causing a PE. The nursing diagnosis that was formulated: Alteration in tissue perfusion, cardiopulmonary, related to possible thrombus as evidenced by sudden onset of acute respiratory distress with oxygen desaturation.

This nursing diagnosis helped the nurse understand the urgency of Mrs. Smith's problem and make the correct recommendations. It allowed him/her to anticipate important and specific background information and assessment findings that the physician would need to understand the urgency of the problem and the need for immediate action.

Physician considerations

- Most physicians have several patients and when you call he/she may be dealing with multiple issues therefore you need to be specific especially with the situation and background.
- Physicians are disease orientated and respond best to specific concrete data.
- If you are requesting a medication or treatment try to anticipate what information related to the situation might be needed, e.g., lab values, allergies, weights, etc.
- Try to have a detailed focused assessment related to the situation, i.e., vital signs, heart sounds, lung sounds, etc.
- If time allows, consider writing out the report in SBAR format before you call the physician or use a pre-written tool if available.

Multidisciplinary education

- SBAR communication techniques should be introduced and utilized in nursing school.
- Physicians should be educated on and utilize SBAR with all members of the health care team.
- Orientation to health care facilities should include SBAR communication techniques for all caregivers, professional and nonprofessional.
- Develop and implement standardized SBAR written tools that can be filled out prior to hands off communication for shift to shift, transfer, and physician reporting.

References

Alfaro-LeFevere, R. (2006) *Applying the Nursing Process a Tool for Critical Thinking*, 6th edition. Lippincott Williams & Wilkins, Philadelphia.

Amato-Vealey, E.J., Barba, M.P. & Vealey, R. (2008) Hands off Communication: A Requisite for Perioperative Safety. *AORN Journal* **88**(5), 763-770.

Eden, T. & Willingham, M. (2007) Can you hear me yet? The importance of effective communication and patient safety. *Oncology Nursing Forum* **34**(2), 517-518.

Joint Commission on Accreditation of Health Care Organizations Patient Safety Goals (2007) Online. Available from http://www.jointcommission.org/standards_information/npsgs.aspx (accessed 3 April 2012).

Nadzam, D. (2009) Nurses' role in communication and patient safety. *Journal of Nursing Care Quality* **24**(3), 184-188.

Glossary

Acute kidney injury: Formerly referred to as acute renal failure, acute kidney failure is a rapid reduction (within 48 hours) in kidney function and a percentage increase in serum creatinine of more than or equal to 50% from baseline.

Analgesics: Medications designed to relieve pain. Pure analgesics do not have an effect on inflammation.

Ankle/Brachial index: A noninvasive test used to identify large vessel peripheral artery disease in lower extremities by comparing the ankle systolic pressure to the highest arm systolic pressure.

Anti-CCP antibodies: Antibodies to cyclic citrullinated peptide (anti-CCP). A positive test for the antibodies is useful for confirming a diagnosis of rheumatoid arthritis. In fact, tests for the antibodies can be positive years before the development of symptoms.

Antiplatelet therapy: Medications that decrease platelet induced blood clotting.

Atherosclerosis: The process of plaque accumulation within the blood vessel.

Arthrocentesis: Aspiration of joint fluid.

Arthroscopy: Visualization of the joint capsule through an endoscope. Aspiration, lavage, and debridement can be done at the same time.

Autoimmune disease: A disease in which the immune system, which is designed to protect the body from foreign invaders, mistakenly sees the body's own tissues as foreign and makes autoantibodies against them, leading to tissue destruction.

Benign: Cancerous growths that are encapsulated, remain localized and are slow growing.

Biologic response modifiers: Genetically engineered medications that help reduce inflammation and structural damage to the joints by interrupting the cascade of events that drive inflammation.

Brawny induration: An area of hardened skin or tissue.

Cancer: A neoplastic disorder that can involve all parts of the body. Cells lose their mechanism to control normal growth and the growth of cells is uncontrolled.

Carcinogen: A physical, chemical, or biological stressor that causes neoplastic changes in normal cells.

Cellulitis: Inflammation of the subcutaneous, loose connective tissue.

Nursing Care of the Hospitalized Older Patient, First Edition. Edited by Terry Mahan Buttaro and Kate A. Barba.
© 2013 John Wiley & Sons, Inc. Published 2013 by John Wiley & Sons, Inc.

Chronic bronchitis: The presence of a cough with sputum production for at least 3 months in each of two consecutive years.

Chronic kidney disease (CKD): A gradual loss of kidney's ability to filter the byproducts of protein metabolism with a decrease in glomerular filtration rate of less than 60 ml/min for 3 months or greater.

Cockroft-Gault: Formula used to calculate glomerular filtration rate (GFR).

Complicated UTI: An infection of the bladder or upper urinary tract associated with a structural defect in the urinary system (i.e., obstruction or stricture) or a metabolic or immunologic issue.

Cystitis: Infection of the bladder.

D-dimer test: A blood laboratory test that assesses blood clotting activity, an elevation may indicate venous thromboembolism or disseminated intravascular coagulation; normally plasma does not contain detectable D-dimer fragments.

Debridement: The removal of devitalized tissue, noted as slough or eschar, from a wound bed in order to promote healing. It can be done by through autolytic, chemical, mechanical, or surgical removal of the tissue.

Disease-modifying antirheumatic drugs (DMARDs): A class of medications used in the treatment of rheumatoid arthritis. DMARDs do more than ease the symptoms of rheumatoid arthritis than some other medications. They often slow or stop the course of the disease to help prevent joint damage.

Dyspnea: The subjective sensation of uncomfortable or difficult breathing.

Embolus: A plug, composed of detached thrombus, which occludes a blood vessel.

Emphysema: Marked, permanent destruction of the alveolar sacs with loss of lung elasticity and air trapping that leads to enlargement of the remaining alveoli.

Erythema: Redness of the skin from capillary dilation.

Erythrocyte sedimentation rate (sed rate): A blood test used to detect and monitor inflammation. It is measured by recording the rate at which red blood cells fall and form sediment at the bottom of a test tube.

Eschar: Tan, black, yellow or brown necrotic devitalized tissue.

ESR: Erythrocyte sedimentation rate, an inflammatory marker.

Exudate: A fluid rich in protein, and cellular elements that seeps out of tissues or blood vessels due to inflammation.

Flare: A period of heightened disease activity. In rheumatoid arthritis, a flare may be characterized by increased fatigue, fever, and painful, swollen, and tender joints.

Forced expiratory volume in 1 second (FEV1): The amount of air which can be forcibly exhaled from the lungs in the first second of a forced exhalation after a maximum inspiration.

Forced vital capacity: The amount of air a person can expire after a maximum inspiration.

Friction: The mechanical force of two surfaces moving across each other; it damages surfaces tissues, causing blisters or abrasions such as, with a boost up in bed.

Full thickness injury: Tissue damage that passes through the dermis extending to deeper tissue layers, and disrupts dermal blood vessels.

Giant cell arteritis: An inflammatory disease of the blood vessels (most commonly large and medium arteritis of the head) and is a form of vasculitis.

Glomerular filtration rate (GFR): Rate that a given compound passes through the glomerulus at a given time.

Granulation tissue: Pink or red, collagen rich tissue composed of connective tissue, new capillaries, fibroblasts and inflammatory cells, that eventually fill an open wound for healing.

Hematoma: Localized collection of extravasated blood confined under the skin in a localized organ or tissue.

Hemoptysis: Blood in the sputum usually derived from the bronchial or lung hemorrhage.

Hemiplegia: Paralysis of one side of the body.

Hypertension: Stage 1 BP >140-159/90-99
Stage 2 BP >160/00

Hypertensive emergency: BP >180/110 with end organ dysfunction.

Hypertensive urgency: BP >180/110 without end organ dysfunction.

Intermittent claudication: Exercise-induced lower extremity pain caused by ischemia that is relieved with rest.

Irrigate: Is the procedure used to wash away bacteria and cellular debris from an open wound.

Jaw claudication: Pain in the jaw that generally occurs while chewing.

Lavage: Washing out (of the joint).

Limb ischemia: Inadequate tissue perfusion of the effected extremity.

Lipodermatosclerosis: Brown smooth discoloration of the skin above the ankles, which is caused by scaring of the skin and fat tissue from long-standing chronic venous insufficiency.

Lupus: A chronic inflammatory condition in which the immune system attacks the skin, joints, heart, lungs, blood, kidneys and brain. Also called systemic lupus erythematosus.

Malignant: Cancerous growths that are not encapsulated and grow in a disorderly, uncontrolled rate.

Metastasis: The transfer of disease from one organ or part of the body to another not directly connected with it.

Modification of diet in renal disease (MDRD): Formula used to calculate GFR.

National Kidney Foundation (NKF) Kidney Disease Outcomes Quality Initiative (KDOQI): Guidelines to assist physicians in identifying the stage of kidney disease and interventions and treatment at each stage.

Nonblacheable erythema: Redness that persists when pressure is applied and removed-usually with a fingertip.

Osteomyelitis: An infection in the bone.

Pandemic: Pandemics happen when a novel influenza virus emerges that infects and can be efficiently transmitted between humans. Animals are the most likely reservoir for these emerging viruses. The last three pandemics, in 1918, 1957 and 1968, killed approximately 40 million, 2 million and 1 million people worldwide, respectively. Although the timing cannot be predicted, history and science suggest that we will face one or more pandemics in this century. Despite annual vaccinations, the US faces a burden of influenza that results in approximately 36,000 deaths and more than 200,000 hospitalizations each year. In addition to this human toll, influenza is annually responsible for a total cost of over $10 billion in the US. http://www.flu.gov/professional/federal/pandemic-influenza.pdf

Partial thickness injury: Tissue damage that is limited to the epidermis and superficial dermis with no damage to the dermal blood vessels.

Peripheral vascular disease: Narrowing of the arteries as a result of progressive atherosclerosis.

Prehypertension: BP 120-139/80-89

Protein C deficiency: Inherent deficiency of the naturally occurring anticoagulant protein c which can increase patient risk for coagulation.

Protein S deficiency: Inherent deficiency of the naturally occurring anticoagulant protein s which can increase patient risk for coagulation.

Purpura: Purple-colored lesions.

Pyelonephritis: Infection of the kidney.

Renal replacement therapy: A modality that is used to remove waste products that have accumulated in the body. Two types of therapy: hemodialysis and peritoneal dialysis.

Reiter's syndrome: Condition characterized by polyarthritis, urethritis, and conjunctivitis.

Rheumatoid factor (RF): An antibody that is present eventually in the blood of most people with rheumatoid arthritis. Not all people with rheumatoid arthritis test positive for rheumatoid factor, and some people test positive for rheumatoid factor, yet never develop the disease. Rheumatoid factor also can be positive in some other diseases.

Shear: The mechanical force that is parallel rather than perpendicular to the skin, which can damage deep tissue such as muscle (tissues attached to bone are pulled one way whereas surface tissue remain stationary).

Slough: Yellow, tan, gray, green or brown avascular tissue.

Staging: A method of classifying malignancies based on the presence and extent of the cancer within the body.

Synovial fluid: A fluid secreted by the synovium that lubricates the joint and keeps the cartilage smooth and healthy. Normally it is clear. Purulent fluid indicates infection.

Synovium: A thin membrane inside the joint capsule that secretes synovial fluid. In rheumatoid arthritis, the synovium is attacked by the immune system.

Temporal arteritis: An inflammatory disease of the blood vessels (most commonly large and medium arteritis of the head) and is a form of vasculitis.

Thrombus: A clot in the vascular system formed from the blood forming factors.

Tachypnea: Rapid breathing.

Uncomplicated UTI: An infection of the bladder.

Undermining: An area of tissue destruction extending under intact skin along the periphery of a wound.

Uremia: An excess accumulation of urea in the bloodstream, a sign of kidney failure or disease.

Urinary tract infection (UTI): Infection of the urinary system.

Vasculitis: Inflammation of the blood vessels. Vasculitis can occur as a complication of rheumatoid arthritis.

Vasculitides: Plural of vasculitis.

Selected Websites for Geriatric Information

Alzheimer's Association	www.alz.org
American Association of Retired Persons	www.aarp.org
American Geriatrics Society	www.americangeriatrics.org
American Society on Aging	www.asaging.org
ANCC Certification	www.nursecredentialing.org
ElderWeb	www.elderweb.com
GeroNurseOnline	www.geronurseonline.org
Gerontological Advanced Practice Nurses Association	www.gapna.org
Gerontological Society of America	www.geron.org
Hartford Institute for Geriatric Nursing	www.hartfordign.org www.consultgerirn.org
National Association of Geriatric Education Centers	www.n-age.org
National Center for Health Statistics	www.cdc.gov/nchs
National Council on Aging	www.ncoa.org
National Gerontological Nursing Association	www.ngna.org
National Institute on Aging	www.nia.nih.gov
Rosalynn Carter Center for Caregivings	www.rosalynncarter.org

Nursing Care of the Hospitalized Older Patient, First Edition. Edited by
Terry Mahan Buttaro and Kate A. Barba.
© 2013 John Wiley & Sons, Inc. Published 2013 by John Wiley & Sons, Inc.

Index

Page numbers in *italics* denote figures, those in **bold** denote tables.

Nursing Care of the Hospitalized Older Patient, First Edition. Edited by
Terry Mahan Buttaro and Kate A. Barba.
© 2013 John Wiley & Sons, Inc. Published 2013 by John Wiley & Sons, Inc.